harwood academic publishers SPECIALIST HANDBOOK

Respiratory
Medicine

Respiratory
Medicine

J. Paul Dilworth

Consultant Physician and Honorary Senior Lecturer, Department of Thoracic Medicine

Royal Free and University College Medical School, London, UK

David R. Baldwin

Consultant Respiratory Physician, Department of Respiratory Medicine

Nottingham City Hospital, Nottingham, UK

Printed in Singapore.

Amsteldijk 166, 1st Floor, 1079 LH Amsterdam, The Netherlands

British Library Cataloguing in Publication Data

A catalogue record for this book is available from the British Library.

ISBN: 90-5823-077-5

Respiratory
Medicine

Contents

Foreword ix

Preface xi

Contributors xiii

1   The Conduct and Interpretation of Pulmonary
     Function Tests   1
     M.D.L. Morgan

2   Thoracic Imaging   29
     Melanie Greaves

3   Invasive Procedures   65
     David R. Baldwin

4   Asthma   81
     Timothy W. Harrison and Anne E. Tattersfield

5   Practical Allergy   107
     Glenis K. Scadding

6   Chronic Obstructive Pulmonary Disease   131
     David M.G. Halpin

7   Chronic Ventilatory Insufficiency and Non-Invasive
     Ventilation   155
     Anita K. Simonds

8   Sleep Apnoea Syndromes   171
     Lesley S. Bennett and Robert J.O. Davies

9   Pulmonary Vascular Disease   199
     Nicholas Morrell

10   Lung Cancer   235
     Jeremy George

11   Pleural Diseases and Techniques   269
     Gerrard Phillips

12   Lung Infections   331
     John T. Macfarlane

13   Tuberculosis   355
     L. Peter Ormerod

14   HIV/AIDS   383
     Michael A. Beckles, Marc C.I. Lipman and
     Margaret A. Johnson

15   Cystic Fibrosis and Bronchiectasis   407
     Diana Bilton

16   Diffuse Parenchymal Lung Disease   423
     Athol U. Wells

17   Occupational Lung Diseases   457
     Robert Niven and Anthony Pickering

18   Radiotherapy and the Lung   495
     J. Paul Dilworth

19 Drug-induced Respiratory Disease (DRD) 499
Simon C.O. Taggart and J. Paul Dilworth

20 Intensive Care 505
Brendan Madden

21 Acute Respiratory Distress Syndrome 527
Brendan Madden

22 Lung Transplantation and Thoracic Surgery 545
Brendan Madden

23 Chest Trauma and Respiratory Emergencies 567
W. Ellis Morgan and David R. Baldwin

24 Chronic Cough 591
Ian D. Pavord

25 Pulmonary Disease in Pregnancy 605
J. Paul Dilworth

26 Perioperative Pulmonary Assessment and Treatment 611
J. Paul Dilworth

27 Physiotherapy 617
Tracey Hughes

28 Flying, Diving and Climbing 639
Kevin Peter McKinlay

29 Palliative Care 645
Andrew Wilcock

30 Teaching, Learning and Assessing 673
Venetia M. France

31 Preparation for Research 679
David A. Lomas and Michael Plotnick

Index 685

Respiratory Medicine

Foreword

There is a gap between the small pocket aid for medical emergencies and the comprehensive fully referenced textbook. This book, the first of a series aimed at the specialist in training, fills the gap admirably and complements both styles of existing text. While the idea of a portable guide to specialist respiratory medicine is not new, previous attempts have all resulted in a pared down version of the big textbook with pathogenesis and the basic science of disease squeezing out details of practical management. Here practice squeezes out theory.

Paul Dilworth and David Baldwin are both typical of the hands on specialist who spends most of his time with patients rather than at his desk or in the library. This experience is well reflected in the way they have persuaded their thirty authors to follow a consistent pattern and keep their contributions practical and relevant. While the practising specialist will still need a big textbook for reference and deeper understanding, the approach taken by this new book provides just about everything needed to run a specialist service. I expect to see it in trainees pockets and on the specialists desks for many years to come.

Professor Duncan Geddes, Royal Brompton Hospital, London

Respiratory Medicine

Preface

The goal of this handbook is to be a pocket size but comprehensive daily practical guide to be carried or kept close at hand. It is not intended that it should compete with larger texts, but should provide all the information that is required to manage the patient at the bedside or in the clinic. The emphasis on practical, diagnostic and management issues is presented in a rapidly accessible form including tables and algorithms. Where more detail is required, the reader is referred by the contributors to suitable reference texts for key papers. The intended readership is trainees and specialists in respiratory medicine.

We are deeply grateful to the many contributors to the text. We have been overwhelmed by their hard work and enthusiasm for the project, despite their busy schedules. We would also like to thank the editors at Harwood Academic Publishers for their patience and flexibility in facilitating the production of this concise text.

J. Paul Dilworth
David R. Baldwin

Respiratory Medicine

Contributors

David R. Baldwin
Consultant Respiratory Physician
Department of Respiratory
    Medicine
Nottingham City Hospital
Nottingham
UK

Michael A. Beckles
Specialist Registrar
London Chest Hospital
London
UK

Lesley S. Bennett
Consultant Chest Physician
Oxford Centre for Respiratory
    Medicine
The Churchill Hospital
Oxford
UK

Diana Bilton
Consultant Physician
Cystic Fibrosis Unit
Papworth Hospital
Cambridge
UK

Robert J.O. Davies
Consultant Physician and
    Senior Lecturer
Oxford Centre for Respiratory
    Medicine
The Churchill Hospital
Oxford
UK

J. Paul Dilworth
Consultant Physician &
    Honorary Senior Lecturer
Department of Thoracic
    Medicine
Royal Free and University
    College Medical School
London
UK

Venetia M. France
Medical School Curriculum
    Development Facilitator
Royal Free and University
    College Medical School
London
UK

Jeremy George
Consultant Physician
Department of Thoracic
    Medicine
Middlesex Hospital
London
UK

Melanie Greaves
Consultant Radiologist
Department of Radiology
Wythenshawe Hospital
Mancheser
UK

David M.G. Halpin
Consultant Physician in
    Respiratory Medicine
Royal Devon and Exeter
    Hospital
Exeter
UK

Timothy W. Harrison
Consultant Physician
Department of Respiratory
    Medicine
Nottingham City Hospital
Nottingham
UK

Tracey Hughes
Senior Physiotherapist
Department of Physiotherapy
Nottingham City Hospital
Nottingham
UK

Margaret A. Johnson
Consultant Physician
Department of Respiratory
    Medicine
Royal Free Hospital
London
UK

Marc C.I. Lipman
Consultant Physician
Department of Respiratory
    Medicine
Royal Free Hospital
London
UK

David A. Lomas
Consultant Physician
Institute for Medical Research
Wellcome Trust
Cambridge
UK

John T. Macfarlane
Consultant Physician
Department of Respiratory
  Medicine
Nottingham City Hospital
Nottingham
UK

Brendan Madden
Consultant Cardiothoracic and
  Transplant Physician
Cardiothoracic Unit
St Georges Hospital
London
UK

Kevin Peter McKinlay
Consultant Chest Physician
North Hampshire Hospital
Basingstoke
UK

M.D.L. Morgan
Consultant Physician
Department of Respiratory
  Medicine and Thoracic
  Surgery
Glenfield Hospital
Leicester
UK

W. Ellis Morgan
Consultant Thoracic Surgeon
Department of Thoracic Surgery
Nottingham City Hospital
Nottingham
UK

Nicholas Morrell
University Lecturer and
  Honorary Consultant
Respiratory Medicine Unit
University of Cambridge
  School of Clinical Medicine
  and Addenbrooke's and
  Papworth Hospitals
Cambridge
UK

Robert Niven
Consultant Respiratory Physician
North West Lung Centre
Wythenshawe Hospital
Manchester
UK

L. Peter Ormerod
Professor of Respiratory
  Medicine
Chest Clinic
Blackburn Royal Infirmary
Blackburn
UK

Ian D. Pavord
Consultant Physician
Department of Respiratory
  Medicine
Glenfield Hospital
Leicester
UK

Gerrard Phillips
Consultant Physician
Department of Respiratory
  Medicine
Dorset County Hospital
UK

Anthony Pickering
Consultant Respiratory Physician
North West Lung Centre
Wythenshawe Hospital
Manchester
UK

Michael Plotnick
Consultant Physician
Department of Pulmonary and
    Critical Care
University of Pennsylvania
USA

Glenis K. Scadding
Consultant Physician in
    Rhinology, Immunology and
    Allergy
Royal National Ear, Nose and
    Throat Hospital
London
UK

Anita K. Simonds
Consultant in Respiratory
    Medicine
Department of Respiratory
    Medicine
Royal Brompton Hospital
London
UK

Simon C.O. Taggart
Consultant Physician
Department of Respiratory
    Medicine
Trafford General Hospital
Manchester
UK

Anne E. Tattersfield
Professor of Respiratory
    Medicine
Department of Respiratory
    Medicine
Nottingham City Hospital
Nottingham
UK

Athol U. Wells
Consultant Physician
Department of Respiratory
    Medicine
Royal Brompton Hospital
London
UK

Andrew Wilcock
Consultant Physician
Haywood House Macmillan
    Specialist Palliative Care
    Unit
Nottingham City Hospital
Nottingham
UK

The Conduct and Interpretation of Pulmonary Function Tests

MDL Morgan

Introduction

The function of the respiratory system is to make sufficient molecules of oxygen available for delivery so that the survival of each cell is assured. It also removes carbon dioxide, one of the major products of cellular respiration. The rapid handling of carbon dioxide gives the lung its role as the major organ involved in the short-term control of acid-base balance. The final delivery of an oxygen molecule to the cell is the result of a number of processes which extract the gas from the atmosphere, transport it to the place of exchange with the blood, ensure its transfer to the circulation and allow its release in the appropriate region. These processes are subject to the variable requirements of the body and can be influenced by neurological control. At the same time they depend upon the co-operation of healthy respiratory muscles and an intact and flexible circulation. Impairment of function can arise from a major disruption of one element of the respiratory system or equally from a combination of less critical failures. The respiratory system has a large reserve of function which can be called upon during exercise or disease. However this also means that there can be considerable covert respiratory disease of which the patient may be unaware. The purpose of lung function measurements is to discover, define and describe these abnormalities.

Modern clinical lung function testing has four main roles:

• contributing to differential diagnosis
• monitoring disease
• assessing therapeutic response
• assessing impairment and disability

The most valuable lung function tests are those of airway function, lung volume and gas exchange. Arterial blood gas analysis, chest wall function and exercise assessment may also have a role in specific circumstances. Readers will also be familiar with some other less commonly used tests which are described separately (see appendix 1). Since many trainees in respiratory medicine are not now automatically exposed to research experience in physiology, this chapter will seek to describe these common tests of lung function and how they can be used to guide clinical practice.

Conduct, Quality Control, Reporting and Reference Values

It is stating the obvious to emphasise that lung function tests can only be useful if they can be relied on to be accurate and reproducible. Their value also increases if they are also standardised and the results can be compared to normal reference values. Most detailed lung function tests are now conducted in hospital laboratories while some simple tests are performed in clinics or primary care. Wherever they are performed, the conduct of the test should adhere to the standards of practice laid down by the appropriate national body or society. In the UK these standards are overseen by the British Thoracic Society (BTS) and the Association of Respiratory Technicians and Physiologists (ARTP) and published in the appropriate documents. Occasional or limited operators outside laboratories are also expected to adhere to the same standards.

The preparation of equipment is an important part of any measurement, and quality control methods are used to ensure standardisation, accuracy and guard against equipment malfunction. Although modern computer controlled equipment may contain quality control routines they also harbour potential hazards since errors may be hidden in the software. Therefore quality control routines should continue to be conducted in all modern laboratories e.g. regular recording of volume, device and gas analyser calibration. Since testing routines involving human subjects can be complex, individual component quality control may be difficult to perform. For this reason the use of a biological control is recommended, particularly for TLCO and exercise measurements. In practice this involves one of the more permanent technicians undergoing the tests on a regular basis.

Laboratories now have an increasing responsibility to patients and staff to maintain infection control. Although the risk of infection from lung function equipment to staff or patients is likely to be small, it should be recognised, especially when dealing with patients with HIV or TB. This is particularly prudent when aerosols are generated (challenge testing or sputum induction). Disposable accessories are available to isolate high risk patients from the equipment and known infection risks should be tested at the end of the day. However since the source of infection risk cannot always be predicted, it is better to impose a strict, generalised, laboratory infection control policy.

The value of lung function tests are enhanced by attractive presentation and sensible clinical reporting. Lung function values in the UK should now be presented in a common format in line with the European Respiratory Society (ERS) recommendations on nomenclature and SI units. The presentation will include the numerical values printed alongside the normal ranges and previous results. Graphical representation of the spirogram and the flow volume loops also aid interpretation as well as demonstrating the technical adequacy of the forced manoeuvres. Reporting of lung function tests may comprise a computerised version, a technical report and clinical commentary (Box 1). The specialist trainee is often asked to supply the latter.

The identification of abnormal lung function depends upon the knowledge of normal values for the served population. Ideally this should be derived from the results from healthy people belonging to the local population. In practice, this is unachievable in most centres so the UK has adopted the ERS compilation of reference values. The regression equations for individual tests are derived from the combination of normal values whose variability appears to depend primarily on age, gender and height. Weight and ethnic background are considered to be minor factors but can sometimes be accounted for if required. The expression of individual test results in relation to the reference values has engendered some debate. The presentation of a value as percent predicted value has some merit in simplicity and many treatment guidelines use this format. The

Box 1   Composition of lung function report

Computerised report	Usually highlight outlying values and classify broad categories (obstruction/restriction)
Technician's report	Should comment on the process factors which may have influenced the results (e.g. recent use of bronchodilator, troublesome cough, poor effort, language difficulties etc).
Clinical commentary	The clinical commentary should not seek to replicate either of these factual reports but should add clinical knowledge to the interpretation for the non-expert recipient. Examples of valuable comments would include discussion of the differential diagnosis, significance of response to treatment, or suggestions for further investigation.

disadvantage of this format is twofold. Firstly half of the normal population will lie below 100% and may be erroneously seen as abnormal. Secondly the actual confidence intervals of normality will vary according to the nature of the test, leading to misinterpretation. A practical solution to this problem is simply to print the test value against the normal range and allow the interpreter to come to their own conclusions. Lastly, the longitudinal monitoring of lung function may not identify relative deterioration or improvement with the normal range or across the span of time. The expression of results as a standardised residual (i.e. the number of standard deviations away from the mean) can address this issue but may also be a difficult concept to grasp, though some laboratories are adopting it.

Airway function

Measurement of airway function, usually patency, is used to diagnose airway obstruction, assess potential for treatment and to monitor progress. It is assessed by the quantification of gas flow or volume. The major divisions of lung volume include tidal volume

(TV) and vital capacity (VC) which can be measured simply. There are several devices for measuring volume including the bellows spirometer (Vitallograph®) and the rolling seal spirometer. Recently, devices which measure flow and differentiate to obtain volume have become popular since they are compact and can produce a flow volume loop. Examples include turbines and pneumotachometers. Slight differences in the sensitivity of these instruments mean that inter-instrument differences may prevent accurate comparison between measurements with different devices.

Most tests of airway patency examine expiratory function and there are three common methods:

- spirometry (FEV_1 and FVC)
- flow-volume curves
- peak expiratory flow rate (PEFR)

Production of the spirogram from a maximum forced expiration from a full inspiration is reliable and provides the forced expiratory volume in one second (FEV_1) and the forced vital capacity (FVC). The slow or relaxed vital capacity (SVC) may produce a larger value in patients with airway obstruction by avoiding premature dynamic airway closure. The presence of airway obstruction is recognised by an FEV_1/VC ratio <75%. Reduction in FEV_1 with relative preservation of FVC indicates and grades airway obstruction: i.e. FEV_1<80% mild, <60% moderate and <40% severe impairment.

Administration of a bronchodilator is an important part of laboratory practice because it can uncover unsuspected airway obstruction and also guide the patient and clinician to effective management. There exists some lack of standardisation in the nature and dose to be administered as well as expression of the results. The maximum bronchodilator response will be obtained with combined nebulised doses of beta-agonist and anticholinergic bronchodilator but this is seldom necessary and the usual practice is to give a beta-agonist by MDI/spacer or nebuliser alone. The additional value of the anticholinergic response is doubtful. There is a significant improvement in FEV_1 if the value rises by >15% and 200 ml.

Simultaneous reduction in both FEV_1 and FVC with an increase in the FEV_1/FVC ratio is called a restrictive defect and usually associated with a reduction in lung volume. This is not graded in the same way as the obstructive pattern. Thus simple spirometry can detect and quantify airway obstruction but it is not able to comment on the cause.

The measurement of the flow volume curve is now commonplace in most hospitals and can provide information about the nature of airway obstruction. In this test the gas flow from a full maximum expiration is plotted against the expired volume as the lung empties. The flow of gas from the lung reaches a peak in about 100msec, the peak expiratory flow (PEF), and then declines linearly until the lung empties. If the measurement is continued into the subsequent full inspiration, a flow-volume 'loop' is produced and can record the inspiratory flow rates. The shape of the expiratory and inspiratory portions are different since in expiration the active expulsion is assisted by the elastic recoil of the lung while inspiratory flow rates are a reflection of airway calibre and respiratory muscle strength only. Something of the nature of the obstruction to the airway can be learnt from the actual and relative values of PEFR, PIFR and other later values of expiratory flow at 50% and 75% of the vital capacity (V50 and V75). For example, the normal ratio of PEF to PIF is 1.3:1, and this would be increased in diaphragm weakness or other inspiratory flow limitation and decreased in

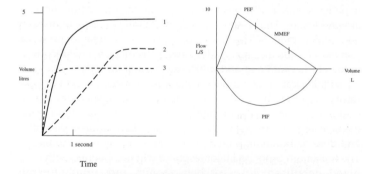

Figure 1.   Schematic views of the spirogram (A) and the flow volume loop (B). In the spirogram (expired volume vs time) 75% of the normal expired volume is achieved within one second (FEV$_1$). This ratio is reduced in the "obstructive" pattern (2) and increased in the "restrictive" pattern.
The flow volume loop is the combination of the maximum expiratory flow volume curve and the maximum inspiratory flow volume curve. The peak expiratory flow (PEF) is larger than the peak inspiratory flow (PIF) and displaced to the left, because of the effect of elastic recoil forces on expiration. The expiratory flow rates decline as the lung empties from the smaller airways this can be observed as the mid expiratory flow rate (MMEF or FEF$_{25-75}$)

expiratory flow limitation. Simple inspection of the loop is often sufficient to distinguish between rigid upper airway obstruction, intraluminal obstruction in chronic bronchitis and asthma, and the pressure-dependent collapse seen in pure emphysema with relative preservation of inspiratory flow rates.

The absolute value of PEF is of less use than the serial measurements which are used to monitor and manage asthma. The use of serial PEF measurements in COPD is not recommended since it may underestimate airway obstruction and also be insensitive to change. To be of value, PEF measurements should also be made to the appropriate standard. If the technique or effort are inadequate then airway obstruction will be overestimated. Recent research has also demonstrated differences in the accuracy of devices which make comparisons or reliance on absolute values unwise. The PEF (l/min) does also have a minor role in the detection of upper airway obstruction by comparison to the FEV_1 (in mls). Values of the ratio of FEV_1/PEF which exceed 8 may point to upper airway obstruction.

Lung volumes

The maximum volume of the lung or the Total Lung Capacity (TLC) cannot be measured directly in life but can be estimated by some methods. This is usually done by dilution of an inhaled tracer gas (helium dilution), by plethysmography (bodybox) or by reconstruction of lung volume from chest radiograph images. These methods measure slightly different things but in most circumstances result in similar values of functional residual capacity (FRC) from which the residual volume (RV) and TLC can be derived. The minor differences reflect the nature of the techniques. Radiographic lung volumes, which are not used routinely, contain gas, tissue and blood volume in the calculation. The plethysmographic lung volumes include all thoracic gas, including pockets that could not be accessed in the course of normal breathing. The helium dilution multi-breath lung volume approaches the plethysmographic value, but may not be equivalent in obstructed patients. The single breath helium dilution lung volume (VA) is used in the estimation of carbon monoxide gas transfer and determines the volume of the lung which is accessible in the course of a ten second breath hold. An idea of the amount of 'trapped gas' can be obtained from the TLC-VA as a further index of obstruction. This subtlety may be particularly useful in assessing emphysematous patients for surgery for bullae or reduction pneumoplasty.

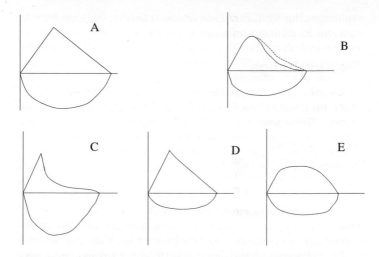

Figure 2. Schematic representations of the configurations of flow-volume loops which can help to characterise the nature of airway obstruction. A) normal pattern, B) airway obstruction in asthma or chronic bronchitis with reduction in all components and some response to bronchodilator. C) In pure emphysema the relatively preserved PEF is followed by a rapid fall in flow rates (pressure dependent collapse) at a long tail of expiratory flow. Inspiratory flow rates appear unaffected. D) Inadequate inspiratory flow in diaphragm weakness or extra thoracic floppy obstruction of the extrathoracic airways (e.g. chondromalacea of the trachea) E) Rigid obstruction of a major airway by external compression or luminal tumour

Usually the nature of the defect of lung function can be predicted from the spirometry but valuable additional understanding can be obtained from the increase in volume, or hyperinflation associated with airway obstruction. Hyperinflation associated with emphysema is expressed to a greater degree in RV than TLC. As a result the RV/TLC ratio is also an important secondary indicator of obstruction (i.e. >40%).

Patterns of volume loss associated with restriction are less characteristic but the gradual changes in volume can be used to monitor diffuse lung disease. The RV can be used here to help distinguish true 'intrinsic' restrictive pulmonary disease from external 'constriction' due to obesity or chest wall disease. In the former there will be a reduction in RV as well as TLC while in constrictive conditions the RV/TLC ratio may rise as the TLC falls and the RV remains constant or elevated.

Gas exchange

There are many causes of the failure of tissue oxygen delivery, but there are only four pulmonary causes of impairment of gas exchange. These are:

- hypoventilation
- interference with pulmonary diffusion
- ventilation/perfusion imbalance
- true pulmonary shunt

The overall competency of gas exchanging ability can be assessed by measurement of blood gases or oximetry. The lung's contribution to the process is more difficult to define and detection of the pulmonary abnormalities of gas exchange require a more subtle approach.

In health, the red blood cells traverse the pulmonary capillaries and are fully oxygenated after about one third of their transit. This usually takes about 100msecs. A reduction of oxygen transfer will occur if the membrane is damaged, if the transit time is increased or if the quantity of available haemoglobin is reduced. It is not possible to measure the uptake of oxygen directly but carbon monoxide can be used to trace its path. Carbon monoxide (CO), when inhaled, moves rapidly across the alveolar-capillary membrane, combines with haemoglobin and is removed by the circulation. This property is exploited by the single-breath transfer test, in which a breath containing a small, known quantity of CO is held for approximately 10 seconds. The amount of CO removed by the lungs in the breath is known as the TLCO; this can be corrected for lung volume by division of the simultaneous VA; when it is termed the coefficient of gas transfer (TLCO/VA = KCO). The TLCO needs to be corrected for haemoglobin concentration if the patient is anaemic or polycythaemic since the calculation will assume a normal value.

Reduction of the TLCO occurs when the overall transfer of gas is impaired by interstitial lung diseases (e.g. ARDS, CFA) or when the available capillary blood volume is reduced by emphysematous destruction or when part of the lung is removed by surgery. The KCO will also be reduced when the quality of lung tissue is impaired (e.g., fibrosis or emphysema) but may be increased when there is proportionately more blood flow to tissue (e.g. pneumonectomy, scoliosis, obesity). Disease processes which pick off lung units progressively (CFA) may retain a normal KCO while the TLCO gradually declines.

The single breath TLCO and VA measurements have become the standard procedure. However, many patients with severe lung disease may not be able to hold their breath for the required 10s. Rebreathing and intra-breath estimates of CO transfer are available but not yet in widespread use.

Interpretation of standard lung function tests

The interpretation of lung function tests is an important skill for respiratory trainees to master and, like the CXR, can be achieved by piecemeal analysis or Gestalt impression. The important principle is that a single test alone may not provide enough information for diagnosis but may subsequently offer a method of monitoring progress. The standard set of lung function tests should include:

- pre and post bronchodilator
- flow-volume loop
- lung volumes (usually He dilution)
- carbon monoxide gas transfer

All these tests should be considered together before coming to a conclusion. Obviously the development of an analytical algorithm is an individual matter but the following approach, based on a series of questions, may be helpful:

- have the tests been conducted to technical satisfaction?
- is the clinical information sufficient? (including smoking and occupational history and Hb)
- do all the tests fit in the normal range?
- if not, is the predominant pattern obstructive, restrictive, constrictive or mixed?
- are the lungs big or small?
- if obstructed, what is the grade of FEV_1
- is there a significant bronchodilator response
- does the flow-volume loop inform about the nature of obstruction?
- is the KCO reduced (in emphysema) or preserved (even elevated) in asthma?

Table 1.   Patterns of abnormality on standard lung function tests

	Asthma*	Chronic bronchitis	Emphysema	Sarcoidosis	CFA	Scoliosis/ Obesity	Cardiac failure
FEV$_1$ (L)	↓	↓↓	↓↓	↓	↓	↓	↓
FVC (L)	n or ↓	↓	↓	↓	↓	↓	↓
FEV$_1$/FVC %	↓	↓	↓	↓ or ↑	↑	↑	n or ↓
TLC (L)	↓	n	↑	↓ or ↓↓	↓↓	↓	↓
RV (L)	n or ↑	↓	↑↑	↓	↓		n or ↑
RV/TLC %	↑	↑	↑↑	n or ↓		↑	↑
TLCO ml/min/kPa	n	↓	↓	↓	↓	n	↓
KCO ml/min/kPa/L	n or ↑	n	↓	n or ↓	n or ↓	↑	↓

* All results in asthma in remission may be normal

- if restricted, is the RV reduced or preserved (↓ in interstitial disease, ↑ in muscle weakness)?
- is the KCO reduced (in interstitial disease) or preserved (in constrictive disease)?
- would any other tests contribute to understanding?
- has the situation improved or deteriorated since previous examinations?

Experience in interpretation is only likely to be gained from trial and error and discussion of the results with an experienced supervisor. The worked examples in the appendix may be helpful.

Chest wall function

The chest wall is the physiological organ which contains the bony structure of the ribcage as well as the respiratory muscles which inflate it. The diaphragm is the major muscle of inspiration but its action is supported by obligatory function of the intercostal and scalene muscles. The smooth expansion of the ribcage depends upon co-ordinated action of these muscles as well as the mobility of all the ribcage joints. Clearly any interference with either the power of the respiratory muscles or the compliance of the ribcage will lead to difficulties. Respiratory muscle weakness may occur in myasthenia, poliomyelitis, and the muscular dystrophies. Reduced compliance of the ribcage (increased stiffness) will be present in patients with scoliosis and following thoracoplasty. The two problems often compound each other when they coexist as for example, in paralytic scoliosis complicating old polio. A reflection of impaired function can be obtained from standard lung function tests which might demonstrate a constrictive picture with reduced TLC (weak inspiratory muscles or decreased ribcage compliance) and elevated KCO and RV (weak expiratory muscles). Specific tests of muscle function are also available.

Global respiratory muscle strength is most easily judged by the peak pressures generated at the mouth by the respiratory muscles in inspiration from RV and expiration from TLC (PIMax and PEMax). The function of the diaphragm can be separated from the other muscles by observing the transdiaphragmatic pressure gradient (Pdi) between the oesophagus and the stomach. This is not usually very convenient and the diaphragm can be also be assessed by X-ray or ultrasound screening, or simply by observing the difference between the standing and lying vital capacity which should be less than 30%. The normal ranges of these tests are rather wide but recently, peak sniff pressure, a purely diaphragmatic action, has demonstrated more reliability.

Apart from the wide range of normality, the other difficulties of respiratory muscle testing are the volitional requirement and the lack of sensitivity to loss of function. Non-volitional testing of the respiratory muscles is possible by electrical or magnetic stimulation but these are not, at present, performed outside specialist units. The clinical testing of the respiratory muscles is most important in the situation of deteriorating function when mechanical support is being considered. Examples include the slow deterioration in muscular dystrophy or the more rapid progression in Guillain Barré or botulism. In the latter conditions, frequent, serial monitoring of the vital capacity or PiMax is recommended. Once the Pimax falls below 30 cm H_2O or the VC below 1 litre, intervention will be required. For patients with more chronic deterioration, nocturnal oximetry can confirm periods of hypoventilation which would justify ventilatory support.

Blood gas analysis

This topic is likely to recur throughout his book, particularly in the discussion of respiratory failure. However, arterial blood gas analysis is a fundamental task of the lung function laboratory as a component of comprehensive lung function testing.

In the laboratory, sampling directly from an artery is often inconvenient and unnecessary. In most situations an arterialised earlobe capillary sample is adequate and does not require medical involvement. Such samples can also be stored on ice for a short period and can therefore be taken in the patients home if necessary.

Blood gas analysis provides information about gas exchange (oxygenation) and also about the acid base status of the body which are not always linked. It is worth remembering that the blood gas analyser only measures PO_2, PCO_2 and pH (or H^+). Other parameters (HCO_3, base excess etc.) are calculated from the Henderson-Hasselbach equation. A very simple analysis of blood gases asks the questions:

- what is the PaO_2? (i.e. is hypoxia or respiratory failure present ($PaO_2 < 8.0$ kPa)
- what is the acid base status?

The examination of acid base status can be performed using the standard Flenley diagram which relates $PaCO_2$ to pH (or H^+)

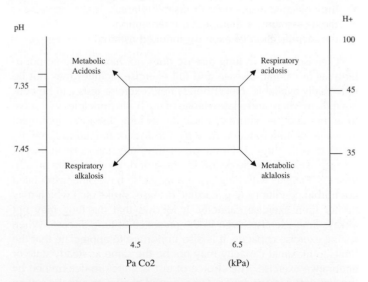

Figure 3. The Flenley diagram helps to interpret blood gas acid base abnormalities by relating the pH or H^+ concentration to the $PaCO_2$. Movement away from the box of normal values would describe the category of abnormality e.g. respiratory acidosis suggests ventilatory failure, metabolic acidosis suggests diabetes or uraemia etc

and describes respiratory and metabolic causes of acidosis and alkalosis.

The practical value of blood gas analysis in the lung function laboratory relates to:

- identification of hypoxia or respiratory failure in patients of uncertain severity
- prescription of LTOT or inflight oxygen
- use of the base excess to warn of nocturnal hypoventilation in vulnerable patients
- identification of blood gas abnormalities during exercise.

Exercise testing

Symptoms of lung disease usually include exertional breathlessness and in the assessment of lung disease the testing of exercise capacity has four major functions:

- the differential diagnosis of exertional dyspnoea
- the objective assessment of disability
- the assessment of therapeutic intervention
- the identification of exercise induced asthma

Exercise testing in lung disease does not have the same popularity as in cardiac disease and full exercise facilities may not be universally available. Nevertheless field exercise tests can be conducted anywhere and a knowledge of the basic principles will serve to understand the nature of disability in lung disease. Impairment (damage) of lung function may lead to loss of function (disability) either directly through limitation of lung mechanics or indirectly through skeletal muscle deconditioning or disproportionate breathlessness. Patients with lung disease may also have other associated co-morbid conditions (e.g. cardiac disease, stroke etc.) which may further limit exercise capacity. It follows that the lung may not always limit exercise, even in the presence of lung disease. When testing exercise capacity, it is also important to appreciate that the limits to maximal capacity may not be the same as steady state or endurance exercise. The choice of test is therefore determined by the aim of the investigation, the required challenge and the setting (field or laboratory).

Field tests of exercise capacity in lung disease generally only record a task performance, usually distance or time, but there is no reason why they should not be enhanced by other additional measurements such as heart rate or breathlessness scores. Examples of popular field tests include the six minute walk (SMWT) and the shuttle walk test (SWT). The SMWT is a self paced test where the subject is asked to walk at their own pace along a corridor with aim of covering as greater a distance as possible. Encouragement is standardised but there is a learning effect which requires 2 to 3 practices before the test is reproducible. The result is expressed as the distance covered in metres in six minutes.

The SWT is a down graded development of the shuttle running test where a patient walks to-and-fro between two cones, 10 metres apart. The pace of the walking is set by an audio signal which increases every minute. The subjects continue to shuttle until they cannot keep up to the pace and the result is also expressed in metres. There are fundamental differences between the two tests since the SWT is a reproducible test of maximal capacity, akin to the laboratory exercise test while the SMWT is less reproducible but perhaps closer to real life activity. Ranges of normal values have not been developed yet for either test but the clinically significant change in SMWT after an intervention is about 55 metres and less in SWT.

The laboratory cardio-pulmonary exercise test remains the gold standard exercise assessment in lung disease. The modern exercise laboratory will contain an exercise platform (cycle ergometer or treadmill), gas analysers for the measurement of oxygen uptake and carbon dioxide elution, and methods of measuring ventilation, heart rate, gas exchange and symptom intensity. The usual protocol for examination in lung disease is the incremental test of maximal capacity with one minute increments of about 10–15 watts. Although this does not reflect real life it does provide an opportunity to assess disability objectively and determine the limiting factors to under performance. Other protocols may be used for specialist purposes. The choice of exercise platform is open but the cycle allows direct measurement of workload and stability while the exercise may be unfamiliar. The treadmill on the other hand offers familiar exercise but is more difficult to control. Repeat measurements should always be made on the same platform. The safety of exercise testing in lung disease is not known precisely since most figures relate to combined cardiac and pulmonary testing. Since patients with lung disease are likely to be limited by respiratory mechanics before they stress their cardiovascular system, then the risks will be lower. Nevertheless, the procedure must be ordinarily supervised by at least two technicians or a doctor in higher risk cases.

As subjects with lung disease exercise, their ventilation (VE), oxygen uptake (VO_2), carbon dioxide output (VCO_2), heart rate (HR) and cardiac output (CO) all increase in a linear fashion. In healthy people, maximal exercise is limited by cardiovascular factors and VO_2 may reach a plateau (VO_{2max}) while anaerobic activity continues for a short time. This is seldom seen in patients with lung disease whose oxygen uptake is truncated prematurely (VO_{2peak}) by reaching the limits of ventilatory capacity. For this reason patients with lung disease may also demonstrate a high or absent anaerobic threshold (AT). Thus the value of the AT (usually identified by the inflection on the VO_2/VCO_2 plot) is rather diminished in lung disease, though it can still serve to discriminate cardiac from pulmonary limitation. At the end of exercise it is important to enquire why people have stopped, in many cases this may be due to dyspnoea but leg fatigue and chest pain may also play a part.

Presentation of exercise data is usually made as:

* a summary sheet of maximal data with normal values
* a graphical presentation of key data (VO_2, VCO_2, VE, VT, Workload, HR, SpO_2)
* tables of the raw data and technical comments

The interpretation of laboratory cardiopulmonary exercise tests may also follow a computer algorithm (usually based on AT) or analytical approach. The former may be difficult in lung disease while the latter is achieved in the same manner as the interpretation of static lung function tests with a series of questions.

* is the exercise a maximum effort?
* does the effort reach the expected normal value?
* how is the effort achieved?
* what limits the exercise?

Indicators of maximum effort include reaching predicted maximum heart rate, VO_{2max}, $R_Q > 1$, or a ventilatory limit. Poor effort is recognised by high heart rate and breathing reserves, variable ventilation and relatively high symptom scores.

Reference values for cardiopulmonary exercise tests exist but are not as well developed as static lung function. As a guide, values of VO_{2peak} of <25 ml/Kg/min are abnormal and <10 ml/Kg/min associated with severe disability. Obviously the expectation of the peak values has to be considered in the light of the potentially elderly and infirm population. The calculation of predicted maximum VE (MVV) has been a subject of controversy but a calculated value of actual $FEV_1 \times 37.5$ is a reasonable approximation.

The pattern of exercise response derived from inspection of the graphs which may demonstrate steep VO_2/VE plots (ventilatory equivalent), steep HR slopes, variable effort etc. This provides the reporter with information about the pathophysiological mechanisms during exercise.

The cause of exercise termination can be identified either by questioning (e.g. chest pain) or by inspection of the data. A ventilatory limit can be assumed if VE_{max} >80% predicted MVV, VT >70% of vital capacity, respiratory rate >50, breathing reserve MVV-VE_{max} <11 litres or an elevated $PaCO_2$. Other respiratory limitation such as oxygen desaturation may also be obvious.

Cardiac limitation can be recognised by high resting heart rate, achievement of maximal predicted heart rate or other cardiac features.

Respiratory physicians are often asked to make an assessment of disability for legal or benefit purposes. This is frequently done from questioning, physical examination and static exercise tests. These methods have proven unreliability, and the relationship between a clinicians estimate or lung function tests, and exercise performance is very poor. Exercise testing provides an opportunity to make an objective estimate of disability. In the rehabilitation setting, field tests will be a convenient and sensitive method to assess disability and demonstrate therapeutic response. In the legal assessment of disability, the closer laboratory examination is probably required.

It is clear that laboratory exercise testing is much more complex than static lung function tests and is not used in the UK as much as other countries. However, the principles of exercise testing are relatively simple and can provide important knowledge to guide clinical practice.

Lung function for specific requests

In addition to the usual lung function requests for diagnostic or monitoring purposes, laboratories are often required to provide specific advice for the following circumstances:

Surgery

There are two common requests for lung function assessment for surgery. Firstly, whether a patient with lung disease is fit for general surgery and secondly is a patient fit enough to have thoracic surgery. In general, the assessment of fitness should be left to the anaesthetist. However, as a guide patients with lung disease will generally tolerate ophthalmic or urology procedures much better than abdominal or thoracic procedures. Overall patients with lung function tests in excess of 50% predicted are likely to manage satisfactorily.

Fitness for thoracic surgery is a different proposition since it may not only damage or remove functioning lung tissue but is also likely to be performed on patients with existing lung disease. In the long term, lobectomy causes little functional loss but pneumonectomy may result in significant disability. In this situation, patients with FEV_1 <50% predicted, (or FEV_1 <1.5l for lobectomy and FEV_1 <2.0l for pneumonectomy) will need careful assessment. This can involve calculation of the postoperative FEV_1 from the number of segments to be removed as well as the demonstration of a basic level of exercise capacity (VO_2 >15 ml/kg/min or equivalent field test). A post operative FEV_1 of >40% predicted normal value and DLCO >40% predicted normal value is required for successful outcome. For borderline patients an exercise test may be needed to discriminate.

Although even an uncomplicated thoracotomy may temporarily reduce FEV_1 by about 500 ml, it is worth remembering that a few thoracic surgical procedures actually improve lung function. Examples of functionally beneficial surgery include transplantation, bullectomy, reduction pneumoplasty and decortication.

Travel

See Chapter 6, page 150; Chapter 26.

Oxygen prescription

LTOT assessment. See Chapter 6, page 148.

Appendix 1. Less common tests of lung function

Bronchial challenge testing

Tests of bronchial responsiveness are usually performed when the diagnosis of asthma requires confirmation. Specific bronchial challenges may be performed to identify specific occupational sensitisers.

More commonly, non specific bronchial challenge testing is conducted to demonstrate hyper-responsiveness. Examples of chemical challenge agents include methacholine and histamine while physical challenges such as exercise and cold air may also reproduce symptoms.

The methodology of chemical challenge involves the inhalation of increasing doses or concentrations of histamine or methacholine until the FEV_1 falls by 20%. This threshold is known as the provocative dose or concentration (PD_{20} or PC_{20}). A value of PC_{20} of <8.0 mg/ml is indicative of bronchial hyperresponsiveness and suggestive of asthma. The value of PC_{20} may alter with remission and relapse of the condition. Sometimes specific airway conductance (S_{gaw}) is used instead of FEV_1 to limit the effect of the forced manoeuvre when the result is expressed as the PC_{35}.

Exercise induced asthma may be uncovered by an exercise challenge in a similar fashion. In this case the subject exercises at a standard level (6 mins in excess of 60% VO_{2max}) while the FEV_1 is measured serially. In this situation, exercise may initially bronchodilate and the measurements must be continued for 30mins after the challenge. Caution should also be applied because exercise challenges in warm, humid, laboratories may not be the same as cold dry air.

Airway mechanics

The quantification of airways resistance could provide a relatively effort independent measure of airway obstruction. The major site of airway resistance is in the upper airway during normal breathing and the resistance (R_{aw}) can be measured by a variety of techniques. The most common are the plethysmographic panting or closed shutter techniques to obtain flow/pressure relationships. Other methods include the multiple interrupter and oscillography which has undergone a recent renaissance. Airways resistance changes with lung volume and therefore it may also be expressed as the reciprocal, corrected for lung volume (the specific conductance, S_{Gaw}).

Pulmonary and chest wall compliance

The pressure-volume characteristics of the lung and the total respiratory system can be plotted to obtain the compliance (stiffness) of the components. In theory stiff lungs would be a feature of fibrosis and distensibility occur in emphysema. Pulmonary compliance (C_L) requires the use of an oesophageal balloon to measure pleural pressure and the pressure-volume curve is obtained in a static or quasi-static manner by controlled expiration. Apart from research there is now very little clinical application for the test.

Respiratory Drive

Respiratory drive cannot be measured directly in man but proxies can be obtained by CO_2 rebreathing and the P0.1 measurement. In the former the subject rebreathes from an anaesthetic bag containing 4% CO_2 while ventilation is monitored. The slope of VE vs PCO_2 indicates respiratory drive. The alternative, non chemical, method involves an interruption to inspiration by a mechanical shutter 0.1 s after the beginning of the breath before any voluntary correction can apply. The inspiratory effort at this point is a reflection of respiratory drive. Once again, these tests only have limited clinical value and caution must be applied since the tests assume normal respiratory muscle function.

MIGET

The multiple inert gas elimination technique is a method for examination of the V/Q relationships within the lung. It involves the intravascular injection of a solution of different gases of varying solubility. The pattern of elution in the expired gas or retention in the blood can describe the V/Q relationships. Obviously this is a highly sophisticated technique which is not yet in regular use.

Regional lung function

It is possible to examine the function of the different regions of the lung by a variety of techniques. Radioisotope imaging of lung for perfusion with [99m] technetium and ventilation with the short half life [81m] Krypton provides topographic regional information. Its also possible to obtain regional anatomical data from endobronchial spirometry and inert gas techniques. These rather specialised examinations require occlusion of a lobe or segment by fibreoptic bronchoscopy followed by spirometry at the mouth. The inert gas techniques examine the expired concentration profiles of insoluble argon and soluble freon sampled by mass spectrometer. The regional techniques, particularly the perfusion scanning have some practical application in planning for surgery.

Imaging

Even plain radiographs of the lung can demonstrate the symmetry and degree of ventilation if taken in inspiration and expiration. Radiographs taken under known conditions of magnification can be used to calculate lung volume. CT and MRI can also demonstrate regional inhomgenieties in ventilation and diaphragm configuration. Ultrasound examination of the diaphragm can describe function and also examine the area of apposition as a function of muscle bulk and geometry.

Single breath nitrogen test

The single breath nitrogen washout test follows the expired concentration of nitrogen following the inspiration of a breath of 100% oxygen. The expired concentration has four phases or slopes. The phase II allows calculation of the anatomical dead space, the slope of phase III reflects the homogeneity of ventilation. The terminal rise in concentration is the phase IV or closing volume of the lung when depend airways collapse. The latter was thought to identify early airways disease but has not fulfilled its promise.

Further Reading

1. Gibson GJ. Clinical Tests of Respiratory Function, 2nd ed. London: Lippincott, Williams and Wilkins 1995

2. Cotes JE. Lung Function Testing, 6th ed. Oxford: Blackwell 1997

3. Hughes JMB, Pride NB. Lung Function Tests: Physiological principles and clinical applications. WB Saunders 1999

4. Kinnear WJM. Lung function tests; a guide to their interpretation. Nottingham University Press 1997

5. West JB. Respiratory physiology: the essentials, 6th ed. Lippincott, Williams and Wilkins 1999

6. Wasserman K, Hansen JE, Sue DY, Whipp BJ, Casaburi R. Principles of exercise testing and interpretation, 3rd ed. Lippincott, Williams and Wilkins 1999

7. Jones NL. Clinical Exercise Testing, 4th ed. Philadelphia: WB Saunders 1997

Key references

1.   Quanjer PH (ed). Standardised lung function testing. *Eur Respir J* 1993;**6**:suppl 16

2.   BTS and ARTP, Guidelines for the measurement of respiratory function. *Respiratory Medicine* 1994;**88**:165–194

3.   ERS task force document. Clinical exercise testing with reference to lung diseases: indications, standardisation and interpretation strategies. *Eur Respir J* 1997;**10**:2662–2689

4.   European respiratory monograph "Clinical exercise testing", Roca J, Whipp BJ, eds. *Pub Eur Respir Soc* 1997;**2**:Monograph 6

Case History 1

A 64 year old female ex smoker with airway obstruction had a full set of lung function tests before (visit 1) and after lung volume reduction surgery (visit 2). Lung volumes were performed by both plethysmography and helium dilution.

	range	mean	Visit 1	post bronchodilator	Visit 2
FEV_1 (L)	1.48–2.74	2.11	0.50	0.73	1.62
FVC (L)	2.09–2.95	2.52	1.72	2.50	3.2
SVC (L)			1.84		
FEV_1/FVC %	71–	77	29	29	51
TLC (L) plethysmography	3.71–5.84	4.77	7.10		5.17
RV (L)	1.2–2.75	1.97	5.27		2.24
RV/TLC %	30–	41	74		43
TLC (L) Helium dilution			5.52		4.48
RV			3.68		1.28
TLCO ml/min/kPa	19.99–23.00	21.5	9.89		11.47
KCO ml/min/kPa/L	4.38–5.37	4.87	2.16		2.88

Comments

The initial results show severe airway obstruction (FEV_1 <40% predicted) with a maximal flow volume loop which is characteristic of emphysema (preserved peak, sudden cut off and relatively unrestricted inspiration).

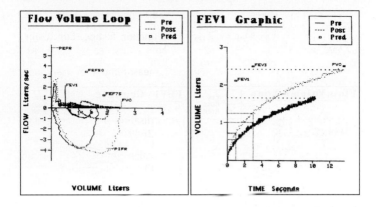

There is a significant bronchodilator response (>15% and >200ml increase in FEV$_1$). Note also the substantial improvement in FVC. Note the longer time of expiration of the spirogram and the deeper inspiratory flow volume curve.

The slow vital capacity (SVC) is bigger than the forced VC.

The lung volumes show gross hyperinflation which is more evident on the plethysmographic measurement. The RV/TLC is very high (RV exceeds predicted TLC). There is approximately 2.52 litres of gas trapping (TLC-VA) indicating inaccessible lung.

Both the TLCO and the KCO are reduced in keeping with loss of pulmonary capillary bed in emphysema.

The pattern of emphysema was heterogeneous and the patient underwent lung volume reduction surgery. Six months later the repeated lung function tests show substantial deflation associated with improvement in airway obstruction and reduction in symptoms. The TLCO is little affected by surgery.

This case demonstrates a typical pattern for emphysema and suggests that the presence of hyperinflation may not have been appreciated from the spirometry alone. Patients with COPD may also have varying degrees of bronchodilator reversibility.

Case 2

A 46 year old woman presented with cough and exertional breathlessness. Clinical examination uncovered a thyroid goitre without a palpable lower border. The chest radiograph showed a retrosternal thyroid.

	range	mean	Visit 1	post bronchodilator	visit 2
FEV$_1$ (L)	2.01–3.29	2.65	2.87	2.84	3.08
FVC (L)	2.37–3.99	3.18	3.39	3.56	3.73
FEV$_1$/FVC %	73–	82	80	83	83
PEF	190–532	361	338	304	494

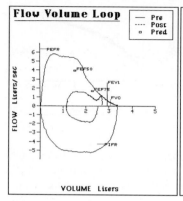

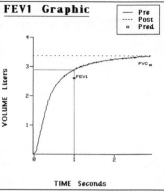

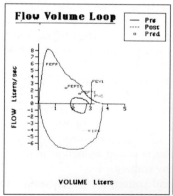

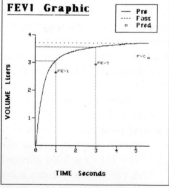

The lung function tests including the flow volume loops were performed before and after retrosternal thyroidectomy. Her symptoms were relieved by surgery.

Comments

Upper airway obstruction may be difficult to recognise on simple spirometry and there is no bronchodilator response.

A suspicion of upper airway obstruction is obtained from the relative loss of peak flow to FEV$_1$. The ratio of FEV$_1$ to PEF (Empey index) is 8.5 and improves to 6.2 after surgery.

The improvement in FEV$_1$ is relatively modest compared to PEF.

The initial flow-volume loop shows characteristic amputation of the peak flow which is restored following surgery.

Case 3

A 62 year old woman presents with progressive cough and breathlessness. The chest radiograph, CT scan and lung biopsy confirm the diagnosis of cryptogenic fibrosing alveolitis. Lung function tests are conducted over a period of two years.

	range	mean	Visit 1	Visit 2	Visit 3	Visit 4
FEV$_1$ (L)	1.4–2.16	1.78	1.84	1.88	1.47	1.47
FVC (L)	1.72–2.58	2.15	2.04	2.18	1.68	1.8
FEV$_1$/FVC %	71–	77	90	86	88	82
TLC (L) helium dilution	3.52–4.71	4.11	2.95	2.95	2.68	2.63
RV (L)	1.36–2.06	1.71	1.22	0.8	0.89	0.83
RV/TLC %	34–	40	41	27	33	32
TLCO ml/min/kPa	17.94–20.94	19.44	8.33	9.86	8.65	6.27
KCO ml/min/kPa/L	4.4–5.39	4.89	3.11	3.69	3.36	2.75

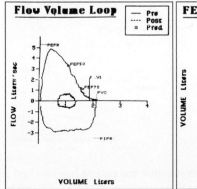
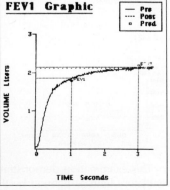

There is an initial restrictive pattern with reductions in spirometry with a high FEV$_1$/VC ratio. In this instance both The TLCO and KCO are reduced at the outset. Sometimes the KCO is preserved. The flow volume loop does not contribute greatly in this case.

After treatment with steroids and azathiaprine there is a slight improvement at visit two.

By visit 3 there has been further restriction which is manifest in the drop in TLC and fall in TLCO.

Two years after diagnosis there has been further decline in lung volumes and gas transfer

The changes in TLC and TLCO from visit 2 to 3 could be variation in the measurement but the visit 4 results confirm the trend.

Case history 4 (exercise test)

A sixty year old man was making a legal claim for disability resulting from COPD resulting from industrial exposure. He is an ex smoker, wt 99 Kg, BMI 33 and FEV1 1.45 (46%).

He underwent a progressive incremental treadmill protocol (Balke) with a constant walking speed of 4 km/hr and increments of 1.5% gradient per minute. Oxygen saturation fell to 90% at peak exercise from a baseline of 96%.

		Predicted	measured	% predicted
VO_{2peak}	Litres/min	3.09	1.67	54
VO_{2peak}	mls/kg/min	32	16.9	
VE	Litres/min	58	59.3	102
HR_{peak}	Beats/min	160	108	68
O_2 pulse	(mls/beat)	19.3	15.5	80
W_{peak}			gradient 7.5% at 4.0kms/hr	
GET (AT)			61% of $VO2_{peak}$	

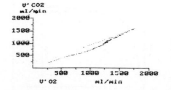 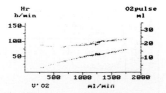

This examination demonstrates that the patient has reached a ventilatory limit as defined by the achievement of VE_{peak} close to predicted VE_{peak} while the heart rate reserve is high and the O_2 pulse is not maximal.

The graphs show a linear rise to a peak in VO_2 without a plateau. There is an inflection in the VO_2/VCO_2 plot at the gas exchange threshold (GET). The heart rate and oxygen pulse plots are shallow and do not reach predicted maximum values.

The subject has achieved a gas exchange threshold (Anaerobic threshold) and an RQ >1 to suggest that effort was maximal.

Peak exercise has therefore occurred after a satisfactory effort and is limited by the respiratory mechanics (i.e. COPD).

Case 5 (exercise test)

Another sixty year old man made a legal claim for disability from COPD resulting from industrial exposure. He is also an ex-smoker, wt 89 Kg, BMI 32 and FEV1 1.85 (62% predicted).

He underwent a progressive incremental treadmill protocol (Balke) with a constant walking speed of 3 km/hr and increments of 2.0% gradient per minute.

		Predicted	measured	% predicted
VO_{2peak}	Litres/min	2.76	1.44	52
VO_{2peak}	mls/kg/min	31	16.2	52
VE	Litres/min	74	38.8	52
HR_{peak}	Beats/min	160	120	75
O_2 pulse (mls/beat)		17.3	12	69
W_{peak}			gradient 12.0 speed 3.0 km/hr	
GET (AT)			not achieved	

In this case the exercise performance was inadequate and no limiting factor is identified. The RQ at end exercise was 0.96 and there are high heart rate and breathing reserves suggesting that there is neither cardiac or pulmonary limitation to exercise.

The VO_2/VCO_2 plot shows no obvious inflection of AT and the heart rate plot is shallow. The subject has therefore failed to demonstrate limiting disability due to unsatisfactory effort.

2

Thoracic Imaging

Melanie Greaves

This chapter provides an introduction to chest imaging for the respiratory physician. Imaging techniques useful in the investigation of thoracic diseases are discussed in Section 1. Basic principles of chest radiographic diagnosis are covered in Section 2. More detailed coverage of specific topics in chest imaging can be found in Section 3.

Section 1: Imaging Techniques for the Investigation of Thoracic Disease

Chest radiography

The standard chest radiographic projection is taken in deep inspiration with the patient positioned upright and the front of their chest positioned against the film cassette. X-rays pass through the patient from back to front, hence this projection is called postero-anterior (PA).

If patients are unable to stand or sit upright by themselves they are imaged either sitting or lying with their backs against the film cassette. If this is the case, the X-ray beam passes from front to back and the projection is called antero-posterior (AP). Usually, the radiographer will write on the film if the projection is AP and if taken erect or supine. If the radiographer has forgotten, AP chest radiographs can usually be identified as the scapulae will overlie the lungs.

PA erect chest radiographs are always preferable to AP chest radiographs for several reasons.

- anterior structures such as the heart are not magnified and distorted
- the scapulae are normally rotated anteriorly so that they do not project over the lungs

Films taken at the patient's bedside are more difficult to interpret as the majority are taken supine or semi-erect. Magnification is greater than on standard PA chest radiographs, small amounts of rotation produce marked distortion of anterior structures and the lung bases are frequently obscured by the anterior diaphragms. Supine and semi-erect positioning alter the distribution of free intrapleural air and fluid and change the size and appearance of pulmonary vessels. Portable examinations should only be requested when there is no feasible way of transporting the patient to the main X-ray department.

Additional projections include:

- lateral. Useful in confirming and localising abnormalities seen on the frontal (PA or AP) chest radiograph or in identifying those behind the heart or diaphragm. Approximately 10% of pulmonary disease is more clearly or exclusively visualised on a lateral radiograph. The standard teaching is to position the abnormal side against the film cassette. In reality, it makes very little difference and routinely a left lateral chest radiograph will be taken.
- oblique radiographs. Occasionally useful in differentiating a small pulmonary nodule from superimposed normal bony and vascular structures
- lateral decubitus radiographs. These are helpful in evaluating the presence, size and mobility of small amounts of intrapleural air or fluid
- apical-lordotic views project the clavicles above the chest and may be helpful in evaluating apical lesions
- chest radiographs in expiration may be required for the detection of tiny pneumothoraces

Fluoroscopy of the chest enables real time imaging of the patient using X-rays and an imaging intensifier. It can be useful for confirming the presence of small nodules but its main application is in the assessment of diaphragmatic motion and to guide interventional procedures.

Table 1.   Common applications of conventional thoracic CT

1.   assessing the equivocal hilum
2.   staging of lung carcinoma
3.   diagnosis and characterisation of mediastinal masses
4.   diagnosis and characterisation of pleural disease
5.   detection of metastatic malignancy
6.   assessment of thoracic aortic disease
7.   guidence for percutaneous thoracic intervention

Chest ultrasound

Ultrasonography is useful in the detection and characterisation of pleural diseases, particularly pleural effusions and is often helpful in guiding pleural and pericardial fluid aspiration, pleural biopsy and drain placement. Occasionally, peripheral lung lesions can be localised for biopsy using this technique.

Computed tomography

Computed tomography (CT) generates a cross-sectional image of the patient with a very narrow (collimated) beam of X-rays. The beam passes through the patient and the intensity of the emerging beam is recorded by electronic detectors. During the examination the beam is rotated around the patient and multiple measurements are made from different angles. The measurements of beam intensity are processed by a computer which reconstructs a digital image representing a thin 'slice of patient'. Unlike plain radiographs, images are produced that are free from superimposition of overlying structures. The thickness of the beam determines the thickness of the image slice. Typically 8–10 mm thick slices suffice but the examination protocol is tailored for individual examinations. The imaging information is displayed as a grey scale image; bone usually appearing white and air dark. It can be manipulated to show soft tissue, lung or bone to best advantage and usually several sets of images are provided for review.

An intravenous injection of iodinated contrast may be given during the examination. This increases the density of blood making it brighter on CT images and enables differentiation of vessels from other structures such as lymph nodes. Common indications for thoracic CT are detailed in Table 1.

Table 2.   Indications for high-resolution CT

1. suspicion of lung disease in the setting of a normal chest radiograph
2. characterisation of lung disease
3. assessment of disease activity
4. localisation of disease for biopsy
5. disease follow-up and assessment of response to therapy

High resolution CT (HRCT) is a modification of conventional CT technique enabling resolution of tiny lung structures. This is achieved primarily by producing 1–2 mm thick slices using short scan times (1–2 seconds). The images are reconstructed with sharper interfaces. This enables visualisation of the lung in a manner comparable to macroscopic evaluation by a histopathologist. This technique is of particular value in the diagnosis of diffuse parenchymal lung disease and bronchiectasis. Indications for HRCT are listed in Table 2 and the clinical utility of HRCT is discussed in Section 3.

Conventional CT scanning can only image a few slices in one breath hold. Recent technical developments in CT scanner technology have enabled continuous scanning with spiral or helical CT. This results in very fast imaging and production of a block or volume of scan data which can be subsequently reconstructed into a similar set of image slices as with conventional CT. Spiral CT has several advantages over conventional CT:

- imaging of a volume of tissue in one breath hold limits problems resulting from respiratory movement and small lesions are less likely to be missed
- the data can be reconstructed into high quality multiplanar and three dimensional images
- fast scanning enables improved contrast enhancement of vessels

Magnetic resonance imaging (MRI)

Patients are positioned within the scanner and exposed to short bursts of radiowaves, called radiofrequency (RF) pulses. This looks at the distribution of hydrogen atoms. An atom of hydrogen has one proton within its nucleus and the motion of these protons is altered by the RF pulses. When returning to their original state the protons emit RF signals of their own. These are detected by the detector coils of the scanner and are processed by the computer before display as a cross-sectional image. MRI has several advantages compared with CT:

- MRI does not use ionising radiation
- images can be produced in any plane
- there is excellent contrast between different soft tissues

MRI is well established in the diagnosis of cardiac, aortic and mediastinal disease. The advantages detailed above should make MRI an ideal modality for imaging the lung parenchyma but unfortunately technical problems (magnetic susceptibility effects and motion) mean that at present it is of little value in imaging lung parenchyma. New pulse sequences are presently being researched that will hopefully expand the role of MRI for imaging the lungs in the future.

Ventilation-perfusion radionuclide lung imaging

Ventilation-perfusion radionuclide lung imaging (V/Q scanning) is used primarily in the diagnosis of pulmonary embolism. The VQ scan is safe and easy to perform with images of lung perfusion and ventilation recorded by a gamma camera. Lung perfusion is assessed by injecting radiolabelled (99m Tc) tiny particles. These lodge in the microvasculature of the lung and the number of particles lodged is directly proportional to the pulmonary blood flow in that region. Subsequently, the patient breaths a radioactive gas (typically krypton 81 or xenon 133) and images of lung ventilation obtained. In PE vessels are typically occluded by emboli resulting in perfusion defects. These areas usually ventilate normally. If this classical picture of ventilation-perfusion mismatch occurs then the diagnosis of PE is made. If the VQ scan is normal then PE can be excluded. Unfortunately many patients with suspected PE have V/Q scans that are non specific and that neither confirm nor exclude the diagnosis. In these patients it may be appropriate to proceed to further investigations. The investigation of pulmonary embolism is discussed further in Section 3.

^{67}Ga scanning

^{67}Ga Citrate may be used as a tumour specific tracer specifically for staging and evaluation of treatment response in Hodgkin's disease and other lymphomas and in bone and soft tissue sarcomas. The sensitivity and specificity of ^{67}Ga studies in non-Hodgkin's lymphoma have been consistently greater than 85% with even better results in Hodgkin's disease. It is of particular use in distinguishing residual disease from post treatment fibrosis in the mediastinum.

Gallium scanning is also potentially useful in assessing the activity of interstitial lung disease particularly sarcoidosis and cryptogenic fibrosing alveolitis and has been shown to predict response to therapy. Unfortunately the level of gallium activity demonstrated does not seem to correlate with clinical outcome. Gallium scanning has several limitations. It is relatively costly and studies take up to 72 hours to perform and interpret. In the evaluation of interstitial lung disease, gallium uptake reverses rapidly during corticosteroid therapy. Although useful in the evaluation of malignancy it is not tumour specific with high concentrations of gallium found in liver, spleen, bone marrow, variable bowel uptake and concentration in abscess and inflammation.

^{99m}Tc-pentetic acid (DTPA) scanning

The clearance of ^{99m}Tc-DTPA is increased in patients with sarcoidosis and other interstitial lung diseases. Unfortunately, cigarette smoking also results in increased clearance of this compound limiting the technique to non-smokers.

PET scanning

See Chapter 10, page 246.

Angiography

An injection of iodinated contrast is given via a catheter that has usually been introduced via a femoral artery or vein and guided to the vessel under examination using fluoroscopy. This technique can be applied to the pulmonary arteries, the coronary arteries and the bronchial arteries. Once the vessel has been accessed and imaged, interventional radiology may play a part in patient treatment. Vessel stenoses can be dilated, embolic materials can be injected to control bleeding and thrombus can be mechanically and chemically broken down.

Section 2: Evaluating Chest Radiographs

Basic interpretation

Although the past 25 years have seen major advances in imaging technology, the chest radiograph remains the standard imaging technique for the initial investigation and follow-up of thoracic disease. It is also one of the most challenging to interpret correctly.

A basic checklist to follow is detailed below:

- check the patient name, the examination date and the side marker
- assess radiographic technique; good quality radiographs allow for visualisation of pulmonary vessels behind the heart and hemidiaphragms and fine lung structures in the lung periphery. Patient rotation can lead to distortion of mediastinal and hilar structures and is present if the medial ends of the clavicles are not equidistant from the spinous processes
- compare with previous chest radiographs. Previous chest radiographs are of primary importance when interpreting current examinations. Subtle abnormalities are much easier to detect with a 'spot the difference technique' particularly for the inexperienced observer
- be methodical in your examination of the chest and evaluate the bony thorax, the soft tissues, the diaphragm, the pleura, the hila, the lungs and the mediastinum
- pay particular attention to areas in which lesions are easily missed; the edges of the film, the lung apices, behind the heart and beneath the diaphragms
- if you see an obvious abnormality be careful not to miss additional less obvious findings

The normal radiographic anatomy of the chest is illustrated (Figures 1 and 2).

Localisation of intrathoracic lesions

The majority of lesions can be easily localised with PA and lateral chest radiographs. The lateral is usually very helpful in localising lesions. If an opacity lies beneath the major fissure then it must lie within the lower lobe. Similarly, if it lies above the major fissure it must lie within an upper lobe or the right middle lobe. If the minor fissure can also be clearly seen, differentiation between an upper and a middle lobe lesion is easy.

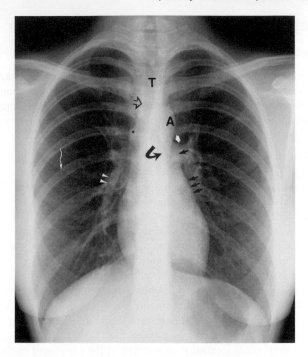

Figure 1. Normal Anatomy
Trachea (T)
Right lateral wall of the trachea (open black arrow)
Azygos arch end on (*)
Aorta (A)
Aorticopulmonary window (short white arrow)
Main pulmonary artery (single black arrow)
Region of the left atrial appendage (triple black arrow)
Left main stem bronchus (curved black arrow)
Right lower lobe pulmonary artery (white arrowheads)
Minor fissure (wavy white arrow)

Localisation of intrathoracic lesions on frontal radiographs is possible in some instances with the aid of the silhouette sign. The basis of the silhouette sign is as follows: An interface is only seen on a plain radiograph when structures of different radiographic density are adjacent to one another. Only four different radiographic densities can normally be appreciated, air (gas), fat, water (soft tissue) and calcium. Use of contrast medium adds a fifth density. Structures that are contiguous and of the same radiographic

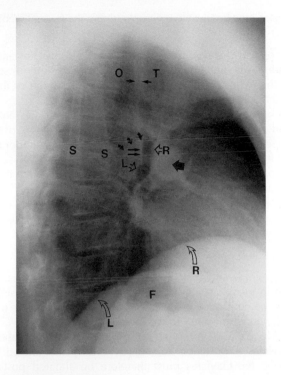

Figure 2. Normal Anatomy
Trachea (T)
Oesophagus (O)
Posterior tracheal wall and anterior oesophageal wall (two opposing arrows)
Right upper lobe bronchus end on (open arrow R)
Posterior wall of the bronchus intermedius (double black arrow)
Left upper lobe bronchus end on (open arrow L)
Posterior wall of the left main pulmonary artery (triple black arrow)
Right pulmonary artery (large black arrow)
Gas in the stomach fundus (F)
Right and left hemidiaphragms (curved open arrows)
Scapulae (S)

density will be inseparable, for example, on a chest radiograph the individual mediastinal organs appear as one grey homogenous mass. The contours of the mediastinum can however be identified as they are bordered by the air density of the lungs. Consolidated or collapsed airless lung will assume soft tissue density, therefore if diseased lung lies next to the mediastinum the normal mediastinal contour will be lost.

- an opacity that obliterates the right heart border lies anteriorly and may be within the right middle lobe, the anterior segment of the right upper lobe, the anterior mediastinum or the right anterior pleural cavity (Figure 3)
- an opacity that obliterates the left heart border lies anteriorly and may be within the lingula, the anterior segment of the left upper lobe, the anterior mediastinum or the left anterior pleural cavity
- an opacity that overlaps but that does not obliterate the heart border is posterior in location and lies in a lower lobe, the posterior mediastinum or the posterior pleural cavity (Figure 4)
- an opacity that obliterates the left hemidiaphragm lies within the left lower lobe

  Additional useful information for localising lesions:

- The right hemidiaphragm on a PA chest radiograph is of little use in localising abnormalities using the silhouette sign as it may be obliterated by disease in the right middle lobe in some individuals and right lower lobe in others
- The lung clearly visualised on a PA chest radiograph above the clavicles is posterior. An opacity clearly marginated by air above the clavicles must therefore be situated posteriorly. Structures that lie anterior to the trachea merge with cervical soft tissues and therefore cannot be clearly seen above the clavicles
- on the lateral radiograph, the vertebral bodies should decrease slightly in density from above to below. Any increase in radiographic density implies additional disease in the lower lobe or posterior mediastinum

Diseases that increase radiographic density

Pulmonary collapse generally means loss of pulmonary volume without significant filling of the alveoli. Collapse may be passive due to extrinsic pressure (for example, adjacent to a large pleural effusion) or be secondary to fibrosis. It most commonly arises from bronchial occlusion (Table 3).

The direct and most reliable signs of volume loss are displacement of the fissures and opacification of the affected lobe.

A

B

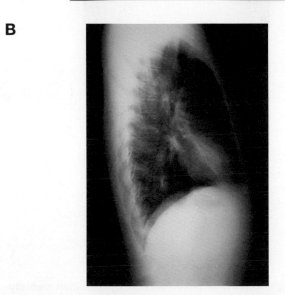

Figure 3. Right middle lobe pneumonia. A, Opacification medially at the right base with loss of the right heart border. B, Consolidation within the right middle lobe is seen overlying the heart

A

B

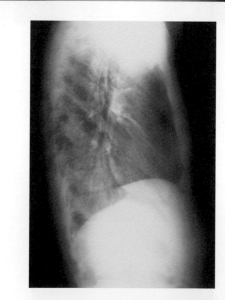

Figure 4. Right lower lobe pneumonia. A, Opacification medially at the right base with preservation of the right heart border. **B,** Consolidation in the right lower lobe is increasing the density of the inferior thoracic vertebral bodies and obliterating the contour of the posterior right hemidiaphragm. An air bronchogram is seen within the consolidated right lower lobe

Table 3.   Causes of collapse

Endobronchial obstruction
1.   tumour (benign, malignant, metastasis)
2.   foreign body (including malpositioned endotracheal tube)
3.   allergic bronchopulmonary aspergillosis
4.   mucus plug

Bronchostenosis
1.   post inflammatory (tuberculosis, sarcoidosis)
2.   post traumatic, post operative

Extrinsic compression
1   lymphadenopathy
2.   aortic aneurysm
3.   mediastinal tumour
4.   enlarged left atrium

There are many indirect specific features of lobar collapse that may be helpful if associated with direct features (Table 4).

- the right upper lobe collapses superiorly and medially. This results in a triangular region of opacification in the right upper lung with elevation of the minor fissure on the frontal radiograph. The trachea may shift to the right and usually, there is some elevation of the right hilum. On the lateral, the upper portion of the right major fissure moves forward and the minor fissure moves superiorly
- the left upper lobe collapses anterosuperiorly; tracheal deviation and left hilar elevation can frequently be identified. On the

Table 4.   Chest radiographic features of lobar collapse

Direct
displacement of interlobar fissures

Indirect
local increase in density
diaphragmatic elevation
mediastinal shift
approximation of ribs
overinflation of the remaining lung
movement or change in contour of a hilum

A

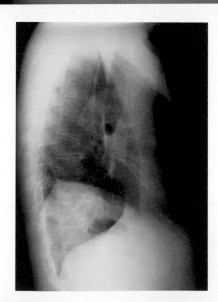

B

Figure 5.   Left upper lobe collapse. A, There is hazy opacification of the left upper thorax with loss of the left heart border associated with marked loss of volume and elevation of the left hemidiaphragm. B, The major fissure is anteriorly displaced and elevated and there is overinflation of the left lower lobe

frontal radiograph the collapsed lobe produces a veil like opacity over the upper left hemithorax with an ill defined lateral border. On the lateral radiograph the major fissure moves anteriorly paralleling the anterior chest wall and the collapsed left upper lobe is seen as a region of increased density anterior to the upper portion of the fissure (Figure 5)

- right middle lobe collapse is diagnosed when the minor fissure is displaced inferiorly and there is loss of definition of the right heart border. It can be very difficult to identify collapse of the right middle lobe on the frontal radiograph but it is much easier to appreciate on a lateral. The minor fissure moves downward and the major fissure moves anteriorly to marginate the triangular density representing the collapsed lobe. The apex of the triangle extends centrally to the hilar area (Figure 6)

- collapse of both lower lobes is similar. They collapse downward, posteriorly and medially toward the spine. The collapsed lobe is seen as a wedge shaped opacity with its apex at the hilum. Left lower lobe collapse results in a triangular opacity behind the heart with obliteration of the left hemidiaphragm; the left heart border remains sharply marginated. On the right, an area of increased opacification can be seen at the right base; the right heart border remaining sharply marginated. On the lateral view the oblique fissure moves posteriorly and the collapsed lobe is seen as a region of increased opacity projected over the lower thoracic spine

Interpretation of chest radiographs can be simplified by identifying basic patterns which can be broadly divided into air-space consolidation, interstitial disease and pulmonary nodules.

Alveolar disease (air-space consolidation). Filling of alveoli with either fluid (pus, oedema or blood) or cells. On radiographs, air-space consolidation is seen as patchy, ill-defined, poorly marginated opacities. Air filled bronchi surrounded by opacified, consolidated lung are visible as dark branching tubes. This finding is called an air bronchogram and is a hallmark of alveolar disease (Figure 7). There are a large number of diseases resulting in alveolar disease that are indistinguishable radiologically and it can be very helpful to assess the time course of the disease. Consolidation that has been present for several weeks without appreciable change usually suggests a different cause than that which has been present only a few days or is evolving rapidly (Table 5).

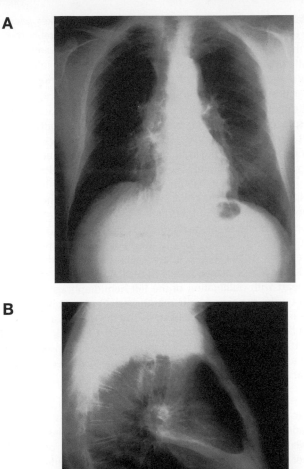

Figure 6.   Right middle lobe collapse. A, Partial loss of the right heart border. B, the collapsed right middle lobe is projected over the heart, bordered anteriorly by the minor fissure and posteriorly by the right major fissure

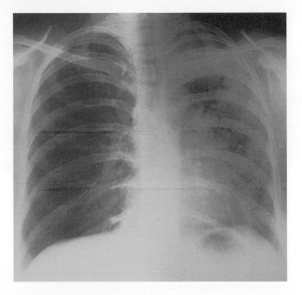

Figure 7. Left upper lobe pneumonia. Left upper lobe consolidation contains a clear air bronchogram

Table 5. Causes of air-space consolidation

Acute
1. pulmonary oedema (cardiogenic and non-cardiogenic-ARDS)
2. pneumonia
3. haemorrhage (contusion, pulmonary embolism, aspiration of blood, bleeding diathesis, anticoagulant therapy, vasculitis
4. Acute radiation pneumonitis
5. Others (acute extrinsic allergic alveolitis, drug reaction etc)

Chronic
1. indolent infections (mycobacterial, fungal, bacterial)
2. neoplasms (bronchioloalveolar cell carcinoma, lymphoma)
3. bronchiolitis obliterans organising pneumonia
4. eosinophilic lung disease
5. pulmonary alveolar proteinosis
6. pseudoalveolar disease (lymphoma, sarcoidosis)

Table 6.   Causes of interstitial disease

Acute

1.   pulmonary oedema (pressure or volume overload)
2.   infection (viral, mycoplasma, pneumocystis carinii pneumonia.

Chronic

1.   idiopathic (cryptogenic fibrosing alveolitis)
2.   collagen vascular disease (rheumatoid arthritis, scleroderma, dermatomyositis, polymyositis, mixed connective tissue disease, Sjögren's syndrome.)
3.   drug toxicity (methotrexate, cyclophosphamide, bleomycin, BCNU etc) and radiation fibrosis
4.   asbestosis
5.   extrinsic allergic alveolitis
6.   infection (post primary TB)
7.   sarcoidosis
8.   lymphangitis carcinomatosis
9.   lymphocytic interstitial pneumonia
10. miscellaneous (tuberose sclerosis, lymphangiomyomatosis, neurofibromatosis, langerhans cell histiocytosis)

Interstitial disease. The interstitium is the connective tissue framework of the lung. It extends out from the hila into the peripheral lung supporting the bronchovascular tree (axial interstitium). It extends beneath the visceral pleura as a fibrous sac from which connective tissue septa extend into the lung (peripheral interstitium), and it also comprises a portion of the alveolar walls. Diseases involving the interstitium typically result in peribronchial thickening and fine lines or a reticular (net-like) pattern on chest radiographs. There are many causes of interstitial disease, many of which cannot be distinguished on chest radiographs. As discussed above, in order to try and limit the differential diagnosis to a manageable number, it is very important to establish if the disease is acute or chronic (Table 6); some diseases have typical distribution patterns that may help limit the differential diagnosis further (Tables 7 and 8).

The most common cause of an acute interstitial pattern is cardiogenic pulmonary oedema; other findings on the chest radiograph may support this diagnosis (cardiomegaly and prominence of upper lobe vessels) (Figure 8). Interstitial disease that is changed little from month to month and associated with volume loss is usually secondary to some form of pulmonary fibrosis (Figure 9).

Table 7.   Causes of upper lobe fibrosis

1.   sarcoidosis (and beryliosis)
2.   tuberculosis
3.   radiation therapy
4.   extrinsic allergic alveolitis (historically, although HRCT has demonstrated predominantly mid lung disease)
5.   ankylosing spondylitis

Table 8.   Causes of lower lobe fibrosis

1.   cryptogenic fibrosing alveolitis
2.   collagen vascular disease
3.   asbestosis
4.   drug toxicity (bleomycin, busulphan, cyclophosphamide etc)
5.   chronic aspiration

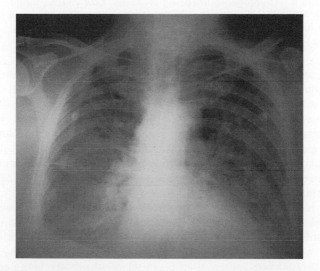

Figure 8.   Acute cardiogenic pulmonary oedema. Peribronchial thickening, subpleural oedema and septal thickening (Kerley A, B and C lines) consistent with interstitial oedema. Additionally, there is patchy alveolar oedema and a small right pleural effusion that is loculating in the minor fissure

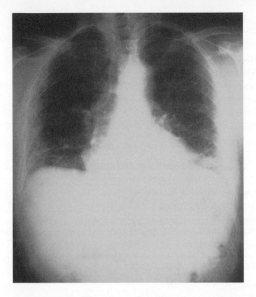

Figure 9. Cryptogenic fibrosing alveolitis. Low volume lungs with interstitial disease that is predominating peripherally and in the lung bases

Occasionally interstitial disease may mimic alveolar disease by compressing the alveoli to such an extent that air bronchograms can be seen. Sarcoidosis and pulmonary lymphoma are both interstitial processes that can produce this 'pseudoalveolar appearance'. The diagnostic limitations of the chest radiograph in chronic interstitial lung disease are well established and without exception, CT, particularly HRCT, has been shown to be more sensitive and specific than chest radiography. The clinical utility of HRCT is discussed in Section 3.

Nodules can range in size from a few millimetres to several centimetres. Again it is very helpful to determine the time course of the disease (Table 9). By convention, nodules greater than 3 cm in maximum diameter are termed masses and the majority of solitary nodules greater than 3 cm represent primary lung carcinoma. There are a large number of causes of multiple pulmonary nodules but metastatic malignancy outnumbers all the others put together.

Table 9. Causes of pulmonary nodules

Acute
1. infections, tuberculosis, viral and fungal
2. septic emboli
3. pulmonary oedema

Chronic
1. pneumoconioses
2. sarcoidosis
3. metastases
4. rheumatoid nodules
5. Wegener's granulomatois
6. lymphoma
7. sub-acute extrinsic allergic alveolitis

Diseases causing decreased opacification or increased lucency of lung

Before definitively diagnosing increased lucency of the lungs a number of other possibilities should be considered. An overexposed radiograph may result in apparently hyperlucent lungs, and rotated radiographs often lead to increased blackening of one side of the film, generally the side toward which the patient is rotated. A previous mastectomy will result in apparent increased lucency of the ipsilateral hemithorax due to the relative lack of soft tissue compared with the other side.

Emphysema is a common cause of increased lucency. Destruction of alveoli and their capillary beds combined with overinflation of the lungs produces a general reduction in lung density. Severe emphysema can usually be diagnosed on a chest radiograph but mild and moderate degrees of this disease are more difficult to detect. Patients with moderate to severe emphysema have increased lung volumes on chest radiographs, although this finding alone is non specific. Flattening of the diaphragms is more helpful. On a PA chest radiograph, the diaphragm is flattened if the highest point of the dome is less than 1.5 cm above a line drawn between the costophrenic angles (Figure 10). Additional findings include an increase in the AP diameter of the chest and an increase in the retrosternal clear space. A reduction in lung markings reflects lung destruction but may be difficult to appreciate and lacks sensitivity.

A

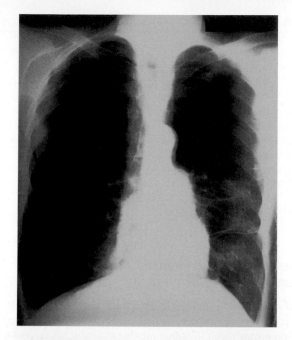

B

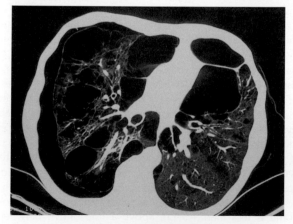

Figure 10.   Severe pulmonary emphysema. A, Grossly
hyperinflated lungs with flattening of the hemidiaphragms and
marked vascular attenuation bilaterally. B, HRCT confirms the
presence of severe emphysema with multiple bullae and clearly
demonstrates the complicating right pneumothorax

HRCT can be used to diagnose and quantify emphysema and is more sensitive and accurate than plain chest radiographs in establishing type and location of disease. Areas of emphysema are clearly seen as focal areas of low attenuation (increased blackness) contrasted with areas of more normal lung. In those patients who present with shortness of breath with a low diffusing capacity and a normal chest radiograph, CT may distinguish emphysema from early interstitial lung disease. CT is also useful in the assessment of severely emphysematous patients for lung transplantation, bullectomy or lung volume reduction surgery.

Pneumothorax. On an upright chest radiograph a pneumothorax usually appears as a well demarcated, visceral pleural line paralleling the thoracic wall. No lung markings are present peripheral to this line and the underlying lung exhibits varying degrees of collapse depending on the size of the pneumothorax.

Pneumothoraces can be difficult to see in supine patients (Figure 11). Air usually migrates to the most non-dependent regions of

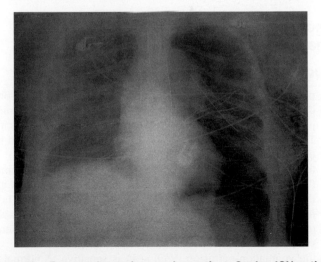

Figure 11. Pneumothorax in a supine patient. Supine ICU patient with a left basal pneumothorax. There is marked depression of the lateral costophrenic sulcus with increased lucency at the left base and clear visualisation of the left heart border and hemidiaphragm. Subcutaneous emphysema is tracking through tissues of the left chest wall. The left intercostal chest drain was situated within the left major fissure. Also note the right pleural effusion that is layering posteriorly and extending into the right major fissure

the chest and therefore, in a supine patient, collects in the anterior, inferior and medial portions of the pleural space. Features that suggest a pneumothorax in a supine patient are:

- deepening of the lateral costophrenic sulcus
- increased lucency of the lung base
- exceptionally clear visualisation of the inferior mediastinal contours
- apparent presence of two diaphragm-lung interfaces

If a pneumothorax is suspected but cannot be definitively diagnosed and the patient cannot be sat upright, consider obtaining a lateral decubitus film with the side of interest placed up. If this fails, CT may be necessary.

Frequently radiologists are asked to comment on the percentage of pneumothorax present. This is difficult to do accurately and it is much more appropriate to consider the effect of the pneumothorax on the individual patient when considering management options.

Section 3: Specific Topics in Thoracic Imaging

Diagnosing pulmonary embolism

1 pulmonary embolism (PE) accounts for 10% of all hospital deaths and is a contributing factor in a further 10%. The clinical presentation of acute PE is highly variable and non-specific. The majority of patients who die of PE are undiagnosed at the time of death

2 the chest radiograph is abnormal in 40–60% of patients. Common findings include, atelectasis with unilateral elevation of the diaphragm, consolidation and small pleural effusions. These findings are however all non-specific. The chest radiograph's usefulness often lies in excluding other causes for the patient's symptoms

3 the ventilation-perfusion (V/Q) scan is sensitive. A normal or near normal VQ scan essentially rules out the diagnosis (negative predictive value of 91%). A high probability scan makes the diagnosis very likely (positive predictive value of 88%). Additionally, concordance between clinical suspicion and VQ scan result improves the predictive value. Unfortunately, approximately 75% of hospitalised patients have indeterminate (intermediate or low probability) VQ scans or discordance

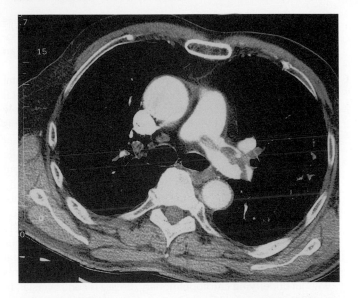

Figure 12. Spiral CT image demonstrating pulmonary thromboembolic disease. Clot is clearly seen within the left main, left upper lobe, left descending and right upper lobe pulmonary arteries

between clinical suspicion and V/Q result. In these patients additional tests are required to confirm or exclude the diagnosis. Compounding this problem is a 25%–30% interobserver disagreement in the interpretation of low and intermediate probability V/Q scans and an 8% mortality in patients with a low probability V/Q scan and limited cardiopulmonary reserve

4   pulmonary angiography remains the gold standard for the diagnosis of PE. This is costly, requires expertise and is not widely available on immediate demand. Although safe and accurate there is a reluctance by many physicians to subject their patients to this invasive procedure

5   fast scanning CT techniques (spiral and electron-beam) have both high sensitivity and specificity for the detection of thrombus to the segmental arterial level (Figure 12). In one of the first prospective studies using spiral CT, Remy Jardin et al. demonstrated a sensitivity of 100% and specificity of 96% for the detection of central pulmonary emboli (to the segmental

level) in 42 patients. Additionally pulmonary infarction has typical appearances on CT. CT can also document non thrombo-embolic abnormalities of the thorax that may provide an alternative explanation for the patient's symptoms

6   although reliable for demonstrating main, lobar and segmental clot, the accuracy of spiral CT for the detection of subsegmental thrombus decreases considerably. Goodman et al. prospectively compared helical CT and pulmonary angiography in 20 patients with unresolved suspicion for PE based on clinical assessment and V/Q scan criteria. CT was 86% sensitive and 92% specific for the detection of acute thrombus to the segmental level, but when subsegmental arteries were included, CT sensitivity dropped to 63%, diagnosing only one of four isolated sub-segmental thrombi. The detection of subsegmental thrombus on pulmonary angiography is also less than perfect. The PIOPED study found 98% interobserver agreement for lobar thrombus using this technique but only 66% agreement for subsegmental thrombus. The significance of subsegmental thrombus in patients without underlying cardiopulmonary disease is controversial. In contrast, subsegmental clot in patients with severe cardiac or pulmonary disease may be associated with significant morbidity and mortality, particularly if the occluded vessels supply areas of relatively normal lung. It has been suggested that lower limb ultrasound combined with spiral CT may prove a safe and cost effective diagnostic strategy for the diagnosis of PE. Further studies are currently being undertaken

Radiological staging of lung carcinoma

1   bronchogenic carcinoma is the most common malignancy in the Western World. It accounts for 34% of all cancer deaths in men and 22% in women

2   once the diagnosis has been established accurate staging is necessary to categorise patients world-wide into prognostic groups for prognosis, treatment and research. The TNM staging system of the American Joint Committee on Cancer is the most widely accepted method of preoperative and postoperative staging of lung carcinoma and was introduced in 1986. This describes the extent of the primary tumour (T), nodal metastasis (N) and metastatic disease (M). It has recently been slightly amended but continues to divide patients with lung carcinoma into five major groups, stages I to IV

3   resection of lung carcinoma still offers the only true means of
     cure and is the treatment of choice for localised non-small cell
     lung cancer. The main task of radiology in conjunction with
     clinical information and pathologic data is to differentiate
     potentially resectable (stages I-IIIa) from unresectable (IIIb-IV)
     disease

4   staging the primary tumour (T staging). The presence of chest
     wall invasion (stage IIb-IIIa) does not preclude surgical resection
     although it usually requires aggressive surgical resection. Plain
     radiographs, CT and MRI findings may be suggestive but it is
     difficult to definitively confirm chest wall invasion unless a large
     chest wall mass or rib destruction are present. Although MRI
     can potentially demonstrate very subtle chest wall invasion it
     can be difficult to differentiate this from inflammatory change
     and this technique probably offers little advantage over CT. MRI
     can however be very helpful in the assessment of superior
     sulcus (Pancoast) tumours (Figure 13). Its ability to image directly

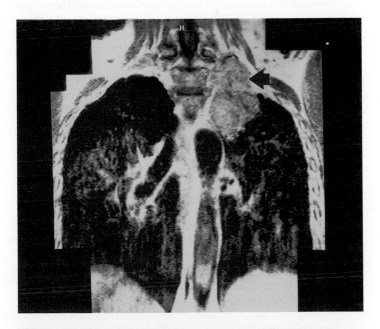

Figure 13. Coronal MRI image of a left Pancoast tumour. It demonstrates chest wall invasion at the left apex that was not identified at CT (arrow)

in coronal and saggital planes allows for accurate assessment of local invasion and brachial plexus and subclavian vessel involvement. Invasion of the mediastinum represents T4 disease and unresectability although some surgeons will operate if only mediastinal fat is involved. Gross mediastinal invasion can usually be detected by both CT and MRI whilst tumours having less than 3 mm contact with the mediastinum, less than 90° contact with the descending thoracic aorta or a preserved fat plain between the tumour and the mediastinum are almost always resectable. In general, it should be remembered that the diagnosis and exclusion of mediastinal invasion by these modalities is unreliable and patients should not be denied surgery on the basis of isolated CT or MRI findings

5   nodal disease (N staging). Metastases to ipsilateral hilar nodes (N1) decrease survival rate but are not a contraindication to surgery. Ipsilateral mediastinal lymph node disease (N2, IIIa) usually precludes surgical resection. Unfortunately, size is the only useful criterion used to distinguish normal and abnormal nodes. The short axis diameter of a node seen on an axial CT image is the best predictor of nodal volume and as such is usually used in staging. The current consensus is that the size of the short axis diameter of a normal mediastinal or hilar node should not exceed 1 cm. This does lead to problems as micrometastases may be found in normal sized nodes and hyperplastic nodes may be enlarged. Reported sensitivities and specificities for CT in the assessment of nodal metastases are variable, reflecting differing methodology and precision of radiologic, surgical and pathologic correlation. McLoud et al. used extensive nodal sampling at thoracotomy and demonstrated a sensitivity and specificity of 64% and 62% respectively. CT is however highly predictive of a negative mediastinoscopy. If no mediastinal or hilar nodes are seen at CT then mediastinoscopy may not be necessary. Any enlarged node detected with CT must be biopsied to confirm metastatic involvement.

6   distant metastasis is M1 disease (stage IV) and unresectable. Radiological investigation of possible metastatic disease is usually based on clinical history, examination and blood indices. CNS metastases are a rare isolated finding in patients with non-small cell lung carcinoma; when present they are associated with an abnormal neurological examination. Patients with skeletal metastases are usually symptomatic or have an elevated alkaline phosphatase suggestive of bone metastases. Radionuclide bone

scanning and plain radiographs will help evaluate this group of patients further. Liver and adrenal metastases are not uncommon and upper abdominal imaging is frequently performed with the staging CT thorax. It should be remembered that 3–5% of the population have nonfunctioning adrenal cortical adenomas. In the absence of other extrathoracic metastases an adrenal mass is more likely to represent an incidental finding

7   there is much interest in the potential role of PET for staging lung carcinoma. The reported sensitivities and specificities of [18]FDG-PET for identifying mediastinal nodal metastases have consistently bettered both CT and MRI, although the combination of [18]FDG-PET and CT provides the best diagnostic accuracy. Total body [18]FDG-PET is similarly impressive in identifying metastatic disease and in assessing disease recurrence. Unfortunately, PET scanners are not widespread in the UK although it is likely that with increasing availability of this technology, optimal staging of lung carcinoma will require some combination of CT and PET.

Clinical utility of high-resolution CT

1   the chest radiograph remains the first line imaging investigation in the diagnosis and follow-up of patients with suspected lung disease. Biopsy proven interstitial disease may however exist in the setting of a normal chest radiograph (10–16%). Chest radiographs are even less sensitive in diagnosing bronchiectasis with 30–50% of patients with proven bronchiectasis having normal chest films. Chest radiographs are also prone to overinterpretation. Between 10% and 20% of patients thought to have interstitial disease on chest radiographs subsequently have normal biopsies

2   HRCT is considerably more sensitive than plain radiography in detecting lung disease (94% compared to 80% respectively). It should be remembered that the sensitivity of HRCT for lung disease is not 100%

3   the diagnostic accuracy of HRCT is superior to that of plain radiographs. It can often be used to limit the differential diagnosis to a few possibilities. Some diseases have such characteristic appearances as to allow a diagnosis to be made in the absence of histologic verification in the appropriate clinical setting. These include sarcoidosis, pneumoconiosis, Histiocytosis X, lymphangiomyomatosis, hypersensitivity pneumonitis, extrinsic

allergic alveolitis, cryptogenic fibrosing alveolitis and lym-
phangitic carcinomatosis (Figures 14–17). HRCT can also allow
a confident diagnosis of both bronchiectasis and emphysema.
HRCT can even differentiate between the causes of end-stage
lung disease

4   HRCT has a sensitivity of 96–98% and a specificity of 93–99%
    for the diagnosis of bronchiectasis and has replaced broncho-
    graphy as the imaging modality of choice

5   HRCT may help evaluate disease activity in patients with diffuse
    lung disease and may be used to follow patients on treatment.
    The identification of disease activity centers on the finding of
    ground-glass opacity. Ground-glass opacity is a non-specific
    term referring to the presence on HRCT of a hazy increase in
    lung density through which the underlying vessels can still be
    seen. In patients with chronic diffuse infiltrative lung disease,
    ground-glass opacity often represents active parenchymal
    infiltration. It may however represent pulmonary fibrosis below
    the limits of HRCT resolution and in general to suggest that
    ground-glass opacity represents active disease it should be
    unassociated with HRCT findings of fibrosis. Wells et al. found
    that the presence of ground-glass opacity and its extent was
    related to prognosis and likelihood of response to treatment.
    Four-year survival and response to therapy was highest in those
    patients with a high proportion of ground-glass opacity

6   HRCT may be useful in the selection of optimal sites for lung
    biopsy. Diffuse interstitial diseases are typically quite patchy in
    distribution with areas of active disease, end-stage fibrosis and
    normal lung. HRCT can direct biopsy to sites of potentially
    active disease.

Interventional chest radiology

1   percutaneous transthoracic needle biopsy may be performed for
    any undiagnosed intrathoracic lesion providing the patient is
    cooperative and there is safe access. Specific indications and
    relative contraindications are detailed in Tables 10 and 11. A
    full blood count and prothrombin time should be obtained
    within 2 weeks of the procedure

2   lesions that can be clearly identified on frontal and lateral
    radiographs are most suited to biopsy using C-arm or biplane
    fluoroscopy. Computed tomography is most useful for lesions
    seen only on a single radiographic view. Ultrasound guidance

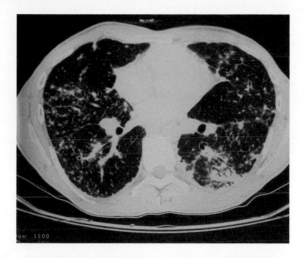

Figure 14. Pulmonary sarcoidosis on HRCT. Multiple small nodules are distributed along bronchovascular bundles, interlobular septa and pleural surfaces. A small focus of apparent consolidation with an air bronchogram in the left lower lobe is secondary to innumerable confluent granulomas

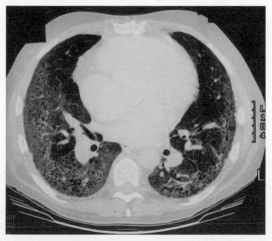

Figure 15. Pulmonary fibrosis secondary to scleroderma. HRCT demonstrates bilateral irregular reticular opacities and honeycombing involving predominantly the lung periphery. These findings are indistinguishable from those seen in cryptogenic fibrosing alveolitis

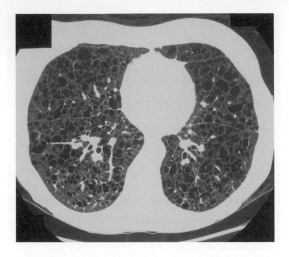

Figure 16.   Lymphangiomyomatosis. HRCT shows multiple thin walled cysts bilaterally that are diffusely distributed throughout the lungs

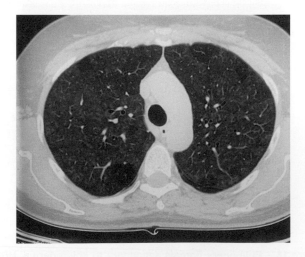

Figure 17.   Subacute extrinsic allergic alveolitis. Multiple ill-defined nodules of ground-glass opacity are seen on HRCT of the upper lobes. The majority of these are centrilobular in location, a typical feature of this disease

Table 10. Indications for percutaneous transthoracic needle biopsy

1. Evaluation of solitary or multiple pulmonary nodules
2. Evaluation of mediastinal and/or hilar masses
3. Staging evaluation of thoracic lesions (pulmonary, mediastinal, hilar, pleural, and chest wall) in the setting of known malignancy
4. Evaluation of focal or multifocal airspace disease for the presence of infection
5. Evaluation of diffuse lung disease in selected patients

Table 11. Contraindications to percutaneous transthoracic needle biopsy

Absolute Contraindications
1. Uncorrectable coagulopathy
2. Lack of patient cooperation or consent
3. Cases in which biopsy results have no effect on patient management

Relative Contraindications
1. Pulmonary artery hypertension (which may increase the risk of hemoptysis or hemorrhage)
2. Poor respiratory reserve (such as may be seen with prior contralateral pneumonectomy)
3. Moderate to severe obstructive lung disease (especially with bullae, blebs, or pneumatoceles along the biopsy path)
4. Intractable cough
5. Suspected vascular lesions or hydatid disease

is usually limited to pleural disease and peripheral pulmonary masses, usually with a broad pleural contact. Needles typically used are fine 20–22G aspirating needles and 14–20G cutting needles

3   pneumothorax is the most common complication with most series reporting an incidence of 5–30%. Chest tube drainage is required in 0–15%. Pneumothorax rates are increased in patients with obstructive airways disease, intractable coughing, small and deep lesions, lengthy procedures, those requiring multiple pleural punctures and cavitary lesions. Haemorrhage has a reported incidence of 0–10%. Systemic air embolism and seeding of the biopsy path and the pleural space are extremely rare

4   fine needle aspiration combined with expert cytopathological opinion yield sensitivities of 95–97% for malignancy. Dif-

Table 12. Indications for pleural drainage

1. Empyema/complicated parapneumonic effusions
2. Diagnosis of small pleural effusions
3. Failed blind pleural tap.

ferentiation between non-small cell and small cell carcinoma is possible in the majority of cases although precise determination of cell types of non-small cell carcinoma can be difficult, particularly in undifferentiated tumours. The diagnosis of lymphoma usually requires cutting biopsy and the definitive diagnosis of benign lesions can be problematic with positive diagnoses ranging from 16–68%. Cutting biopsy is again more helpful in these patients than aspiration biopsy

5   indications for pleural drainage procedures are detailed in Table 12. Typically ultrasound or CT are used for guidance. A 10–12 F catheter is usually sufficient for serous collections whereas 12–28 F catheters are required for thick, purulent or bloody material. Fibrinolytic therapy with streptokinase or urokinase may be necessary to enhance drainage of empyema or complicated effusions and reported success rates range from 62–94%. Intrapleural administration of 80–100 000 units of urokinase in 100 ml of saline for several hours may facilitate drainage and obviate surgery

6   image guidance may also be useful for insertion of pneumothorax drainage catheters either for spontaneous pneumothorax or loculated pleural air collections

7   CT, fluoroscopy or ultrasound may be useful to guide drainage of a lung abscess if conservative medical therapy has failed. Whilst some patients may require surgical resection, closed drainage is a reasonable alternative. Care is taken to avoid traversing normal lung with the drainage catheter to minimise the risk of haemothorax, pneumothorax, empyema or broncho-pleural fistula formation

8   although surgical resection remains the treatment of choice, percutaneous topical aspergilloma treatment may be performed by direct needle injection or following imaging guided catheter placement. Amphotericin B is the most commonly used agent and is delivered either as a liquid or a paste. Most authors report immediate cessation of haemoptysis although the mycetoma does not always completely resolve

References

1. PIOPED investigators. Value of the ventilation/perfusion scan in acute pulmonary embolism. Results of the prospective investigation of pulmonary embolism diagnosis (PIOPED). *JAMA* 1990;**263**:2753–2759

2. Remy-Jardin M, Remy J, Wattinne L, Giraud F. Central pulmonary thromboembolism: diagnosis with spiral volumetric CT with single breath hold technique-comparision with pulmonary angiography. *Radiology* 1992;**185**:381–387

3. Glazer HS, Kaiser LR, Anderson DJ et al. Indeterminate mediastinal invasion in bronchogenic carcinoma: CT evaluation. *Radiology* 1989;**173**:37–42

4. McLoud TC, Bourgouin PM, Greenberg RW et al. Bronchogenic carcinoma: Analysis of staging in the mediastinum with CT by correlative lymph node mapping and sampling. *Radiology* 1992;**182**: 319–323

5. Padley SPG, Adler B, Müller NL. High-resolution computed tomography of the chest: current indications. *J Thorac Imaging* 1993;**8**: 189–199

6. Leung AN, Miller RR, Müller NL. Parenchymal opacification in chronic infiltrative lung diseases: CT pathologic correlation. *Radiology* 1993;**188**:209–214

7. Wells AU, Rubens MB, du Bois RM, Hansell DM. Serial CT in fibrosing alveolitis: prognostic significance of the initial pattern. *AJR* 1993;**161**:1159–1165

8. Webb WR, Müller NL, Naidich DP. High-resolution CT of the lung. Lippincott-Raven 1996

Further Reading

Goodman LR, Curtin JJ, Mewissen MW et al. Detection of pulmonary embolism in patients with unresolved clinical and scintigraphic diagnosis: Helical CT versus angiography. *AJR* 1995;**164**:1369–1374

Patz EF Jr. Imaging lung cancer. *Semin Oncol* 1999;**26** (5 Suppl 15): 21–26

3

Invasive Procedures

David R Baldwin

Introduction

Becoming proficient in the performance of clinical procedures depends not only on manual dexterity and a lot of practice but also on the local facilities and expertise in procedures and a sound theoretical knowledge of the technique. When learning a new procedure, it is advisable to seek out those trainers who are highly skilled and learn by an apprenticeship. To make the most of this, one should be familiar with the principles rather than attempting to learn with no prior reading. This section provides an overview of the essential knowledge required for learning the techniques commonly performed by respiratory physicians: bronchoscopy with associated procedures and pleural procedures including medical thoracoscopy.

Bronchoscopy

Rigid bronchoscopy

Most respiratory physicians are familiar with fibreoptic bronchoscopy but relatively few perform rigid bronchoscopy regularly. Those that do perform rigid bronchoscopy do so as part of other procedures, such as cryotherapy or laser therapy where the better control of the airway with respect to bleeding and removal of large particles is an advantage. Rigid bronchoscopy is almost always performed under general anaesthetic and is, therefore, a longer and more involved procedure. The view obtained with the rigid bronchoscope is more limited than that given by the fibreoptic bronchoscope and, therefore, fibreoptic bronchoscopy has mostly replaced rigid bronchoscopy as a diagnostic procedure. Thoracic Surgeons often perform rigid bronchoscopy and many use the procedure as a way of assessing the mobility of the airways to give some indication of operability of tumours. Generally, computed tomography and mediastinoscopy are more important in assessing operability.

Fibreoptic bronchoscopy

What follows is a relatively detailed description of the procedure to provide a guide but it is acknowledged that there are many variations and one should develop preferences which work best. Bronchoscopy can be performed with the patient lying flat and the bronchoscopist behind (the position for rigid bronchoscopy) or, as is more often the case now, with the patient lying on a couch with their legs horizontal and the trunk at approximately 45°. In this position, the neck muscles should be relaxed by placing a pillow behind the patients head. One of the most important aspects is preparation of the patient and in particular paying attention to allaying anxieties as far as is possible. This may be facilitated by the use of a pre-medication such as an oral benzodiazepine. Most procedures, however, are pre-medicated immediately before bronchoscopy with either an intravenous benzodiazepine or an opiate. Many bronchoscopists give atropine one hour to the procedure (0.6 mgs). The authors preference to use a combination of 1 to 4 mgs IV midazolam and 250 mcgs to 1 mg of alfentanil (the latter given in 250 to 500 mcgs boluses during the procedure). The midazolam provides amnesic properties and the alfentanil is a potent antitussive and very short acting. Topical anaesthesia may be provided by introducing lignocaine gel into the nose prior to the procedure and/or spraying the oropharynx with 10% lignocaine. Anaesthesia to the vocal cords is provided by direct spraying of 2–4% lignocaine onto the vocal cords or alternatively by cricothyroid puncture, an injection of 2–4 mls of 4% lignocaine. Cricothyroid injection requires practice. The needle (21 gauge) is inserted into the cricothyroid membrane at 90° to the skin. Air is first aspirated and then with the needle firmly held onto the syringe, lignocaine injected rapidly and the needle immediately removed before the patient coughs. If the needle is left in place, the patient may cough and cause injury to the posterior wall of the trachea. Before introducing the bronchoscope, the focus should be checked and, if using a video system, the colour balance and depth of field should be checked. The fibrescope may be introduced through the nose or, if this is not possible, then through the mouth using a mouth guard. The patient should be reassured at this stage and constantly throughout the procedure. Once through the nose, the posterior oropharynx is inspected and the vocal cords are checked for symmetrical movement by asking the patient to say "ee". When anaesthetising the vocal cords, 3 × 2ml aliquots of 2% lignocaine are usually used. The bronchoscope should not be advanced through the cords until there is only a minimal response to an aliquot of lignocaine. The bronchoscope tip is then advanced through the vocal cords without touching them and normally 2 ml aliquots of 2% lignocaine are sprayed onto the carina and in the right and left bronchial trees. A thorough Inspection of the bronchial tree is then carried out followed by sampling.

Pathological appearances

A reference to a suitable atlas of bronchoscopy is given at the end of the chapter but there is no substitute for experience.[1] Notes should be made of the nature of mucosal inflammation, the presence of secretions and their nature. Pigment or nodularity in the endobronchium or the presence of suspected tumour. Anatomical variation is common but occasionally there may be additional bronchi which may have pathological relevance.

Sampling techniques via fibreoptic bronchoscope

Cytological samples are obtained by two methods in common use: Bronchial washing and bronchial brushing. The former is best obtained at the beginning of the procedure since any bleeding which may be caused will reduce the quality of the sample. The area to be sampled is identified and the bronchoscope introduced close to that area. 10–20 mls of normal saline is introduced and aspirated. The sample may then be sent for both cytology and bacteriology. A bronchoscopic brush may be used to scrape the surface of a suspect lesion and then is immediately wiped onto a slide which is then fixed with formalin spray. Cytology samples can also be obtained by transbronchial or transtracheal needle aspiration (see later).

Bronchial biopsies

If possible, a direct biopsy of a lesion should be obtained avoiding

Table 1. Notes on common bronchoscopic procedures

Sampling technique	Indication	Technique	Common pitfalls	Sample preparation
Bronchial wash	Cytology, microbiology	Advance bronchoscope to desired area. Inject 5–20 mls of normal saline and aspirate immediately.	Excessive trauma to airway thus giving heavy blood staining.	None.
Bronchial brush	Cytology	Advance sheathed bronchial brush to suspect lesion. Advance brush. Work back and forth over lesion. Retract brush. Remove sheathed brush from bronchoscope.	Can cause marked haemorrhage. Care needed with sample processing.	Slides prepared immediately and fixed.
Protected bronchial brush	Bacteriology	Review with nurse assistant instruction on packaging. Advance protected brush to site of lesion. Advance inner sheath distally. Advance brush distally. Retract brush to inner sheath. Retract inner sheath. Withdraw brush from bronchoscope.	Confusion with operation of protected brush.	Advance inner sheath and cut off inner sheath with brush inside into sterile container.
Bronchial biopsy	Sampling of abnormal lesions	Advance biopsy forceps to lesion. Open forceps and firmly close.	Haemorrhage — beware carinal or tracheal lesions. Excessive angulation of the bronchoscope preventing forceps closure.	Biopsies either placed in 10% formol saline or first on a piece of card according to preference of laboratory.

Table 1. Continued

Sampling technique	Indication	Technique	Common pitfalls	Sample preparation
Transbronchial lung biopsies				
a) With fluoroscopic control	Interstitial lung disease. Peripheral nodule. Focal parenchymal lung disease. Diffuse infective lung disease.	Identify area to be biopsied on chest x-ray and other images available. The patient should have had a platelet count, prothrombin time and partial thromboplastin time. Identify segment to be biopsied. Advance forceps along bronchoscope and screen patient with fluoroscopy. If possible take biopsies from the lateral segment of the right lower lobe. Advance forceps until they stop at periphery of lung (patient may complain of some discomfort). Withdraw forceps 2 cms, open forceps. Ask patient to inspire and then expire and breath hold. Advance forceps 5–10 mm and close. Withdraw forceps slowly. Keep watching for signs of haemorrhage. Repeat procedure until three good biopsies have been obtained (only biopsy from one lung to avoid danger of bilateral pneumothoraces).	Failure to advance along a bronchus — reposition forceps until they advance easily to the periphery of the lung. Pneumothorax, haemorrhage (may indicate a proximal biopsy). It is possible to obtain transbronchial biopsies from patients on mechanical ventilation but the chances of producing a pneumothorax are greater and, therefore, it is best to use fluoroscopic control.	Biopsies are placed directly into 10% formol saline or if for bacteriology, directly into 1 ml of normal saline.

Table 1.   Continued

Sampling technique	Indication	Technique	Common pitfalls	Sample preparation
b) Without fluoroscopic control	As for a)	Identify segment. Advance forceps along bronchial tree — they should pass easily. Withdraw biopsy forceps 2 cms. Open forceps. Ask patient to inspire and then expire and breath hold. Advance forceps 5 mm. Close forceps. Ask patient if they have any pain — if they do, open forceps and re-position. Withdraw forceps slowly.	As for a)	As for a)
Broncho alveolar lavage [5,6]	Investigation of suspected pulmonary infection, particularly in immuno-compromised hosts; investigation of possible neoplastic disease.	a) Lavage for diagnosis of infection. Identify area of suspected infection using chest x-ray and other imaging. If disease is diffuse, use right middle lobe. Advance bronchoscope to desired segment and gently wedge tip into segment. Instil 50 mls of normal saline at 37°C and aspirate using gentle suction. Use two further aliquots of 50 mls with aspiration in between. Aspirate from first sample can be sent separately as a "bronchial wash" and the second two aspirates pooled as the bronchoalveolar lavage.	Failure to provide an adequate wedge leading to excessive coughing and a contaminated sample. Trauma to the airways producing a blood contaminated sample. Wedging bronchoscope against side of the airway resulting in failure to aspirate fluid. Excessive suction pressure producing airway collapse. Excessive wedge pressure producing kinking of the airway and failure to aspirate.	It is important to inform the laboratory that the sample is on its way.

Table 1. Continued

Sampling technique	Indication	Technique	Common pitfalls	Sample preparation
	Investigation of interstitial lung disease; research.	b) Lavage for research purposes and investigation of interstitial lung disease. Advance tip of bronchoscope to desired segment and wedge. Instil 50 mls of normal saline at 37°C and aspirate. This sample is discarded as a bronchial wash. Exchange trap and tubing for siliconised tubing and glassware. Instil 3 further 50 mls aliquots of warm normal saline with aspiration between. Suction may be by gentle hand suction or suction limited to 100 cms of water.	As for a)	The sample may be buffered to pH 7 and should be immediately cooled. A sample is taken for a total cell count and cytospin preparations for a differential cell count. Further processing may be performed with flow cytometry.
Transtracheal/ transcarinal needle aspiration	Paratracheal or subcarinal suspected neoplasia.	Identify on CT scan area to be sampled. Familiarise with the instructions on packaging of transcarinal needle. Insert needle sheath into bronchoscope. Advance needle through tracheal or carinal wall and aspirate. Withdraw needle. Withdraw sheath and then place sample directly onto slide.	Failure to hit desired location.	It is best if a cytologist is present in the bronchoscopy suite and can immediately examine the sample for malignant cells. If there are no malignant cells, then the procedure may be repeated.

any areas which are obviously necrotic. Biopsies should be placed directly into preservative or may be first placed on a small piece of filter paper according to the preference of the laboratory. When there is tumour visible, a diagnosis is obtained in about 90% of cases.

Transbronchial lung biopsies

Transbronchial lung biopsies may be used to aid diagnosis in parenchymal lung disease or to sample peripheral nodules. Many physicians use fluoroscopic guidance although there have been several studies which have shown that the diagnostic yield for interstitial lung disease is similar. Radiographic screening during transbronchial lung biopsy reduce the instance of pneumothorax of 2.9% to 1.8% in a British survey of 231 physicians performed in 1983. It is generally recommended that the procedure be taught using fluoroscopy. Otherwise, it is difficult to appreciate the exact location of the forceps within the lung and how the forceps behave when they are advanced distally and into lung parenchyma. The technique has to be modified slightly if not using the aid of fluoroscopy. Table 1 indicates the technique in brief and common pitfalls.

Complications of bronchoscopy[2,3]

The incidence of complications from fibreoptic bronchoscopy is low. The incidence of cardiac dysrhythmias is directly related to the degree of hypoxaemia. Continuous monitoring with a pulse oximeter is, therefore, recommended and the administration of supplementary oxygen where indicated. Some physicians recommend that bronchoscopy should not be performed in patients with an FEV_1 of 1.0 litres, but this is not a universal practice. Additional procedures raise the complication rate. Transbronchial biopsy carries a higher mortality rate (0.12% compared with 0.04% for standard bronchoscopy) and a greater major complication rate of 2.7% (0.12% for a standard bronchoscopy). Major complications were those deemed to have threatened life. Bronchoalveolar lavage increases the incidence of post bronchoscopy fever from around 10% to up to 50% of patients. The incidence of fever is directly related to the volume of fluid instilled into the lungs.

　　Cross infection is a potential complication. There are clear guidelines for disinfection practices for fibreoptic bronchoscopes. 2% glutaraldehyde remains the disinfectant of choice. Standard sterilisation process includes immersion for 20 minutes but for mycobacteria, the immersion time must increase to 60 minutes. It is generally recommended that the bronchoscopist and other bronchoscopy staff should be protected by wearing a gown, gloves, mask and preferably eye protection for all procedures. In practice, however, many Units do not do this and only wear mask and eye protection for high risk patients.

Endobronchial therapy[4]

Palliative therapy for lung carcinoma is the main indication for endobronchial therapy. The techniques consist of various ways to resect tumour, stenting and brachytherapy. Table 2 summarises the techniques and gives their advantages and disadvantages.

See also Chapter 10, page 257–262.

Medical thoracoscopy[7,8]

Thoracoscopy was first performed by the Swedish physician Jacobeus in 1910. Before the use of chemotherapy for pulmonary tuberculosis, thoracoscopy was used in a variety of different procedures. There has been a revival in thoracoscopy following the move to minimally invasive surgery — initially abdominal and later video assisted thoracic surgery (VATS). It is important at the outset to distinguish between VATS and medical thoracoscopy. The former is the domain of the Thoracic Surgeons and is used to perform advanced procedures such as wedge lung resections, lobectomy and even pneumonectomy. Medical thoracoscopy, on the other hand, is in most centres used for diagnostic purposes with the addition of other procedures depending on the local expertise. With some Units performing more and more advanced procedures, the dividing line between medical thoracoscopy and VATS can be a little blurred. This section will describe medical thoracoscopy and some of the less advanced procedures. Table 2 shows the indications for medical thoracoscopy.

Procedure

There are two principle variations in procedure. Firstly some prefer to perform the procedure under general anaesthetic whilst others use local anaesthetic and sedative and secondly some use a rigid thoracoscope and others more expensive video assisted equipment

Table 2.   Endobronchial therapy[4]

Name of technique	Method	Comment
Brachytherapy	Best performed in the radiotherapy suite and requires a clinical oncologist and radiotherapy physicist. During fibreoptic bronchoscopy, a plastic after-loading catheter (1.5m length is best) is passed through the tumour and the bronchoscope removed. A marker wire is inserted into the catheter. A chest X-ray is taken and used to plan the area to be irradiated, having made a careful note of the proximity of the tumour to the carina (visible on X-ray). The patient is transferred to the afterloading suite	Generally used after first trying external beam radiotherapy. Can be used after a response to external beam as a second, radiation limiting procedure. May cause haemotysis. Most effective if the catheter is passed through the tumour but can still be effective if catheter is wedged into tumour. May be repeated. May be preceded by laser therapy, facilitating passage through tumour
Laser	Usually performed through a rigid bronchoscope under general anaesthetic. Special training is needed in the use of the laser. Laser is administered through the fibreoptic bronchoscope via a fibre optic catheter. Tumour vaporised with 1 sec bursts.	Main complication is bleeding which can occasionally be fatal. Tissue damage extends beyond the visible area depending on energy used and requires caution. Endobronchial fires avoided by reducing FiO_2 to 0.40
Cryotherapy	A cryotherapy probe is inserted through the fibrescope under local anaesthetic and used to freeze tumour. Dead tissue is removed and often requires more than one bronchoscopy.	A time consuming procedure, requiring more than one bronchoscopy. Good safety profile
Electro cautery	Latest method is to use the electrocautery probe under local anaesthetic. Similar technique to laser.	Latest reports indicate that this method is tolerated under local anaesthetic. May be combined with brachytherapy. Less expensive than laser
Surgical debridement	Performed by thoracic surgeons through a rigid bronchoscope under general anaesthetic. Tumour is removed with forceps and bleeding stemmed with electrocautery	Rapid relief of endobronchial obstruction. Requires thoracic theatre time (expensive)

similar to that used in VATS. If a general anaesthetic is used, it is not necessary to intubate the patient and some anaesthetists prefer to employ a laryngeal mask. Local anaesthetic is preferred by some because an anaesthetist is not required but generally one has to accept a less complete examination of the hemithorax. Local anaesthetic is given in a similar fashion to that when inserting an intercostal drain and an opiate and benzodiazepine are used in combination for the sedative. In both methods, oxygen is given during the procedure and there is continuous oximetry and electrocardiographic monitoring.

Equipment

Rigid thoracoscopy

The equipment required for rigid thoracoscopy includes the thoracoscope itself which is inserted through a trocar. The trocar should be 5–7mm in diameter — larger trocars can be difficult to manipulate through narrow intercostal spaces and can cause pain when the procedure is done under general anaesthetic. The trocar allows air to enter the chest cavity but can be made air tight using a detachable rubber stopper. If electro-cautery is to be used, the trocar must be electrically insulated. The telescopes, which are part of the thoracoscope, can be straight viewing or set at a oblique angle of 50°. Forceps fit around the telescopes and can be used to extract large pleural biopsies. The rest of the equipment essential for rigid thoracoscopy is listed in Table 3.

Thoracoscopy should be performed in an operating room or clean endoscopy suite. There should be adjustable aspiration equipment available and simple anaesthetic equipment with full resuscitation apparatus. There should be good overhead lighting. All staff should be fully versed with the procedure. All equipment must be sterilised.

Thoracoscopy technique[5]

Thoracoscopy may be performed using one port of entry (a relatively uncomplicated procedure) or with up to two further ports for introduction of instruments or when changing the site of the telescope, to improve the view. Whether under local or general anaesthetic, the procedure for a single port insertion is the same, except for the administration of local anaesthetic to the skin and intercostal space.

Table 3.   Indications and comments on Medical Thoracoscopy

Basic indications

Indications	Comment
Diagnosis	When fluid cytology and blind pleural biopsy fail to achieve a diagnosis (30–40% of cases) the diagnostic rate of medical thoracoscopy is 95–98%.
Spontaneous pneumothorax	In cases which persist despite chest drainage or in those cases where pleurodesis is indicated, provided that the apical blebs are no larger than 1–2 cms in diameter, talc pleurodesis may be performed and this has been shown to achieve a success rate of 95%. Where leaking bullae are visible, it is advisable for the leak to be coagulated prior to talc pleurodesis. 2–4 mls maximum of talc are required.
Talc pleurodesis for malignant pleural effusion, Chronic persistent pleural effusion due to cardiac disease or liver cirrhosis etc	This is successful in over 90% of cases. The talc must be asbestos free and sterilised in an autoclave prior to use. 6–8 mls of talc are needed since much is lost through the suction drain.

Advanced indications

Indications	Comment
Lung biopsy	At the larger medical thoracoscopy centres, lung biopsy is carried out safely using coagulating forceps for the diagnosis of interstitial lung disease, granulomatous disease etc. Also peripheral lung lesions may be biopsied using this technique.
Purulent pleurisy and empyema	Skilled personnel may successfully section adhesions and gently debride the pleural cavity before placement of a drain.
Sympathectomy	The sympathetic chain is adjacent to several large vessels and, therefore, specific training is required for this procedure.
Pericardial window	Special training required. Useful for some forms of chronic pericardial effusion.

The patient is placed in the lateral position with the arms raised to shoulder level and placed comfortably on a soft support. A point is selected between the third and sixth intercostal space, local anaesthetic administered and an incision made of 1.5 cm. There is then blunt dissection down to the pleural surface. It is some centres practice to induce a pneumothorax the day before the procedure and confirm this by chest radiography. Many have found simple dissection down to the pleural surface sufficient. If there is pleural fluid this will usually be apparent. Air can be let into the chest cavity during the blunt dissection and a finger can confirm that the lung is away from the point of dissection. The trocar is then inserted and the obturator can be removed. Further air may be let into the chest or alternatively pleural fluid could be aspirated at this stage. The telescope is then gently inserted, initially very cautiously to establish where the lung is and whether there are any adhesions. In order to examine as much of the pleural cavity as possible, the lung should be allowed to deflate. A systematic examination of the pleural surface is then carried out. If only one point of entry is used there is the limitation that the pleura at the point of entry cannot be examined and the apex and paravertebral space may be difficult to see. A thorough knowledge of the intrapleural cavity anatomy should be revised before attempting this procedure. If a CT scan is available then the point of entry may be varied from the anterior to the midclavicular line to obtain a better view and facilitate biopsies. Pleural biopsies should only be taken from parietal pleura. Biopsies should generally be limited to areas of parietal pleura over the ribs. This reduces the risk of damaging the neurovascular bundle. Large biopsies can often be obtained by gently dissecting off an area of the pleura with the biopsy forceps and then extracting these through the thoracoscope. Attempting lung biopsies (which involves visceral pleural biopsies) should only be undertaken after training with coagulation forceps. At the end of the procedure, a chest drain is inserted and the air removed by underwater seal. In many institutions, the chest drain is removed as soon as the lung has re-inflated, usually before the patient comes off the operating table. In others the chest drain is left in situ for an hour or two and then removed before the patient is discharged home. This of course depends on the details of the procedure and it is customary for the patients to have more prolonged chest drainage when a lung biopsy has been performed.

Complications of thoracoscopy[7]

Early thoracoscopy was associated with some rather dramatic and (rarely) fatal complications including rapid development of subcutaneous emphysema or mediastinal emphysema. These however can be avoided by inserting a chest drain at the end of the procedure. Other reported complications including sudden death from induction of a pneumothorax and air embolism, are extremely rare at present. In one series of 8,000 examinations there was only one fatality. Another series of 4,301 cases, the death rate was 0.09% and this series included more invasive thoracoscopy than most physicians would attempt. With all procedures it is important to perform them within ones capability. The important complications, largely preventable, are: pulmonary perforation due to careless introduction of the trocar; transient hypotension or tachyarrhythmia (the chances are reduced by avoiding contact with the pericardium); and contamination of the entry tract with tumour cells. The latter is an important complication and may be remedied by prophylactic radiotherapy.

Infectious complications: 10–20% of patients show a slight fever after thoracoscopy and 2% of patients develop a mild bronchitis. A further 2% develop some local infection at the wound site but this almost always resolves quickly with antibiotic therapy. Complications can be minimised by ensuring the patient is not hypoxic when breathing room air, has normal coagulation and does not suffer from serious ischaemic heart disease. Postponing thoracoscopy until after infective illnesses have resolved is a useful precaution.

References

1. Wang K-P, Mehta AC. Flexible bronchoscopy. Bronchoscopy Atlas. Oxford: Blackwell Science

2. Simpson FG, Arnold AG, Purvis A, Belfield PW, Muers MF, Cooke NJ. Postal survey of bronchoscopic practice by physicians in the United Kingdom. *Thorax* 1983;**41**:331

3   Credle WF, Smiddy JF, Elliott RC. Complications of fibreoptic bronchoscopy. *Am Rev Respir Dis* 1974;**109**:67

4. Macha H-N, Loddenkemper R. Interventional bronchoscopic procedures: endobronchial radiotheapy, laser therapy and stent implantation. European Respiratory Monograph: Vol 1 No 1: p332–360

5. Klech H, Pohl W. Technical Recommendations and Guidelines for bronchoalveolar lavage. European Working Party Report. *Eur Respir J* 1989;**2**:561

6. The BAL Cooperative Group Steering Committee. Bronchoalveolar lavage constituents in healthy individuals, ideopathic pulmonary fibrosis and selected comparison groups. *Am Rev Respir Dis* 1990; **141**:s169

7. Boutin C, Viallat JR, Aelony Y. Practical Thoracoscopy. Heidelberg: Springer Verlag 1991

8. Brant HJ, Loddenkemper R, Mai J. Atlas of daignostic thoracoscopy. Gerorg Thieme Verlag 1985

4

Asthma

Tim W Harrison and Anne E Tattersfield

Introduction

Asthma is rare in rural third world countries but becomes increasingly common as societies become more affluent and urbanised. In the United Kingdom some 15% of children and at least 5% of adults have asthma. There is strong evidence that the incidence and prevalence of asthma and other atopic diseases has increased over the past three decades but the cause of this increase is not clear. Although genetic factors are important for the development of asthma the time scale of changes in prevalence suggests that environmental factors are playing an important role. There appears to be something about the lifestyle of the more affluent countries that causes the development of asthma in genetically susceptible individuals. Various environmental factors have been proposed including increased exposure to allergens, indoor and outdoor air pollution, pet ownership, diet, hygiene, infections and immunisations but as yet no specific agent has been unequivocally identified as being responsible for the increase in prevalence.

The widespread lay view that air pollution is responsible for the increased prevalence of asthma is in fact contrary to most of the evidence. For example, asthma prevalence was higher in West Germany compared to East Germany after the Berlin wall came down despite much higher concentrations of particulates and sulphur dioxide in the latter. This doesn't exclude a role for motor vehicle air pollution but the high prevalence of asthma in New Zealand and in the Isle of Skye in Scotland would argue against that, as would the lack of important urban rural differences in most surveys. There is evidence to suggest that air pollution may make asthma worse, however.

Asthma is now recognised as a chronic inflammatory disease of the airways. The main histological features are airway epithelial damage, an inflammatory reaction characterised by eosinophils, lymphocytes and mast cells, increased numbers of mucus secreting goblet cells, deposition of collagen below the basement membrane and smooth muscle hyperplasia and hypertrophy. Persistent chronic inflammatory changes may lead to permanent structural changes and fixed airway obstruction although why this occurs in some patients but not others is not clear. The recognition that asthma is primarily an inflammatory disease has led to the widespread use of anti-inflammatory agents particularly inhaled corticosteroids as first line treatment.

Asthma imparts a major burden on health services. The total annual costs of asthma are estimated to be as much as £686 million per annum in the UK.[1] These costs include direct costs defined as resources consumed, such as drugs and devices and medical, nursing and hospital costs, and indirect costs that include resources that are lost, such as time off work and premature retirement or death.

The number of deaths from asthma varies considerably from country to country and it has varied over time within countries. In England and Wales asthma deaths increased markedly during the early 1960s. This increase was most marked in younger patients, in whom the mortality rate increased two to fourfold, and the increase coincided with a high-dose preparation of isoprenaline being available over the counter. The number of deaths started to rise again more gradually in the early 1980s peaking in 1988 at around 2000 per year. This increase was mainly in older age-groups and was probably mainly due to increased recognition of asthma rather than chronic bronchitis as a cause of death in this age group — so called diagnostic transfer. Since then asthma deaths have been falling and are currently around 1500 per year in England and Wales.

Asthma deaths are not homogeneous and different factors may be responsible. There is reasonable presumptive evidence that the epidemic of deaths in the 1960s was related to excessive use of β-agonists and the same may be true of a second epidemic in New Zealand in the 1970s following the introduction of the less selective β-agonist fenoterol. Outside these epidemics controlled studies have identified factors associated with death from asthma. These include a long history of asthma, marked peak flow varia-bility, under-use of corticosteroids, pyschosocial problems and a previous admission with acute severe asthma, particularly if ventilated or life-threatening features were present.

Most asthma deaths occur in patients who present late, despite prolonged symptoms. Poor patient education, underestimation of severity by patient or doctor, under-treatment and inappropriate treatment have all been implicated. Occasionally fatal attacks occur very rapidly with little time for intervention but this is relatively uncommon.

Clinical Features

History

The patient's history is extremely important. Often it is highly characteristic of asthma but it is important to look for symptoms that are atypical. The diagnosis should be questioned if there are unusual factors particularly if there are features suggestive of hyperventilation or upper airways obstruction which might be due to a tumour, foreign body or vocal cord dysfunction. Consider if there is disparity between symptoms and objective measures of lung function or if the response to therapy is inappropriate. In older patients, asthma may need to be distinguished from smoking related chronic obstructive pulmonary disease which may coexist with asthma.

When asthma has been diagnosed it is important to try to identify possible aetiological and provoking factors (Table 1), assess the disease severity and explore the patient's views and concerns about asthma and its treatment.

Examination

The findings on clinical examination range from being completely normal to chest deformity, severe wheeze and use of the accessory muscles of respiration. The features of severe or life threatening asthma, including tachycardia, silent chest, cyanosis, feeble respiratory effort and exhaustion, must be recognised and acted upon. One of the main purposes of the clinical examination is to exclude atypical signs such as localised or unilateral wheeze, inspiratory stridor or crepitations.

Investigations

The number and type of investigations depend on the degree of

Table 1. Factors that can provoke asthma attacks

Smoking	
Upper respiratory tract infections	mainly viral
Allergens	eg pollen, house dust mite, pets
Exercise	particularly children and in cold air
Work related	irritants and specific sensitisers (see Table 2)
Pollution	
Drugs	eg aspirin, β-blockers (including eye drops) and as part of an anaphylactic response to other drugs
Food and drinks	eg dairy produce, alcohol, peanuts, orange juice
Additives	eg metabisulphate, tartrazine, monosodium glutamate
Medical conditions	rhinitis, gastroesophageal reflux
Hormonal	Pre-menstrual exacerbations, pregnancy

certainty that the diagnosis is asthma and on its severity. The diagnosis of asthma requires evidence of airways obstruction which is variable over time or is reversible with pharmacological agents. Patients with mild but clear cut asthma may not require any investigations other than a measure of peak expiratory flow, before and after a β-agonist, or during an attack of asthma. Patients with more severe asthma should undergo spirometry ideally before and after a β-agonist and peak flow monitoring over at least a week to determine the variability and pattern of their airflow obstruction. Possible investigations include:

- peak flow monitoring   Used to determine diurnal variation, asthma severity, pre-menstrual exacerbations, occupational factors and response to treatment
- full blood count   A high eosinophil count is in keeping with asthma; a very high count is characteristic of allergic

bronchopulmonary aspergillosis, Churg-Strauss syndrome or tropical eosinophilia

- chest radiograph

  Indicated if allergic bronchopulmonary aspergillosis is suspected and to exclude other pathologies particularly in older patients who have smoked

- intradermal skin tests

  Used to determine sensitivity to common allergens though usefulness is limited since around 40% of the general population have positive skin tests and potential to remove common allergens is limited. A positive skin test to aspergillus should alert to the possibility of allergic bronchopulmonary aspergillosis

- bronchial challenges

  Most patients with asthma show increased non-specific bronchial reactivity to agents such as methacholine. The tests have limited sensitivity and specificity for the diagnosis of asthma but are sometimes helpful when there is diagnostic doubt. Protocols for testing sensitivity to metabisulphate, tartrazine, aspirin and certain occupational sensitisers are available but require experienced personnel

- exercise test

  Useful particularly in children when the diagnosis is uncertain and who are normal when seen. In asthma peak flow falls maximally 5–10 minutes after exercise particularly if performed in cold air

- sputum analysis

  If not produced spontaneously, sputum can be induced by inhalation of hypertonic saline. The procedure can cause bronchoconstriction and requires pre-treatment with a β-agonist. It can be used to assess airway

inflammation but its role in everyday
patient management is not yet clear

- laryngoscopy   Can be useful in diagnosing vocal
                                  cord dysfunction.
- bronchoscopy   May be indicated to exclude an
                                  upper airway lesion and very
                                  occasionally for bronchial biopsies
                                  if diagnosis is in doubt

Asthma syndromes

Asthma is a feature of allergic bronchopulmonary aspergillosis and
Churg-Strauss syndrome. Although both are uncommon the correct
diagnosis is important for management and prognosis.

Allergic bronchopulmonary aspergillosis

Allergic bronchopulmonary aspergillosis (ABPA) is one of several
diseases caused by *Aspergillus fumigatus*. Following inhalation of
spores the fungus proliferates in the bronchial tree provoking an
antibody reaction (probably a combination of type 1 and type 3
hypersensitivity reactions) with the production of specific IgE and
IgG antibodies. Specific antibodies combine with *Aspergillus* antigen to produce immune complexes which damage the bronchial
walls and initiate an eosinophilic infiltration in the distal lung. The
airways become occluded with eosinophilic plugs that are heavily
infiltrated by *Aspergillus* hyphae and which can cause the distal
lung to collapse. Repeated damage from these immunological reactions leads to bronchiectasis which is often proximal and in the
upper lobes. Bronchiectasis causes additional clinical problems for
patients with ABPA.

The clinical picture is of asthma with recurrent exacerbations,
particularly in the autumn and winter, often associated with tenacious secretions and radiological evidence of lobar or segmental
collapse or transient peripheral shadowing. The diagnostic features
include:

- asthma (almost invariably)
- recurrent pulmonary infiltrates
- eosinophilia; usually 1.0–3.0×10^9/l
- positive skin prick tests to *Aspergillus fumigatus* (100%)
- precipitating antibodies to *Aspergillus fumigatus* (>90%)
- elevated serum IgE

- *Aspergillus fumigatus* and bronchial casts in sputum
- proximal bronchiectasis.

The main aim of therapy is to suppress the immunopathological response to *A. fumigatus* and thereby prevent the development of bronchiectasis. For mild disease inhaled steroids control the asthma and are likely to reduce the number of acute episodes, although this is unproven. Exacerbations should be treated with prednisolone 40–60 mg/daily and this may need to be continued for several weeks until lung function has returned to previous values. In patients with more severe disease long-term oral corticosteroids are needed and regular treatment (e.g. prednisolone 10 mg/day) may be more beneficial than intermittent treatment. Higher doses of prednisolone are required for acute exacerbations. When there is evidence of airways collapse physiotherapy and/or bronchoscopy may be required to remove impacted mucus. Long-term follow-up is generally recommended to monitor lung function and optimise corticosteroid treatment as disease progression can occur without symptoms.

Specific antifungal therapy has been disappointing although benefit was seen in a double-blind study of itraconazole.[2] N-acetyl cysteine and DNase therapy are unproven but may be worth a trial in patients with difficult disease.

Churg-Strauss syndrome (allergic granulomatosis)

In the Churg-Strauss syndrome severe asthma is associated with hypereosinophilia (usually greater than $1.5 \times 10^9/l$) and necrotizing granulomatous inflammation. Considered to be a variant of polyartritis nodosa, it usually starts with adult onset asthma with or without rhinitis followed by tissue and peripheral blood eosinophilia and a life threatening phase of systemic vasculitis. The mean age of onset of asthma was 35 years in one study followed by vasculitis at 38 years, although asthma may precede vasculitis by many years. Eosinophilic infiltrates in the lungs give rise to non-cavitating bilateral nodular or confluent shadows on the chest radiograph. Other features include coronary arteritis and myocarditis, ulceration and perforation of the gastrointestinal tract, erythema, purpura and nodules on the skin and a peripheral neuropathy. Patients are often atopic and approximately 70% have positive antineutrophil cytoplasmic antibodies (predominantly p-ANCA). There are recent case reports of a Churg-Strauss-like syndrome following the use of macrolide antibiotics and leukotriene antagonists although whether these are causal is not yet clear. Otherwise the trigger(s) for the Churg-Strauss syndrome is unknown.

Diagnosis is based on clinical features, eosinophilia and positive antinuclear cytoplasmic antibodies. Early treatment is important to prevent life-threatening complications. High doses of oral corticosteroids normally bring the disease under rapid control and are usually adequate as sole treatment. Refractory or relapsing disease may require additional cytotoxic treatment with cyclophosphamide.

Occupational asthma

See also Chapter 17, page 459.

Aetiology

Occupational asthma is the term used to describe asthma due to sensitisation to specific substances in the work place. It usually occurs *de novo* although patients with pre-existing asthma may also become sensitised to agents at work. Occupational asthma does not include asthma made worse by irritants at work although this is also very important. The term reactive airways dysfunction syndrome (RADS) has been introduced to describe patients who develop symptoms and persistent non-specific bronchial hyperreactivity after a single exposure to high levels of an irritant such as chlorine gas or anhydrous ammonia which may occur following an industrial accident. The original cases of RADS were based on patients history alone as re-exposure to low levels of the incriminating agent did not reproduce the symptoms. Much less is known about the pathogenesis and outcome than with the other types of occupational asthma.

More than 200 agents capable of causing occupational asthma have been reported but most cases are due to a more limited number. The agents can be classified into high and low molecular weight compounds (Table 2). High molecular weight compounds such as flour and proteolytic enzymes usually induce asthma through an IgE-dependent mechanism. Some low molecular weight agents such as acid anhydride and platinum also causes IgE-dependent responses by acting as haptens although the majority of low molecular weight compounds such as isocyanates work through a non-IgE-dependent mechanism, which is as yet unidentified. Agents that induce asthma by non-immunological mechanisms are mostly irritant gases, fumes or chemicals.

Table 2.   Some of the commoner causes of occupational asthma

High molecular weight compounds	Examples	Occupations
Animal-derived antigens	Small mammals	Animal handlers, vets, laboratory technicians
Insects	Grain mite, locusts	Farmers, laboratory workers
Plant products	Wheat, rye, gluten Latex Henna	Bakers Healthcare workers Hairdressers
Biological enzymes	*Bacillus subtillis* Papain, pepsin	Detergent industry Laboratory packaging, pharmaceutical industry
Seafood proteins	Oysters, prawns, crabs	food processors
Low molecular weight compounds		
IgE-dependent		
Acid anhydrides	phthalic and trimellitic anhydride	Used in alkyd and epoxy resins for paints, varnishes, plastics and adhesives
Metals	Halogenated platinum salts, cobalt	Platinum workers and hard-metal grinders
IgE-independent		
Diisocyanate combinations	TDI, HDI and MDI (polyurethane)	Foams, coating for electrical wiring, car paints and adhesives
Wood dusts or bark	Western red cedar Reactive dyes	Sawmill workers, joiners Dyeing, textile workers
Amines	Secondary, tertiary and quaternary amines	Rubber, cosmetic and hair dyes
Glutaraldehyde		Health care workers
Drugs	Penicillins Salbutamol intermediates	Pharmaceutical and healthcare workers

NB Some of the sensitisers occasionally cause problems in non-occupational situations such as when small mammals are kept as pets. Adapted from reference[3].

Diagnosis

A low threshold of suspicion is the key to diagnosing occupational asthma. It is an important cause of late onset asthma and needs to be considered in every case of adult-onset asthma or worsening of asthma in adult life. Atopy and individuals who smoke appear to be at increased risk of asthma due to some IgE-inducing agents. The latency period between first exposure and onset of symptoms depends on the sensitising agent and varies from weeks to years. Once sensitised, re-exposure to very low concentrations of the agents can provoke symptoms. There may be associated rhinitis, conjunctivitis and urticaria and symptoms often improve when subjects are away from work although this may take several days. If the patient is still working documentation of objective changes in lung function is highly desirable and two hourly peak flow recordings throughout the day for several weeks can be very useful. Spirometry or bronchial reactivity testing before, during and after exposure can be helpful, as can skinprick tests and specific IgE tests for certain sensitisers eg laboratory animals, insects, platinum salts. Specific inhalation challenge tests of the likely sensitisers are rarely required. They are not without risk and when required need to be performed in specialised centres. Appropriate controls are required to separate a specific response to a sensitising agent from a non-specific response to withdrawal of treatment prior to the test. Patients may be sensitised to more than one agent.

Management

Decisions about work are extremely important and should be made by someone with knowledge and experience of occupational asthma. Early diagnosis of occupational asthma and removal from exposure are the most important factors in determining the long-term outcome. Patients should normally be withdrawn from any contact with the causal agent. Patients with normal lung function may be allowed occasional exposure to the sensitising agent (e.g. small mammals) as long as they wear protective gear. For other sensitisers (e.g. isocyanates) subjects can be exquisitely sensitive and should not work anywhere in the vicinity.

Employers who are shown to be negligent can be sued for damages and in some countries an employee can claim for disability payments. In the UK, for example, if work has involved contact with one of the substances listed in leaflet NI 237 within the last 10 years the employees are entitled to claim for Disablement Benefit.*

Asthma Management

Aims

The approach to asthma management has changed over recent years with an increased emphasis on patients managing their own asthma as much as possible and an increased involvement of specialised respiratory nurses in general practice and hospitals. The overall aim of management is to ensure that patients are able to live as normal a life as possible at present and in the future. To facilitate this patients should be encouraged to take some responsibility for their asthma management. The patient's knowledge and perception of the disease and treatment should be determined so that any exaggerated or inappropriate fears and anxieties can be allayed.

There is evidence that patients with asthma are less fit than they should be and patients should be encouraged to be as active as possible. Identifying well known sportsmen and women who have asthma may encourage young people to be active.

Non-drug treatment

Education

Patients require a clear explanation of their symptoms and diagnosis. A clear understanding of the underlying inflammatory disorder and approaches to treatment should improve compliance with medication and self-management.

Preventative measures

Factors that provoke or exacerbate asthma can sometimes be reduced. Smoking has an adverse effect on lung function and increases the risk of developing occupational asthma. Passive cigarette smoke is an airway irritant which should be avoided. People with asthma should avoid dusty work environments and young people should be advised to try to avoid jobs associated with occupational asthma

---

*Patients should complete form BI 100(OA) available at Social Security Offices.

whenever possible since options for change may be limited later in life.

Allergen avoidance may be possible when discrete agents such as a pet can be identified. More commonly, however, patients are sensitive to many aeroallergens, including the ubiquitous house dust mite. Attempts to reduce the numbers of house dust mite have shown some evidence of clinical efficacy in a few studies but the methods used, such as liquid nitrogen, are difficult to apply and cannot as yet be considered suitable for general use. Whilst awaiting the results of trials currently in progress we advise patients with troublesome nocturnal asthma despite prophylactic treatment to minimise soft furnishings in the bedroom and consider covering their mattress with allergen impermeable covers. When there is a reluctance to remove soft toys their allergen content can be reduced by a few hours in the deep freeze.

Evidence of intolerance to foods such as dairy products or peanuts or food additives such as metabisulphate or tartrazine should be sought and can be confirmed by careful challenge testing in the laboratory using established protocols. Trial exclusion of food groups may be worthwhile in patients with severe asthma.

Immunotherapy

Allergen immunotherapy has been used to treat allergic asthma for over 70 years and although widely used in many parts of the world its role remains controversial. A meta-analysis of 20 double-blind controlled trials showed a small but significant improvement in asthma control with allergen immunotherapy but this small benefit has to be balanced against reactions to immunotherapy which can be fatal. In the UK, the Committee on Safety of Medicines has concluded that immunotherapy should not be used in patients with asthma except for hypersensitivity to wasp and bee venoms as these reactions can be life-threatening. The injection of allergen genes has shown evidence of efficacy in mice and rats but whether it will be a useful and safer approach is unknown.

Complementary medicine

Many patients have tried or wish to try alternative or complementary medicine for asthma but there have been few good clinical studies of its effectiveness. Benefit has been seen in some studies with yoga and acupuncture, for example, but it has been small in relation to that expected from pharmacological treatments.

If patients wish to try alternative approaches they should be advised to continue their normal treatment at least until any benefit can be assessed.

Drug treatment

Self management

To achieve good asthma control with minimal side effects careful thought needs to be given to the type of drug and the dose and route of administration. Patients should be taught to assess the severity of their asthma preferably by measuring their peak expiratory flow and most can then adjust their treatment according to the fluctuations in asthma control. This approach provides maximum therapeutic benefit with minimal risk of adverse effects from treatment. Many patients now have personal management plans which summarise their asthma treatment and give guidelines for the patient to adjust their treatment so that their peak flow recordings remain within agreed limits.

Inhaler devices

Most asthma treatment is prescribed via the inhaled route because this provides maximum lung availability with minimal adverse effects. Unfortunately none of the many devices available for inhalation is ideal for all patients and experience shows that one of the commonest reasons for treatment failure is poor inhaler technique. The metered dose inhaler remains the cheapest option and is acceptable provided patients receive careful instruction and their inhalation technique is checked at intervals and shown to be satisfactory; otherwise pulmonary deposition from a metered dose inhaler can be very poor. The addition of a large volume spacer offers several advantages including a reduced need for co-ordination between inspiration and activation of the inhaler, greater lung deposition and less oropharyngeal impaction of drug, which in the case of inhaled steroids, can lead to candidiasis and systemic side effects. For these reasons large volume spacers are recommended for high dose inhaled steroids by metered dose inhaler.

Chlorofluorocarbon (CFC) metered dose inhalers are currently being replaced with CFC-free inhalers. This can be associated with differences in particle size and therefore airway distribution which could influence both efficacy and systemic activity for a given dose. This may not be important for bronchodilators but it is relevant to the long term safety of inhaled steroids. Unfortunately because of the large number of different inhalers used to deliver inhaled steroids it is difficult to predict the net effect of changing to CFC-free products.

Breath actuated and dry powder inhalers may help overcome many of the problems of co-ordination associated with metered dose inhalers but still require careful instruction and demonstration. Special device aids are available for patients with arthritis, for example, and can be individually tailored by respiratory nurses.

Chronic stable asthma

International guidelines on asthma management provide a logical approach to management for the great majority of patients with asthma. The main features are a stepped approach to treatment and emphasis on patient self-management. The recommendations are a consensus based on a combination of evidence and clinical experience. Table 3 shows the main steps of the British Guidelines for adults and school age children. The majority of patients in the

Table 3.   Summary of the management of chronic asthma in adults and schoolchildren (from the British Guidelines)[5]
The percentage of patients with asthma on each step from a community population in Nottingham is given at the bottom (8% were taking no treatment).

step 1	step 2	step 3	step 4	step 5
Occasional use of relief bronchodilators	Low dose inhaled steroid **or** cromoglycate **or** nedocromil sodium	High dose inhaled steroids **or** low dose with an inhaled long-acting β-agonist	High dose inhaled steroid and regular bronchodilators (inhaled long-acting β-agonist, theophylline, ipratropium or oxitropium, oral β-agonists, cromoglycate or nedocromil)	Addition of regular oral steroids
54%	22%	11%	4%	1%

community are on steps one and two as shown in a survey in Nottingham (data in Table 3). Rather than reproduce the British Guidelines we have highlighted some of the more important points:

Gaining disease control

The initial aim of treatment for symptomatic patients should be to gain control of the disease rapidly. For most patients a medium dose of an inhaled corticosteroid, eg beclomethasone or budesonide 800 μg or fluticasone 400 μg/day, is a reasonable starting dose. Patients with more severe asthma may be better started at a higher initial dose or with a short course of oral corticosteroids. Once control is achieved treatment is reduced to the minimum required to maintain control. The advantage of this approach is that the patient is aware that the treatment works; a potential disadvantage is that patients may remain on unnecessarily high doses of inhaled corticosteroids unless care is taken to avoid this.

Place of inhaled corticosteroids

Inhaled steroids are very effective in improving asthma control and in allowing oral corticosteroids to be withdrawn in patients with more severe asthma. As a consequence they are widely used and in many patients will be taken for many decades. The long term balance of benefit and risk from inhaled steroids needs therefore to be considered. Local adverse effects such as candidiasis and dysphonia can be a nuisance but are not serious and can be reduced by mouth rinsing and by using a large volume spacer or dry powder device to reduce oro-pharyngeal impaction. All inhaled corticosteroids have some systemic activity due to absorption from the lung and to a variable extent from the gastrointestinal tract. The amount of systemic activity depends on the dose but also on which steroid and which delivery device is used. The extent to which this activity causes clinically important adverse effects is still unclear. A small effect on bone density after one or two years may become important if the drugs are taken for 30 years.

There is little evidence to say when prophylactic therapy should be introduced. The guidelines suggest that it should be started once a bronchodilator is required more than once daily. Some patients use bronchodilators rarely, however, despite persistently abnormal lung function. This may be because they are poor perceivers of bronchoconstriction or because they curtail their activities to those they can do comfortably. Such patients may feel considerable benefit from the introduction of an inhaled corticosteroid whereas others may question the need for regular treatment. At present we have no good evidence that inhaled steroids alter the long term outcome of asthma and when they are stopped lung function rapidly returns to pre-treatment values.

There is much debate over the comparative efficacy and systemic activity of the available inhaled corticosteroids (beclomethasone dipropionate, budesonide and fluticasone propionate). All three show similar efficacy although this is achieved with half the dose of fluticasone propionate because it is approximately twice as potent. Due to differences in first pass metabolism the contribution of gastrointestinal absorption to the total systemic effect is greatest with beclomethasone dipropionate. Gastrointestinal absorption can be reduced by using a large volume spacer or a dry powder device. Oral bioavailability is less with budesonide and fluticasone propionate (9% and 1% respectively) and most of their systemic activity results from pulmonary absorption. Comparative studies of systemic effects of the inhaled steroids are difficult to interpret because of the differences in drug doses, inhaler devices and the outcome measures but budesonide and fluticasone propionate probably have the preferable safety profile especially at high dose.

Place of long-acting β-agonists

The inhaled long-acting β-agonists provide effective bronchodilatation over 12 hours without the peaks and troughs seen with regular short-acting β-agonists. In long term studies they have provided continuous bronchodilatation, symptom relief, improved quality of life and a reduction in exacerbations whereas regular short acting β-agonist have differed little from placebo. With regular treatment there is no evidence of a rebound increase in bronchial reactivity or fall in FEV_1 when the long-acting β-agonists are stopped although their protective effect against exercise-induced bronchoconstriction is reduced. Predictable β-agonist side effects can limit their use and salmeterol occasionally causes transient bronchoconstriction following inhalation, presumably due to the propellant and because it has a relatively slow onset of action.

For patients not controlled on a low dose of inhaled steroid the choice, according to the British guidelines, is between increasing the dose of the inhaled steroid or adding a long-acting β-agonist.

Both can be effective but there is some evidence to suggest that adding a long-acting β-agonist may be better for patients with symptoms whereas a larger dose of inhaled steroid may be better for patients with frequent exacerbations.

Other prophylactic drugs

Sodium cromoglycate and nedocromil sodium have a similar pharmacological profile. They attenuate bronchoconstriction induced by antigen and a wide variety of indirectly acting stimuli including exercise and cold air. In the clinical setting they appear to be equivalent to a low dose of inhaled corticosteroid probably between 200 and 400 mg budesonide or beclomethasone per day. Both drugs are very safe but their limited efficacy and requirement for inhalation four times daily limits their use.

Other bronchodilators

For patients who continue to have symptoms despite reasonable doses of a regular inhaled steroid a long acting β-agonist should be tried first followed by the other drugs outlined in step four of the British guidelines. These should be tried sequentially and only continued if clear benefit is demonstrated.

Ipratropium and oxitropium bromide are fairly non-specific muscarinic antagonists, inhibiting vagally mediated bronchoconstrictor activity on airway smooth muscle. Their onset of action is relatively slow (75% maximum at 15 minutes and around 1 hour for maximal effect) and although effective if given alone they usually add little when taken in addition to large doses of a β-agonist.

Theophylline relaxes bronchial smooth muscle probably through phosphodiesterase inhibition. Bronchodilatation increases linearly as serum theophylline concentrations increase above 5 μg ml^{-1} but toxic effects become common with serum concentrations above 25–30 μg ml^{-1}. Ideally serum concentrations (pre-dose) should be measured at intervals because theophylline has a narrow therapeutic window and a number of important drug interactions. There is interest in the effect of adding lower doses of theophylline (serum concentrations below 10 μg ml^{-1}) to low dose inhaled steroids. At these concentrations theophylline causes few adverse effects although the improvement in lung function has been less than that achieved with the addition of a long-acting β-agonist.

New treatments

Leukotriene receptor antagonists and 5 lipoxygenase inhibitors are the first new class of anti-asthma drugs to become available for 25 years. They inhibit the bronchoconstrictor response to various challenges including allergen, exercise and cold air in the laboratory and are particularly effective against aspirin-induced bronchoconstriction in aspirin-sensitive patients. In clinical studies to date they have produced modest improvements in lung function and symptoms with a decrease in asthma exacerbations, and appear to be equivalent to between 200 and 400 µg inhaled beclomethasone dipropionate. More information on their effects compared with other treatment, particularly inhaled corticosteroids, and when used in combination with other treatments is required to determine their place in asthma management.

Severe asthma

Special considerations

It has been estimated that the 10% of patients with the most severe asthma consume around 50% of the total resources and much time in hospital is taken up with these patients. Before considering further treatment options it is worth asking some specific questions:

- *is the diagnosis correct?* — Severe asthma can be mimicked by other conditions such as smoking related chronic airways obstruction and vocal cord dysfunction
- *is the patient compliant with treatment?*
- *are there any avoidable precipitating or aggravating factors?* — e.g. foods or food additives, pre-menstrual exacerbations or gastroeosophageal reflux
- *has an occupational sensitiser been overlooked?*
- *does the patient have allergic bronchopulmonary aspergillosis or the Churg-Strauss syndrome?*
- *are other factors relevant?* — Patients with severe asthma may have associated psychological problems and some become dependent on the health service. When this occurs alternative therapeutic strategies may be required although these have been poorly studied

Oral corticosteroids

Around 1% of patients with asthma are taking oral corticosteroids continuously for asthma and most have or will have adverse effects from them. It is important therefore to ensure that the dose of oral steroids is adjusted to the minimum required to achieve reasonable control of symptoms and that the patient is taking appropriate inhaled treatment including a reasonable dose of inhaled corticosteroid. Most patients require a maintenance dose of 2.5 to 10 mg prednisolone (or equivalent) daily to control their asthma. Few patients require higher doses and those that do require careful assessment.

Long term oral steroids are associated with many adverse effects but two are highlighted because they are, to some extent, potentially preventable.

Osteoporosis. Patients on long term oral corticosteroids or those requiring frequent courses are at increased risk of osteoporosis. All patients should be given general advice to help prevent osteoporosis including advice on smoking cessation, regular weight bearing exercise and a diet containing adequate calcium and vitamin D. Hormone replacement therapy should be considered for postmenopausal women. Patients with established osteoporosis may benefit from specific therapy with calcium and vitamin D or bisphosphonates. Bone mineral density can be used to guide treatment. Our practice is to obtain a baseline measurement of bone mineral density after 6 months or less of oral corticosteroid treatment and treat according to the algorithm shown in Figure 1.

Infections. Immunosuppression by systemic steroids can lead to severe and sometimes fatal infections including chickenpox and measles. Patients taking oral steroids who have not had chickenpox are at risk of severe infections and must be told to seek urgent medical attention if they are exposed to an infected patient. Specific IgG antibodies should be checked urgently and if negative they should be given passive immunisation with immunoglobulin preferably within three days of exposure and not later than seven days. Immunocompromised patients exposed to measles should be given human normal immunoglobulin within 96 hours. Testing measles antibody is not recommended because it will delay treatment and previous immunisation or low levels of measles antibodies do not guarantee immunity in the immunocompromised.

Steroid sparing agents

Although any effective asthma treatment can be considered as a steroid sparing agent this term is usually reserved for agents with

I. **Ensure patient is having optimal treatment to ensure minimal dose of oral corticosteroids**

II. **Bone mineral density scan if:**
    - oral corticosteroids >6 months
    - <6 months if other major risk factors: – menopause <45 years
        - underweight
        - previous low impact fracture
        - family history of osteoporotic fracture under 60 years old

III. **If bone mineral density is low consider other causes:** check full blood count, erythrocyte sedimentation rate and biochemical profile including thyroid function tests.

IV. **Management according to bone mineral density/T-score***

T-score > –1   **A**

Normal

General advice
regular weight bearing exercise
stop smoking
dietary advice
consider HRT for post-menopausal women

T-score –1 to –2.0   **B**

General advice as in **A**
calcium and vitamin D
eg. Calcichew D3 2 tabs od
(1000 mg Ca Carbonate + 400 IU vit D)
consider HRT for post-menopausal women

If patient has had a low impact fracture treat as for osteoporosis

---

T-score < –2.0   **C**

osteoporosis

General advice as in **A**
HRT – for post menopausal women unless contraindication
biphosphonate – treat for 3+ years

Consider specialist referral

V. **Follow up – repeat bone mineral density after 1–2 years if still on oral steroids.**
    T-score = difference in standard deviations between patients' bone mineral density (BMD) and reference mean BMD at age of peak bone mass for race and sex.

Figure 1.   Prevention of steroid-induced osteoporosis
Guidelines for patients with asthma/COPD who are taking oral corticosteroids

anti-inflammatory or immune modulating activity. Steroid sparing agents may be considered for patients requiring high doses of oral steroids or where adverse effects are causing problems. There is evidence of benefit from cyclosporin A, gold and methotrexate although their steroid sparing effects in the short term have been only modest. The reduction in prednisolone achieved is usually around 5 mg per day (range 0 to 9.5 mg per day in different studies).[6] These drugs have their own serious adverse effects which need to be borne in mind and their use requires careful monitoring (see Table 4).

Alternative pharmacological options are limited to the same drugs (corticosteroids and bronchodilators) either at higher dose or via a different route of administration. Some patients benefit from nebulised β-agonists and anti-cholinergic drugs. Terbutaline can be given as a continuous subcutaneous infusion (3–12 mg per 24 hours diluted in normal saline) but skin abscesses, tremor, palpitations, cramps and hypokalaemia can be a problem and, like nebulised budesonide, it has not been evaluated in a controlled clinical trial in adults.

Corticosteroid resistance

A small number of patients with asthma are 'corticosteroid resistant,' possibly representing one end of a continuous spectrum of corticosteroid responsiveness. In corticosteroid resistance patients are able to respond to other drugs such as β-agonists and in this respect it can be differentiated from severe asthma where patients may respond poorly to all drugs. True insensitivity to corticosteroids is very uncommon but needs careful assessment to avoid treatment with high doses of corticosteroids.

The mechanism of corticosteroid resistance is not known. The effects of exogenous glucocorticoid on the hypothalamic-pituitary-adrenal axis and on osteocalcin suppression is normal in these patients and they appear to run a similar risk of developing steroid side effects. The amount of activated glucocorticoid receptor available for interaction with DNA may be reduced possibly due to increased levels of the pro-inflammatory transcription factor activating peptide 1 (AP-1).[7]

Specific problems

Asthma may be particularly troublesome at certain times such as during exercise, at night and premenstrually. This is usually an

Table 4. Steroid sparing agents

Agent	Efficacy	Comment, side effects and monitoring
Gold — intramuscular	Evidence for reduced inhaled but not oral steroid requirements.	Some evidence for steroid sparing effects but high incidence of adverse effects — stomatitis, dermatitis, proteinuria.
Gold — oral	Steroid sparing effects in one study.	Monitor urine, full blood count* before each injection or monthly for oral gold.
Cyclosporin A (2.5–5 mg/kg/day in two doses)	Improved asthma control and steroid sparing properties in two studies.	Some evidence for steroid sparing effects but significant adverse effects — hypertrichosis, hypertension and renal impairment. Check blood pressure and urine dipstick every visit. Monitor creatinine and (trough) cyclosporin levels initially every 1–2 weeks (every 2–3 months when stable). Annual 24 hour creatinine clearance and cervical smear. Advise to avoid sun exposure Many important drug interactions.
Methotrexate (15 mg once weekly)	oral steroid sparing efficacy in 5 studies, no effect in 6. Overall benefit in meta-analysis.	Variable efficacy; nausea and anorexia can be problematic. Monitor liver function tests and full blood count* every 2–4 months of therapy. Avoid concurrent non-steroidal anti-inflammatory drugs.
Hydroxychloroquine	2 small studies — no effect in one, some benefit in the other open study	No good evidence of efficacy
Colchicine	Improved symptoms and bronchodilator use but not lung function in one small study	No good evidence of efficacy
Troleandomycin	Improved lung function and steroid sparing properties in several studies	Efficacy probably secondary to reduced metabolism of methylprednisolone so no net advantage. Steroid-like adverse effects.
Azathioprine	one small study — no efficacy	No good evidence of efficacy
Intravenous immunoglobulin	Improved lung function and steroid sparing effects in 1 small study	No good evidence of efficacy

*including differential white cell count

indication that asthma control is less than ideal, in which case adding or increasing regular prophylactic treatment may be the most appropriate treatment. If asthma is otherwise well controlled but specific problems remain the following treatment may help:

- *exercise-induced asthma.* Inhalation of a β-agonist or sodium cromoglycate a few minutes before exercise should be tried first. A leukotriene antagonist or a long-acting β-agonist may help although some tolerance may be seen
- *nocturnal asthma.* A long acting β-agonist or slow release theophylline with the later should be tried before retiring to bed (see also section on preventative measures)
- *premenstrual asthma.* Around one third of pre-menopausal women with asthma find that their asthma deteriorates slightly before or during menstruation. A few women have more disabling problems which may be helped by intramuscular progesterone; liaison with a gynaecologist is recommended.

Asthma in pregnancy

Not only do doctors need to know about asthma in pregnancy but asthmatic patients will want information about the effect of asthma and asthma treatment on pregnancy and the effects of pregnancy on their asthma. They can be reassured that pregnancy, does not usually cause particular problems for patients with asthma. In many patients asthma remains largely unchanged during pregnancy; though about a quarter show some deterioration and a quarter improve.

A large prospective study compared the outcome of pregnancy in 824 women with asthma and 678 control women and the results were very reassuring. No significant relationships were identified between major congenital malformations and exposure to β-agonists, theophylline, sodium cromoglycate, corticosteroids, antihistamines or decongestants. Oral corticosteroids were associated with twice the risk of pre-eclampsia but no other independent associations were observed between asthma or asthma medication and adverse perinatal outcomes. Nevertheless using the inhaled route for drug delivery reduces blood levels and has even clearer advantages during pregnancy. It is important to ensure that patients understand that the dangers of uncontrolled asthma to the foetus exceed any possible effects of the drugs. Acute asthma should be treated in the normal way with oxygen, nebulised β-agonists and systemic corticosteroids.

Post-natal women can breast feed since breast milk contains only minute concentrations of inhaled drugs and only a small fraction of prednisolone is secreted in breast milk. Theophylline may cause a problem with irritability in the infant.

Acute severe asthma

Assessment

Acute severe asthma should be considered as a largely preventable disease. Patients admitted to hospital with severe asthma frequently give a history of poorly controlled symptoms over the preceding few days or more suggesting that had appropriate action been taken earlier the attack might have been aborted.

The priority in managing acute severe asthma is to make a quick but accurate assessment of severity and initiate appropriate treatment within minutes of presentation. Acute severe asthma is very frightening and patients require reassurance and a calm but efficient environment. Objective measurements should include peak expiratory flow rate, heart and respiratory rate and an assessment of the patient's ability to talk in sentences, paying special attention to the presence of any features of acute severe or life threatening asthma (see Table 5).

Patients with life threatening asthma may not be distressed and they may demonstrate all the features listed; the presence of any should alert the doctor. Arterial blood gas concentrations should be measured on all patients with an oxygen saturation <92% when breathing air, on all patients on oxygen therapy and if there is a suspicion of inappropriate hyperventilation or vocal cord dysfunction.

Treatment

Immediate management for a severe exacerbation should include 40–60% oxygen, salbutamol 5 mg or terbutaline 10 mg nebulised with oxygen, and either prednisolone 30–60 mg or intravenous hydrocortisone 200 mg. Hydrocortisone has no pharmacological advantage over prednisolone unless the patient is vomiting or unable to take oral medication but if a patient is very unwell it may be sensible to give the first dose by the intravenous route. A chest radiograph is indicated if a pneumothorax is considered possible but only after initiation of treatment.

Most patients will start to improve following initial treatment. They should continue with oxygen, oral steroids (e.g. prednisolone

Table 5.   Recognition and assessment of severe asthma in hospital

Features of severe asthma
- PEF <50% of predicted or previous best value
- Unable to complete sentences in one breath
- Respiration >25 breaths per minute
- Pulse >110 beats per minute

Life threatening features
- PEF <33% of predicted or previous best value
- Silent chest, cyanosis, or feeble respiratory effort
- Bradycardia or hypotension
- Exhaustion, confusion or coma

Blood gas markers of a very severe, life threatening attack:
- High $PaCO_2$
- severe hypoxia: PO_2 <8 kPa irrespective of treatment with O_2
- Low pH

NB: Patients with a mild to moderate asthma attack usually have a low arterial $PaCO_2$. A normal $PaCO_2$ in conjunction with arterial hypoxaemia suggest that asthma is deteriorating.

30 mg daily) and nebulised β-agonist four hourly reducing to six hourly. Progress must be carefully monitored and should include twice daily peak expiratory flow recordings in all patients and arterial blood gas measurement if there is deterioration.

If the patient fails to improve or subsequently deteriorates the following can be added: inhaled ipratropium 0.5 mg, intravenous aminophylline 250 mg over 20 minutes followed by 500 μg kg^{-1} hour^{-1} (unless the patient is taking oral theophylline) or intravenous salbutamol or terbutaline 250 μg over 10 minutes. If life threatening features are present the patient should be transferred to an intensive care unit. Further deterioration or a tiring patient are indications for endotracheal intubation and ventilation.

Antibiotics. Asthma exacerbations are often triggered by viral infections — there is no evidence that antibiotics help. Broad spectrum antibiotics should be reserved for patients with presumptive evidence of bacterial infection such as a pneumonic changes on a chest radiograph.

Sedatives are absolutely contraindicated in the management of acute asthma.

Discharge

Once the patient is recovering it is important to try to identify the cause of the acute attack and the need for admission to hospital. If the deterioration was gradual were appropriate measures taken to pre-empt the attack? If the attack occurred suddenly were there any avoidable precipitating factors such as aspirin ingestion or contact with pets? Admission to hospital is another opportunity for asthma education and to review treatment compliance and inhaler technique. Most patients who die from asthma have previously been admitted to hospital with acute severe asthma.

Patients should not normally leave hospital until they have been on their discharge medication for at least 24 hours, their peak flow is greater than 75% of previous best or predicted and peak flow diurnal variability is less than 25%. Patients should be discharged on inhaled and oral corticosteroids which should be continued at high dose until asthma control, ideally judged by peak expiratory flow, has returned to normal. Early communication with the patient's general practitioner and follow up in a respiratory clinic within four weeks should be standard management.

References

1. Barnes PJ, Jonsson B, Klim JB. The costs of asthma. *Eur Respir J* 1996;**9**:636–642

2. Stevens DA, Schwartz HJ, Lee JY, Moskovitz BL, Jerome DC, Catanzaro A, Bamberger DM, Weinmann AJ, Tuazon CU, Judson MA, Platts-Mills TAE, DeGraff AR. A randomized trial of itraconazole in allergic bronchopulmonary aspergillosis. *N Engl J Med* 2000; **342**:756–762

3. Chan-Yeung M, Malo J-L. Aetiological agents in occupational asthma. *Eur Respir J* 1994;**7**:346–371

4. Hsu C-H, Chua K-Y, Tao M-H, Lai Y-L, Wu H-D, Huang S-K, Hsieh K-H. Immunoprophylaxis of allergen-induced immunoglobulin E synthesis and airway hyperresponsiveness *in vivo* by genetic immunization. *Nature Med* 1996;**2**:540–544

5. The British Guidelines on Asthma Management. *Thorax* 1997;**52**:S1–S21

6. Hill JM, Tattersfield AE. Corticosteroid sparing agents in asthma. *Thorax* 1995;**50**:577–582

7. Barnes PJ, Pedersen S. Efficacy and safety of inhaled corticosteroids in asthma. *Am Rev Respir Dis* 1993;**148**:S1–S26

Practical Allergy

Glenis K Scadding

Introduction

This chapter deals with both asthma and rhinitis since now that evidence exists for rhinitis as a predisposing factor, exacerbating factor and therapeutic avenue for asthma, respiratory physicians should consider the whole of the respiratory tract.

The major allergic diseases (asthma, eczema, rhinitis), have all shown a dramatic increase in prevalence over the past few decades. Both environmental and genetic factors are important in allergy. Epidemiological studies demonstrate an association with an affluent western lifestyles. The major environmental influences are probably relevant very early in life, with early infections such as hepatitis A and a crowded living environment decreasing the chances of becoming atopic. Theoretically this is via interferon gamma, a Th-1 cell cytokine (vide infra), which promotes IgG and decreases IgE production. The difference between gut flora in western society compared to poorer countries has been noted, it may be that this is the major relevant factor. Other environmental influences such as increased allergen exposure to housedust mite and pet dander in warm, carpeted, centrally heated, poorly ventilated homes and urban pollution such as diesel exhaust particles may play a part.

The allergic reaction begins with the phase of sensitisation. Allergen contact occurs usually at a mucosal surface and allergen is taken up by antigen presenting cells (of the macrophage series), broken down into peptides which are expressed on the cell surface in the groove of the HLA-DR molecule. In this fashion they are recognised by a T-lymphocyte which in an atopic individual is of the Th-2 type and produces cytokines such as IL4 and IL5. B-lymphocytes which also recognise the antigen are induced to form antibody of the IgE class. B-cell switching to IgE production has been demonstrated in the nasal mucosa. Locally produced IgE antibody is rapidly and avidly taken up by local mast cells and held on the cell surface by the high affinity Fc epsilon R1 receptor so that the antigen combining site is available for further antigen (allergen) contact.

Allergic sensitisation does not always result in allergic disease. The reasons for this are as yet unknown. However in many cases subsequent contact with the same allergen results in mast cell degranulation and mediator release. This results in immediate symptoms such as itching, running and sneezing in the nose; wheezing, coughing and shortness of breath in the chest. This phase of the reaction is most often seen when allergen contact is intermittent such as with animal allergy in non pet owners or seasonal allergy (e.g. hayfever). It is easy to diagnose.

With chronic allergen exposure or very large exposure a late phase results. This consists of inflammation involving eosinophils and other cells including lymphocytes, mast cells and basophils. The major symptom is chronic obstruction with hyper-reactivity in both nose and chest. This is a more difficult diagnostic problem and

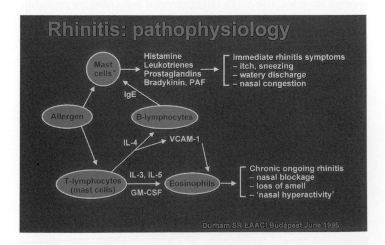

Figure 1.   Diagrammatic representation of the early and late phase responses. Courtesy of Professor S. Durham, Nat. Hrt + Lung Institute

Nasal	Running (ant/post)
	Sneezing/itching
	Blocking

2 of 3 symptoms for >1 hour/day for > 2 weeks

Figure 2.   Definition of rhinitis

such chronically obstructed patients are frequently misdiagnosed as non-allergic since the acute symptoms are largely absent (Figure 1).

In asthma there is epithelial shedding and exposure of sensory nerves, which when stimulated can cause symptoms such as cough and wheeze, either directly or via tachykinin release. In rhinitis the epithelium remains intact but nerve stimulation by mediators occurs and results in reflex sneezing and secretion.

Allergy in Clinical Management of Asthma and Rhinitis

Whereas the majority (probably more than 80%) of children with asthma are atopic this figure is lower in adult asthmatics. However since the late phase response can be prominent in chronic disease, underlying allergic factors can be missed therefore an allergy history and skin prick testing are advisable in all asthmatics. Patients with late onset disease should be questioned about aspirin and NSAID sensitivity, including a question on when they last took any of these medications.

The definition of rhinitis is clinical (Figure 2). Rhinitis suffers can largely be divided into 'runners/sneezers' with predominantly immediate allergic reactions and 'blockers' with mainly late phase inflammation. Similarly not all allergic asthmatics have obvious exacerbations of their disease in response to allergen, but this may become apparent if they are alerted to the possibility of allergy and monitor symptoms and peak flow.

History

This should include the features mentioned in Figure 3. A questionnaire which the patient can fill in whilst waiting to be seen is often helpful.

1   Major presenting symtom that bothers the patient.

2   Other relevant symptoms

3   Diurnal/seasonal/environmental variations in the above

4   Past history of atopic disease
    • milk allergy in infancy
    • atopic dermatitis
    • asthma
    • rhinitis

5   Family history of atopic disease

6   Environment: home/work/hobbies (eg: carpets, central
    heating, pets, bedding, furry toys, cigarette smoke etc)

7   Diet including any food addictions/dislikes including any
    oral and/or gut reactions to food.

8   medication used: which
                       for how long
                       how used
                       any reactions to drugs (aspirin/NSAIDs,
                       beta-blockers etc)

Figure 3.   Allergy history

Examination

The external facial appearance of the allergic individual can provide several clues. A transverse allergic crease occurs in many
patients due to nasal rubbing. Other facial features are mouth
breathing, dark circles under the eyes and an additional crease
beneath the eye, eczema on the cheeks and a high arched palate.
Internal examination of the nose is easily achieved with the fibreoptic scope or failing that with an otoscope. The allergic nose is
frequently pale, bluish and oedematous with watery rhinorrhoea.
However the mucosa may be reddened if nasal sprays are in use
or if there is additional infection. The major examination points are
detailed in Figure 4.

Investigations

Skin prick testing with aqueous extracts of allergens is simple, cheap

1. Physical Appearances:
    (a) external: atopic eczema
                    other rashes (eg) urticaria
                    allergic crease/salute
                    allergic facies
                    mouth breathing: nasal: external deviations
                    bridge collapse/alar collapse

    (b) airway: septal deviation/perforation
                    colour of mucosa
                    wetness
                    presence/absence of secretions (eg)
                        muco pus
                        crusting/blood
                    presence/absence of polyps

    (c) throat: presence of tonsils
                    post-pharyngeal islands of lymphoid tissue
                    postnasal drip

    (d) ears: otitis externa
                    state of eardrums

    (e) chest: usual examination including: wheezing at rest
                    and on forced expiration

Figure 4.   Allergy examination

and quick (Figure 5). Provided inhalant allergens only are used and intradermal testing is avoided, then there is no risk of anaphylaxis. Use of a negative control — saline — and a positive control — histamine phosphate — is mandatory. The major allergens are housedust mite, cat, dog and grass pollen, using these approximately 95% of allergic patients can be diagnosed. Other useful allergens include tree pollens (a UK 3–tree mix is available), for those individuals with early seasonal symptoms, other pet allergens such as budgie feathers and moulds such as aspergillus. Food allergens are less reliable and may cause anaphylaxis; RAST tests (vide infra), can be substituted.

It is safer to avoid skin prick testing in those with a past history of anaphylaxis or with moderate to severe eczema (where it may cause scratching, irritation and disease exacerbation). Patients on antihistamines will give unreliable results as will those on high doses of oral corticosteroids. About 5% of the population have

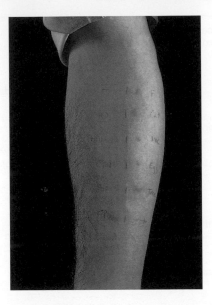

Figure 5. Skin prick testing
With only a few aqueous allergen extracts such as housedust
mite, grass pollen, cat and dog together with a negative saline
and a positive histamine most respiratory atopics can be
diagnosed. Aqueous extracts of relevant allergens together with a
positive control (histamine) and a negative control (saline) are
placed on the skin and are pricked gently into the epidermis with
a skin prick test needle, using a skin prick test lancet, with a
fresh one for each test. After one to two minutes the area can be
blotted with clean tissue. The test results are read at 15 minutes
and weal sizes of 3mm > the negative control are regarded as
positive. These must be interpreted in the light of the history.
Abnormalities such as large weals at all sites (dermagraphism) or
failure of all tests including histamine suggest the need for an
alternative such as blood testing for specific IgE

dermagraphism with responses to skin pricking alone. In these cases
the substitution of radio-allergo sorbent testing (RAST), on serum is
available. This is no more sensitive than skin prick testing and is
expensive and the result is delayed. However RAST testing is useful
for allergens which are not frequently tested in clinic. A total IgE
level can be done at the same time but is relatively unhelpful since
it is within normal limits in approximately 50% of patients with
allergic asthma and rhinitis.

1.	Allergen identification and avoidance
2.	Pharmacotherapy
3.	Immunotherapy
4.	Surgery

Figure 6. Management of respiratory allergy

The results of skin prick and RAST testing must always be interpreted in the light of the patients history. False positive results can occur (although these indicate sensitisation and a proportion of patients later develop disease), false negative results are also possible especially with a short history. The final arbiter is local allergen challenge which needs to be undertaken in a specialist department with objective airway monitoring.

The demonstration of eosinophils in nasal smears or in sputum is relatively simple and can be used both in diagnosis and in monitoring progress. Nasal smears should be taken from both nostrils since the results can differ (possibly because there is a nasal cycle with one nostril being patent for 4 to 6 hours whilst the other is largely resting). Eosinophils of >10% of the cell content are found in allergic rhinitis and also in the non-allergic rhinitis with eosinophilia syndrome (NARES). This is as yet poorly understood but may be a precursor of nasal polyposis and/or aspirin sensitivity. It could represent the T-cell IL5 eosinophil arm of the allergic response. Eosinophils are also found in 'allergic-type' nasal polyposis and in vasculitides such as Churg-Strauss syndrome.

Nitric oxide levels in exhaled air are simply measured by chemi-luminescence. In untreated allergic rhinitis levels are usually elevated above the normal range of 500 to 800ppb. Interestingly in allergic-type nasal polyposis levels are low and are decreased proportional to the extent of polypoid disease. Pulmonary levels are usually <10ppb but are elevated in inflammation from any cause (as in the nose). The use of nitric oxide monitoring to decide whether pulmonary inflammation exists or whether chest symptoms are entirely secondary to upper respiratory tract disease is under investigation.

Management

Basic management strategies for allergic rhinitis and asthma are detailed in Figure 6.

Aeroallergens:
Perennial: house dust mite, cat, dog Seasonal: tree and grass pollens, mould spores
Occupational:
Biological: flour, laboratory animals, latex etc Chemical: Isocyanates, acid anhydrides, colophony etc (low molecular weight)
Drugs:
Aspirin, NSAIDs, antihypertensives, oral contraceptive pill, hormone replacement therapy

Figure 7. Allergen avoidance

Allergen Avoidance

Management of patients with asthma and rhinitis should always include identification and, where possible, avoidance of causal factors. The commonest cause of perennial rhinitis and asthma symptoms are sensitivity to housedust mite and domestic pets. Important seasonal causes include pollen allergy (tree pollen in Spring time, grass and weeds during the Summer), and mould spores during the late Summer and Autumn months.

Occupational allergens may provoke perennial symptoms and it is therefore essential to ask whether symptoms are work related and whether they improve at weekends and whilst on holiday. There is strong evidence that good housedust mite avoidance measures improve asthma both from patients at altitude, in hospital or in low allergen, specially ventilated homes. A careful drug history should always be taken (see Figure 7). Food allergy is a rare cause of asthma and rhinitis. It is usually accompanied by other allergic manifestations such as oral or gastrointestinal symptoms, rash or anaphylaxis.

Housedust mite avoidance

Housedust mites are found in mattresses, pillows, carpets, bed covers and soft furnishings throughout the home. Well-insulated, centrally heated homes provide optimal conditions for mite growth.

Mattress/bedding barrier intervention has been shown to reduce mite allergen levels and improve clinical symptoms of both asthma and rhinitis. There is also evidence of reduction of bronchial hyper-reactivity. In addition regular vacuuming of carpets and soft furnishing with a vacuum cleaner which has a filter before the exhaust is

1. Encase mattress, pillows* and quilt in impermeable covers.

2. Wash all bedding in the hot cycle (55 to 60°) weekly.

3. Replace carpets with linoleum or wood flooring.
   – if they cannot be removed treat with acaricides or tannic acid regularly.

4. Minimise upholstered furniture — replace with leather furniture.

5. Keep dust-accumulating objects in closed cupboard.

6. Use a vacuum cleaner with integrated HEPA filter and double thickness bags.

7. Replace curtains with blinds or easily washable (hot cycle), curtains.

8. Hot wash/freeze soft toys.

* Recent reports have shown use of non-feather pillows was associated with wheezing and that synthetic pillows harbour more housedust mite allergen per pillow than feather ones, possibly because the casing on feathers is more tightly woven

Figure 8.   Housedust mite avoidance measures

recommended, plus where possible, use of alternative cork, vinyl or hardwood floors. The major housedust mite avoidance measures are shown in Figure 8.

Animal allergens

The major cat allergen (Fel-d-1), is a salivary protein which is preened onto the fur where it dries into flakes which becomes airborne as minute (<2.5mu), particles which remain airborne for many hours and are very respirable. Families with atopic members should be advised against having furred or feathered pets in the home. Where pet removal is not possible advice can be given to keep the animal out of the bedroom at all times and confine it either outside or to the kitchen and garden. Vigorous prolonged water-based cleaning measures are needed to remove pet allergen from the home. Washing the cat or dog once weekly may help to reduce airborne allergen levels. Once an animal goes it should not be replaced.

Animal dander remains in the home for several months after the removal of the pet.

Pollen avoidance

This is more difficult but certain measures such as keeping windows shut in cars and buildings, in the latter especially as evening approaches and pollen descends as the air cools.

Wrap-around sunglasses may reduce eye symptoms. Pollen filters can be obtained for cars which do not already have them in place.

Patients should be advised to avoid walking in open, grassy spaces particularly in the evening when pollen counts are at their highest.

If possible a holiday by the sea or abroad during the major part of the allergen season (for grass this is usually the last 2 weeks in June), can be helpful.

Pharmacotherapy

Allergic rhinitis

If allergen avoidance is impossible or fails to control symptoms then drugs will be needed. The major drugs used in rhinitis and their effects on various symptoms are detailed in Figure 9. The mainstay of treatment, as with asthma, is topical corticosteroids which are effective against all nasal symptoms including nasal congestion and blockage in the majority of sufferers. Drops should be used in the head upside down position and are thought to be more effective in nasal polyposis and in sinus obstruction since they can reach the ostiomeatal complex. Sprays should be used standing upright with the head tilted forwards, sniffing hard is not recommended since this pulls the solution directly to the postnasal space.

Short courses of oral corticosteroids may be needed for very severe symptoms, for example when blockage is such that nasal sprays are ineffective or when the nose is full of polyp tissue. Patients with no contra-indications should take the minimal effective dose usually 0.5mgs per kg per day in a single dose with food for 5 days, and this should be combined with intranasal therapy.

Depot intra-muscular corticosteroids are not recommended as the dose is not controllable and local and systemic side can occur.

	ITCH/SNEEZE	DISCHARGE	BLOCK	SMELL
Topical decongestant	–	–	+++	+
Oral antihistamine	+++	++	+/-	–
Topical antihistamine	+++	++	+/-	–
Ipratropium bromide	–	+++	–	–
Topical cromoglycate	+	+	+/–	–
Topical corticosteroids	+++	+++	++	+
Oral corticosteroids	+++	+++	+++	++

Figure 9. Pharmacotherapy of allergic rhinitis

It is preferable to use intranasal corticosteroids plus an oral antihistamine and to use occasional oral corticosteroids for days when symptoms are very severe.

Sodium Cromoglycate

This weak anti-inflammatory needs to be used several times a day in order to be effective. This raises problems with compliance and major place is in the treatment of young children for whom it is first line treatment. Cromoglycate or nedocromil sodium eye drops are helpful in the prophylaxis of allergic conjunctivitis.

Antihistamines

These are particularly effective against immediate symptoms of sneezing, itching and rhinorrhoea, but have little effect on nasal blockage. Oral antihistamines have the advantage of also acting on eye, palatal and throat itching.

The first generation of oral antihistamines have sedative and psychomotor effects and are best avoided. Second generation ones produce less sedation and psychomotor impairment and are equally effective.

Many antihistamines have been shown to have some weak anti-inflammatory effects in vitro. The relevance of these in vivo is not yet fully known, however both ketotifen and cetirizine appear to have the potential to reduce subsequent development of asthma in children with severe atopic dermatitis. Recently a year of regular terfenadine in children reduced upper respiratory tract symptoms and visits to the doctor by about 50%.

Decongestants

Systemic decongestants are of doubtful value and have serious side effects such as raised blood pressure in the elderly and hyperactivity in small children. Topical decongestants can be helpful in the short term (eg, when starting treatment with nasal sprays to open up the nose to aid eustachian tube function during flying and in otitis media with effusion to reduce ear pressure and pain). Prolonged use (over a week) carries the danger of rebound nasal blockage and rhinitis medicamentosa.

Ipratropium bromide

This helps patients with watery rhinorrhoea and is mainly used in patients with true vasomotor rhinitis where there is thought to be an imbalance between the sympathetic and parasympathetic nervous systems. Several doses should be taken when symptoms are worse — usually early in the mornings — and only 1 or 2 doses taken later in the day. This usually produces control without excessive nasal dryness. Prolonged use occasionally results in complete remission.

Leukotriene receptor antagonists (LTRAs)

These have some effects in rhinitis mainly on congestion and mucus secretion. Their actions appear to be additive to those of antihistamines.

There are few trials as yet but our experience with montelukast in nasal polyposis, particularly in aspirin sensitive patients, suggests that montelukast can help reduce polyp size and restore the sense of smell when used in addition to topical corticosteroids. Unfortunately not all patients experience any benefit, possibly due to leukotriene receptor polymorphism. There is some evidence for anti-inflammatory activity of these drugs in asthma with reduced sputum eosinophilia and a gradual rise in pulmonary function over several weeks. Similarly there is a trend for a gradual improvement in nasal polyposis seen over weeks. Thus a trial of therapy lasting about a month is needed.

Summary

Pharmacotherapy should always be combined with allergen avoidance where possible. Careful attention should be paid to the type and dominance of the patients symptoms and drugs used alone or in combination to match the symptom profile.

The importance of regular prophylactic medication, even in the absence of symptoms, requires emphasis. Treatment failure should always provoke a review of compliance.

The possibility of steroid loading in patients with allergy at more than one site, particularly in children with asthma, eczema and rhinitis, should always be borne in mind[8]. Certain evidence suggests that topical corticosteroid in the nose may have more effect on bronchial hyper-reactivity than the same dose delivered to the lungs. This, if true, suggests that it is important always to treat concomitant rhinitis in patients with asthma.

If regular treatment has been unsuccessful then the diagnosis should be reviewed and the need for alternative treatment (e.g. surgery or immunotherapy should be considered.

Immunotherapy

At present this is reserved for the small group of subjects who despite regular use of medication and allergen avoidance continue to have marked symptoms. It is for pollen sensitive patients who fail to respond to conventional treatment that allergen injection immunotherapy retains a place at present in the UK. Careful patient selection is essential. Subjects should give a clear history of seasonal symptoms with a corresponding skin prick test or RAST. Patients with multiple allergies or with other immunological or medical diseases are specifically excluded. In the United Kingdom patients with chronic asthma, even mild disease, are at present specifically excluded.

The mechanism of immunotherapy is largely unknown but recent research suggests that it involves tolerisation of T-lymphocytes.

The efficacy of immunotherapy has been demonstrated in seasonal allergic rhinitis caused by grass pollen, ragweed and birch. There are also studies suggesting efficacy in housedust mite and animal dander perennial rhinitis.

- Unilateral nasal problems
- Nasal perforations, ulceration or collapse
- Sero-sanguinous discharge
- Crusting high in the nasal cavity
- Recurrent infections
- Periorbital cellulitis

Figure 10. Features of rhinitis which suggest ENT referral

Safety

Allergen injection immunotherapy always involves a risk of eliciting severe systemic reactions, even death. Following a Committee of Safety of Medicine report allergen immunotherapy in the United Kingdom largely ceased outside a few specialist centres. The Committee expressed concern about the number of deaths from severe bronchospasm and anaphylaxis which were almost exclusively confined to patients with asthma. The recommendation that injections should be given only where facilities for resuscitation are available and that patients be kept under medical observation for 1 hour after each injection has been made. This, together with the fact that regular injections initially at weekly intervals, renders compliance with treatment difficult with patients and physicians. Safer methods of immunotherapy such as nasal and sublingual application of allergen peptides are under investigation.

The Place of Surgery

The treatment of rhinitis is essentially medical with surgical help in selected cases where this fails. Surgery can be used for diagnosis (nasal biopsy), for improving nasal function by correction of anatomical deformity or by removal of polyps or improvement of sinus drainage. The development of rigid endoscopes in order to gain a good view of the middle meatus and the ostiomeatal complex have helped in the diagnosis and treatment of chronic rhinosinusitis and of nasal polyposis. Surgery can be performed in the nose using these (endoscopic sinus surgery = FESS). Figure 10 shows those features which suggest ENT referral.

In patients with chronic ethmoiditis where anatomical variations of the middle meatus cause localised disease by obstructing sinus drainage, functional endoscopic sinus surgery is frequently helpful. Since the ostiomeatal complex is easily blocked by a small amount of swelling it follows that allergic rhinitis may be complicated by secondary infection and patients with chronic or recurrent infective rhinosinusitis should be tested for underlying factors such as allergy or immune deficiency.

Further information is available from the BSACI Rhinitis Management Guidelines — third edition available by post from: Mrs Susan Duff, BSACI Secretariat, 66 Weston Park, Thames Ditton, Surrey KT1 0HL.

Anaphylaxis and Anaphylactoid Reactions

The term anaphylaxis (from the Greek 'without protection'), was coined by Portier and Richet in 1902. They attempted to immunise dogs to sea anemone venom, unwittingly sensitising them so that they subsequently died when injected with a previously non-lethal dose. Anaphylaxis now refers to a systemic immediate hypersensitivity reaction caused by IgE mediated release of mediators from mast cells and basophils. Anaphylactoid reactions are clinically similar but are not mediated by IgE.

Incidence

Although the true incidence is unknown an estimate of 3 cases per 10,000 hospital patients was published in 1973. A more recent report from Munich suggested 9.79 cases per 100 000 population in 1995.

The major causative agents are listed in Figure 11.

Typical manifestations usually occur within a few minutes of allergen contact, but can be delayed and are occasionally biphasic. Usually multiple organ systems are involved (see Figure 12), however Sampson has pointed out that in fatal and near fatal reactions to food the only clinical manifestation may be collapse and cyanosis.

Anaphylaxis tends to be more frequent in adults for drug induced reactions and is reportedly more frequent in females for drug reactions such as latex, aspirin and muscle relaxants, but in males for Hymenoptera venom. Orally administered allergens are less likely to produce severe reactions. Gaps in administration of drugs may predispose to reactions, however the longer the interval the less likely the recurrence for many allergens. Atopy is a risk factor

Drugs: penicillin, anaesthetic agents, hormones
Insect stings
Foods: peanuts, seafood
Latex
Animals
Plants
Chemicals
Exercise
Vibration
Osmotic effects of intravenous solutions
Idiopathic

Figure 11.   The major causes of anaphylaxis/anaphylactoid reactions

Usually multiple organ systems involved
Skin   93%
CVS   89%
Respiratory tract   40%
G-I tract   7%

Of 502 patients reacting to intravenous drugs peri-operatively

The reaction is more likely to affect the upper airway and alimentary tract if the allergen has been eaten.

Figure 12.   The frequency of occurrence of signs and symptoms of anaphylaxis

for anaphylaxis for foods, exercise, radio contrast media and latex as well as idiopathic anaphylaxis but is probably not a risk factor for insulin, penicillin and Hymenoptera reactions.

Mechanisms

The initiating mechanisms of anaphylaxis and anaphylactoid reactions are shown in Figure 13. In many patients multiple inflammatory pathways such as the complement cascade, the kinin system and

Anaphylaxis
1. IgE-mediated — food, drugs, insect venom, some cases of exercise.

Anaphylactoid:
1. Direct release of mast cell mediators — drugs idiopathic, exercise, cold and sunlight.
2. Disturbances in arachidonic acid metabolism — aspirin NSAIDs
3. Immune complexes — gammaglobulin, IgG anti IgA, dextran
4. Cytotoxic — transfusion reaction to cellular elements
5. Direct complement activation — radio contrast media, dialysis membranes (?) protamine reactions
6. Activation of contact system — dialysis membranes and radio contrast material

Figure 13.   Mechanisms of anaphylaxis and anaphylactoid reactions

also various parts of the coagulation pathway also become activated.

Differential diagnosis

The commonest condition mimicking anaphylaxis is vaso-vagal collapse, however in this there is no skin reaction such as urticaria or flushing and bradycardia occurs rather than tachycardia which is usual in anaphylaxis. Other possible diagnoses include the flushing syndromes such as carcinoid, restaurant syndromes which occur in response to monosodium glutamate (MSG), ingestion of rotten fish, (usually tuna or mackerel) can cause scombroidosis with flushing, itch and urticaria, nausea, vomiting and diarrhoea due to the histamine-like chemicals produced in the fish. In addition there are syndromes in which excess histamine production occurs such as urticaria pigmentosa, systemic mastocytosis and hydatid cyst.

Hereditary angioeodema due to C1–esterase inhibitor depletion or malfunction can present with laryngeal oedema, abdominal pain and a rash. Some females have progesterone — related anaphylactic episodes at the relevant stage of their menstrual cycle. Patients with recurring and chronic urticaria rarely suffer anaphylaxis or anaphylactoid episodes, with the exception of patients with hyper-immunoglobulinaemia-E. Various non-organic diseases such as panic attacks and vocal cord dysfunction syndrome can mimic anaphylaxis.

Immediate treatment:
1. Check airway, breathing and circulation — start cardio-respiratory resuscitation if needed and remove from further allergen contact (tourniquet proximal to injection/sting).
2. Epinephrine (adrenaline) 1/1000 — 0.3 to 0.5ml sc/im adult. 0.01mgs/kg or 0.1 to 0.3ml sl/im child. May need repeating in 15 minutes.
3. Volume replacement — 1 to 2 litres IV colloid rapidly in adults — may need repeating.

Over 50% of patients respond to the above measures.

Further treatment if needed:
1. Antihistamines
2. Beta-2 agonists
3. Vasopressors
4. Corticosteroids
5. Aminophylline
6. Glucagon (for patients on beta-blockers)
7. Atropine

Transfer to hospital with observation after for 2 hours for mild cases, 24 hours for severe episodes.

Investigation — take blood (20mls), at 1, 3 and 8 hour intervals for mast cell tryptase, specific IgE (RAST), complement, [2 EDTA bottles (5mls each), plus 1 serum bottle (10mls).]

Allergy referral

Figure 14. Management of acute anaphylaxis

Management of the acute event

This is detailed in Figure 14. Prompt recognition and treatment with adrenaline are essential. The Medihaler-Epi device has been withdrawn from production in the UK so sublingual adrenalin is no longer easily available. Patients at risk should be taught to carry their own injectable adrenalin in the form of a Epi-pen device which delivers 0.3mls of 1/1000 solution. This may be insufficient for a large adult and so two should be supplied to each patient.

Other preventive measures include medic alert bracelets and necklaces to be worn by the patient at all times and the discontinuation of beta-blockers, angiotensin converting enzymes (ACE inhibitors), monoamine-oxidase inhibitors and certain tricyclic antidepressants where possible in patients with a history of anaphylaxis. If patients are required to undergo a procedure or to take an agent which places them at risk then either pre-treatment with corticosteroid and antihistamines should be considered or a low dose provocation test employed with consideration of desensitisation where possible.

Investigation of the acute episode to confirm the diagnosis and to identify the allergen can be undertaken by taking blood samples as specified above. Any food remaining or regurgitated can be used in the investigation of specific IgE. Otherwise relevant factors from the history should determine the tests employed.

Post-mortem determination of specific IgE and serum tryptase may be useful in establishing anaphylaxis as the cause of death in patients who have died suddenly and unexpectedly. Blood needs to be taken within 15 hours.

Bee and Wasp Venom Allergy

Allergic reactions to insect stings are reported by approximately 1% of adults in Europe, with about 40 deaths per year occurring in the USA and between 16 and 38 in France.

Stinging insects belong to the Hymenoptera order which contains apids, bees, vespids (wasps and hornets), and formicids (fire ants). In the UK the relevant species are the honeybee and the wasp.

Reactions can be divided into immediate and delayed. Immediate local reactions are normal and consist of pain, redness and swelling at the sting site. Large local reactions may involve swelling and erythema of most of an arm and leg, but all signs and symptoms are contiguous with the sting site. Systemic reactions are generalised and involve signs or symptoms at a site remote from the sting. Toxic reactions are non-immunologic but are caused by multiple stings within a short period of time. The signs and symptoms are identical to systemic reactions but are caused by vaso-active amines in the insect venom, rather than release of mediators following IgE-allergen interaction.

Delayed reactions usually consist of progressive swelling and erythema at the site of the sting, but can include serum sickness-like reactions, glomeralonephritis, myocarditis or Guillain-Barre acute syndrome. These are rare.

Therapy

Large local reactions to stings are best treated with ice compresses and time, although anti-histamines and glucocorticoids are usually prescribed in addition.

Systemic reactions to stings are treated as for anaphylaxis from any other cause (see preceding pages). In all cases of anaphylaxis the patient or parent should receive instructions on future avoidance of insects, an emergency kit containing epinephrine and an allergy referral.

Desensitisation

Only patients with systemic reactions should be considered for venom immunotherapy. A diagnosis needs to be made with a careful clinical history followed by skin prick testing which is more sensitive than the alternative RAST testing. Lyophilised preparations of honeybee and wasp venom are commercially available. Venom immunotherapy should be considered in persons who have experienced a systemic reaction to an insect sting and who have positive puncture or intradermal skin tests to venom with a concentration of 1mcg/ml or less. Medical indications are strongest in adults with life threatening reactions to stings who are at 50% to 60% risk of a subsequent systemic reaction on further allergen contact. The indications are weakest in children who have experienced only cutaneous angioeodema or urticaria, they have an approximately 10% risk of future systemic reactions. Individuals with large local reactions have only a very small risk of anaphylaxis after future stings and therefore should not undergo skin testing or measurement of venom specific IgE.

Immunotherapy schedules vary from the ultra rapid which reaches the targeted maintenance dose of 100mcgs in a few hours to much slower schedules which take weeks to build up to top dose. Once reached it is usual to continue administration for 3 to 5 years. Venom specific IgE and IgG levels are not helpful in determining the cessation of therapy. Patients who have received immunotherapy have a protection rate of approximately 98%.

Food Allergy

Allergic reactions to food are less commonly the cause of respiratory tract disease than are reactions to inhalant allergens.

Food allergy can be immediate (occurring within an hour of ingestion), or delayed. Immediate food allergy is almost always associated with oral symptoms such as burning or itching or soreness of the mouth or throat, this may be followed by nausea or vomiting or by urticaria, angioeodema, rhinitis, wheezing or even anaphylaxis. The responsible allergen can usually be identified from the history, especially if the reaction is repeated. Confirmation can be by skin prick or RAST testing, the latter is safer where anaphylaxis has occurred. These have an accuracy of around 70%.

Cross-reactivity exists between certain foods and inhalant allergens (eg) the birch-apple syndrome in which patients who are sensitive to birch tree pollen experience oral symptoms on eating apples, hazelnuts and sometimes other soft fruits such as cherries, nectarines etc. This occurs in approximately 1/3 of birch sensitive patients. The reaction is thought to be directed against profilin which is a common component. Other cross-reactivities occur between latex, banana, avocado, chestnut and sometimes pineapple.

Delayed food reactions are more problematical and tend to occur to common frequently eaten foods which make identification difficult. The mechanisms are unknown but IgE is probably not involved and therefore skin prick testing and RAST testing is inappropriate. The diagnosis is usually made by allergen avoidance and re-introduction, frequently this involves restriction of several dietary elements such as cow's milk and wheat and should be undertaken with the help of a dietician and preferably with some objective monitoring such as peak flow. If this open testing identifies a possible allergen then double-blind, placebo-controlled challenges are recommended in theory, but are difficult to undertake in practice and are usually reserved for research procedures.

Reactions to food additives are less common than is popularly supposed. However asthmatic patients are more sensitive than non-asthmatics to the sulphur dioxide which can emanate from sodium metabisulphate which is a common preservative often sprayed onto salad displays. Patients who are aspirin/NSAID sensitive may also exhibit reactivity to additives such as tartrazine (E102), and other coal-tar derived colourings and some preservatives (vide infra).

Aspirin Sensitivity

The classic history is a non-allergic rhinitis which progresses to a polypoid rhinosinusitis with the subsequent development of asthma and aspirin sensitivity. The latter can be exquisite such that 1 tablet can lead to a life-threatening asthma attack. Aspirin challenge can be undertaken in the hospital setting with full resuscitatory facilities to hand either orally or topically using lysine aspirin which is a truly soluble form. Nasal challenge using 8mcgs of lysine aspirin intranasally with monitoring of the nasal airway by acoustic rhinometry has proved to have a sensitivity and specificity of around 90% and has not provoked severe bronchospasm in any of the 80 patients tested thus far. The mechanism of aspirin sensitivity is unknown. Immunohistology shows plentiful eosinophils and mast cells, many of the latter being degranulated. Levels of leukotriene E4 are elevated in urine and leukotriene sensitivity is increased in these individuals. It is assumed that cylo-oxygenase inhibition with mast cell arachidonic acid being metabolised largely via the lipoxygenase pathway is relevant, although the initial cause of mast cell degranulation is unknown since IgE is rarely demonstrable.

Management

Aspirin sensitive patients should be instructed in the avoidance of all aspirin and NSAID medications. Approximately 50% of them appear to react to salicyates in medication and diet too as well as additives and preservatives. Dietary salicyate is highest in herbs and spices which should be avoided.

Oral desensitisation by incremental dosing with aspirin has been reported as helpful. The doses needed are high and gastrointestinal symptoms usually result. Topical nasal desensitisation with lysine aspirin has been attempted, but results were variable.

The advent of leukotriene receptor antagonists, which should be used in addition to inhaled and topical glucocorticosteroids, should prove helpful in this group of patients. However in patients treated thus far the response if variable with some deriving very significant benefit but others remaining completely unchanged. This probably reflects the fact that leukotriene receptors are polymorphic.

Further Reading

Scadding GK. Treating Asthma: Don't Forget the Nose. *Canadian Journal of Allergy and Clin Immunol* 1999;**4**(5):238–243

Meyers DA, Bleecker ER. In: Middleton, Rees, Ellis, Franklin Adkunson Jr, Younginger & Busse, eds. Genetics of Allergic Disease Allergy Principals and Practice, 5th Edition, Vol 1, Chapter 4, p 40–45. St Louis: Mosby 1998

Holgate ST. Asthma Genetics — Waiting to Exhale. *Nat Genet* 1997; **15**:227–229

Stachan D, Sibbald B, Weiland S, Ait-Khaled N, Anabwani G, Anderson HR et al. World-wide variations in prevalence of symptoms of allergic rhinoconjunctivitis in children: the International Study of

Asthma and Allergies in Childhood (ISAAC). *Pediatr Allergy Immunol* 1997;**8**(4):161–176

Aberg A. Asthma and Allergic Rhinitis in Swedish Conscripts. *Clin Exp Allergy* 1989;**19**:59–63

Devalia JL, Rusnak C, Herdman ML et al. Effect of nitrogen dioxide and sulphur dioxide on airway response of mild asthmatics to allergen inhalation. *Am Journal Resp Critcare Med* 1994;**344**:1668–1671

Sporik R, Holgate ST, Platts-Mills TA et al. Exposure to housedust allergen (Der.p.1) and the development of asthma in childhood; a prospective study. *N Engl Journal Med* 1990;**323**:502–507

Young S, Le Souef PN, Geelhoed GC et al. The influence of family history of asthma and parental smoking on airway responsiveness in early infancy. *N Engl Journal Med* 1991;**324**:1168–1173

Bjorksten B, Kjellman N-IM, Zieger RS et al. In: Middleton, Rees, Ellis, Franklin Adkunson Jr, Younginger & Busse, eds. Development of prevention of allergic disease in childhood in allergy principles and practice, 5th Edition, Chapter 58, p 816–837. St Louis: Mosby 1998

Strachan DP, Carey IM. Home environment and severe asthma in adolescence: a population based case control study: *Brit Med Journal* 1995;**311**:1053–1056

Butland BK, Strachan DP, Anderson HR. The home environment and asthma symptoms in childhood: two population based case control studies 13 years apart. 1997;**52**:618–624

Kemp TJ, Siebers RW, Fishwick D, O'Grady GB, Fitzharris P, Crane J et al. Housedust mite allergen in pillows. *Brit Med Journal* **313**:916

Scadding GK. Controlling the problems caused by steroid loading. Prac: 5th Edition 1998

Durham S, Scadding GK. Immunology of the nasal mucosa. In: Jones AS, Phillips DE and Hilger FJM, eds. Diseases of the Head, Neck, Throat and Ears, Chapter 45. London: Arnold 1998

Bousquet J, Lockey RF, Malling HJ et al. WHO Position Paper — Allergen Immunotherapy: Therapeutic Allergy 1998

Scadding GK. Pharmacological Modulation of the Allergic response: different mechanisms of action. *Allergy* 1999;**Sup 54**:39–42

Barnes PJ, Pedersen S, Busse WW. Efficacy and safety of inhaled corticosteroids. *Amer Journal Respir Critcare Med* 1998;**157**:S1–S53

Sampson H et al: Fatal and near fatal reactions to food. *NEJM* 1992; **327**:80–84

6

Chronic Obstructive Pulmonary Disease

David MG Halpin

Introduction

Definition

Chronic obstructive pulmonary disease (COPD) is now the pre-ferred designation for a group of conditions variously known as chronic airflow limitation (CAL), chronic obstructive airways dis-ease (COAD), chronic obstructive lung disease (COLD), chronic bronchitis and emphysema. The last two are specific conditions with distinct clinical or pathological features but there is consider-able overlap with the substantially irreversible airflow limitation that characterises COPD.

COPD is a chronic slowly progressive disease characterised by airflow obstruction that shows minimal diurnal or day to day vari-ation. Variability of airflow limitation is not dichotomous and in practice there is a spectrum ranging from complete irreversibility to the complete reversibility seen in asthma. There is thus some over-lap between COPD and chronic asthma.

British, American and European guidelines on the management of COPD have been published.[1-3]

Epidemiology

COPD accounts for over 25 000 deaths in England and Wales each year: approximately 6.5% of all male deaths and 4% of all female deaths. The burden of disease is however considerably greater. Morbidity from COPD is high and patients are frequent users of primary and secondary care facilities. As many as 1 in 8 hospital admissions may be due to COPD and consultation rates in General Practice are 2–4 times higher than those for angina.

Aetiology

Cigarette smoking is unquestionably the major aetiological factor for COPD. There is a clear dose response relationship between total tobacco consumption and the risk of developing COPD as well as the severity of the disease; however, not all smokers will develop COPD and susceptibility factors, possibly genetic, are also important. Alpha-1 antitrypsin deficiency is associated with the development of emphysema in non-smokers but the risk is substantially higher in smokers. Environmental dust has also been suggested to be important for certain groups of workers (particularly coal miners) but this remains controversial.

Pathology

The pathological changes of COPD are complex and correlate poorly with the physiological abnormalities.[4] Chronic bronchitis (i.e. chronic mucus hypersecretion) is associated with an increase in the volume and number of submucosal glands and the number of goblet cells in the mucosa. Emphysema is defined by the pathological changes that occur as "a condition of the lung characterised by abnormal, permanent enlargement of airspaces distal to the terminal bronchiole accompanied by destruction of their walls and without obvious fibrosis". The distribution of the abnormal airspaces allows the classification of emphysema into panacinar, centriacinar and paraseptal. Panacinar emphysema may be found in the upper or lower lobes but in α-1 antitrypsin deficiency is generally maximal at the base. Centriacinar emphysema is commonest in the upper zones of both upper and lower lobes and has a closer relationship to cigarette smoking than panacinar disease. Bullae are areas of emphysema larger than 1cm in diameter which are locally overdistended. Bronchioles and small bronchi derive some of their structural integrity from the attachment of surrounding alveolar walls that act like guy ropes to hold open the airway. In the presence of emphysema it has been suggested that some of this support is lost and airflow limitation develops.

Thirty years ago it was shown that the site of airflow obstruction was the small peripheral airways.[5] Pathologically, however, the changes in these airways are subtle, especially when compared to other conditions associated with small airways obstruction such as bronchiectasis. Possible causes of small airway obstruction include: the loss of alveolar attachments discussed above; decrease lung recoil (see below); increased surface tension as a result of replacement of surfactant by inflammatory exudate; occlusion of the lumen by exudate; oedema and inflammation of the mucosa; and bronchoconstriction.

Pathophysiology

Decreased maximal expiratory flow and impaired gas exchange are fundamental to the pathophysiology of COPD. As discussed above the reason for the development of small airways obstruction is still not clear; however, it is undoubtedly limitation of flow in these airways that leads to the reduction in expiratory flow. The effects of static airway narrowing due to intrinsic disease are exacerbated by loss of lung recoil so that flow limitation develops at lower driving pressures and flows.

Changes in the static pressure-volume (PV) curve of the lungs are partly responsible for the changes in lung volumes seen in patients with COPD. The characteristic changes are an increase in static compliance, reduction in static transpulmonary pressure (P_L) at standard volume and decreased P_L at TLC. This reduction in lung recoil pressure leads to an increase in the lung volume at the neutral position (i.e. relaxation volume Vr) which is in part responsible for the increase in FRC. Loss of lung recoil pressures also results in airway closing pressures developing at larger lung volumes and thus an increase in RV. Decreased dynamic compliance also leads to the development of hyperinflation. Dynamic hyperinflation develops when the severity of airflow limitation is such that the duration of expiration is insufficient to allow the lungs to deflate to relaxation volume prior to the next inspiration.

The increase in functional residual capacity (FRC) greatly increases the work of breathing and also means that unlike the situation in normal individuals, the end-expiratory elastic recoil pressure in the lung is positive. This pressure has been termed auto PEEP or intrinsic PEEP ($PEEP_i$)[6] and in stable patients with COPD may reach 7–9 cmH_2O, increasing to up to 13 cmH_2O in exacerbations. When $PEEP_i$ is present the onset of inspiratory muscle activity and inspiratory flow are not synchronous; flow only begins when the negative pressure generated by the muscles exceeds

$PEEP_i$. Thus $PEEP_i$ acts as an inspiratory threshold load, further increasing the elastic work of breathing.

In COPD both the force of contraction generated by the inspiratory muscles and the mechanical load against which they are required to act are abnormal. The inspiratory load is increased as a result of the increased respiratory impedance and the force of contraction is reduced as a consequence of the effect of hyperinflation altering the mechanical advantage of the muscles (both intercostal and diaphragmatic), malnutrition and, in some cases, respiratory muscle fatigue. Inspiratory muscle dysfunction is central to the development of hypercapnia. $PEEP_i$ also increases the load on the inspiratory muscles and has also been shown to correlate with the development of hypercapnia.

Pulmonary artery hypertension is the most important cardiovascular complication of COPD and it is associated with a poor prognosis. The normal pulmonary circulation is a low-pressure low-resistance system with low vasomotor tone. The considerable increases seen in cardiac output with exercise do not lead to significant increases in pulmonary artery pressure because they are associated with recruitment of under-perfused vessels, particularly at the lung apex. In hypoxaemic patients with COPD characteristic changes occur in peripheral pulmonary arteries: the intima of small arteries develops accumulations of smooth muscle; and muscular arteries develop medial hypertrophy. These structural changes may be more important in the development of sustained pulmonary hypertension than hypoxic vasoconstriction. Pulmonary thrombosis may also develop, possibly secondary to small airway inflammation.

Clinical Features

Symptoms

Patients with mild airflow obstruction are usually asymptomatic, but as COPD develops patients become progressively more symptomatic. The relationship of symptoms to different levels of physiological abnormality and the rate of progression can be very variable. Most patients have smoked at least 20 cigarettes per day for at least 20 years before they develop symptoms; however, airflow obstruction may develop sooner and if this is detected progression to symptomatic COPD may be prevented by stopping the patient smoking.[7] The identification of these pre-symptomatic individuals presents a challenge for health promotion programmes. The introduction of spirometry into primary care may allow smokers to be screened for airflow limitation but unless more effective smoking cessation programmes are developed this approach is likely to remain time consuming and relatively ineffective.

When patients do first develop symptoms these are usually mild and intermittent.[8] The most common symptoms at this stage are: cough, especially in the mornings; breathlessness on moderate to severe exertion; and recurrent winter 'chest infections', i.e. periods of increased breathlessness associated with increased production of sputum, which may be purulent. In 75% of patients with COPD cough is one of the first symptoms: preceding or developing simultaneously with breathlessness.

Patients with moderate COPD invariably have some symptoms, but again the spectrum is wide and includes: cough and sputum production; breathlessness on moderate exertion (e.g. walking up hills); wheeze; typical exacerbations with increased breathlessness and purulent sputum;

Patients with severe COPD are almost always breathless on minimal exertion, and often their sleep is disturbed by breathlessness. They generally cough, especially in the mornings and frequently wheeze. In addition they may have symptoms of complications such as peripheral oedema. Historically, patients have been divided into *blue bloaters* and *pink puffers*: the latter maintain relatively normal blood gases through a drive to breathe that can be extremely distressing. The former are patients who are hypoxaemic and hypercapnic as a result of a resetting of their regulatory centres and no increased drive to breathe. They frequently have peripheral oedema as a reflection of pulmonary hypertension and cor pulmonale. In practice these are extremes of a spectrum and most patients lie somewhere in the middle. There is no firm relationship with the predominance of airflow obstruction or emphysema.

The BTS guidelines describe the 'COPD escalator' (Box 1) which reflects the progressive increase in symptoms as lung function worsens and the increased number of treatments required.

Breathlessness is the symptom associated with the worst prognosis, the greatest disability and the greatest loss of lung function over time. Patient's breathlessness can be assessed clinically by asking about exercise tolerance. In particular it is useful to record how far they can walk on the flat and how many flights of stairs they can climb without stopping. Patients with more severe breathlessness should be asked about whether they are breathless when

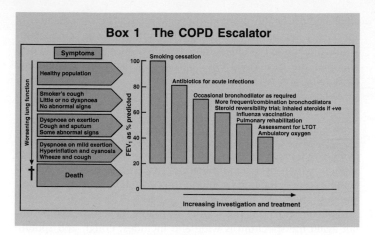

Box 1   The COPD Escalator

washing, dressing or eating. Severe breathlessness correlates well with an FEV_1 less than 30% predicted and a VO_2max less than 15 ml/kg/min; however, psychological factors are also important in determining the level of breathlessness.

Chest pain is also a common symptom in patients with COPD. This may be due to associated conditions such as ischaemic heart disease or acid reflux, but may also be due to the disease itself, possibly as a result of intercostal muscle ischaemia or raised intrapulmonary pressure as a result of air trapped in poorly ventilated parts of the lung.

Exacerbations

Exacerbations are a feature of COPD at all stages in the natural history of the disease. They may be associated with one or more of the following symptoms: increased breathlessness; increased sputum volume; increased sputum purulence; increased wheeze; chest tightness; peripheral oedema. The majority of exacerbations are probably viral in origin. As discussed below, bacteria can be cultured in sputum from patients with COPD at most stages of their illness whether or not they have an exacerbation and their role in the pathogenesis of exacerbations remains controversial. The differential diagnosis includes: lobar pneumonia; pneumothorax; left ventricular dysfunction; pulmonary embolism; and bronchogenic carcinoma.

Pulmonary hypertension & Cor pulmonale

The term cor pulmonale is frequently used to describe the clinical picture of peripheral oedema and an elevated venous pressure in patients with respiratory failure. Strictly speaking it refers to right ventricular hypertrophy and dysfunction secondary to elevated pulmonary artery pressures. In practice, this is frequently a consequence of hypoxic pulmonary vasoconstriction and does lead to the development of peripheral oedema.

Additional features in history

The clinical history of all patients with COPD should include a detailed smoking history. Patients should be asked at what age they started smoking, their tobacco consumption during the time they were smoking and when they stopped smoking (if they have). The smoking history is often conveniently expressed as total pack years, taking 'a pack' as 20 cigarettes per day; however, cigarette yields vary considerably and thus self-reported estimates of tobacco usage are at best an approximation.

The history should also include a detailed occupational history as well as a detailed past medical history stretching back to childhood. Many patients are labelled as having COPD when their history reveals other conditions such as bronchiectasis. In the future patients with bronchopulmonary dysplasia following neonatal ventilation may form an important subgroup of adults with fixed airflow obstruction and as with airflow obstruction of other specific aetiology it is important that these patients are not mis-diagnosed as having COPD.

Clinical signs

The findings on clinical examination in patients with COPD are as variable as the symptoms. Examination is generally normal in patients with asymptomatic or mild disease. In patients with moderate disease there may be signs of hyperinflation (depressed liver, loss of cardiac dullness, reduced cricosternal distance, increased AP diameter of chest) and wheezes or abnormally quiet breath sounds may be heard. There is a very poor correlation between the clinical signs and the severity of airflow obstruction.

In patients with severe disease the findings on examination may include: signs of hyperinflation (as above), wheezes, quiet breath sounds, peripheral oedema, elevated venous pressure, central cyanosis, right ventricular heave, loud pulmonary second sound, tricuspid regurgitation, signs of hypercapnia (flapping tremor, bounding pulse, drowsiness), and weight loss or cachexia.

Investigations

Spirometry

Assessment of the severity of airflow obstruction by spirometry should be central to the management of patients with COPD. Measurement of the peak expiratory flow (PEF) is frequently misleading: it often underestimates the severity of the airflow obstruction and frequently shows little variation during exacerbations. The BTS guidelines propose a classification of COPD into mild moderate and severe based on FEV_1 (Box 2).[1] A normal FEV_1 effectively excludes the diagnosis of COPD but a normal PEFR does not. Significant day to day or diurnal peak flow variability of more than 20% may suggest a large reversible component to the airflow obstruction but at low absolute values the spontaneous variability in PEFR may exceed this value.

Box 2   Classification of COPD

- **Mild COPD**
  FEV_1 60–79% of predicted with an FEV1/FVC ratio < 70%
- **Moderate COPD**
  FEV_1 40–59% of predicted
- **Severe COPD**
  FEV_1 < 40% predicted

Radiology

The plain chest radiograph is frequently unremarkable in patients with stable mild disease. As such it contributes little to the diagnosis but its role lies in excluding other diagnoses such as a bronchogenic carcinoma. It may show single or multiple bullae, but may be surprisingly normal in patients with significant emphysema as assessed by gas transfer measurements or by CT. In patients with exacerbations, plain chest radiographs are again principally useful for excluding other causes of the patient's symptoms such as lobar pneumonia or pneumothorax. Follow-up films are only indicated if there is a serious deterioration in the patients existing symptoms or if new symptoms develop.

CT is good at showing the presence of emphysema but is only rarely clinically indicated for this purpose. Examples of its use are as part of a work up for bullectomy, lung reduction surgery, or single lung transplantation, and to confirm the presence of emphysema in young patients with isolated low gas transfer measurements (e.g. α1-antitrypsin deficiency).

Reversibility testing

Spirometry will not diagnose COPD it will merely show the presence of airflow obstruction. Reversibility testing is central to making the diagnosis of fixed or substantially irreversible airflow limitation. In practice there is a spectrum of reversibility that overlaps with asthma. Reversibility can be assessed acutely with short-acting bronchodilators or over a period of weeks with oral or inhaled corticosteroids.

Reversibility testing with bronchodilators should be carried out in a way that ensures that a failure to respond is not because the dose is too low. For this reason it is best to use nebulised drugs and both beta agonists such as salbutamol or terbutaline and anticholinergics should be used either sequentially or in combination. Tests should be performed when patients are clinically stable and free of infection. The patient should not have taken a short acting bronchodilator in the previous 6 hours, a long acting beta agonist in the previous 12 hours or a sustained release theophylline preparation in the previous 24 hours. The response should be assessed by measuring the pre- and post-trial FEV_1. An increase in FEV_1 that is both more than 200ml and more than 15% of the pre-test value is the recommended threshold for establishing reversibility.[1,8] The post-test FEV_1 also gives information about prognosis[9] and is useful in defining a benchmark against which the success of therapy can be judged. A negative result does not mean that patients will not derive symptomatic benefits, in terms of perception of breathlessness and increases in walking distance, from treatment with bronchodilators.

Reversibility testing with corticosteroids should be carried out in all patients with moderate and severe disease and the BTS guidelines suggest that it should also be carried out in patients with mild disease who need to use their bronchodilators more than once per day.[1] FEV_1 should be measured before and at the end of a course of oral steroids. Opinions differ about the dose and duration of therapy required. The BTS guidelines recommend 30mg prednisolone daily for 2 weeks, but some clinicians continue the trial for up to 4 weeks. Inhaled steroids can also be used, but in this case the trial should continue for 6 weeks with doses equivalent to 1000mg beclomethasone per day. The criteria for a positive response are the same as for trials of bronchodilators and a rise in FEV_1 of more than 200ml is associated with a better prognosis over 5 years. Again, if the trial is positive, the post trial FEV_1 provides a benchmark for future management. Some patients report a subjective improvement following steroid therapy but do not show a significant increase in their FEV_1. Such patients should not be considered as having a positive response and should not continue on oral corticosteroids. Failure to respond to a steroid trial when clinically stable does not mean that patients should not receive steroids during an exacerbation.

Pulse oximetry and arterial blood gas tensions

Pulse oximetry can be used to assess hypoxaemia at rest and on exertion in patients with stable disease and during exacerbations. If the SaO_2 is more than 92% in patients with stable disease measurement of arterial blood gas tensions is probably not required. If the SaO_2 ≤92% arterial blood gas tensions should be measured and measurement of arterial blood gasses should be considered in all patients with an exacerbation as their $PaCO_2$ may be abnormal even if their SaO_2 is normal.

Electro- & echocardiography

The ECG is useful for detecting ischaemic heart disease and arrhythmias but is relatively insensitive for detecting right ventricular hypertrophy. ECG criteria for ventricular hypertrophy are modified by hyperinflation of the lungs.

Echocardiography is a useful way of identifying right ventricular hypertrophy and dilatation; however, hyperinflation increases the retrosternal air space thus making satisfactory transthoracic studies difficult. Where available, trans-oesophageal echocardiography increases the proportion of satisfactory examinations. Pulmonary artery (PA) pressure can be estimated using echocardiography in a number of ways. The blood velocity in the main PA can be used to estimate the PA pressure and the interval between the onset of RV ejection and peak velocity correlates well with the mean PA pressure. In patients with tricuspid regurgitation, the addition of the mean right atrial (RA) pressure to the peak systolic gradient between the RA and RV yields the systolic pulmonary artery pressure.

Haematology

Identification of anaemia and polycythaemia is useful in the management of patients with COPD. Patients with a haematocrit > 47% in women or > 52% in men should be investigated for hypoxaemia, including at night, before attributing the finding to their COPD. Venesection should be considered if the PCV is greater than 60% in men or 55% in women; however the evidence for its benefits in terms of improved exercise performance and reduced risk of vascular events is limited, as is evidence regarding the duration of benefit.

Sputum culture

Routine sputum culture is of no value in the management of patients with stable COPD. Sputum is frequently colonised with bacteria such as *Haemophilus influenzae* whose identification, in itself, is not an indication for antibiotic therapy.

Management

Stopping smoking

Stopping patients smoking is the single most effective way of altering he outcome in patients at all stages in COPD.[9,10] This is as true for presymptomatic patients with airflow obstruction as it is for patients with severe disease. Those who continue to smoke will continue to lose FEV_1 at an accelerated rate, and although lost function cannot be regained, those who stop smoking will deteriorate more slowly[7,11] and derive more benefit from therapies such as oxygen.

Advice about stopping smoking (Box 3) should be given at every opportunity and is effective in those with high motivation.[12] Overall the reported success rates of anti-smoking strategies is between 10 and 30%.

Box 3   Advice to smokers regarding smoking cessation

- **Preparation**
  Make a positive decision and list reasons for quitting.
  Get the support of family and friends and set a target date.
  Have realistic but not negative expectations about the difficulty.
  Know that most relapses occur in the first week after quitting.

- **Switch Brands**
  Switch to a brand that is distasteful and that is low in tar and nicotine prior to the target date.

- **Cut down the number of cigarettes**
  Smoke only half of each cigarette.
  Postpone the lighting of the first cigarette each day by 1 hour.
  Smoke only during the odd or even hours of each day.
  Remember that cutting down is not a substitute for quitting.

- **Don't smoke automatically**
  Smoke only the cigarettes that you really want.
  Don't empty ashtrays.
  Make yourself aware of each cigarette you smoke by using the opposite hand or putting the packet in an unusual location.

- **Make smoking inconvenient**
  Buy one packet at a time.
  Stop carrying cigarettes at work or at home.

- **Make smoking unpleasant**
  If used to smoking in company only smoke alone.
  Whilst smoking isolate yourself from others and focus on the negative effects of smoking.
  Collect all the butts in a large glass container.

- **Prepare for the target day**
  Practice going without cigarettes.
  Think of quitting in terms of one day at a time.

- **On the day of quitting**
  Throw away all cigarettes and matches, and hide ashtrays and lighters.
  Make a list of things you would like to buy, price them in terms of packets of cigarettes and put the money aside to buy these presents.

Keep very busy on the target day.
Remind family and friends that this is the big day.
Buy yourself a treat or do something special to celebrate.

- **Immediately after quitting**
Develop a clean, fresh, non-smoking environment around you.
Spend as much time as possible in environments where smoking is not permitted.
Drink large quantities of water and fruit juice.
Avoid drinks that you associate with smoking.

- **Avoid temptation**
Instead of smoking after meals clean your teeth or go for a walk.
For the first 1–3 weeks avoid situations you strongly associate with smoking.
Until confident about having stopped, limit socializing to activities where smoking is not allowed.

- **When tempted**
Keep oral substitutes handy.
Learn to use relaxation techniques.
Never allow yourself to think it won't hurt.

- **Find new habits**
Do things that make smoking difficult.
Do things that require the use of hands.

Based on advice from the National Cancer Institute

Drug therapy

Bronchodilators

Bronchodilators are the mainstay of pharmaco-therapy for COPD. The structural changes in the airways prevent these drugs returning airway calibre to normal and clinically relevant improvements in FEV_1 may be too small to identify against the background day to day variation. Inhaled agents are preferred to oral because of the reduction in systemic side effects. Beta agonists act directly on bronchial smooth muscle to cause bronchodilation whereas anti-cholinergics act by inhibiting resting broncho-motor tone. Both classes of drugs act synergistically to reduce airway resistance and reduce hyper-inflation.

As discussed above, single dose bronchodilator reversibility tests are important in the assessment of patients with COPD; however, they do not predict the symptomatic benefit that patients may obtain from bronchodilator therapy. Bronchodilators may increase FEV_1, FVC or exercise tolerance independently, but an increase in FVC does not correlate well with an improvement in symptoms.

Short-acting beta agonists

Beta agonists are the most widely used bronchodilators for COPD. The dose response relationship for salbutamol in patients with largely or completely irreversible COPD is almost flat. The time to peak response is slower than in asthmatics and the side-effect to benefits ratio is such that there is little benefit in giving more than 1mg salbutamol. Patients who do not have a significant spirometric response may still benefit in terms of an increased exercise tolerance.

Long-acting beta agonists

The physiological effects of long acting beta agonists are similar to the short-acting agents but their duration of action is around 12 hours c.f. 4 hours. Salmeterol has a slow onset of action, but eformoterol acts within minutes.

Although the data are still limited some patients with COPD undoubtedly get symptomatic benefit. Current guidelines suggest that their use should be restricted to patients who have shown a clear response to short-acting drugs.

Anti-cholinergics

Cholinergic nerves are the main neural bronchoconstrictor pathway in the airways and the resting tone is increased in patients with COPD. Cholinergic effects on the airway are mediated by muscarinic receptors and these also mediate effects on mucus secretion. Anti-cholinergic drugs produce significant bronchodilatation and, unlike the situation in asthmatics, are approximately equipotent with beta agonists. Although their onset of action is slower than the short acting beta agonists, the duration of bronchodilation may be up to 8 hours. Optimal bronchodilation with ipratropium is achieved at around 80mg, a dose higher than is often used in practice.

Patients may respond to a combination of beta agonists and anticholinergics but current guidelines suggest that this is reserved for patients who fail to get adequate symptom relief from single agent therapy.

Delivery systems

As with asthma, delivery of the drugs to the lungs is an essential part of pharmacotherapy. When considering delivery devices co-existing problems, such as arthritis, must be taken into account. Pressurised metered dose inhalers (pMDIs) are cheap but unless used with large volume spacers give poor pulmonary deposition and as many as three quarters of patients with COPD are unable to use them correctly. Dry powder devices are more expensive but can be used successfully by up to 90% of patients and thus may be significantly more cost-effective. Elderly patients are less able to use pMDIs than younger patients and develop a poor inhaler technique more rapidly. It is essential to check inhaler technique at every opportunity and re-instruct as necessary.

Nebulisers

Most patients with COPD can be adequately treated with inhalers but a few derive additional benefit from higher dose bronchodilator therapy delivered by nebuliser.[13] Compressors to drive nebulisers are relatively cheap, but the drug costs are high and patients may experience more severe systemic effects. Studies comparing equivalent doses of bronchodilators given by inhaler or nebuliser in patients with stable COPD have been inconclusive but as other therapeutic options are limited many physicians have a low threshold for recommending nebulised therapy in patients who report symptomatic benefit.

The BTS nebuliser guidelines make recommendations about the assessment of patients for nebuliser therapy (Box 4).[14] There is no consensus about whether patients benefit most from regular or as required nebulised bronchodilator therapy.

Box 4   Nebulised Bronchodilator Assessment

- Determine maximum objective and subjective response to a hand-held inhaler that the patient can use.
- Assess steroid reversibility
- If still symptomatic assess response to high dose bron-

chodilator (1mg terbutaline or 400ug salbutamol) from same device

- If poor or no-response assess response to nebulised bronchodilators
  - Instruct patient in use & supervise first dose
  - Assess FEV1 or peak flow response
  - If >15% improvement continue with domiciliary therapy
  - If <15% improvement but symptomatic benefit use clinical judgement
  - Do not continue with domiciliary therapy if any other outcome
- Advise patients to use therapy as needed, up to 4 times per day
- Arrange to follow-up patients by out-patient or respiratory nurse specialist review

Theophyllines

The mechanism of action of theophylline remains uncertain but despite this they remain widely used in COPD. Their primary effect is generally assumed to be relaxation of airway smooth muscle; however, at therapeutic concentrations it has little direct bronchodilator effect.

Despite the efficacy of beta agonists and anti-cholinergics there is still a place for theophylline. The availability of formulations giving stable plasma concentrations for 12 to 18 hours facilitates their use, but even in patients with stable COPD their bronchodilator effect is modest. Some patients do appear to get symptomatic benefit despite insignificant changes in lung function. Like long acting beta agonists their principal role is the control of nocturnal symptoms. The therapeutic index of theophyllines is narrow and some patients experience significant side effects even when the plasma levels are in the therapeutic range. This, together with their interaction with many other drugs, makes careful monitoring of plasma levels essential. For most patients a measurement of plasma theophylline concentrations 8–10 hours following a single oral dose will be sufficient to predict maintenance requirements and a repeat measurement 1–2 weeks later will confirm that the plasma concentration is in the therapeutic range. Thereafter monitoring is not necessary unless there has be a change in concomitant medication or the patient's condition that would lead to altered theophylline clearance.

Corticosteroids

Although inflammatory changes are present in the airways of patients with COPD, the role of corticosteroids remains controversial. At best, trials of oral corticosteroids in patients with stable disease have shown improvements in a small subset (15–40%); however, this may be achieved at considerable cost in terms of side effects and at present there is no means of predicting those who will respond. Less than half of those patients who show objective improvements with oral therapy maintain the improvement on inhaled corticosteroid therapy. Nevertheless, current guidelines recommend that patients showing a good response to oral corticosteroids should be maintained on the equivalent of 800mcg budesonide per day and patients with substantial reversibility should be treated along similar lines to asthmatics.

Uncontrolled retrospective studies have suggested that oral corticosteroid therapy can slow the decline in FEV_1 but there is insufficient evidence to recommended this in all patients and so far studies have failed to show a similar effect of inhaled steroids. Inhaled steroids do appear to reduce the number of exacerbations and slow the decline in health status in more severe patients, although uncertainties still remain about the dose required, whether particular sub-groups do better and what the long-term consequences of such treatment would be.

Other treatment modalities

Vaccination

Although there have been no studies specifically in patients with COPD vaccination against respiratory pathogens is thought to be of benefit. Annual influenza vaccination is recommended for all patients with COPD.[16] It is now also common to vaccinate patients against the pneumococcus using the polyvalent capsular polysaccharide vaccine.

Pulmonary rehabilitation

Pulmonary rehabilitation is an increasingly popular option for patients with moderate to severe COPD.[15] Rehabilitation aims to prevent deconditioning and allow the patient to cope with their disease. Most programmes are hospital based and comprise individualised exercise programmes and educational talks, but a major component is the sharing of experiences amongst participants and their spouses. Pulmonary rehabilitation is effective. It leads to small improvements in lung function, but there are frequently much greater improvements in exercise tolerance and quality of life measures. Rehabilitation may also reduce hospital readmission rates.

Oxygen

Long term oxygen therapy (LTOT) in patients with resting hypoxaemia leads to significant improvements in survival, less polycythaemia, reduced progression of pulmonary hypertension and improvements in neuropsychological health. LTOT appears to reduce short term mortality related to the pulmonary circulation but long term mortality remains high and is inversely related to the FEV_1 suggesting that it is due to the severity of airflow obstruction.

LTOT prescription should be based on hypoxaemia demonstrated when the patient has been stable for 4 weeks and on maximal medication. Patients with a $PaO_2 < 7.3$ kPa and an acceptable $PaCO_2$ (see Hazards of Oxygen Therapy below) should receive LTOT. Patients with a PaO_2 between 7.3 and 8.0 kPa should also receive LTOT if there is evidence of pulmonary hypertension, peripheral oedema or nocturnal hypoxaemia.[16]

LTOT is usually provided from an oxygen concentrator prescribed by the GP in England & Wales and chest physicians in Scotland. To get full benefit patients must use LTOT for at least 15 hours a day but patients may get additional benefits from using it for longer periods. Most patients need a flow rate of between 1–3 l/min. The purity of the oxygen declines above 3 l/min and if higher flow rates are required it is necessary to use two concentrators connected in parallel. Oxygen is usually delivered to the patient via nasal cannulae but the transtracheal route can be used for patients with severe nasal problems or refractory hypoxaemia.

Patients prescribed LTOT should not continue to smoke because smokers do not appear to get benefit and the obvious dangers of fire and explosion.

Ambulatory Oxygen Therapy can improve exercise tolerance, quality of life and compliance with LTOT. Currently portable cylinders are the only source of ambulatory oxygen available in the UK. These are heavy, have a limited capacity, providing only 2 hours at 2 l/min, and cannot be refilled in the patient's home. Oxygen conserving devices, which restrict the flow of oxygen to the inspiratory phase of respiration are now available and these can prolong the effective life of the cylinder. Weight for weight, liquid oxygen provides longer treatment and can be refilled at the patient's home, but it is not available in the UK.

There are no agreed criteria for ambulatory oxygen therapy. Documented desaturation on an exercise test and relief of symptoms or improvement in walking distance are commonly used to assess patients' needs.

Intermittent Oxygen Therapy. It is common practice to prescribe as required oxygen therapy for use by patients who do not meet the criteria for LTOT. The principal indication is breathlessness, often following exertion, which is relieved by oxygen and which is associated with a fall in SaO_2. There are no guidelines about the use of such treatment and no data to support or refute its use, but many patients do appear to benefit.

Hazards of Oxygen Therapy. CO_2 retention may preclude oxygen therapy in patients with COPD. Depression of the hypoxic drive to breathe leads to hypercapnia, acidosis and CO_2 narcosis. Some CO_2 retention is tolerable and depending on the initial value, rises in the $PaCO_2$ of up to 1 kPa may be safe. Theoretically prolonged exposure to high concentrations of oxygen may lead to pulmonary toxicity related to the generation of free radicals but in practice this is rarely a problem. Fire and explosion are real dangers and there have been many reports of patients starting fires, usually by lighting a cigarette whilst wearing nasal cannulae. Patients and their families and carers must be warned not to smoke in the vicinity of the oxygen.

Surgery

Surgery may be of value in patients with severe hyperinflation due to localised bullous disease. By removing single large bullae or areas containing multiple smaller bullae hyperinflation can be reduced and pulmonary mechanics improved, leading paradoxically to significant improvements in FEV_1. The success of surgical techniques for bullectomy have been improved considerably in recent years by the introduction of bovine pericardial strips to butress suture/staple lines. Patient selection is crucial and many centres require patients to have undertaken a programme of pulmonary rehabilitation as well as being on maximal medical therapy before considering them for surgery.

Lung transplantation has been used successfully in young patients with emphysema related to α-1 antitrypsin deficiency but the procedure is not without morbidity and mortality and is currently limited by donor organ availability.

Psychological aspects

Many patients with COPD are depressed often as a result of the isolation and physical limitations that their disease brings. Antidepressant drugs are frequently beneficial, but psychological assessment and therapy can also be of considerable value.

COPD and air travel

Aircraft cabins are not usually pressurised to sea level and patients with compensated COPD at sea level may experience significant hypoxaemia when flying. Patients may become breathless, wheezy or develop chest pain and on long flights right heart failure may develop. Most aircraft are pressurised to between 5 000 and 7 000 feet, but a worst-case scenario of 8 000 feet is generally used when assessing patients. Patients with COPD who are contemplating air travel can be assessed by either hypoxic inhalation testing or by using regression equations. During an hypoxic challenge patients are given an FIO_2 of 15.1% (equivalent to the PO_2 of air at 8 000 feet) for a minimum of 15 minutes and their ECG and blood gases are assessed. Regression equations predict an individuals response based on the observed responses of a group of patients with similar characteristics who have been exposed to hypoxia. They have the advantage of being easy to use but do not allow assessment of symptoms at a given PaO_2.

Management of Exacerbations

Acute exacerbations occur in patients at all stages of their disease but are most common in those with severe disease. As discussed above, they are manifest as worsening of existing symptoms and patients frequently state that they have an "infection". Many exacerbations are related to infections both viral and bacterial but other causes such as pneumothorax, cardiac dysfunction, pulmonary emboli and tumours should be considered.

Many patients can be managed at home but others need hospital treatment and the BTS COPD guidelines give guidance on factors affecting the decision about where to treat patients.[1]

Management of patients in hospital should include the taking of a history, including specifically: details of the patient's best recent exercise tolerance; current therapy; time course and symptoms of the recent deterioration; social situation and the presence of carers at home; previous admissions; and an adequate smoking history (particularly if this is a first presentation).

Relevant signs include pyrexia, purulent sputum, wheeze, tachypnoea, use of accessory muscles, peripheral oedema, cyanosis, drowsiness, tremor and a CO_2 flap.

Immediate investigations should include arterial blood gasses (ensuring the inspired oxygen concentration is recorded), a chest radiograph and an ECG. A full blood count should be sent and urea and electrolyte concentrations measured. The patient's FEV_1 should be recorded as soon as practicable.

Initial treatment should include oxygen therapy to achieve a PaO_2 of at least 6.6 kPa without a significant rise in the $PaCO_2$ or the development of significant acidaemia (pH < 7.26). Until the arterial blood gas tensions are known patients should receive 24% or 28% oxygen via a Venturi mask. Once the blood gas tensions are known oxygen therapy should be adjusted accordingly. It is not uncommon to find significant hypercapnia in patients brought in by ambulance as a result of high concentration oxygen therapy during transfer and stabilisation with an appropriate FIO_2 often allows the patient to correct this themselves. If the patient is hypercapnic or acidotic the blood gas measurement must be repeated within 1 hour to determine whether the values are stable, improving or deteriorating. If the patient is not hypercapnic the adequacy of oxygenation can be assessed with pulse oximetry.

Nebulised bronchodilators should be given on arrival and at frequent intervals thereafter. For moderate exacerbations either salbutamol (2.5mg or 5mg) or ipratropium (250µg or 500µg) may be used but both should be used for patients with severe exacerbations. If the patient is not responding to inhaled bronchodilators intravenous aminophylline may be used (0.5mg/kg/h) but care should be taken in patients receiving oral methylxanthines, antibiotics such as macrolides or ciprofloxacin or other drugs which alter its clearance. Plasma theophylline levels should be monitored on a daily basis.

Antibiotic use in exacerbations of COPD is controversial but some studies have shown benefits. The BTS COPD guidelines recommend that antibiotics should be given if two of the following three features are present: increased breathlessness, increased sputum volume or increased sputum purulence. The most common pathogens identified in patients at the time of exacerbations are *Haemophilus influenzae, Streptococcus pneumoniae* and *Moraxella catarrhalis*, but these organisms can also be isolated from the sputum of patients with stable disease and their role in causing exacerbations is still unclear. Other pathogens such as *Chlamydia pneumoniae* may also be important. Antibiotic choice will depend on local policies, but intravenous antibiotics are not usually required unless there are features of an acute pneumonia. In general amoxycillin 500mg tds, clarithromycin 500mg bd or trimethoprim 200mg bd taken orally is adequate for most patients.

The role of systemic corticosteroids is also unclear, although most patients admitted with an exacerbation do receive 30–40mg prednisolone for 7 to 14 days. Oral steroid therapy is certainly of value if the patient is already on maintenance steroid therapy or has previously shown reversibility to steroids. Steroids should be discontinued after the acute episode unless the patient has shown a clear response that has not reached a plateau. In this case steroid therapy should be continued until maximum improvement has been achieved, when oral steroids should be withdrawn if possible.

Patients should be given diuretics if the venous pressure is elevated or if there is peripheral or pulmonary oedema.

Assisted ventilation

Non-invasive positive pressure ventilation (NIPPV) or intermittent positive pressure ventilation (IPPV) via an endotracheal tube should be considered in patients with hypercapnic respiratory failure. In the absence of other organ system failure, and provided that patient does not have large volumes of secretions and is able to co-operate, NIPPV is the treatment of choice. However, if this is not available or if the patient is not suitable, IPPV should be considered. The outcome of patients requiring IPPV is better than generally thought, particularly by anaesthetists, and misconceptions about the difficulty of weaning patients or about long term survival should not be allowed to affect the decision about intubation. When considering assisted ventilation the aetiology of the exacerbation, the patient's previous exercise tolerance and quality of life, and the presence of co-morbidities must be considered. The decision to initiate or withhold ventilation should be made by a senior physician, preferably one with prior knowledge of the patient. A small proportion of the patients treated with NIPPV require continuing support once they have recovered from the exacerbation and domiciliary ventilation is supported by a few specialist centres in the UK.

Doxapram may help to get a patient through an episode of acute respiratory failure due to a reversible cause if NIPPV is not available.

References

1. BTS Guidelines for the management of chronic obstructive pulmonary disease. *Thorax* 1997;**52**(Suppl 5):S1–S28

2. American Thoracic Society. Standards for the diagnosis and care of patients with chronic obstructive pulmonary disease. *Am J Respir Crit Care Med* 1995;**152**:S77–S121

3. Siafakas NM, Vermeire P, Pride NB, Paoletti P, Gibson GJ, Howard P et al. Optimal assessment and management of chronic obstructive pulmonary disease (COPD). *Eur Respir J* 1995;**8**:1398–420

4. Lamb D. Pathology. In: Calverley PMA, Pride NB, eds. Chronic obstructive pulmonary disease. London: Chapman and Hall 1994

5. Hogg JC, Macklem PT, Thurlbeck WM. Site and nature of airway obstruction in chronic obstructive lung disease. *N Eng J Med* 1968;**278**:1355–60

6. Pride NB, Milic-Emili J. Lung Mechanics. In: Calverley PMA, Pride NB, eds. Chronic obstructive pulmonary disease. London: Chapman and Hall 1994

7. Fletcher C, Peto R. The natural history of chronic airflow obstruction. *BMJ* 1977;**1**:1645–8

8. Quanjer PH. Standardised Lung Function Testing. Official Statement of the European Respiratory Society. *Eur Respir J* 1993;**6**(Suppl 16):5–40

9. Traver GA, Cline MG, Burrows B. Predictors of mortality in COPD. *Am Rev Respir Dis* 1979;**119**:895–902

10. Doll R, Peto R, Wheatley K, Gray R, Sutherland 1. Mortality in relation to smoking: 40 years observations on male British doctors. *BMJ* 1994;**309**:901–10

11. Anthonisen NR. The Lung Health study: effects of smoking intervention and the use of an inhaled anticholinergic bronchodilator on the rate of decline of FEV. *JAMA* 1994;**272**:1497–505

12. Golding JF. Smoking. In: Brewis RAL, Corrin D, Geddes DM, Gibson GJ, eds. Respiratory Medicine. London: WB Saunders 1995

13. Gross NJ, Petty TL, Friedman M, Skorodin MS, Silvers GW, Donoghue JF. Dose response to ipratropium as a nebulised solution in patients with chronic obstructive pulmonary disease. *Am Rev Respir Dis* 1989;**139**:1188–9 1

14. British Thoracic Society. Current best practice for nebuliser treatment. *Thorax* 1997;**52**(Suppl 2):S1–106

15. Fishman AP. Workshop summary: Pulmonary rehabilitation research. *Am J Respir Crit Care Med* 1994;**149**:825–833

16. Department of Health. *Domiciliary oxygen therapy service. Drug tariff Part X*. London: HMSO 1990

7

Chronic Ventilatory Insufficiency and Non-Invasive Ventilation

Anita K Simonds

Introduction

Arterial PO_2 and PCO_2 and pH are kept within a narrow physiological range despite a diversity of challenges placed on the respiratory system. Normal values of blood gases are maintained by a feedback system from central and peripheral chemoreceptors and mechanoreceptors to the ventilatory pump. In essence, a balance is maintained between ventilatory drive, the capacity of the respiratory system and applied load. It follows that ventilatory failure will occur if ventilatory drive is insufficient, ventilatory capacity is markedly reduced, or load is increased. Where this balance is precarious, minor alterations to the status quo such as a decrease in ventilatory drive and intercostal muscle activity during sleep, or a mild increase in bronchospasm during an acute exacerbation of COPD, will precipitate ventilatory failure. Factors affecting ventilatory control mechanisms, capacity and load i.e. the work of breathing are shown in Table 1. By contrast, hypoxaemic *normocapnic* or *hypocapnic* respiratory failure is caused by gas exchange and gas transfer derangement, for example in the acute respiratory distress syndrome, massive pulmonary embolism, and pulmonary oedema. These insults do not usually provoke ventilatory pump dysfunction until the patient is in extremis.

Table 1.   Factors affecting ventilatory pump function

⇓ Ventilatory drive	⇑ Load	⇓ Capacity
Sleep	Airflow obstruction	Respiratory muscle
Sleep fragmentation	Hyperinflation	weakness due to:
Hypercapnia	Chest wall deformity	Myopathies
Congenital	Lung fibrosis	Muscular dystrophies
hypoventilation	Pulmonary oedema	Hypoxaemia, acidosis
syndromes	High metabolic rate	Hypercapnia
Brainstem lesions	Sleep (increased	Endocrinopathy
e.g. CVA	upper airways	Hypophophataemia
	resistance)	Hyperinflation
		Fatigue
		Disuse atrophy
		Sleep (decreased
		intercostal muscle tone)

Pathophysiology

Chronic obstructive airways disease (COPD) is characterised by airflow obstruction, hyperinflation and loss of alveolar/capillary bed. The degree of emphysema is indicated by the extent of reduction in gas transfer factor and can be confirmed radiologically by CT scan. Hypoxaemia is caused by ventilation perfusion (V/Q) mismatch, alveolar hypoventilation and diffusion defect. The pink puffer (emphysema)/blue bloater (chronic bronchitis) categorisation of COPD patients is somewhat artificial, but individuals at each end of the spectrum are clinically obvious. CO_2 retention in the blue bloater patient can be seen as an adaptation to the increased work of breathing, whereas in the pink puffer patient chronic hypercapnia is a sign of end stage disease.

COPD patients with hypoxaemia when awake will develop further desaturation during sleep and on exercise, although the degree of nocturnal hypoxaemia is difficult to predict from daytime wake values. Sleep-related desaturation, most pronounced during the rapid eye movement (REM) stage, occurs as a result of a further decrease in alveolar ventilation due to reduction in intercostal, accessory and pharyngeal postural muscle tone, coupled with loss of cortical drive to breathe, and a lesser degree of V/Q mismatch. Individuals with daytime hypercapnia will show a further rise in PCO_2 during sleep.

Hyperinflation reduces the efficiency of the inspiratory muscles, which are already loaded by airflow obstruction. It has been assumed that respiratory muscle fatigue is an important cause of ventilatory failure in COPD. This remains unproven and it seems more likely that compensatory changes occur to prevent the development of respiratory muscle damage (e.g. resetting of hypercapnic drive, alternation of use of muscle groups). However, the ability of the diaphragm to generate negative intrathoracic pressure is reduced in COPD, and further decreased by acute on chronic hyperinflation. Ventilatory drive is usually normal or high in normocapnic COPD patients, but secondary depression of hypercapnic drive by raised CSF bicarbonate levels occurs leaving some chronically hypercapnic patients primarily reliant on hypoxic drive. It is this group of patients who develop uncontrolled hypercapnia on high flow oxygen therapy and who should be treated with controlled oxygen therapy (24 or 28%).

Restrictive Disorders

Neuromuscular and chest wall diseases that are commonly associated with chronic ventilatory insufficiency are shown in Table 2. In patients with respiratory muscle weakness a reduction in lung volumes is caused by a combination of loss of distending force and a secondary decrease in the compliance of the lung and chest wall. Vital capacity is predominantly affected, with a lesser impact on total lung capacity and variable effects on functional residual capacity. Bilateral diaphragm weakness will cause a 15–20% fall in vital capacity on assuming the supine position from standing. Recurrent aspiration due to bulbar weakness, or atelectasis may complicate the picture.

Thoracic idiopathic scoliosis is the commonest cause of chest wall deformity. It is associated with a purely restrictive ventilatory defect (unless the patient has smoking-related lung disease), but those with acquired chest wall disease due to thoracoplasty, plombage, or old artificial pneumothoraces for TB often have an additional component of airflow obstruction due to airway distortion. Parenchymal lung disease is rare in congenital chest wall disease. As it is easier to squeeze air rather than blood from the restricted thoracic cavity, gas transfer coefficient (gas transfer factor divided by accessible alveolar volume) is almost always supra normal in idiopathic scoliosis. Low values suggest pulmonary hypertension, or independent lung pathology.

Table 2.   Examples of chest wall and neuromuscular diseases associated with chronic cardiorespiratory decompensation

Chest wall disease
Early onset idiopathic thoracic scoliosis
Congenital scoliosis e.g. associated with neurofibromatosis,
Klippel-Feil syndrome, congenital heart disease.
Paralytic scoliosis e.g. due to poliomyelitis
Thoracoplasty
Plombage
Artificial pneumothorax, oleothorax
Fibrothorax

Congenital neuromuscular disease
Myopathies: nemaline
          Acid maltase deficiency (Pompe's disease)
          Mitochondrial myopathy
          Centronuclear, minimal change

Muscular dystrophies: Duchenne
               Congenital
               Limb girdle, Facio scapulo humeral
               Emery-Dreifuss

Spinal muscular atrophy
Hereditary sensory motor neuropathy
Dystrophia myotonica

Acquired neuromuscular disease
Cervical cord lesions
Phrenic nerve injury
Polymyositis
Myasthenia gravis
Guillain Barre syndrome
Brainstem lesion
Motor neurone disease

Acute Exacerbation of Ventilatory Insufficiency

Clinical features

In COPD patients the first episode of ventilatory failure is usually precipitated by an acute chest infection. The individual will present with increased breathlessness, cough and sputum production, variable wheeze and cyanosis. Marked hypercapnia and hypoxaemia will provoke confusion, a flap and often sleep disturbance, with a sensation of claustrophobia and panic.

Arterial pH on admission with an acute exacerbation is a key prognostic factor, although increasing age and uraemia are also adverse features. The mortality rate for the acute episode ranges from 12–20%, but is highest in those with a pH of less than 7.26 (equivalent to hydrogen ion concentration of more than 55 nmoles per litre)[1]. A recent survey of patients admitted with an acute exacerbation of COPD showed that the mean age was 68 years and around 20% of patients were significantly acidotic. A US study has shown that while an arterial PCO_2 on admission of >7.3 kPa is associated with a moderate in-hospital mortality, it is predictive of a substantial risk of death after discharge (33% at 6 months, 49% at 2 years).

Management of acute exacerbations of COPD

Hospital admission is likely to be required for patients who have severe symptoms, an altered level of consciousness, increased cyanosis, or who are unable to cope at home. The aim is to treat the underlying cause of the exacerbation and improve arterial pH and PO_2, without precipitating a rise in PCO_2. Clinical assessment should immediately establish the degree of ventilatory adequacy and the presence of cor pulmonale, with the aid of arterial blood gas measurement, chest X-ray, peak flow rate and spirometry, together with full blood count and biochemistry screen. Controlled oxygen therapy via a Venturi mask (24% or 28%), nebulised bronchodilator, antibiotics, corticosteroids in selected patients, chest physiotherapy, and a diuretic for patients with cor pulmonale should be used as outlined in the British Thoracic Society (BTS) guidelines[2]. Progressive hypercapnia and acidosis in the face of optimum standard therapy is an indication for ventilatory support (see below). The likelihood of reversibility of the illness precipitating the acute decompensation, the patient's pre-existing quality of life, and his/her wishes and those of the family regarding the level of intervention should always be taken into account, and a summary of these discussions recorded in the medical notes.

Acute Ventilatory Failure in Other Obstructive Lung Disease

In-patients with bronchiectasis of any aetiology, including cystic fibrosis, hypercapnia is a feature of advanced disease and usually occurs initially during an acute infective exacerbation. Vigorous sputum clearance with the aid of intensive physiotherapy, antibiotics as indicated by sputum culture results, bronchodilator and steroid therapy should be employed, as appropriate. In status asthmaticus, CO_2 retention is an indicator of severe decompensation with imminent cardiorespiratory collapse. Management should include urgent ventilatory support.

Acute Ventilatory Failure in Restrictive Disorders (Chest Wall and Neuromuscular Disease)

Some chronic neuromuscular disorders (e.g. motor neurone disease, acid maltase deficiency, nemaline myopathy) may present for the first time with ventilatory failure. Other neurological illnesses also characterised by an acute presentation with ventilatory insufficiency include Guillain-Barre syndrome, polymyositis, brain stem cerebrovascular events and encephalitis. Even in severely affected patients respiratory muscle strength can be assessed with non-invasive tests (vital capacity, mouth pressures, cervical magnetic resonance studies, diaphragm screening) and invasive tests such as determination of transdiaphragmatic pressure. Serial measures of vital capacity are the easiest method of monitoring progress at the bedside. Every effort must be made to secure a definitive diagnosis for prognostic and therapeutic purposes by obtaining a neurology opinion, EMG studies, cervical spine views, plus muscle biopsy and screening blood tests, where indicated. A minority of causes will respond to specific treatment (Table 3), but in these and others cases supportive measures will also be required.

Most acute exacerbations in restrictive patients are caused by a chest infection and require treatment with antibiotics, controlled oxygen therapy and efficient physiotherapy. The latter is particularly crucial in those with poor cough ability and sputum retention.

Non-invasive Ventilation in Acute Ventilatory Failure

Both negative pressure and positive pressure ventilatory techniques can be used effectively to control ventilatory failure in those who meet appropriate criteria. As negative pressure ventilation is only

Table 3. Causes of respiratory muscle weakness amenable to specific treatment

Condition	Treatment
Myaesthenia gravis	Anticholinesteases Immunosupression in some cases
Polymyositis	Immunosupression
Endocrinopathy e.g. Hypothyroidism Acromegaly	Thyroxine Pituitary surgery, Bromocriptine etc.
Drug induced myopathy e.g. due to steroids, lipid lowering drugs, vincristine, amipdarone	Withdrawal of drug

performed in specialist centres this account will concentrate on nasal intermittent positive pressure ventilation (NIPPV) which is more widely available.

Acute Hypercapnic Exacerbations of COPD[3,4]

Non-invasive ventilation is an attractive proposition in acute ventilatory failure due to COPD as complications related to intubation such as nosocomial pneumonia and tracheal injury can be avoided, and the patient is able to eat, drink and communicate normally. However, not all cases are suitable for NIPPV, and there is an inevitable failure rate (around 10–20%). Most centres using NIPPV experience a learning curve.

At least four randomised controlled trials of standard therapy versus NIPPV in addition to standard therapy have been carried out. Three of these have demonstrated a better outcome with NIPPV including more rapid correction of arterial pH and blood gases, a reduced need for intubation, decreased mortality and a reduction in hospital stay. Only one study has shown no improvement over and above standard therapy. In the largest study mortality was reduced from 29 to 9% using NIPPV and most of the deaths in the standard therapy group were related to complications of intubation. Findings from the studies of NIPPV in acute COPD including the

Table 4. Overview of trials of NIPPV in acute exacerbations of COPD

Author Reference	Study	n	Entry pH	Entry PCO_2	Time NIV	Post pH	Post PCO_2	Vent	Success rate %
Meduri Chest 1991; 100:445	Open	18	7.29	9.5	25hr	7.37	7.2	P/F	72
Vitacca Int Care Med 1993;19:450	Open	13	7.25	11.4	69	7.40	7.5	V/F	77
		16	7.29	10.1	57	7.35	8.0	P/F	87
Fernandez Int Care Med 1993;19:456	Open	14	7.19	12.1	8	7.31	8.8	P/F	79
Brochard N Engl J Med 1990;1523	Retrospec	13	7.29	8.5	7.6	7.40	6.3	P/F	76
Bott Lancet 1993; 341:1555	RCT	60	7.348	8.6	7.6	7.376	7.3	V/N	83
Kramer AJ RCCM 1995;151;179	RCT	31	7.27	10.7	14.4	*	8.9	P/N	91
Brochard N Engl J Med 1995;333:817	RCT	85	7.27	9.3	>6hr	7.31	9.1	P/F	74
Barbe Eur Resp J 1996;9:358	RCT	24	7.33	7.9	2×3h for 3 days	7.37	7.2	P/N	No difference

RCT: Randomised controlled trial n-number of subjects
Vent –Ventilator V- Volume preset P- Pressure preset
M- Mask N-nasal mask F-facemask
Time NIV- Duration of NIPPV in hours
No difference = no difference in outcome compared to standard therapy

randomised controlled trials are shown in Table 4. Keenan et al[5] have carried out a meta-analysis of NIPPV in acute ventilatory failure. In COPD patients the combined results show a relative risk reduction in mortality of 69% (95% CI 35–86%), and for intubation of 65% (CI 45–78%). Subgroup analysis indicates better results in COPD compared to non-COPD patients. It is clear that any advan-

Table 5.   NIPPV: Criteria for implementation and contraindications in acute COPD

1. Progressive hypercapnia and pH <7.35 in patient receiving optimal medical therapy.
2. No imminent need for intubation
3. Cardiovascular stability
4. Patient able to co-operate
5. No upper airway problems limiting application of mask

Contraindications
1. Coma or severe confusional state
2. Haemodynamic instability
3. Severe bulbar weakness
4. Excessive bronchial secretions
5. Ventilatory support likely to be futile because of extent of chronic disease/co-morbidity, or irreversible nature of event precipitating respiratory failure

tage from NIPPV accrues from intervening early to prevent the need for intubation. NIPPV should therefore be considered in a COPD patient in whom hypercapnia and acidosis are progressing despite maximal conventional therapy. A figure of pH of less than 7.26 is quoted as a indication for assisted ventilation in the BTS guidelines[2], but earlier introduction when pH is <7.35 is probably advisable, if conventional measures have failed. NIPPV is likely to be preferable to doxapram in this situation, but the latter can be used where NIPPV is unavailable. Indications for starting NIPPV are shown in Table 5.

Factors suggestive of a good outcome with NIPPV are an improvement in pH and PCO_2 after one hour of NIPPV, and good compliance. Poor prognostic features are severe acidosis and hypercapnia on initiation of therapy, pneumonic consolidation on chest radiograph, and a severe confusional state which limits co-operation. Before starting NIPPV a clear management plan should be established, including a decision as to whether the patient should be intubated and conventionally ventilated in the event of NIPPV failure.

Acute NIPPV in Restrictive Disease[4]

NIPPV has been extended to patients with chest wall and neuromuscular disease. Here too, results are encouraging, but there have been no randomised controlled studies, as groups of restrictive patients tend to be more heterogeneous. Bulbar incompetence is an obvious contraindication to NIPPV in those with neuromuscular disease. Uncontrolled hypercapnia and acidosis are the indication for NIPPV. In general, if the criteria in Table 5 are fulfilled a trial of NIPPV should be considered before embarking on intubation and conventional ventilation. It should be remembered that chest wall and neuromuscular patients are more likely than COPD patients to develop progressive CO_2 retention on oxygen therapy, so that arterial blood gas tensions should be monitored carefully.

Weaning

NIPPV can also be used to wean ventilator-dependent patients and is particularly suited to those with a significant chronic component to their cardiorespiratory disease[4]. To ensure suitability for weaning using NIPPV a number of criteria should be fulfilled. These include:

- normal or near normal bulbar function
- ability to breathe spontaneously for at least 5–10 minutes
- haemodynamic stability
- functioning gastrointestinal tract

In several studies NIPPV has been shown to speed the weaning process, and one randomised controlled study has shown a survival advantage in COPD patients, although this work needs to be confirmed. Patients who deteriorate on the waiting list for heart/lung or lung transplantation can use NIPPV as a 'bridge' until transplant organs become available. The outcome in transplant recipients treated with NIPPV is no worse than those who did not require ventilatory support preoperatively, and is definitely preferable to intubation and ventilation. The main obstacle to bridging a patient in this way is the scarcity of transplant organs.

Chronic Ventilatory Failure

Patients present with symptoms of daytime fatigue, reduction in exercise tolerance, breathlessness, headaches, sleep disturbance, and features of cor pulmonale. It is possible to predict those who are at high risk of ventilatory failure (Table 6).

In COPD ventilatory failure is unusual if FEV_1 is more than around 800mls. If FEV_1 exceeds a litre then other contributory causes should be considered such as obstructive sleep apnoea or

Table 6.   Indicators of high risk of cardiorespiratory failure

Chest wall disease:
   early onset idiopathic scoliosis (age less than 5 years)
   Vital capacity less than 30% predicted
   Additional respiratory muscle weakness
   High thoracic curve

Neuromuscular disease:
   Respiratory muscle strength less than 30% predicted
   Additional thoracic scoliosis
   Disease with progressive potential e.g. Duchenne muscular dystrophy,
   motor neurone disease
   Associated cardiomypathy e.g. Acid maltase Deficiency, Duchenne muscular dystrophy

respiratory muscle weakness. A good history will elicit symptoms of obstructive sleep apnoea such as persistent loud snoring, witnessed apnoeas and daytime somnolence, or characteristic features of respiratory muscle weakness (e.g. breathlessness on lying flat). In patients with neuromuscular or chest wall disease, respiratory failure becomes likely once vital capacity and respiratory muscle strength fall below 30% predicted. Relevant investigations should include pulmonary function tests, arterial blood gas measurement, a sleep study, and assessment of respiratory muscle strength where muscle weakness is suspected. Maximum static inspiratory and expiratory mouth pressures (PI and PE max) are a useful screening tool, although measurements depend on patient cooperation. Values below 80 cmH_2O should be followed up by more detailed studies including measurement of trans-diaphragmatic pressure and assessment of phrenic nerve activity using direct stimulation in the neck or cervical cord magnetic stimulation, if clinical suspicion is high.

   ECG and echocardiogram are helpful to gauge left ventricular function and the presence of pulmonary hypertension and right heart strain.

General Management

Advice regarding smoking cessation, nutrition and attainment of ideal body weight are essential. Bronchodilator and steroid responsiveness should be investigated and treated appropriately in COPD patients[2]. Care should be taken to ensure that patients are able to use inhaled drug delivery systems efficiently. There is now clear evidence that pulmonary rehabilitation programmes containing an exercise component are effective in improving exercise tolerance and quality of life in COPD patients, and these are likely to be beneficial in restrictive groups, too. Hypercapnic patients should not be excluded from rehabilitation programmes.

Domiciliary Long Term Oxygen Therapy (LTOT)[2]

LTOT is gold standard treatment in COPD patients who fulfil the criteria:

PaO_2 < 7.3 kPa in a steady state period

LTOT can also be prescribed in stable patients with a PaO_2 between 7.3 and 8.0 kPa in the presence of either polycythaemia, peripheral oedema, pulmonary hypertension or nocturnal SaO_2 < 90% for at least 30% of the night.

Patients should use LTOT 16 hours a day via a concentrator. Employed appropriately LTOT should reduce mortality, but does not significantly improve the quality of life. Surveys continue to show that oxygen therapy is under-prescribed and underused. No survival benefit is seen in COPD patients with a PO_2 in excess of 8 kPa.

Transplantation and Lung Reduction Surgery

Selected patients with endstage lung disease due to cystic fibrosis, pulmonary fibrosis, pulmonary hypertension, congenital heart disease and emphysema may be suitable for heart-lung or single/double lung transplantation. Transplant centres have an upper age limit and individuals with co-morbidity such as renal impairment are unsuitable. One year survival figures for double lung transplant and single lung transplant are around 90% and 70%, respectively. It seems that patients with emphysema survive longer than those with endstage pulmonary fibrosis on the waiting list. The main limitations to outcome are a deficiency in donor organs and obliterative bronchiolitis. The former may be helped by the development of live donor lobe transplant programmes.

Lung reduction surgery has recently been introduced for emphysema patients. Early studies suggest that the benefits of an increase in FEV_1, gas exchange and exercise tolerance are obtained as a result of a reduction in dynamic hyperinflation and increase in elastic recoil. Randomised controlled studies of the technique are now in progress. Hypercapnia is a contra-indication to lung reduction surgery in most centres.

Domiciliary Non-invasive Ventilation for Chronic Ventilatory Failure[6]

Restrictive disorders

Domiciliary non invasive ventilation has been available for neuromuscular patients for many decades, originally in the form of negative pressure techniques (e.g. cuirass, iron lung, pneumojacket). Before the introduction of home ventilatory support patients with early onset scoliosis died in middle age, and many individuals with congenital neuromuscular disease succumbed to ventilatory failure in childhood or adolescence. NIPPV has now superseded negative pressure ventilation and some centres use the variant of mouth intermittent positive pressure ventilation (MIPPV). Longitudinal studies from France and the UK show a five year survival in patients presenting in ventilatory failure who receive NIPPV is 80% in those with idiopathic scoliosis, 90% in those with previous tuberculous lung disease and 100% for patients with old poliomyclitis[6]. Health-related quality of life is good and many individuals are able to return to work.

Progressive neuromuscular diseases

Any intervention in-patients with progressive disease should aim to palliate symptoms and improve quality of life and survival where possible, without burdening the individual and protracting the terminal phase. Judged by these standards, NIPPV improves survival in Duchenne muscular dystrophy (five year survival > 70% in some centres) and patients receiving NIPPV judge their quality of life as acceptable. Selected patients with motor neurone disease and early respiratory muscle involvement may also derive benefit particularly if they have symptoms of nocturnal hypoventilation and sleep disturbance, in the absence of severe bulbar involvement. There is no evidence that NIPPV can prevent the development of ventilatory failure in normocapnic patients. Contrary to some accounts, NIPPV can be used successfully in children with neuromusculo-skeletal disease[6].

COPD

Whereas the role of domiciliary NIPPV in chronic ventilatory failure due to restrictive disorders is well established, NIPPV remains controversial in COPD patients. Several uncontrolled and crossover studies suggest that in COPD patients with marked hypercapnia and severe nocturnal hypoventilation, NIPPV + LTOT produces a greater improvement in arterial blood gases and quality of life than LTOT alone. However, the results of randomised controlled studies are awaited. In the meantime it has been argued that it may be reasonable to consider domiciliary NIPPV in motivated COPD patients in whom daytime arterial PCO_2 is greater than 8 kPa and nocturnal PCO_2 excedes 9 kPa while receiving controlled oxygen therapy[7].

Practical Aspects of NIPPV[6]

Nasal ventilators can be classified into pressure and volume preset models. An example of a pressure preset machine is the Nippy and volume preset machines include the Lifecare PLV-100, BromptonPAC and Monnal models. The pressure preset group incorporates bilevel pressure support models such as BiPAP (Respironics), VPAP (Resmed) and DP90 (Taema) ventilators. Newer modes such as proportional assist ventilation (PAV) are being explored, but the indications for these are not yet established. Theoretically, volume preset ventilators cope better with changes in airway resistance and thoracic impedance than pressure preset machines, but the latter are more effective in compensating for leaks and may be safer for patients at risk of pneumothorax. In practice, familiarity with the performance of the ventilator so that optimum results are obtained, is just as important. No study has shown that any one type of ventilator is superior, but care should be taken to match the equipment performance to the patient's ventilatory requirements. Inspiratory pressures of around 10–25 cmH_2O or flow rates of 0.7–1.0 l/second are required for the average adult and should be titrated to arterial blood gas levels. Entrained oxygen should be added if arterial oxygen saturation cannot be increased to 90% or higher using NIPPV alone. The addition of low levels of expiratory positive airway pressure (EPAP) (e.g. 2–5 cmH_2O) may be helpful in COPD patients and those with atelectasis or left ventricular dysfunction.

Table 7.   Basic steps for starting NIPPV

1. Ensure patient suitability for NIPPV (Table 5).

2. Assemble equipment away from the bedside to check it is functioning correctly.

3. Explain to the patient what you are going to do. Select a well-fitting mask. Consider a full facemask if the patient is confused.

4. Entrain oxygen therapy into the mask or circuit if PaO_2 is < 7.0 kPa. Start at a flow rate of 1–2 l/minute.

5. Pressure preset ventilator: Use a starting inspiratory pressure of around 12–20 cmH_2O. If expiratory pressure available do not set > than 5 cmH_2O. Volume preset ventilator: aim for a tidal volume of 8-12 mls per kg.

6. Use the ventilator in triggered ie. assist control (spontaneous timed) mode. Set trigger at most sensitive setting.

7. Average inspiratory time is around 0.8–1.0 seconds, but titrate to patient comfort.

8. Always monitor SaO_2 continuously and check arterial blood gas tensions after 30–60 minutes of NIPPV.

9. Aim to correct the respiratory acidosis, initially stabilise $PaCO_2$, and then gently reduce hypercapnia in the presence of an improved PaO_2.

10. If $PaCO_2$ levels remain high, increase inspiratory positive pressure by 2 cmH_2O increments or raise tidal volume.

11. Don't expect immediate correction of $PaCO_2$. This should be beginning to fall after 1 hour and will probably correct optimally over the next 24-48 hours.

12. Encourage the patient to use NIPPV as much as possible, especially over night for the first 48 hours. Aim to use for a minimum of 6 hours/day.

13. Protect the nasal bridge and watch out for nasal bridge pressure sores. If these develop swap to a better fitting mask, bubble mask (Resmed) or nasal plugs. Granuflex (ConvaTec Ltd) or Spencodermal pad (Spenco Medical UK Ltd) skin dressings may help.

It is imperative that the mask is comfortable and fits well. Nasal masks are usually preferred for domiciliary use, but for a confused patient or individuals with nasal blockage, a full facemask is helpful. Variants on the theme include nasal plugs (Adams circuit, Puritan Bennett or nasal seals, Healthdyne).

Basic steps for the novice in setting up NIPPV are given in Table 7, and further details are given elsewhere[6]. However, it is always advisable to get advice from a more experienced team member, as the success of the technique will depend, in part, on the operator's skills.

For patients receiving home ventilation, final ventilatory settings should be established by overnight monitoring of transcutaneous PCO_2 and arterial oxygen saturation before discharge. A home care package should be provided which includes service and maintenance of the ventilatory equipment in the home, provision of disposables, and access to emergency medical treatment[6]. This is best organised by centres which have experience in home ventilatory care.

Suggested Reading

Jeffrey AA, Warren PM, Flenley DC. Acute hypercapnic respiratory failure in patients with chronic obstructive lung disease: risk factors and use of guidelines for management. *Thorax* 1992;**47**:34–40

BTS Guidelines for the management of chronic obstructive pulmonary disease. *Thorax* 1997;**52**:Supplement 5

Wedzicha JA. Non-invasive ventilation for exacerbations of respiratory failure in chronic obstructive pulmonary disease. *Thorax* 1996; S35–39

Ambrosino N. Non-invasive mechanical ventilation in acute respiratory failure. *Eur Respir J* 1996;**9**:795–807

Keenan SP, Kernerman PD, Cook DJ et al. Effect of noninvasive positive pressure ventilation on mortality in patients admitted with acute respiratory failure: a meta-analysis. *Crit Care Med* 1997;**25**:1685–92

Simonds AK. Non-invasive respiratory support. Chapman & Hall 1995

Sivasothy P, Smith IE, Shneerson JM. Mask intermittent positive pressure ventilation in chronic hypercapnic respiratory failure due to chronic obstructive pulmonary disease. *Eur Respir J* 1998;**11**:34–40

8

Sleep Apnoea Syndromes

Lesley S Bennett and Robert JO Davies

Introduction

Obstructive sleep apnoea and its variants are by far the commonest causes of sleep disordered breathing. Increasing recognition of these conditions in recent years has led to a rapid expansion in research, improving our understanding of the epidemiology and pathophysiology of this condition and leading to an abundance of new sleep study techniques. This chapter describes the different sleep apnoea syndromes and leads on to a discussion of the diagnosis, differential diagnosis and management of each.

Prevalence

Obstructive sleep apnoea (OSA) is an extremely common phenomenon, but exactly how common can appear confusing. This confusion is predominantly due to the use of different methods and thresholds for detecting respiratory events in different studies (illustrated in Figure 1). When these factors are considered, the published studies are reasonably consistent with about 5% of adult men having some detectable obstructive sleep apnoea (OSA). The prevalence in women is one tenth of this. Only about one in five of these individuals has significant associated daytime sleepiness (sleep apnoea syndrome).[1] Thus, OSA is much like many other common disorders such as asthma; minor detectable respiratory disturbances are extremely common, but only a small subset of those with detectable disturbances require treatment.

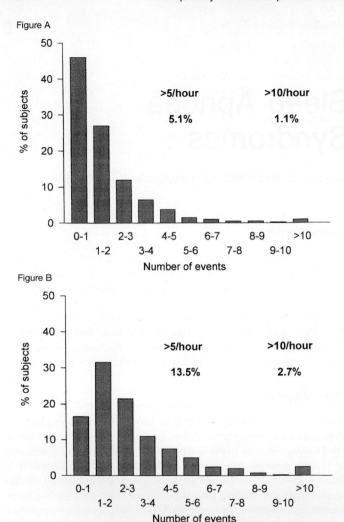

Figure 1. This figure demonstrates how changing methodology for identifying sleep apnoea alters disease prevalence in normal men drawn from an Oxfordshire village. Figure A shows the prevalence of ≥ 4% oxygen saturation dips in 893 normal men. Figure B shows the effect of changing the definition of an oxygen saturation dip ≥ 3%. Also shown is the percentage of subjects above two arbitrary thresholds (>5 and >10 events per hour)

Pathophysiology

The critical event in obstructive sleep apnoea is the narrowing and collapse of the pharyngeal airway with the onset of sleep. Pharyngeal muscular activity declines at sleep onset, reducing pharyngeal patency, and so precipitating airway collapse in patients with an anatomically narrowed airway (see below). The collapse can be complete (apnoea) or partial (hypopnoea, when snoring is characteristically present). The resulting airflow obstruction increases respiratory effort that sometimes leads to pleural pressures of down to -80cm H_2O. After a variable period (from a few seconds to over one minute) arousal from sleep occurs with a return of upper airway muscular activity and hence the opening of the airway. The trigger for arousal is probably multifactorial, but the detection of increased respiratory effort by pleural and/or pharyngeal receptors is probably the most important. Arousal from sleep may only last a few seconds, after which sleep is resumed, the airway collapses, and the cycle is repeated. The sleep disruption produced by this cycle results in inefficient sleep and hence daytime hypersomnolence.

Since it is the collapsibility of the pharynx that predisposes to airway collapse, any factor that prejudices this balance will tend to precipitate snoring and OSA. These factors can be categorised into four groups:

- *anatomical factors reducing airway calibre.*
  These include the amount of soft tissue outside the airway (particularly fat deposits but also muscle mass) and within the airway (tonsilar/adenoidal tissue, pharyngeal mucosal thickness, pharyngeal tumours, etc.) and the bony structure of the face and skull
- *factors reducing pharyngeal muscle tone.*
  These include, age, alcohol and sedative intake, nerve and muscle weakness (causes of both pharyngeal and the rarer laryngeal sleep apnoea)
- *factors decreasing negative inspiratory intra-pharyngeal pressure.*
  Particularly nasal obstruction
- *factors decreasing the sleeping drive to breathe and hence neural drive to the upper airway.*
  These include sleep deprivation (which has a positive feedback link with OSA), hypothyroidism (which also has anatomical effects), and hypocapnia (such as occurs at altitude)

Of all of these factors, the anatomical abnormalities are overwhelmingly the most important.

The Clinical Assessment of Obstructive Sleep Apnoea

Definition

The original definitions of the sleep apnoea syndrome were very specific with an arbitrary number of respiratory events (apnoeas and hypopnoeas) required per hour of sleep to confirm a diagnosis (apnoea/hypopnoea index (AHI)). As our understanding of the disease has progressed, this index is no longer ideal for defining sleep apnoea and for grading its severity for two important reasons. First, it relates poorly to the daytime symptoms of sleepiness (the main indication for treatment) and second, snoring alone without apnoeas, hypopnoeas or hypoxaemia, can cause sleep disturbance, resulting in symptoms of 'classical' sleep apnoea. As there is such a wide spectrum of severity, a single diagnostic cut-off point above which breathing is 'abnormal' is misleading. A clinical definition of sleep apnoea syndrome is more appropriate; for example, significant daytime symptoms (e.g. sleepiness) in conjunction with evidence of sleep-related upper airway obstruction and sleep disturbance.[2]

History

Excessive daytime somnolence

The predominant symptom of sleep apnoea syndrome is daytime sleepiness which is the main indication for treatment with nasal continuous positive airway pressure (nCPAP). In the early stages, hypersomnolence may only be noticeable during boring activities, but as the condition worsens the onset of irresistible sleep can occur during talking, driving and occasionally even eating. It may have been progressive over many years and may not be perceived by the patient as abnormal. It is only following successful treatment that the extent of the problem is sometimes realised. Direct questioning such as 'are you ever sleepy during the day?' will not reveal sleepiness under these circumstances, but situational questions such as 'do you fall asleep reading or watching television?' may do. The Epworth Sleepiness Scale is based on such questions and is a useful, verified way to simply estimate the degree of sleepiness (Figure 2). When assessing sleepiness it is important to distinguish between excessive somnolence (the overwhelming desire to sleep) and tiredness, lethargy and lack of energy. Sleepiness is characterised by irresistible sleep onset in inappropriate situations, the other symp-

Epworth sleepiness scale

Name:...

Date:...

Your age (Yr)............................   Your sex (Male = M/Female = F)...

How likely are you to doze off or fall asleep in the situations described in the box below, in contrast to feeling just tired?

This refers to your usual way of life in recent times.

Even if you haven't done some of these things recently try to work out how they would have affected you.

Use the following scale to choose the most appropriate number for each situation:-

> 0 = would never doze
>
> 1 = Slight chance of dozing
>
> 2 = Moderate chance of dozing
>
> 3 = High chance of dozing

Situation	Chance of dozing
Sitting and reading	
Watching TV	
Sitting, inactive in a public place (e.g. a theatre or a meeting)	
As a passenger in a car for an hour without a break	
Lying down to rest in the afternoon when circumstances permit	
Sitting and talking to someone	
Sitting quietly after a lunch without alcohol	
In a car, while stopped for a few minutes in the traffic	

Thank you for your cooperation

Figure 2.   The Epworth Sleepiness Scale

Table 1. Symptoms of obstructive sleep apnoea

Most common	Less common	Rare
Loud snoring	Reduced libido	Enuresis
Excessive daytime sleepiness	Nocturnal sweating	Recurrent arousals/insomnia
Restless sleep	Morning headaches	Nocturnal cough
Unrefreshing sleep	Choking sensation at night	Symptomatic oesophageal reflux
Nocturia		
Apparent personality changes		
Witnessed apnoeas		

toms are typified by a loss of 'get up and go' but not unwanted sleepiness. Excessive sleepiness is often due to those disorders such as OSA that cause recurrent arousal from sleep (pathological sleep fragmentation) and respond to treatment of the underlying cause. Lethargy and tiredness, etc. (as characterised by the 'post viral' syndrome) is rarely due to sleep fragmentation and almost never improved by interventions aimed at correcting sleep fragmentation.

Snoring

Snoring is virtually universal in OSA and is a reliable marker of upper airway obstruction. It is useful to obtain a history from the partner who may have noticed restless sleep and/or witnessed apnoeic pauses, followed by sudden loud snoring.

Table 1 lists the symptoms of sleep apnoea syndrome including common and rarer manifestations. The history should also include alcohol intake and drug use since sedation aggravates OSA.

Examination

The value of a physical examination is limited when assessing for the possibility of OSA and it is the history of sleepiness and snoring which is likely to be the main indication for a sleep study. It is important to look for causes of OSA that may be medically or surgically correctable. The pharynx should be examined to look for encroaching structures such as tonsils or soft tissue tumours and any features suggesting acromegaly or hypothyroidism should be observed. If there is associated airway obstruction there may be respiratory failure. Micrognathia and retrognathia are also risk factors for OSA and if severe may rarely be managed surgically.

Investigations

A sleep study is essential to establish a diagnosis of OSA before commencing treatment. Snoring and daytime sleepiness are both common and not always linked. The aim of the sleep study is to identify whether OSA or an increase in upper airway resistance is present and whether this is responsible for substantial sleep disturbance.

What should a sleep study include?

Important information required from a sleep study is the amount and pattern of snoring, the degree of respiratory obstruction and the severity of any associated sleep fragmentation. It is also necessary to be able to exclude periodic limb movements (see below). There are many different physiological signals that can directly or indirectly provide this information and there is no evidence to suggest that any one collection of signals is optimal. No single signal can produce all the necessary information and a 'montage' of several is needed. Much attention is often paid to which is the 'best' system, but in reality the training and experience of the interpreting physician are overwhelmingly more important. The relative merits of two combat aircraft are of little importance if the pilot cannot fly!

Pulse oximetry alone is an inadequate test for diagnosing sleep apnoea[6]. It may have role for investigating patients at the extreme ends of the spectrum where the clinical prior probability of the presence of significant OSA is either very high or very low (Figure 5 top panel). However, widespread use of oximetry for all patients is insufficient, particularly if the sleep study scorer is inexperienced and unaware of the potential pitfalls. Oximetry alone does not identify sleep disturbed by hypopnoeas or snoring that do not produce falls in oxygen saturation. In addition, other sleep disorders causing daytime sleepiness (e.g. periodic limb movements) will be missed and the recurrent desaturations of Cheyne-Stokes breathing may be confused with OSA.

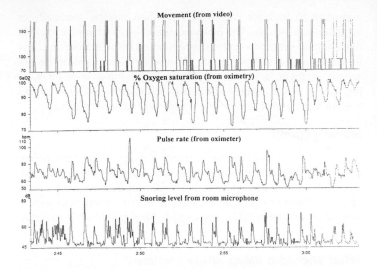

Figure 3. A twenty minute sleep study tracing in a patient with OSA using oximetry and automated video analysis. It shows recurrent arousal from sleep (movement and rise in pulse rate) associated with each fall in oxygen saturation. The fourth line shows the snoring level

Video recordings. The combination of video and sound recordings are useful for subtleties of disturbed breathing which are not evident on any other secondary index — for example the characteristic sound of pharyngeal opening at the end of an obstructive apnoea in a patient with relatively little snoring. The video signal can also be processed to detect body movements as a marker of sleep fragmentation and snoring can be measured as an indirect marker of upper airway partial collapse. An illustration of data drawn from an oximetry and automated video analysis is shown in Figure 3.

Direct measures of breathing. Movements of the ribcage and abdomen, and airflow at the nose and mouth (usually recorded from a thermistor) allow the direct recording of breathing pattern, but are mildly uncomfortable for the patient and may therefore disturb sleep.

The sleep electroencephalogram and sleep stage scoring. Recordings of the sleep electroencephalogram (EEG), combined with records of eye movements and the electromyogram, allow the

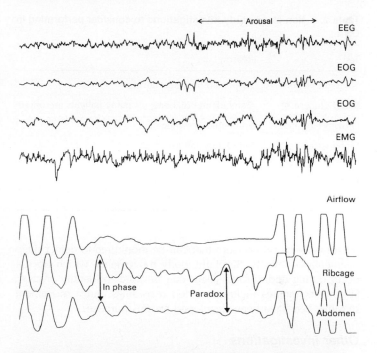

Figure 4.   One minute tracing of an obstructive sleep apnoea. Airflow is initially In phase with rib-cage and abdomen movements (point A). When airflow ceases as a results of upper airway obstruction, inspiratory efforts progressively increase. Paradoxical movement of the ribcage and abdomen occurs during frustrated inspiratory efforts (point B). Just prior to the resumption of airflow, the EEG shows a minor transient arousal from sleep that opens the upper airway. A similar sleep study tracing for central apnoea would show no attempted inspiratory effort from the ribcage and abdomen transducers during the apnoea

most direct estimation of sleep stage and fragmentation. The scoring of these traces is immensely time consuming and for the majority of cases is no more clinically useful than other simple markers of sleep disturbance[7,8] (see below). An example of a sleep recording using both the EEG and direct measures of breathing is shown in Figure 4.

Other markers of sleep fragmentation. At arousal from sleep there is generalised autonomic activation, with consequent rises in

Table 2.   Non-sleep study investigations to consider performing in OSA

Test	Reason
Thyroid function	Suspected hypothyroidism
Blood glucose	Coincidental diabetes (as many patients are obese)
Growth Hormone	Suspected acromegaly
Blood gases (if SaO_2 < 95%)	Ventilatory failure
Haemoglobin	Suspected polycythaemia
Pulmonary function	Airflow obstruction

heart rate or blood pressure that can be monitored to detect sleep fragmentation events. Similarly, body movements, which do not occur during undisturbed sleep, can be used to identify arousal. Several techniques including video recordings and a movement sensitive bed have been developed for this purpose.

Other investigations

If there is clinical suspicion of an associated or causal condition, investigations to consider performing are shown in Table 2. Thyroid function tests are probably the most important particularly in women, in whom sleep apnoea is less common and because some of the features of OSA are similar to hypothyroidism. If ventilatory failure is present then blood gases are checked before and shortly after commencing nCPAP.

Management

Given the wide spectrum of severity of this condition, management is not based solely on the results of sleep studies but is flexible and depends on symptom severity and complications.

Conservative management

If obstructive sleep apnoea is mild or only minimally symptomatic then the patient is unlikely to want nCPAP. Advice should be given for simple measures that can be taken to improve snoring and mild

Table 3.   Treatment options for mild to moderate obstructive sleep apnoea

Avoid sleeping on back	Bolsters, or a tennis ball in a pocket on the back of pyjama top
No alcohol after 18.00 hours	Improves pharyngeal muscle tone
No sedatives	Improves pharyngeal muscle tone
Stop smoking	Improves nasal patency and reduces pharyngeal congestion
Lose weight	Very difficult to achieve
Maintain nasal patency	Elevate bedhead, nasal steroids, nasal surgery
Move jaw forward during sleep	Mandibular advancement device
Tonsillectomy	If tonsils are significantly enlarged

OSA (Table 3). In the milder group, sleep disruption is often only present while lying supine or after taking substances that reduce pharyngeal muscle tone (alcohol, sedatives). Clearing a semi-blocked nose may reduce snoring induced arousals but is unlikely to help in severe OSA. Nasal steroids and anticholinergics are often beneficial here although sometimes nasal surgery is required. A nasal splint may help a small percentage of patients with anterior nasal valve collapse.

In mild cases, quite small amounts of weight loss can be effective, but usually the results of weight loss programmes are disappointing even when an anorectic drug is used. In particular, patients with severe OSA find it difficult to lose weight, probably due to the detrimental effects of sleep deprivation on will-power and daytime activity.

Various drugs have been tried in OSA but with little effect and their role is of doubtful significance. Tricyclic antidepressants have been suggested to reduce symptoms and reduce upper airway obstruction during sleep, although well-controlled studies have found no benefit. Protryptiline may also increase upper airway muscle activity relative to diaphragmatic drive, but whether this is of value in OSA is not known. If tricyclic antidepressants do have a place in the management of OSA it is in the management of the mildly affected patient only. Theophylline and acetazolamide have both been tried in OSA with no useful effect.

Mandibular advancement devices

The recent development of dental appliances (or mandibular/jaw advancement device) has provided an alternative treatment option to patients with mild to moderate sleep apnoea whose symptoms are not severe enough to warrant nCPAP. These devices, worn only at night, open up the retroglossal space by holding the tongue and/ or mandible forward. They range in complexity from a simple gum shield (similar to anti-tooth grinding devices) to elaborate devices that can vary the degree of mandibular protrusion. Most appliances are fitted by dentists under the supervision of a respiratory sleep clinic. Common side-effects include an aching jaw and impaired proprioception of the lower jaw for a couple of hours after the device has been removed. A recent study from Vancouver showed their dental appliance to work adequately in many patients with mild to moderate sleep apnoea, but they are unlikely to be satis-factory in severe sleep apnoea and it is not yet clear how best to identify which patients will benefit most from these devices.

Nasal continuous positive airway pressure

For patients with severe symptomatic OSA by far the most effective treatment is nasal continuous positive airway pressure (nCPAP).[3] It immediately and completely corrects upper airway obstruction (snoring, hypopnoeas and apnoeas) (Figure 5) and hence it corrects the consequent sleep disruption. It has been shown to reduce sleepiness, measured both subjectively (using the Epworth Scale) and objectively in subjects with a wide range of sleep apnoea severity (Figure 6). In a randomised controlled trial of nCPAP versus oral placebo there were statistically significant improvements in daytime sleepiness in the group treated with nCPAP.[4] In contrast to surgical treatment options, nCPAP can be given on a 'trial' basis and withdrawn if there is no improvement in symptoms or if treatment is not tolerated.

Starting nasal CPAP

Nasal CPAP is a cosmetically unappealing treatment and ensuring adequate patient education prior to its commencement is beneficial in reducing anxiety and improving long-term acceptance. Once the decision has been made to commence nCPAP, the prescribing physician should carefully explain what is wrong and the aims of

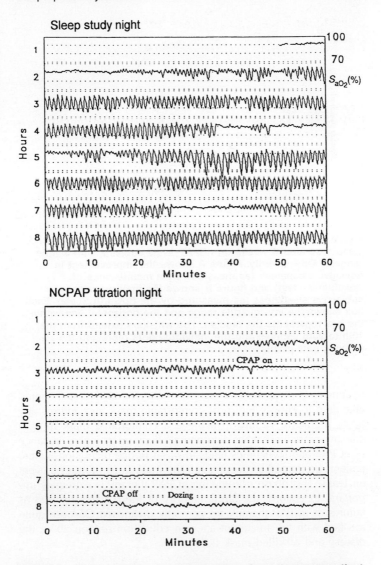

Figure 5. Two separate overnight tracings from the same patient with severe obstructive sleep apnoea. The top panel is before treatment and the bottom panel is on the first night of nCPAP. Once an adequate pressure has been established, the apnoeas and consequent dips in oxygen saturation are abolished

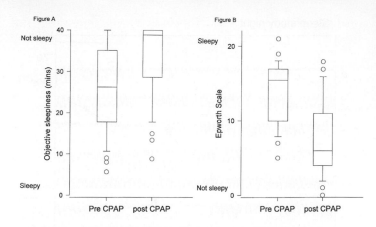

Figure 6. Box and whisker plot to show the improvement in sleepiness after 4 weeks on nCPAP in 39 subjects with a wide range of OSA severity. Figure A shows the improvement in objective sleepiness (as measured by a maintenance of wakefulness test) and figure B shows the improvement in subjective sleepiness (as measured by the Epworth Scale). Each box shows the interquartile range and the horizontal line within the box represents the median. The whiskers extend from the 10th to 90th centiles and the individual dots represent the outlying data points

treatment. Prior to the first night of treatment, skilled staff should take time to choose the most comfortable mask and address any acute problems. Failure to achieve a comfortable mask fit with effective mask air seal has detrimental effects on patient acceptance of nCPAP and sometimes leads to nasal bridge ulceration, where patients are forced to over-tighten the mask attempting to prevent air leaks. This phase of initiating nCPAP therapy is extremely important. In Oxford, the large majority of the patients referred as failures of nCPAP therapy for correctly diagnosed OSA are quite satisfied with the treatment after an education session about the disease and a skilled mask fitting.

NCPAP pressure titration

It is not known exactly what nCPAP pressure is 'optimal' and whether it benefits the patient to have all his snoring and subtle flow limitation corrected. A pragmatic approach is to select the pressure that controls all snoring and associated arousals from sleep. This may result in a marginal over-estimation of the nCPAP pressure requirement, but it does allow for the inevitable night to night variability in upper airway resistance due to sleeping posture, alcohol intake, etc. Automatically self adjusting nCPAP machines are now available that detect apnoea, hypopnoea, snoring or airflow limitation and adjust the pressure accordingly. These are useful for nCPAP pressure titration since they avoid the need for technical staff to supervise an all night nCPAP titration. The following day, the pressure trace is reviewed, together with respiratory event data and arousal markers, and the minimum pressure required to control upper airway related sleep fragmentation is selected for long term treatment. For continuing treatment, there is no evidence that these self adjusting nCPAP machines (which are considerably more expensive) are better tolerated or more effective at controlling OSA than fixed pressure machines, and are therefore not currently recommended for long term use.[5]

Patient follow-up

Throughout treatment and, in particular, at the start of treatment, it is vital that patients have access to experienced staff, so that any physical or technical problems can be addressed promptly. Some common technical problems encountered at the start of nCPAP treatment are listed in Table 4 and the importance of having staff skilled in managing such problems should be emphasised. For this reason both American Sleep Disorders Association and the Royal College of Physicians recommends that a nCPAP service is best run from a specialist centre.[6] Patients on long-term nCPAP are reviewed annually to monitor compliance and provide electrical safety checks of equipment.

Deciding to continue nCPAP

The decision to prescribe nCPAP, is based on the severity of daytime sleepiness and impairment of quality of life. In a subject with severe sleep apnoea, daytime sleepiness is improved after the first night and certainly after one week. If improvements in these symptoms are not seen then either nCPAP is failing in some way (inadequate pressure, mask leakage, poor compliance, claustrophobia, etc.) or the original symptoms are not due to obstructive sleep apnoea. Here the differential diagnosis should be reconsidered and the

Table 4.   Some common problems encountered at the start of nCPAP treatment

Problem	Recommendation
Soreness on the nasal bridge	Loosen straps or change strap position on headgear Use nasal foam bridge pads Change make of nasal mask or try nasal cushions to deliver nCPAP
Claustrophobia	Emphasise importance of breathing through nose Reassurance — stress there is no need to keep mask on for whole night at start of treatment Try nasal cushions to deliver nCPAP
Mask leaks	Lift mask off face and settle again Tighten head straps Ensure no nasal congestion Change size/make of nasal mask
Mouth leaks	Chin support
Nasal congestion and sneezing	Steroid aqueous nasal spray Ipratropium bromide nasal spray Humidifier (hot or cold) if persistent problems
Machine noise	Place machine in cupboard or box (do not obstruct air intake) Increase length of tubing so machine is further away Ear plugs

possibility of having overlooked central sleep apnoea (Cheyne-Stokes breathing), periodic movement of the legs, narcolepsy, poor sleep hygiene, depression, etc. should be reviewed.

The financial debate for treating sleep apnoea can be justified by the fact that patients with untreated sleep apnoea are unable to drive which often leads to unemployment. A nCPAP machine at present costs approximately £300 and can be expected to last at least 5 years (and usually a lot longer). Annual maintenance of the machine and provision of additional masks, tubing etc. cost approximately £150 per annum — so the cost for 5 years of treatment, including machine, would be £1250. This compares favourably with the cost of treating other chronic diseases.

Surgical Treatment

The appeal of surgical treatments for OSA is they offer a definitive treatment, compared to the possible lifetime need for nasal nCPAP. They are, however, not uniformly successful and should be only be recommended in a small number of carefully selected cases. Since few OSA patients require surgery, small centres will not accumulate much experience and therefore most OSA patients considering surgery should be reviewed in a specialist centre.

Tracheostomy

Tracheostomy is a highly effective treatment for OSA although there are many associated complications and repercussions for the patient's lifestyle. The use of nCPAP has diminished the role of tracheostomy in the management of sleep apnoea syndrome, but it should still be considered in very selected cases, most commonly for patients with life threatening ventilatory failure who have failed a thorough trial of nCPAP.

Nasal surgery

Nasal surgery has only a very limited part to play in the treatment of severe OSA. If there is partial pharyngeal collapse with snoring then upstream nasal resistance may be contributing and in this situation improving nasal patency can be useful. Sometimes this is necessary before nCPAP can be effective.

Uvulopalatopharyngoplasty (UPPP)

Uvulopalatopharyngoplasty (UPPP) is an operation designed to increase the volume of the pharynx by resecting pharyngeal wall tissue and the soft palate. It involves resection of the uvula, part of the soft palate and redundant tonsilar tissue. It has significant morbidity (particularly peri-operative pain and nasal fluid regurgitation which affects up to 20% of patients) and an occasional mortality. It also makes subsequent nCPAP treatment less tolerable. Data on the effectiveness of UPPP in sleep apnoea syndrome is variable. Most studies show that about 50 per cent of patients show a 50 per cent reduction in their apnoea index at one year (compared to >90% with nCPAP). Because of this variability in outcome, attempts have been made to discover the predictors of improvement with UPPP but these have also produced conflicting results. It is impossible, at present, to give confidant guidance on selection procedures and its current role in the management of sleep apnoea syndrome is therefore small. The consensus approach is to consider UPPP for OSA only in non-obese patients without retrognathia and who cannot tolerate nCPAP.

Maxillo-facial surgery

There have been various other experimental surgical approaches to OSA. Attempts to advance the hyoid bone to enlarge the space behind the tongue have not proved to be successful in the long-term. Some success has been obtained in highly selected patients by advancing both the mandible and the maxilla.

Gastroplasty

This operation is occasionally used for very obese patients. It produces an inextensible pouch at the top of the stomach so that over-eating leads to regurgitation. Although surgery on such obese patients can be hazardous, the effect on weight and OSA is often dramatic.

Consequences of Obstructive Sleep Apnoea

Sleep deprivation

Most complications are secondary to sleep deprivation. The sleepiness of sleep apnoea syndrome may be seen as disinterest and can lead to employment problems and marital disharmony. The driving accident rate in patients with sleep apnoea syndrome seems to be between 5 and 10 times normal and there are good data showing that OSA patients perform poorly on simulated driving tests. Sleepiness while driving is probably under-reported because individuals fear the loss of their driving licence. It is surprisingly common for patients completing the Epworth Sleepiness Scale (Figure 2) to score a maximum three for every situation except the final question relating to driving which they score at zero.

Driving regulations

In the UK, the Driver and Vehicle Licensing Agency (DVLA) regulations state that driving must cease if the driver is excessively sleepy (from any cause). Group 1 drivers (ordinary licence holders) with a diagnosis of sleep apnoea syndrome should notify the DVLA, but can drive provided their sleepiness is controlled by treatment. Group 2 drivers (public service and heavy goods vehicles) should cease driving until it has been confirmed by a specialist that their condition is adequately treated. In the USA, the Department of Transportation makes similar recommendations, but the legal obligation of the treating physician varies from state to state with either mandatory or permissive (at physicians discretion) reporting of patients with sleep apnoea syndrome and consequent impairing driving ability.

Daytime ventilatory failure

Approximately 10% of patients with severe OSA develop daytime hypercapnia and cor pulmonale. This complication usually only develops in the presence of coincident lower airway obstruction due to COPD or asthma or very severe obesity (causing a restrictive respiratory defect). The airways obstruction may not be particularly severe and when assessing patients with lung disease and hypercapnia disproportionate to the impairment in their lung function, it is always worth considering the presence of coexistent OSA.[10] In such cases arterial CO_2 should return to normal when the OSA is treated with nCPAP.

The acute haemodynamic effects of OSA

The acute effects of OSA on nocturnal blood pressure are due to both increasing respiratory effort and arousal from sleep.[11] Each frustrated inspiratory effort lowers the intrathoracic pressure, which is transmitted along the arterial tree as swings in systolic blood pressure (pulsus paradoxus). The overall mean blood pressure may rise a little across the apnoea but the main rise occurs with the arousal from sleep that occurs at the end of the apnoea. This lasts about 10–20 seconds. Thus, there is a very characteristic beat-to-beat blood pressure profile which is virtually diagnostic of OSA (Figure 7).

The long-term cardiovascular consequences of OSA

The long-term effects of OSA on the systemic circulation and vascular risk remain a subject of heated debate. The acute haemodynamic responses discussed above elevate nocturnal blood pressure, but whether this alone leads to systemic vascular damage

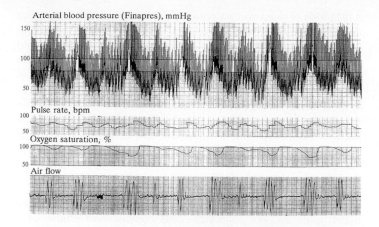

Figure 7.   Five minute recording of blood pressure, pulse rate, oxygen saturation and airflow to show the effect of OSA on blood pressure. The large rises in blood pressure with the end of each apnoea are due to brief arousal from sleep and the transient dips are due to frustrated inspiratory efforts (pulsus paradoxus)

is unproved. Patients with OSA also have a high prevalence of daytime systemic hypertension, but how much of this is due to the disease itself and how much is due to the confounding central obesity and smoking which are common in adult sufferers of this disease has proven very difficult to disentangle. At present we are lacking the carefully designed studies needed to show if snoring and OSA are truly an independent risk factor for cardiovascular morbidity and mortality.

Out-patient Assessment

A suggested algorithm for the assessment of patients with snoring or sleep apnoea is shown in Figure 8 and the following is a guide to what should be included in the out-patient letter to the GP or referring consultant:

- an outline of the patient's main problem (most commonly either snoring or daytime sleepiness). This is important as these symptoms are central to the decisions regarding management
- an assessment of severity of daytime sleepiness including an opinion on fitness to drive

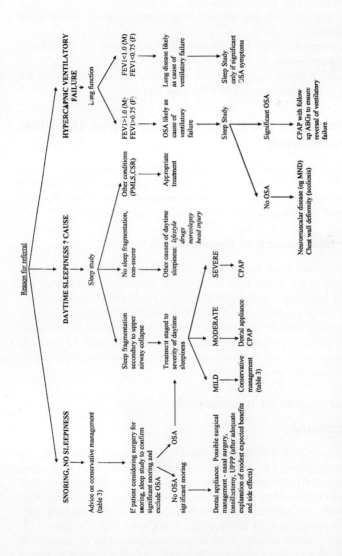

Figure 8. Suggested algorithm for the assessment of patients with snoring or sleep apnoea according to the patient's primary complaint

- any complications of disease such as respiratory failure
- an assessment of aetiological factors, including obesity, tonsilar hypertrophy and retrognathia
- a comment on the severity of abnormality seen on the sleep study
- treatment advice e.g. conservative management, mandibular advancement device, nCPAP etc
- advice given to the patient, including advice for driving for group 1 and group 2 drivers (see above)

Differential Diagnosis of Excessive Daytime Somnolence

Daytime hypersomnia is one of the two main symptoms of sleep apnoea syndrome, therefore an understanding of other causes of this symptom is important. Most commonly this is due to effects of lifestyle (extrinsic causes) rather than a specific disorder.

Extrinsic causes of hypersomnia

Rotating shift work (particularly when the sleep period is brought forward to an earlier time of day) and inadequate sleep time e.g. due to job, offspring etc. will inevitably lead to daytime sleepiness. CNS stimulant drugs (nicotine and caffeine) can suppress or fragment sleep, and alcohol produces a rebound alertness as the blood levels fall and the sedative effects wear off. This leads to the early morning wakening of a hangover and secondary sleepiness due to an inadequate period of sleep.

Other causes of hypersomnia

Narcolepsy

This condition is a disorder of rapid eye movement (REM) or dream sleep regulation and is much less common than obstructive sleep apnoea. The prevalence of classical narcolepsy is about 1 in 40 000. The usual presenting symptom is overwhelming daytime sleepiness, although, in contrast to sleep apnoea syndrome, the daytime naps can be restorative. It is invariably associated with cataplexy, the sudden onset of general muscle weakness provoked in response to an exciting event or emotion. The ability to elicit a good history of cataplexy is therefore an essential skill for the respiratory sleep physician! Cataplexy is characterised by a sudden development of muscle weakness, triggered by an emotional stimulus (typically laughing at a joke). The weakness may be partial and affect the legs ("I go weak at the knees") or arms ("I dare not carry a drink at a party in case someone tells a joke"). Slurring of the voice and myoclonic twitching of the face in association with this are particularly characteristic. The patient will often not freely volunteer a history of these rather peculiar symptoms and it should be sought. Other narcoleptic features are: paralysis on waking from sleep, often associated with intense fear, above average dream recall and hallucinations at sleep onset. These features are only supportive of the diagnosis and not diagnostic. In particular, sleep paralysis is an occasional symptom in otherwise normal subjects.

Narcolepsy has the highest human leukocyte antigen (HLA) association of any disorder and 98% of all Caucasian narcolepsy patients have HLA DQB*0602 (DQ6). Unfortunately, this antigen is present in approximately 23% of the normal population and so is only useful in excluding, and not confirming, a diagnosis. The HLA association of narcolepsy is significantly weaker in West Indian ethnic groups.

The treatment of narcolepsy is largely beyond the remit of this book but includes: regular daytime prophylactic naps, tricyclic antidepressants and CNS stimulant drugs.

Period Movement of the Legs (PMLS)

In this disorder, recurrent brief movements of the legs, or less commonly the arms, causes recurrent arousal from sleep. When severe, this sleep fragmentation has the same effect as that of sleep apnoea syndrome and presents with daytime sleepiness. Milder PMLS may present with poor and disturbed sleep (as can mild OSA) where the arousals interrupt continuous sleep without occurring sufficiently frequently to precipitate daytime sleepiness. If sleep apnoea and PMLS are both present it can be difficult to know whether the movements are due to arousal from sleep or are causing it. This can be determined by a trial of nCPAP. If the movements are secondary to arousals triggered by airway incompetence they will cease when airway patency is maintained with nCPAP. The prevalence of PMLS increases with age and it is often asymptomatic, when it is of no significance. If treatment is needed, clonazepam is effective, working by suppressing the arousals from sleep and increasing sleep related muscle relaxation.

Post-traumatic hypersomnia

Traumatic brain injury (stroke, neurosurgery, accidental injury) may be followed by a period of excessive daytime somnolence which can persist. It is a diagnosis of exclusion in association with a relevant brain injury and successful treatment is difficult.

Recurrent hypersomnia (Kleine-Levin Syndrome)

This is a rare condition characterised by recurrent episodes of hypersomnia (lasting a few days to a few weeks) in male adolescents associated with binge-eating and hyper-sexuality. The condition gradually improves and the ultimate prognosis is said to be good.

Idiopathic hypersomnia

This progressive disorder is essentially a diagnosis of exclusion in a patient with unquestionable sleepiness with no other cause found. The presentation is similar to narcolepsy but with no features of cataplexy, sleep paralysis or sleep onset dreaming.

Variants of Sleep Apnoea

Snoring

Many subjects with pharyngeal collapsibility causing snoring do not have recurrent arousal from sleep in association with this. There is usually no history of daytime sleepiness and the main aim of treatment is to reduce snoring. Conservative approaches to this problem are discussed above (conservative management) and shown in Table 3. If these are unsuccessful then a dental device will reduce the snoring and may prevent it completely. If there is an obvious problem with a partially obstructed nasal airway, corrective nasal surgery may offer some improvement.

Uvulopalatopharyngoplasty (UPPP) may also be performed for snoring although, as discussed above, it is difficult to predict the patients for whom this operation is likely to be successful. UPPP is unlikely to cure snoring and early data show that, on average, measured snoring volume is reduced only by about 25%.

Snoring induced arousals

In some snorers, the increase in inspiratory effort required to breathe through a partially collapsed pharyngeal airway will, on occasions, lead to arousal from sleep and sleep fragmentation. These subjects have very few dips in oxygen saturation, apnoeas or hypopnoeas, but may have daytime sleepiness due to disturbed sleep. Treatment for this is similar to obstructive sleep apnoea and depends on the severity of daytime sleepiness. A staged approach is best, trying simple conservative measures initially or a dental device. If these measures are unsuccessful then symptoms will respond to nCPAP.

Central supine variant of OSA

This variant of obstructive sleep apnoea tends to occur in subjects with less severe sleep apnoea. There is usually a history of snoring and daytime sleepiness suggestive of OSA but the sleep study may show apnoeas without continuing respiratory efforts when supine. More typical snoring or sleep apnoea is usually present in a lateral position. The supine central variant of OSA can be recognised using the sleep study video by a characteristic airway opening noise heard at the end of each apnoea. The physiology of this condition is thought to be due to an inhibition of respiratory drive by pharyngeal collapse in the supine posture. Interestingly, topical anaesthesia of the pharynx reverses this phenomenon — producing typical sleep apnoea. Therefore, it is assumed that sensory afferents from the pharyngeal mucosa are important in triggering this response. Treatment with nCPAP corrects this abnormality.

Laryngeal sleep apnoea

This rare variant of sleep apnoea occurs when upper airway obstruction during sleep is due to laryngeal closure secondary to denervation, rather than pharyngeal collapse. There may be a history of inspiratory stridor during sleep and a story from the patient/partner of 'not ordinary snoring' is worth pursuing. Other symptoms include daytime hypersomnolence, morning headaches and confusion, sometimes with hypercapnia. Causes may be central e.g. Shy-Drager syndrome, Arnold-Chiari malformation and syringobulbia, or peripheral e.g. damage to the laryngeal nerves during thyroid surgery.

Nocturnal laryngeal spasm

The history is usually very suggestive of this diagnosis which is most commonly due to nocturnal acid reflux onto the vocal cords causing acute stridor. The patient suddenly awakes from sleep in a panic, unable to breathe with characteristic stridorous breathing. Symptoms usually take 2 or 3 minutes to settle. Treatment is aimed at controlling gastro-oesophageal reflux with antacids and conservative measures such as raising the head of the bed.

Paediatric Aspects of Obstructive Sleep Apnoea

Obstructive sleep apnoea can occur in children and is usually caused by enlarged tonsils or enlarged adenoids. Rarer causes include micrognathia (Pierre Robin syndrome), craniosynosostoses (Creuzon's and Apert's syndrome), mucopolysaccharidoses (Hunter's and Hurler's syndromes), obesity (Prader-Willi syndrome) and Down's syndrome. Sleepiness does affect these children but their symptoms are often less specific than in adults, for example hyperactivity, bad behaviour, poor school performance, enuresis and restless sleep. Tonsillectomy is nearly always curative where tonsilar enlargement is the cause and can be helpful even if there is an alternative explanation such as a craniosynostosis. The beneficial effects of tonsillectomy in childhood sleep apnoea on behaviour and functioning have been confirmed in one controlled trial.[12] With some of these rarer causes of childhood OSA, tonsillectomy is inadequate and nCPAP or more complex maxillo-facial surgery may be required.

Central Sleep Apnoea

The problems discussed above relate to the consequences of sleep-induced narrowing of the upper airway. This section considers sleep-induced apnoeas where the problem appears to be unstable or reduced ventilatory drive during sleep.

Primary failure of ventilatory drive

Congenital absence of respiratory drive mechanisms (Ondine's Curse*) is extremely rare and usually presents in the first weeks of

---

* Ondine is a mythical wood nymph who cursed her mortal lover to be unable to don anything without thinking of her (and hence to breathe while asleep) when he allowed his amorous attentions to wander in her absence.

life with cyanosis and seizures particularly during sleep. Treatment is very difficult and respiratory stimulants are usually ineffective. Assisted respiration may be required, particularly at night.

Secondary failure of ventilatory pump

This is caused by inefficiency of the respiratory pump and includes neuromuscular weakness or chest wall disease (polio, motor neurone disease, scoliosis, thoracoplasty, etc.). Patients hypoventilate as the respiratory drive falls with sleep, particularly during REM sleep. This leads to daytime ventilatory failure. Nocturnal ventilatory support reverses the respiratory failure and corrects sleep disruption. This subject is covered in more detail in Chapter 7.

Unstable Ventilatory Drive

The fall in overall ventilatory drive at sleep onset can destabilise the complex control of respiration. Periodic or Cheyne-Stokes breathing occurs when the feedback loop controlling respiration has an excessive gain or delay.[13] Contributing factors include excessive central drive levels (CNS disease), circulatory delay (heart failure), hypoxaemia, hypocapnia, and arousal from sleep (high altitude). Many cases are asymptomatic, but sometimes symptoms develop which include daytime sleepiness and restless sleep, as well as symptoms of the primary causative disease. Sleep studies show apnoeas without continuing respiratory effort and breathing shows the classical waxing and waning of ventilation. Treatment is unjustified in the absence of symptoms. For patients with symptoms the first intervention is optimal control of heart failure, but where symptoms persist, overnight oxygen, acetazolamide and even nCPAP have been advocated. The evidence that the first two options are effective is debatable. Nasal CPAP improves the haemodynamics of heart failure and so may help, but is often badly tolerated on a long term basis.

Further Reading

1. Davies RJO, Stradling JR. The Epidemiology of Sleep Apnoea. *Thorax* 1996;**51**(suppl 2):S65–70

2. McNamara SAG, Grunstein RR, Sullivan CE. Obstructive sleep apnoea. *Thorax* 1993;**48**:754–64

3. Sullivan CE, Issa FG, Berthon-Jones M, Eves L. Reversal of obstructive sleep apnoea by continuous positive airway pressure applied through the nares. *Lancet* 1981;**1**:862–5

4. Engleman HM, Martin SE, Deary IJ, Douglas NJ. Effect of continuous positive airway pressure treatment on daytime function in sleep apnoea/hypopnoea syndrome. *Lancet* 1994;**343**:572–575

5. Grunstein RR. Sleep-related breathing disorders: 5 – Nasal continuous positive airway pressure treatment for obstructive sleep apnoea. *Thorax* 1995;**50**:1106–13

6. Practice parameters for the indications for polysomnography and related procedures. *Sleep* 1997;**20**:406–422

7. Douglas NJ, Thomas S, Jan MA. Clinical value of polysomnography. *Lancet* 1992;**339**:347–350

8. Bennett LS, Langford BA, Stradling JR, Davies RJO. Sleep fragmentation indices as predictors of daytime sleepiness and nCPAP response in OSA. *Am J Respir Crit Care Med* 1998;in press.

9. Royal College of Physicians working party (S Semple JG, N Douglas and J Stradling). Sleep apnoea and related conditions: recommendations for service provision. London: Royal College of Physicians 1993

10. Chaouat A, Weitzenblum E, Krieger J, Oswald M, Kessler R. Pulmonary hemodynamics in the obstructive sleep apnea syndrome. Results in 220 consecutive patients. *Chest* 1996;**109**:380–6

11. Working group on OSA and hypertension: Carlson J, Davies R, Ehlenz K, Grunstein R, Hedner J, Podszus T, Sinoway L, Stradling, JR, Telakivi T, Zwillich C. Obstructive sleep apnea and blood pressure elevation. What is the relationship? *Blood Pressure* 1993;**2**: 166–182

12. Ali NJ, Pitson D, Stradling JR. Sleep disordered breathing: effects of adenotonsillectomy on behaviour and psychological functioning. *Eur J Pediatr* 1996;**155**:56–62

13. Khoo MCK, Gottschalk A, Pack AI. Sleep-induced periodic breathing and apnea: a theoretical study. *J Appl Physiol* 1991;**70**:2014–24

9

Pulmonary Vascular Disease

Nicholas Morrell

Introduction

At birth, with closure of the ductus arteriosus, the entire cardiac output must pass through the lungs. The pulmonary circulation becomes vital to the survival of the organism by regulating delivery of deoxygenated blood to the alveolar capillaries where gas exchange occurs. The structure of the pulmonary circulation is dictated by certain constraints. Firstly, red blood cells must be allowed adequate time in the alveolar capillary for haemoglobin to bind oxygen. Secondly, since the gas exchange barrier is thin, alterations in blood flow must be achieved without any great increase in capillary hydrostatic pressure. Thirdly, to optimize arterial oxygenation, regional perfusion must be closely matched to regional ventilation. The normal pulmonary circulation, therefore, is a high-flow, low pressure vascular bed that can accommodate large increases in cardiac output with relatively little increase in pulmonary arterial pressure. At rest the normal pulmonary arterial pressure is approximately 1/5 of systemic arterial pressure, or about 25/15mmHg, with a mean of 17mmHg.

Pulmonary Hypertension

Pulmonary arterial hypertension is defined as a mean pulmonary artery pressure in excess of 25mmHg at rest or 30mmHg on exercise. Generally, there are three main causes of an increased pulmonary arterial pressure (P_{PA}); these are

- an increased pulmonary vascular resistance (PVR)
- increased pulmonary blood flow (CO = cardiac output)
- raised left atrial pressure (P_{LA}), or pulmonary artery wedge pressure.

These factors are related by the following equation:

$$PVR = \frac{P_{PA} - P_{LA}}{CO}$$

Table 1 lists the conditions that lead to pulmonary hypertension by alteration of these factors.

Table 1. Classification of pulmonary hypertension

Increased pulmonary vascular resistance
Primary pulmonary hypertension
Chronic hypoxia
    chronic lung disease
    thoracic musculoskeletal disease
    residence at high altitude
Pulmonary embolism
    thromboembolism
    foreign body embolism from intravenous drugs
    amniotic fluid embolism
    tumour embolism
Collagen and autoimmune diseases
    SLE
    mixed connective tissue disease
    CREST syndrome
    rheumatoid arthritis
Sickle cell disease
Pulmonary vascular toxins e.g. appetite-suppressants, rape-seed oil
HIV infection
Arteritis e.g. Takayasu's disease
Parasitic lung disease e.g. schistosomiasis
Hepatic cirrhosis
Pulmonary haemangioendotheliomatosis

Increased pulmonary blood flow
Ventricular septal defect (VSD)
Double outflow right ventricle (DORV)
A-V canal
Truncus arteriosus

Table 1.   Continued

Aortopulmonary defect
Patent ductus arteriosus
Transposition of the great arteries with left to right shunt
Double inlet ventricle
Tricuspid atresia with large VSD
Atrial septal defect (ASD)
Ostium primum
Common atrium
Hemianomolous pulmonary venous drainage
Total anomalous pulmonary venous drainage
Pulmonary atresia with large congenital systemic collaterals

Elevated pulmonary venous pressure
All causes of left ventricular failure
Congential heart disease
    congenital pulmonary venous stenoses
    obstructive anomalous pulmonary venous drainage
    cortriatrium
Mitral valve disease
Aortic valve disease
Left atrial myxoma
Left atrial thrombus
Pulmonary veno-occlusive disease
Venous thrombosis secondary to neoplastic disease

Primary Pulmonary Hypertension

Epidemiology

Primary, or idiopathic, pulmonary hypertension (PPH) is rare with an annual incidence of approximately 1 per 500 000 in Europe and the US. This gives an estimated incidence of about 50 new cases per year in the UK. It tends to affect women (F:M sex ratio = 2.3:1), especially in the reproductive years and is a progressive, often fatal disorder with a mean survival of only 2.8 years from diagnosis.

Aetiology

The underlying cause of PPH remains unknown but a number of environmental and genetic factors may contribute to the pathogenesis. Recent studies have shown a clear association with appetite suppressant drugs, particularly of the fenfluramine/dexfenfluramine group, though this association was originally noted in the 1970's with the amphetamine-like, aminorex fumarate. There is also an association with the ingestion of Spanish toxic rape seed oil. An immunogenetic basis for the condition is suggested by the association with certain HLA markers (HLA-DR3, DRW52,DQW2). Antinuclear antibodies occur in 30–40% of patients. There is a familial form of the disease (approximately 6% of all cases) with autosomal dominant inheritance with incomplete penetrance. Recent family studies have localized the gene to the long arm of chromosome 2.

It is likely that endothelial cell dysfunction contributes to the pathogenesis, since there is evidence for a deficiency of endothelial derived vasodilators such as nitric oxide and prostacyclin, and an increase in the vasoconstrictors endothelin-1, serotonin, angiotensin II and thromboxane A_2.

Pathology

The pathological finding in cases of unexplained pulmonary hypertension is primary plexogenic arteriopathy. Appearances include increased muscularisation of small (<200μm diameter) arteries and thickening or fibrosis of the intima, both of which contribute to vascular obliteration. In more severe cases dilatation of small arterioles is seen, and sometimes fibrinoid necrosis. The most characteristic lesion is the plexiform lesion (200–400mm diameter) which consists of a plexus of capillary-like channels adjacent to a small pulmonary artery. These changes, although typical, are not pathognomonic of PPH, since they may also be observed in cases of severe secondary pulmonary hypertension, such as that due to congenital heart disease. The diagnosis of PPH, therefore, remains one of exclusion on clinical grounds.

Clinical features

A summary of the main points to elicit when taking a history from a patient with unexplained pulmonary hypertension is given in Table 2.

Symptoms

The main symptoms are dyspnoea, chest pain and syncope. The disease usually follows an insidious course with mild symptoms of exertional dyspnoea often being ignored by the patient. Delay in

Table 2. Unexplained pulmonary hypertension: important points in the history

Country of origin e.g. schistosomiasis, toxic substances, high altitude, sickle cell
Family history of pulmonary hypertension or unexplained "cardiac" death
Obstetric history e.g. miscarriages and abortions
Contraceptive pill
Cigarette smoking and pack years
Alcohol consumption
Previous episodes of jaundice
Appetite-suppressant drugs
Past history of venous thromboembolism
Symptoms of connective tissue disease e.g. Raynauds phenomenon
Thyroid disease
HIV risk factors
Recent viral illness

diagnosis frequently occurs because the patient is labelled as having some other lung disease. The severity of dyspnoea can be graded according to the New York Heart Association (NYHA) functional class (Table 3). As expected, patients with NYHA grade III-IV have a poorer prognosis than patients in grade I-II. Syncope is an ominous sign, usually reflecting severe right ventricular dysfunction. Other symptoms related to right ventricular failure include lassitude, abdominal swelling from ascites and ankle swelling. Small haemoptyses may occur in the later stages. There is an association with Raynauds phenomenon.

Signs

The patient is often tachypnoeic at rest. Peripheral cyanosis is common due to a low cardiac output reflected in cold extremities, tachycardia and a low volume pulse. Central cyanosis occurs later

Table 3. New York Heart Association functional classification of symptoms

Class I	Cardiac disease without dyspnoea on ordinary effort
Class II	Minor limitation of activity by dyspnoea
Class III	Marked limitation of activity by dyspnoea
Class IV	Dyspnoea at rest or on minimal exertion

as pulmonary gas exchange deteriorates, or right to left shunting occurs through a patent foramen ovale. The jugular venous pulse is usually elevated with a prominent 'a' wave, reflecting the increased force of right atrial contraction, or if tricuspid regurgitation is present, a large 'V' wave. A left parasternal heave may be present. On auscultation, a right ventricular third heart sound, often with an (atrial) fourth heart sound may be heard. With significant pulmonary hypertension, forceful closure of the pulmonary valve leads to an accentuated, often palpable, pulmonary arterial component of the second heart sound. A soft systolic murmur of tricuspid regurgitation is often present increasing during inspiration, though the murmur may sometimes be due to flow across the pulmonary valve. A diastolic murmur due to pulmonary regurgitation is sometimes heard. Jaundice, ascites and peripheral oedema may be present.

Investigation

The investigation of the patient with suspected PPH involves 1) the exclusion of other underlying causes of pulmonary hypertension (Table 2) and 2) an assessment of the severity of the disease for prognosis and treatment. Investigations useful in identifying the aetiology of newly diagnosed, unexplained pulmonary hypertension are listed in Table 4. A general outline for evaluation and treatment of patients with PH is shown in Figure 1.

Blood tests

Routine bloods, including full blood count, ESR, clotting and biochemistry should be performed to exclude any coexisting or associated diseases. Liver and renal function may be disturbed in advanced disease. Hypo- and hyperthyroidism are reported associations. Autoantibody screen should include ANA and ENAs to exclude underlying collagen vascular disease. Although an unusual cause of isolated pulmonary hypertension, evidence for vasculitis should be sought from antineutrophil cytoplasmic antibodies (ANCA). Since there is an increased incidence of unexplained pulmonary hypertension in HIV positive patients (0.5%), this diagnosis should be considered.

Chest X-ray

The most common finding on chest x-ray (CXR) is enlargement of the proximal pulmonary arteries. The enlarged pulmonary trunk

Table 4.   Investigation of the patient with unexplained pulmonary hypertension

Full blood count/film/differential
Hb electrophoresis
Urea and electrolytes
Liver function including gamma GT
Thyroid function
Thrombophilia screen
    Antithrombin III
    Protein C
    Protein S
    Factor V Leiden
    Anti-cardiolipin antibody
    Lupus anticoagulant
CMV deaff
Autoantibodies
    RhF
    ANA
    ENAs
    anti-dsDNA
    anti-cardiolipin IgG and IgM
    anti-SM/anti-SCL/anti-SS
    complement C3,C4,CH50
    ANCA
Serum angiotensin converting enzyme
Hepatitis screen
HIV test

Urine microscopy
Chest X-ray
ECG
Pulmonary function tests
Exercise tests with saturation monitoring
    e.g. 6 minute walk, cycle ergometry, ventilatory exercise test
Arterial blood gases on air
Ventilation-perfusion lung scan
Echocardiogram
High resolution and spiral CT
Abdominal ultrasound ?cirrhosis
Diagnostic cardiac catheterization

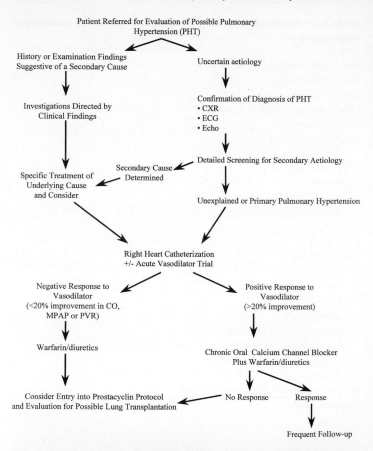

Figure 1. General outline for evaluation and treatment of patients with pulmonary hypertension

causes a prominent convexity between the aortic knuckle and the upper left border of the heart. The proximal right and left main pulmonary arteries are enlarged, sometimes mistaken for hilar lymphadenopathy, and peripheral pruning of the pulmonary vascular pattern occurs, giving rise to increased peripheral radiolucency. On the other hand in pulmonary hypertension caused by high flow from a left to right intracardiac shunt the lung fields may appear plethoric, though with the advent of severe pulmonary hypertension and shunt reversal (Eisenmenger's syndrome) vascular pruning supervenes. If heart failure is present the heart may be enlarged and enlargement of the right atrium can be seen. The appearance of the lung fields may provide clues to underlying parenchymal lung disease.

The electrocardiogram

In symptomatic PPH the electrocardiogram is abnormal in about 90% of cases. The ECG typically shows right axis deviation and right ventricular hypertrophy. Tall peaked P waves in the right precordial and inferior leads denotes right atrial enlargement. Right bundle branch block (RBBB) is common.

Other clues to the presence of underlying cardiac disease include bifid P waves in V1 in mitral stenosis. Right bundle branch block asociated with an rsR' pattern in V1 suggests an ostium secundum atrial septal defect, whereas RBBB with a leftward axis in a young patient points to an ostium primum atrial septal defect.

Lung function tests

Measurements of spirometry and diffusing capacity are essential. In PPH the lung volumes (FEV_1 and VC) are usually normal or mildly reduced, with often marked impairment of the TL_{CO} and K_{CO}.

Arterial blood gases

Arterial hypoxaemia is a feature of pulmonary hypertension secondary to lung disease or thromboembolic disease. An elevated PCO_2 points to underlying airflow obstruction rather than a primary vascular disease. Patients with PPH may show only mild degrees of resting hypoxaemia early in the course of the disease. However, with progression of the disease severe hypoxaemia supervenes with further deterioration on exercise. Failure of the oxygen saturation to normalize when breathing 100% oxygen points to the presence of an intracardiac shunt.

Nocturnal oxygen saturation monitoring

Patients with normal daytime oxygen saturation may develop significant nocturnal hypoxaemia if they suffer from obstructive sleep apnoea (OSA). Although it is unusual to develop pulmonary hypertension secondary to pure OSA, the incidence is increased in patients with co-existing obstructive airways disease.

Ventilation-perfusion lung scan

In PPH the pattern of ventilation is usually normal though small patchy perfusion abnormalities may be present. In thromboembolic pulmonary hypertension there are larger segmental perfusion defects indistinguishable from the pattern of acute pulmonary embolism. The chronic nature of the changes can be demonstrated by the failure of the perfusion defects to resolve after two weeks on anticoagulants.

Echocardiography

Two-dimensional echocardiography in conjunction with Doppler techniques can be used to detect the presence and direction of intracardiac shunts and an estimate can be made of the severity of pulmonary hypertension provided that tricuspid regurgitation is present. The velocity of the tricuspid regurgitant jet can be calculated using Doppler allowing the systolic pulmonary artery pressure to be calculated. A qualitative assessment of right venticular function can also be made. Classically, there is dilatation of the right sided chambers and ventricular and septal hypertrophy. Paradoxical septal movement may be apparent.

CT Thorax

A spiral computerized tomographic (CT) scan and a high resolution CT scan with the patient prone are recommended. The spiral contrast-enhanced CT will detect proximal pulmonary arterial obstruction suggestive of acute or chronic thromboembolic disease. The high resolution scan will pick up unsuspected parenchymal abnormalities, such as fibrosis.

Right heart catheterization

Right heart and pulmonary artery catheterization are carried out 1) to assess the severity of pulmonary hypertension, 2) to determine whether the elevated pressure is due to elevation of pulmonary artery wedge pressure, 3) to exclude left to right shunts, 4) to assess vasoreactivity and predict response to treatment, and 5) to visualize pulmonary artery anatomy by contrast angiography.

i. **Measurement of severity of pulmonary hypertension** Right heart catheterization is essential in all patients with suspected PPH. This allows confirmation of the diagnosis of pulmonary hypertension, exclusion of occult congenital heart disease, and gives important prognostic information. Measurements are usually made with a Swan-Ganz catheter inserted through the internal jugular route with the tip positioned in a descending branch of the pulmonary artery. Measurements are made of mixed venous oxygen saturation (SvO_2), pulmonary arterial pressure (P_{PA}), right atrial pressure (P_{RA}), cardiac output (CO) and the approximation of left atrial pressure (P_{LA}), pulmonary artery wedge pressure. This allows the calculation of pulmonary vascular resistance (PVR) using the same equation as shown above. Cardiac index (CI) is calculated by dividing CO by the body surface area in m^2. Generally, a mean P_{PA} of 85mmHg or more, and a cardiac index of $2l/min/m^2$ or less are associated with a poor prognosis. An SvO_2 of <63% is associated with a 3 year survival of only 17%, whereas SvO_2 of ≥63% is associated with a 55% survival over the same time period.

ii. **Vasodilator trial** Although breathing 100% oxygen has traditionally been part of an acute vasodilator trial it is of limited usefulness in patients with PPH. With oxygen, the pulmonary artery pressure may fall slightly because the cardiac output falls, with no change in pulmonary vascular resistance. A more important test is to determine whether the pulmonary vascular resistance falls in response to a vasodilator such as prostacyclin or nifedipine. Many centres favour a titrated prostacyclin infusion to assess vascular reactivity, since a significant fall in pulmonary vascular resistance (>30%) seems to predict the acute and chronic response to calcium channel blockers. Alternatively, intravenous adenosine is also advocated for acute assessment of vasodilatation or inhalation of nitric oxide.

iii. **Pulmonary arterial angiography** Contrast angiography should be considered in all patients in whom a diagnosis of chronic thromboembolic pulmonary hypertension is suspected, especially if referral for heart-lung transplantation or thromboendarterectomy is being considered. In primary pulmonary hypertension angiography shows enlarged central arteries and tapering of peripheral vessels. In pulmonary hypertension secondary to chronic pulmonary emboli, signs suggestive of organized and recanalized chronic thromboemboli are seen.

Open lung biopsy

This is rarely indicated. Specific circumstances in which biopsy may be helpful are to confirm a diagnosis of veno-occlusive disease, or some other rarity such as schistosomiasis or pulmonary haemangio-endotheliomatosis.

Management

The management of patients with PPH is difficult, since the disease primarily affects young women, with a poor prognosis, for which presently there is no cure. All patients with suspected PPH are best referred to a specialist centre for initial assessment and follow-up. Such centres will have experience with initiating continuous intra-venous prostacyclin and expertise in the critical timing of heart-lung transplantation. Most of the debilitating symptoms of progressive pulmonary vascular obliteration stem from right ventricular failure and reduced cardiac output. The primary aim of medical manage-ment is to improve cardiac output by reducing pulmonary vascular resistance. In some patients there is a significant degree of reversible vasoconstriction, hence the use of vasodilators. However, it is now thought that long term use of some vasodilators may also reverse some of the structural remodelling of hypertensive pulmonary ar-teries.

The specific treatments are as follows:

Oxygen therapy

This is usually aimed at relief of symptomatic hypoxaemia, which may be worsened on exercise. Generally, strenuous exercise should be discouraged, since this can greatly increase right ventricular work by increasing pulmonary arterial pressure.

Diuretics

These may be helpful in patients with right heart failure and periph-eral oedema or ascites. However, they should be used cautiously to avoid an abrupt fall in right ventricular filling pressure, which may lead to systemic hypotension and renal failure. Renal function should be monitored regularly.

Vasodilators

A number of different vasodilators have been tried in the treatment of pulmonary hypertension. No vasodilator is specific for the pul-monary circulation, though some (e.g. nitric oxide and prostacyclin) can be inhaled, and all may produce a more profound fall in systemic rather than pulmonary arterial pressure. In some patients this may be catastrophic, with systemic hypotension leading to an increased cardiac output and acute worsening of pulmonary hypertension resulting in right ventricular failure. The danger of vasodilators in these patients necessitates an acute trial of therapy in the catheter lab as outline above. The most successful vasodilators are the calcium channel blockers such as nifedipine and diltiazem. About 25% of patients with PPH respond acutely with a marked fall in pulmonary vascular resistance and have a dramatically improved survival (95% at 5 years) compared with patients who do not respond (55% at 5 years). The recommended dose of calcium channel blocker is much higher than that usually recommended for the treatment of systemic hypertension or angina (e.g. 720mg diltiazem daily).

Anticoagulation

All patients with primary or severe secondary pulmonary hypertension should be anticoagulated in the absence of contraindications. Studies have shown that treatment with warfarin improves survival in patients with PPH, especially in patients who do not respond to calcium channel blockers. In these patients, warfarin increased the 5 year survival from 31% to 47%. The INR should be maintained between 2 and 3. In patients with thromboembolic pulmonary hypertension the INR should be between 3 and 4.

Prostacyclin

Prostacyclin is a naturally occurring metabolite of arachidonic acid produced mainly by the vascular endothelium. It is a vasodilator and inhibits platelet aggregation. Prostacyclin can cause an acute fall in pulmonary vascular resistance when infused into the pulmonary artery of patients with PPH, though again its effects are not selective for the pulmonary circulation. If long term treatment with prostacyclin is considered, it must be given by continuous central infusion, usually via a Hickman catheter, since the half-life of the drug is only 2 minutes. Patients must be capable of changing their own infusion pumps. Side effects include diarrhoea and abdominal cramps, jaw ache, flushing and headaches. Interestingly, recent trials have shown that long term continuous intravenous prostacyclin improves survival and lowers pulmonary artery pressure in patients with PPH even in patients who exhibit no acute fall in pulmonary arterial pressure.

Lung transplantation

In the majority of PPH patients standard medical therapy will not halt or reverse the course of the disease and lung or heart-lung transplantation (HLT) offers the only hope of survival. In the UK, the majority of patients with PPH receive HLT, though advances in single lung and double lung transplantation will make these operations desirable, since the native right ventricle has a great capacity for recovery. In patients with PPH the timing of transplantation is crucial and a number of systems have been proposed to aid in the decision of when to recommend the operation. The objective indices at right heart catheterization which suggest a poor prognosis and should prompt immediate referral to a transplant surgeon are a right atrial pressure >6mmHg, a cardiac index of <2.8l/min/m2, and a pulmonary artery oxygen saturation of <63%.

Generally, survival after HLT for PPH is worse than for parenchymal lung disease. The mean 1 year survival in the UK is 61% at 1 year, and a 4 year survival of 39%. Death is usually due to anastomosis failure, infection or acute rejection in the early postoperative period, or the development of obliterative bronchiolitis, which affects 30% of patients in the long-term.

Secondary Pulmonary Hypertension

Causes

The commonest identifiable causes of pulmonary hypertension are alveolar hypoxia, pulmonary venous hypertension, or increased pulmonary artery flow in congenital left to right shunts. Some of the specific causes are listed in Table 1. Whatever the underlying condition, the development of secondary pulmonary hypertension is associated with an increased morbidity and mortality. Treatment is rarely directed specifically at secondary pulmonary hypertension, but at the underlying cause. Exceptions are pulmonary hypertension associated with the collagen vascular diseases such as scleroderma, and chronic thromboembolic pulmonary hypertension. As many as 40% of patients with scleroderma develop pulmonary hypertension, and it is frequently the cause of death in these patients. In this setting, treatment should be given as for primary pulmonary hypertension. In patients with chronic thromboembolic pulmonary hypertension, in addition to anticoagulation, patients should be considered for pulmonary thromboendarterectomy, which may be dramatically successful in selected patients.

Cor pulmonale

The WHO definition of cor pulmonale is right ventricular hypertrophy secondary to disease of the respiratory system. It should be remembered that this is a pathological diagnosis, and does not refer to the clinical entity of fluid retention in the face of hypoxaemia, for which it is commonly misused. Indeed the cause of fluid retention in hypoxic COPD is far from clear, and although right heart failure can occur in severe cases or during acute exacerbations, the majority of stable COPD patients with peripheral oedema have a normal or elevated cardiac output. Strictly speaking, cor pulmonale may result from any lung disease, (for a list see Table 5) but the commonest cause seen by the respiratory physician will be that secondary to chronic obstructive pulmonary disease (COPD), accounting for 90% of cases of cor pulmonale.

The true prevalence of pulmonary hypertension secondary to COPD is not known since right heart catheterization is seldom performed in these patients, though small studies have estimated the prevalence at between 5 and 40% in severe COPD. However, Doppler echocardiography now offers the opportunity to investigate larger numbers of patients. The prevalence of patients fulfilling the criteria for long-term oxygen therapy, who are most at risk of developing pulmonary hypertension, was estimated to be 0.3% of the population over the age of 45 around the area of Sheffield. Extrapolating to the United Kingdom as a whole this represents about 165,000 people who are in a "high risk" group for pulmonary hypertension secondary to COPD.

The presence and severity of pulmonary hypertension in patients with COPD clearly correlates with increased mortality. However, the extent to which pulmonary hypertension *per se* contributes to patient morbidity and mortality, independent of the degree of airflow obstruction, is still unclear. Generally the degree of pulmonary arterial hypertension in COPD is mild, though pressures may increase markedly during acute exacerbations, on exercise and during nocturnal desaturations.

Management of cor pulmonale in COPD

Currently, vasodilators have no established place in the management of pulmonary hypertension in COPD. The mainstay of treatment continues to be diuretics and long-term oxygen therapy. The benefit of more selective pulmonary vasodilators such as inhaled nitric oxide awaits further clarification.

Table 5.   Causes of cor pulmonale

Chronic obstructive pulmonary diseases
chronic bronchitis
emphysema
chronic asthma
cystic fibrosis
obliterative bronchiolitis
bronchiectasis

Diseases of the chest wall
neuromuscular diseases
      motor neurone disease
      myopathy
      bilateral diaphragmatic paralysis
kyphoscoliosis
thoracoplasty

Pulmonary fibrosis
sequelae of pulmonary tuberculosis
sarcoidosis
pneumoconiosis
drug-related lung diseases
extrinsic allergic alveolitis
connective tissue diseases
idiopathic interstitial pulmonary fibrosis

Obstruction of extrathoracic airways
Obstructive sleep apnoea
Tonsilar and adenoidal hypertrophy in children

Respiratory falure of central origin
central alveolar hypoventilation
obesity-hypoventilation syndrome

Pulmonary Embolism

Introduction

Pulmonary embolic disease is extremely common. Autopsy series from hospital populations have shown the presence of grossly visible embolism in up to 20% of patients. Recent studies have shown that pulmonary embolism (PE) was not suspected prior to death in up to 70% of patients in whom it was subsequently found to be the major cause of death. It has been estimated that the average district general hospital serving a population of 200,000 can expect to diagnose 50 cases of pulmonary embolism annually. The clinical diagnosis of PE without consideration of the results of special investigations can be likened to tossing a coin. Some clinicians continue to adopt this hit and miss approach, while others act inappropriately on the results of special investigations, such as ventilation-perfusion (V/Q) scans. Overdiagnosis of the condition can be just as dangerous as failing to make the diagnosis, because treatment with anticoagulants is associated with a significant risk of major haemorrhage. However, the eccentric management of these cases is both dangerous and unnecessary, since there are now large numbers of sound clinical studies on which a rational approach to PE diagnosis can be based, even in more difficult cases. An appreciation of the risk factors for venous thrombosis and an awareness of the circumstances in which prophylaxis can prevent many episodes is perhaps even more important

Predisposing factors

Table 6 summarizes the risk factors for PE and deep vein thrombosis (DVT). Over 90% of PEs arise from the deep veins of the legs and evidence suggests that it is virtually always proximal thrombosis (i.e. above the knee), that can result in embolism. However, 15% of below knee DVTs can propagate to the proximal veins and become a potential source of embolus. Most clinicians at present would probably not anticoagulate on the finding of thrombus confined to the calf veins, but would perform a Doppler ultrasound examination of the popliteal veins after a few days to ensure the absence of proximal extension.

An appreciation of the risk factors for PE helps to form a clinical judgement of the likelihood of PE, since one or more predisposing factors are found in 80–90% of patients. The commonest risk factors are prolonged immobilisation, a past history of venous thromboembolism, and recent surgery or fractures, particularly of the lower limb. The risk increases in direct proportion to the number of risk factors present.

Increased awareness of abdominal or lower limb orthopaedic surgery as considerable risk factors for venous thromboembolism has led to widely adopted preventive measures. For example major abdominal surgery (general anaesthesia lasting for more than 30 minutes) without prophylaxis is associated with a 7% incidence of

Table 6.   Major risk factors for venous thromboembolism

Surgery
    major abdominal/pelvic surgery
    hip/knee surgery
    postoperative intensive care

Obstetrics
    pregnancy/puerperium

Cardiorespiratory disease
    congestive heart failure
    myocardial infarction

Prolonged immobilization (bed rest ≥5 days)
    fracture
    stroke/spinal cord injury

Malignancy
    abdominal/pelvic
    advanced/metastatic
    concurrent chemotherapy or hormonal therapy

Thrombotic disorders
    factor V Leiden mutation
    lupus anticoagulant
    protein C and S deficiency
    antithrombin III deficiency

Miscellaneous
    Age ≥40 years
    Obesity
    Previous DVT or PE
    Multiple trauma
    Varicose veins

proximal DVT and 1.6% incidence of PE. Other high risk operations include coronary artery bypass, surgery for gynaecological malignancy, and major urological procedures. Lower extremity orthopaedic operations carry a particularly high risk. In patients undergoing elective hip surgery without prophylaxis the incidence of proximal DVT is about 20%, with a PE incidence of 5–10%. The incidence is even higher in patients undergoing knee replacement surgery. Over 90% of DVTs occur on the operated side.

The risk of venous thromboembolism associated with use of the oral contraceptive pill remains very small. The risk was higher in older preparations containing higher doses of oestrogen, and although the relative risk with current low dose formulations is about 2–4 times that in controls, the absolute risk remains small. It should be remembered that this is still considerably less than the risk of venous thromboembolism associated with pregnancy and the puerperium.

Increasingly important among risk factors is the recognition of prothrombotic disorders of coagulation. These include lupus anticoagulant, protein C and S deficiency, and antithrombin III deficiency. The factor V Leiden mutation (a substitution of arginine for glycine at amino acid position 506) is a recently described polymorphism in the factor V gene, conferring resistance to activated protein C, and is the commonest inherited cause of an underlying predisposition.

Which patients should be investigated for an underlying predisposition to venous thrombosis?

Venous thrombosis is so common that a search for an underlying cause in all patients presenting with DVT or PE is impractical. The Factor V Leiden mutation is so common in the general population that the value of routinely screening for this mutation in patients presenting with a first episode remains uncertain. However, young patients and patients with recurrent DVT/PE should be screened, especially in the absence of another readily identifiable risk factor e.g. postoperative, or trauma. The clinical setting may point to an associated diseases such as malignancy, nephrotic syndrome, myeloproliferative disease or inflammatory bowel disease. Although cancer is 2–3 times more likely to manifest in the 2 years following apparently idiopathic DVT, the risk is not sufficient to warrant intensive investigation, unless there are clues in the history and clinical examination.

Diagnosis of PE

Clinical features

It is well established that symptoms, clinical signs, and results of initial investigations such as serum enzymes, chest radiography, blood gases and ECG have neither sufficient sensitivity nor specificity to enable the diagnosis of PE to be confirmed or excluded. However, all the foregoing should be performed since they may suggest an alternative diagnosis. The differential diagnosis is wide but will include myocardial infarction, left ventricular failure, pericarditis, dissecting aneurysm, pneumothorax, pneumonia, and lobar collapse.

In a large study of patients with proven acute PE and no pre-existing cardiopulmonary disease the most common symptoms at presentation were dyspnoea (73%), pleuritic chest (66%) pain and cough (37%). Haemoptysis occurs in only about 10% of patients. Crushing central chest pain may occur, but uncommonly. The most common signs found in patients with PE are tachypnoea of 20/min (70%), crackles (51%), and tachycardia of >100/min (30%). Other signs which have been described are a 4th heart sound, an increased pulmonary component of the second heart sound, pyrexia of unknown origin, wheeze, pleural rub and cyanosis.

This clinical information helps to decide whether the diagnosis of PE should be entertained, but does not allow the differentiation of PE from other conditions, since there is no difference in the frequency of these signs and symptoms in patients with other acute respiratory diseases, compared to those with PE. However, a diagnosis of PE is extremely unlikely in the absence of dyspnoea, tachypnoea, or pleuritic chest pain, one or a combination of which occurs in 97% of patients with PE. As the foregoing applies to patients with no pre-existing cardiopulmonary disease it is obvious that clinical signs will be considerably less useful in the diagnosis of PE in patients with pre-existing chronic heart or lung disease.

The clinical presentation of PE

Patients with acute PE can be divided into 4 groups based on clinical presentation (Table 7):

1) *Circulatory collapse.* Patients present with hypotension or syncope. There may be overt signs of right ventricular failure with jugular vein engorgement. The ECG commonly shows the typical changes of right ventricular strain: an S wave in lead I, a Q wave in lead III, and T wave inversion in lead III with or without T wave inversion over the right ventricle (leads V_1 to V_3). Right bundle branch block is also common. Acute onset of atrial fibrillation with PE occurs rarely. Blood gas analysis shows marked hypoxaemia often with hypocapnia induced by hyperventilation. The degree of hypoxaemia roughly correlates with

Table 7. Main clinical presentations of pulmonary embolism

	Collapse, previously well	Pulmonary haemorrhage	Isolated dyspnoea	Collapse, poor reserve
Frequency	5%	60%	25%	10%
Pulmonary artery occlusion	Extensive	Small/ moderate	moderate/ large	small/ moderate
Examination	Acute right heart starin	May have localising signs	Tachypnoea	Unhelpful
Chest radiograph	Usually normal	Often suggestive	Usually normal	May be suggestive
ECG	Often acute right heart starin	Normal	Non-specific changes	Unhelpful
Arterial gas tensions	Markedly abnormal	May be normal	Usually abnormal	Unhelpful

the degree of vascular obstruction. A metabolic acidosis may be present if the cardiac output is severely compromised. This presentation of PE is a medical emergency, since 90% of patients with fatal embolism die within the first 1–2 hours after the event, the majority of which fall into this group. Urgent echocardiography (see below) may confirm acute right heart dysfunction.

2) **Pulmonary haemorrhage.** This group presents with pleuritic pain and/or haemoptysis. Since a relatively small cross-sectional area of the pulmonary vascular bed is occluded the ECG is usually normal, apart from a sinus tachycardia. Chest X-ray abnormalities are common such as linear atelectasis, parenchymal infiltrates, or a raised hemidiaphragm. A wedge-shaped, pleurally based opacity is well described but rare. It should be remembered that in patients with no pre-existing cardiopulmonary disease presenting with acute PE that the CXR is abnormal in 84% of patients. A small pleural effusion may also be present. Arterial blood gas tensions may be normal.

3) **Isolated dyspnoea.** Acute unexplained breathlessness in a patient with predisposing factors should always raise the possibility of acute PE. The chest X-ray is often normal and the ECG may show sinus tachycardia and non-specific T wave abnormalities.

4) **Collapse, with poor cardiopulmonary reserve.** This refers to patients with poor cardiopulmonary reserve due to pre-existing severe heart or lung disease. A small embolus can lead to rapid decompensation which is difficult to distinguish on clinical grounds from a deterioration in their underlying condition. Clearly, the results of investigations are often unhelpful in making the diagnosis in this group, and the V/Q scan is frequently non-diagnostic (see below).

The importance of assessing clinical likelihood of PE

The results of the large Prospective Investigation of Pulmonary Embolism Diagnosis (PIOPED) study have demonstrated that a clinical assessment of the likelihood of PE can be helpful in the interpretation of the results of special investigations such as the V/Q scan. This is particularly true when the clinical assessment and V/Q scan are concordant. For example the prevalence of proven PE in patients with a low or very low probability V/Q scan and a high clinical probability (more than 2 risk factors) was 21% in the PIOPED study, whereas patients with this V/Q classification and no risk factors had only a 4% chance of having proven PE. Unfortunately, patients with concordant V/Q and clinical probabilities represents a minority of patients with suspected PE (about 20%), and the large majority of patients will require further evaluation to confirm or refute the diagnosis.

It is worth considering here the common clinical setting of the young person in casualty, often a woman on oral contraceptives, who presents with isolated pleuritic chest pain. Such patients frequently get admitted and heparinised until further investigations can be organised. In a review of these patients it was found that the probability of PE is vanishingly small if there are no risk factors for venous thromboembolism and the patient is either (i) aged under 40 or (ii) has a respiratory rate of <20/min plus a normal chest radiograph.

Confirmation of the diagnosis

The V/Q lung scan

The V/Q lung scan remains the pivotal investigation in the diagnosis of pulmonary embolism. It should be performed within 24 hours of the onset of symptoms because delay leads to partial resolution of defects and makes interpretation more difficult. The perfusion lung scan is performed with macroaggregates of human serum albumin (MAA) or microspheres, labelled with 1.5 to 4 mCi of technetium-99m (^{99m}Tc). The injection of radionuclide-labelled MAA (10–60μm in diameter) leads to embolization in the small pulmonary arterioles. The most uniform distribution of isotope within the lungs is achieved by slow intravenous injection over several respiratory cycles with the patient in the supine position. The patient can then be scanned, preferably sitting, by a gamma scintillation camera. The seated position allows optimal patient mobility for obtaining multiple views and may afford better visualization of the lung bases. Severely ill patients may have to be scanned supine. The most commonly performed views include anterior and posterior and right and left posterior oblique, though lateral views may also be helpful.

The ventilation scan was originally developed in an attempt to increase the specificity of the perfusion scan in the diagnosis of pulmonary embolism, since defects associated with PE should not disturb local ventilation, whereas diseases that result in local alveolar hypoxia, e.g. asthma and chronic bronchitis, will tend to affect ventilation *and* perfusion via the mechanism of hypoxic pulmonary vasoconstriction. However, acute pulmonary embolism may disturb local ventilation, such as when infarction or haemorrhage occur, or rarely when bronchoconstriction is induced by airway hypocapnia or release of bronchoconstrictors such as serotonin from platelets. A variety of techniques are available to perform the ventilalation scan. Most departments in the UK use the radioactive gas krypton-81m (^{81m}Kr) or ^{99m}Tc-DPTA aerosol. The radioactive gas, xenon-133 (^{133}Xe), is less widely used these days since although it can give important information regarding local ventilation, it gives less optimal images for comparison with ^{99m}Tc perfusion images. Although based on sound physiological principles, evidence from recent prospective clinical trials suggests that the ventilation scan adds little to the diagnostic utility of the perfusion scan.

An Evidence-based Approach to Diagnosis of Pulmonary Embolism

Interpretation of the lung scan

The interpretation of the V/Q scan has evolved in complexity over the years since its introduction, based upon correlations with angiographic findings. The most sophisticated criteria are those

Table 8.   Modified PIOPED criteria for interpretation of V/Q scans

Probability	Criteria
High	>1 large V/Q mismatch 1 large plus >1 moderate V/Q mismatch >3 moderate V/Q mismatch
Intermediate	1 large V/Q mismatch <4 moderate V/Q mismatch 1 matched V/Q defect plus normal chest radiograph
Low	1 V/Q mismatch plus normal chest radiograph >1 matched V/Q defects plus some normal Q, plus normal chest radiograph small Q defect(s) plus normal chest radiograph non-segmental Q defects (e.g. small pleural effusion, cardiomegaly, enlarged mediastinal structures, raised hemidiaphragm)
Normal	no V/Q defects present; Q exactly outlines the shape of the lungs on chest radiograph

modified by the recent PIOPED study (Table 8). In these criteria an assessment of the number and size of perfusion defects, and the presence of V/Q mismatch allows a V/Q scan to be classified as normal or assigned high, intermediate, or low probability for pulmonary embolism. A current good quality chest radiograph is essential for proper interpretation. Essentially there are two V/Q scan results which enable rational decisions to be made regarding management (Figure 2):

1) a **high probability V/Q scan** indicates acute pulmonary embolism in about 90% of cases. Patients with this scan result should be considered to have acute PE and be anticoagulated unless there are clear contraindications, or there is a reason to suspect a false positive scan. The commonest causes for a false positive V/Q scan are listed in Table 9. A common catch is the presence of a single large mismatched perfusion defect involving an entire lobe or lung; here the diagnosis is more likely to be proximal bronchial carcinoma with vascular obstruction.

2) a **normal V/Q scan** effectively excludes significant pulmonary embolism and an alternative explanation should be sought for the patient's symptoms. These patients should not be anti-

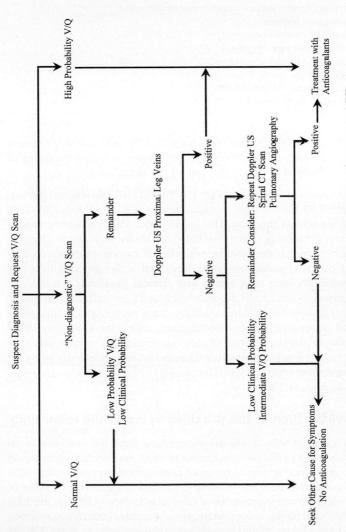

Figure 2. Diagnostic algorithm for the management of suspected PE

Table 9.   Causes of a false positive V/Q scan for acute PE

Previous pulmonary embolism
Chronic thromboembolic pulmonary hypertension
Pulmonary oedema
Bronchial carcinoma
Lymphangitis carcinomatosis
Pulmonary fibrosis e.g. sarcoid, fibrosing alveolitis, radiation
Vasculitis
Arteriovenous malformation
Non-thrombotic emboli

coagulated. Patients with suspected PE but normal V/Q scans followed up over several months have no higher incidence of subsequent PE than the rest of the population.

Unfortunately only about 10–15% of patients referred for suspected PE have a high probability lung scan, and about 15–30% have a normal lung scan. This leaves about 55–75% of patients with a low probability or intermediate probability scan result. One further group can probably be regarded as having an extremely low incidence of pulmonary embolism, that is the group with a **low probability lung scan and a low clinical likelihood** (i.e. no risk factors). In this group the incidence of PE overall is about 4%. It would seem reasonable to withhold anticoagulation in this group and perform no further investigations, unless the clinical situation changed. The large group of patients remaining should be regarded as having **a non-diagnostic V/Q scan** and further investigations are mandatory, since the actual incidence of PE in this group as a whole is as high as 30%.

Investigation of the proximal veins of the lower limb

In a patient with a non-diagnostic lung scan the next step is an assessment of the proximal veins of the lower limb, which should be performed within 24 hours of presentation. Approximately 70% of patients with acute PE have thrombus in the proximal veins of the legs even in the absence of clinical evidence of DVT. In the 30% who have no demonstrable proximal thrombus the clot is assumed to have broken off and embolized in the majority. In about 10% of patients the thrombus has arisen from elsewhere, though this is usually clinically obvious, for example renal vein or subclavian vein thrombosis. Demonstration of deep vein thrombosis in the proximal leg veins warrants anticoagulation and since the treatment is virtually identical no further studies are necessary.

Ascending contrast venography. Venography was until recently widely considered to be the "gold standard" for assessment of the deep veins of the lower limb. However, it is moderately invasive, often uncomfortable, and technical failures preclude an adequate examination in up to 20% of cases. Relative contraindications include contrast sensitivity and pregnancy. Even with nonionic contrast media, an iatrogenic DVT rate of 8% has been reported. Despite these problems contrast venography remains the most reliable method for detecting DVT in the calf veins, though many clinicians would elect not to treat these anyway.

Doppler ultrasound. The present method of choice for detection of suspected DVT in the lower limb is a combination of compression ultrasound and colour Doppler imaging. Several recent controlled trials have demonstrated that ultrasound has a 95% sensitivity and a 98% specificity for the detection of proximal thrombus using contrast venography as the gold standard. Outcome analysis of patients with suspected DVT has shown that the risk of adverse sequelae following a negative ultrasound investigation is less than 0.5% (or less than the risk of contrast-induced DVT in patients undergoing contrast venography). The limitations of ultrasound are that it is very operator-dependent and the ability to detect DVT in calf veins is probably less than contrast venography.

Continuing down the diagnostic pathway, we are now left with patients with non-diagnostic lung scans (except those with concordant low clinical and V/Q scan probability for PE) without evidence of proximal lower limb DVT. This group still represents between 30–60% of all patients referred for V/Q scanning. Traditionally it would be recommended that, since the probability of PE remains unacceptably high (up to 20%) in this group, that these patients should be referred for pulmonary angiography. However, in practice a number of options are available to the clinician, including:

1) using the clinical probability of PE to decide on further action. If the clinical probability is low in the face of an intermediate probability V/Q scan it may be reasonable to withhold treatment if Doppler ultrasound is negative.
2) If the clinical likelihood is intermediate or high and the V/Q scan is low or intermediate probability it is reasonable to repeat

the Doppler ultrasound at intervals looking for evidence of extension of clot into the proximal leg veins. One such strategy is to repeat the ultrasound 2–3 times over the next 2 weeks.
3) perform spiral CT to exclude central or segmental emboli
4) if the service is available and any doubt remains, pulmonary angiography should be performed.

Spiral computed tomographic (CT) scanning

Spiral or helical CT enables most or all of the thorax to be rapidly scanned during a single breath hold with simultaneous intravenous contrast injection. Where available its speed and accessibility make it an attractive alternative to conventional pulmonary angiography. Studies of the correlation with angiography have shown that it has good sensitivity (90%) and specificity (92%) for central or segmental thrombus, though smaller emboli in subsegmental arteries are not reliably visualized. The technique has not yet been as exhaustively investigated as the V/Q scan and Doppler US, thus further evaluation is necessary before definitive statements can be made about its place in the diagnosis of PE. For example, what is the clinical outcome in untreated patients with a negative spiral CT? In the meantime CT could be placed before pulmonary angiography in the diagnostic algorithm, on the basis that if it were positive, angiography would be unnecessary. If it were negative, angiography should be an option in those patients in whom clinical suspicion remains high.

Pulmonary angiography

There is no basis for withholding pulmonary angiography on the grounds that it is a dangerous investigation. Contrary to popular belief, the associated mortality is less than 0.5%, almost all confined to severely ill patients. The complication rate is no greater in elderly individuals. Despite this, only 15% of British radiology departments offer a pulmonary angiography service, and even in those centres, only a small number are performed per year. A negative angiogram excludes PE, although the test is not without problems of interpretation and inter-observer disagreement. The two most reliable signs on angiography are the finding of filling defects in the contrast stream, and abrupt "cut off" of contrast. During the procedure full resuscitation procedures should be available and ITU should be informed if the patient is hypotensive. The internal jugular approach is recommended over the subclavian and femoral approach, to avoid pneumothorax and dislodging clot, respectively. To reduce the volume of non-ionic contrast needed and to reduce the length of time of the procedure, injection of contrast can be confined to the most abnormal area on the V/Q scan and the investigation can be halted as soon as clot is visualized.

Other tests

Plasma D-dimers. This breakdown product of cross-linked fibrin has been proposed as a negative predictor of PE or DVT. Values are rarely in the normal range (< 500ng/ml) for patients with active thromboembolic disease. Unfortunately, a raised D-dimer level has low specificity for venous thrombosis because many common diseases other than embolism give rise to high levels e.g. DIC, pregnancy, malignancy, inflammation, liver disease. However, there is accumulating evidence that a negative d-dimer test (< 500ng/ml) excludes significant venous thrombosis with a negative predictive value of 94–100%, though this is highly dependent on the assay system used (ELISA or latex agglutination assay). One recent study, using the SimpliRED rapid latex agglutination assay, (Egermayer et al. 1998) found that the predictive value of a negative d-dimer for exclusion of PE was 99%. As experience is gained with the appropriate assay, d-dimer measurement may have a useful role in the initial assessment of patients with suspected acute PE and DVT, as shown in the algorithm in Figure 3.

Echocardiography. In patients with major proximal PE, echocardiography can establish the diagnosis as well as exclude common differential diagnoses such as myocardial infarction, aortic dissection and pericardial tamponade. The main signs on 2-D echocardiography are right ventricular dilatation and hypokinesis, pulmonary artery enlargement, and abnormal septal movement. Other pre-existing causes of pulmonary hypertension such as COPD or congestive cardiac failure may make interpretation difficult. In addition, clot may be visualized in the right heart or main pulmonary arteries. This investigation probably has a place in the rapid assessment of the hypotensive patient with suspected massive PE when urgent thrombolysis is being considered. Its availability and the skill of the operator will probably dictate its use in this situation.

Magnetic Resonance Imaging. This investigation has been shown to have a high degree of sensitivity and specificity for the detection

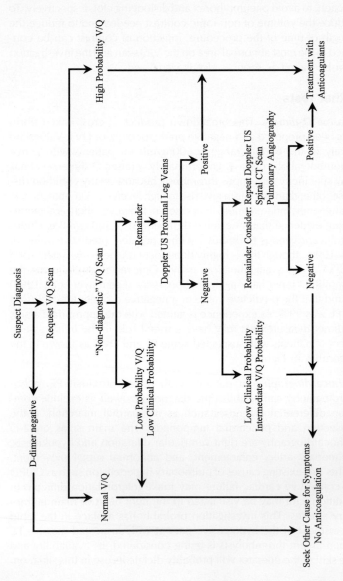

Figure 3.   Flow chart for investigation of stable patient with suspected acute PE

of pelvic and lower limb DVT. Although it is not widely available, and not a currently accepted method for imaging PE, MRI is under investigation as a potential non-invasive one-stop investigation for the patient with DVT and/or PE.

The role of the follow-up V/Q scan

Follow-up V/Q scans in patients who have had acute PE are probably not necessary in the majority of patients. However there are a few circumstances where follow-up scanning is indicated. The rate of recovery of pulmonary perfusion following acute PE depends on the severity of the embolism, the presence of pre-existing cardiopulmonary disease and the patient's age. Mild cases may show complete resolution within a few days. In severe cases one third will have persistent perfusion defects at one year. Overall 16% of patients fail to achieve 90% resolution of the perfusion scan, or 28% of patients with pre-existing cardiopulmonary disease. Generally, any resolution that occurs on the V/Q scan occurs within 3 months. Therefore, a follow-up V/Q scan, if it is to be performed, is particularly useful 3 months after the acute PE. The following are examples of circumstances in which a repeat study may be useful:

1) to establish a new baseline in a patient at high risk of recurrent embolism. In a patient with previous PE the decision as to whether a defect represents an acute embolic event is greatly aided by the availability of a convalescent scan for comparison.
2) to investigate failure of resolution of clinical symptoms. In a patient whose clinical symptoms are slow or fail to resolve a repeat V/Q scan may show evidence of further embolism despite adequate anticoagulation, or raise the suspicion of an alternative diagnosis if defects persist.
3) to look for patients at risk of chronic thromboembolic pulmonary hypertension. A very small proportion of patients with acute PEs (estimates vary between 0.1 and 1%) fail to resolve emboli and may develop chronic thromboembolic pulmonary hypertension. However, there is no data to suggest that this sort of screening leads to better outcome. Indeed, the majority of patients found to have chronic thromboembolic pulmonary hypertension give no preceding history of acute PE.
4) as a diagnostic tool to retrospectively confirm that a perfusion defect was due to acute PE. In theory a perfusion defect that improves over the space of a few days on anticoagulant treatment

is more likely to represent acute thromboembolism than one of the causes of a "false positive" lung scan. However, it can be seen in Table 9 that some of the conditions listed also have the capacity to resolve within the same time frame and this approach has never been tested in a clinical trial.

Treatment

General supportive measures

Hypoxaemia should be treated with high percentage inspired oxygen. If the patient is shocked intravenous colloid should be given whilst monitoring central venous pressure. Right atrial pressure should be allowed to remain high (15–20mmHg) to ensure maximal right heart filling. Analgesics should be given for severe pleuritic pain, but opiates are best avoided as they are vasodilators and may precipitate cardiovascular collapse.

Anticoagulation

Anticoagulation remains the mainstay of treatment for PE and has been shown to reduce the incidence of fatal recurrent embolism. However, treatment with heparin and warfarin is accompanied by a significant risk of major haemorrhage (3–5%). This risk should always be borne in mind when deciding whether or not to anticoagulate a patient with suspected venous thromboembolism. Furthermore, early studies of anticoagulant treatment for PE probably overestimated the mortality of untreated patients (approximately 30% mortality) since they included patients with relatively severe disease. The present day mortality from recurrent PE in untreated patients is unknown, but is probably less than 10%.

Heparin

Heparin should be started immediately, unless contraindicated, in patients with a high or intermediate clinical suspicion of PE, pending the results of further investigations. If the clinical suspicion is low (i.e. no risk factors, or other diagnoses likely) then anticoagulation can be postponed whilst further investigations are organised. Low molecular weight heparin given by subcutaneous injection has recently been shown to be as effective as continuous intravenous unfractionated heparin in the treatment of submassive pulmonary embolism. In addition, it has the advantage of requiring no labo-

Table 10. Recommended drug treatment for PE

	initial treatment	further treatment
Intravenous thrombolysis		
rtPA	100mg in 2 hr	
Streptokinase	250,000 units in 20 min	100,000 units/hr for 24 hr
Urokinase	4400 IU/kg in 10 min	4400 IU/kg/hr for 12hr
Intravenous unfractionated heparin		
Standard	5000–10000 IU bolus	1300 IU/hr infusion
Weight-adjusted	80 IU/kg bolus	18 IU/kg/hr infusion
Low molecular weight heparin		
tinzaparin (Innohep)	175 IU/kg daily	
Warfarin	5–10 mg daily for 2 days	1–10 mg daily

ratory monitoring since the dose is calculated according to the patient's weight. The choice between these two heparins will depend on local prescribing policies. The doses of heparin used in the treatment of PE are shown in Table 10. With intravenous unfractionated heparin the goal is to achieve an activated partial thromboplastin time (APTT) between 1.5–2.5x the upper limit of normal as soon as possible. This is more likely to be achieved by using the weight adjusted dose shown in Table 10. The APTT should be rechecked 4–6 hours after starting treatment, or after a dose adjustment. Thereafter it can be checked daily. Heparin should be continued for 4 or 5 days until adequate maintenance anticoagulation with warfarin is achieved.

Warfarin

Warfarin should be started as soon as the diagnosis of PE is confirmed. The aim is to achieve an international normalised ratio (INR) within the therapeutic range of 2.0–3.0. The current recommendation is that anticoagulation with warfarin should be maintained for 3 months following a first episode of venous thromboembolism.

However, a number of studies have indicated that 6 weeks treatment is adequate in patients in whom there is no continuing risk factor for thrombosis e.g. in a patient following abdominal or orthopaedic surgery. Recurrent thromboembolism in the absence of a recurrent or new risk factor should be treated with long term anticoagulation. Patients with thrombophilia may require lifelong anticoagulation after a first episode of venous thromboembolism and should be referred to a haematologist for further assessment.

Thrombolysis

Thrombolysis should be considered in acute massive PE in patients with systemic hypotension. Traditionally, pulmonary angiography has been considered mandatory prior to the use of thrombolysis. However, in the appropriate clinical setting a high probability V/Q scan, or a positive spiral CT provide sufficient confirmatory evidence to justify its use. Indeed, if the patient is *in extremis* with high clinical suspicion of PE, such as clinical signs of right ventricular failure or echocardiographic evidence, then thrombolysis should be considered. Thrombolysis is equally effective when given via a peripheral vein, or via a pulmonary artery catheter. There is evidence that thrombolysis may be effective at reducing clot burden when given for up to 14 days after acute massive PE.

The rationale for thrombolysis is that the cardiac output from the right ventricle is so compromised by the burden of thrombus in the pulmonary arteries that these patients are in danger of dying from acute right ventricular pressure overload. Thrombolysis is known to clear emboli and restore pulmonary perfusion, and reduce right ventricular pressure more rapidly than heparin alone. Although early trials of thrombolysis in PE failed to demonstrate a significant survival advantage, few patients with massive PE were included. Thus the risks of haemorrhage outweighed any advantage in the group as a whole.

The currently recommended protocols for thrombolysis are shown in Table 10.

Invasive procedures

Pulmonary embolectomy is rarely indicated since thrombolysis is as effective as embolectomy in patients with massive PE. A number of percutaneous transvenous techniques have been developed in an attempt to avoid open surgical embolectomy in patients who have not responded to thrombolysis after one hour, or in whom thrombolysis is contraindicated. The techniques are usually undertaken by an interventional radiologist or cardiologist and consist of sucking out clot with a catheter, or simply attempting to breaking up the clot with vigorous movement of the catheter tip, known as catheter tip dispersion.

Inferior vena caval filters are not widely used in the UK compared with the USA. They should be considered in patients in whom anticoagulants are contraindicated, and for patients with recurrent embolism despite adequate anticoagulation.

Postoperative PE

In the postoperative period PE needs to be differentiated from other common postoperative pulmonary complications such as atelectasis and pneumonia. The diagnosis of acute massive PE should always be considered in the surgical patient who collapses whilst mobilising after a prolonged period of bed rest. The decision to anticoagulate pending the results of investigations must be weighed against the risks of major haemorrhage in each case. Low molecular weight heparins are associated with a lower risk of bleeding and are therfore the initial anticoagulant of choice in this setting.

Pregnancy and PE

Suspected acute pulmonary embolism occurring during pregnancy or in the early post-partum period poses a few special problems. The investigation of PE during pregnancy is essentially the same as for other patients. A chest X-ray can be performed with abdominal shielding. If PE is suspected clinically then a V/Q scan should be performed. Many nuclear medicine departments reduce the dose of ^{99m}Tc for perfusion studies, though such precautions may not be necessary. Nursing mothers should avoid breast feeding for 15 hours after the V/Q scan. Other non-invasive studies of the proximal leg veins may provide confirmatory evidence for venous thromboembolism.

Treatment with warfarin is contraindicated throughout pregnancy because the drug crosses the placenta and is associated with fetal abnormalities, particularly in the first trimester. Heparin, on the other hand, does not cross the placenta and is treatment of choice during pregnancy. The introduction of single daily subcutaneous injections of low molecular weight heparin for treatment of PE or DVT make this the most convenient option during pregnancy. Alternatively, twice daily subcutaneous injections of unfractionated heparin can be given, but this requires monitoring of the APTT. During prolonged treatment with heparins thrombocytopaenia and osteoporosis may occur, but these risks seem to be less with low molecular weight heparin. Thrombolysis is not contraindicated during pregnancy for acute massive PE. In the immediate post-partum period, anticoagulation and thrombolysis may be contra-indicated for acute PE, since the risk of major haemorrhage is high. Under these circumstances, consideration should be given to the use of an inferior vena caval filter to prevent further potentially fatal embolism.

Bibliography

1. British Thoracic Society, Standards of Care Committee. Suspected acute pulmonary embolism: a practical approach. *Thorax* 1997; **52**(supplement 4)

2. Morice AH. Clinical Pulmonary Hypertension. London: Portland Press Ltd 1995

3. Peacock AJ. Pulmonary Hypertension: A Handbook for Clinicians. London: Chapman and Hall 1996

4. Stein PD, Saltzman HA. Venous thromboembolism. *Clinics in Chest Medicine* 1995;**16**(number 2)

5. Rich S, Kaufmann E, Levy PS. The effect of high doses of calcium-channel blockers on survival in primary pulmonary hypertension. *N Engl J Med* 1992;**327**:76–81

6. Worsley DF, Alavi A. Comprehensive analysis of the results of the PIOPED study. *J Nucl Med* 1995;**36**:2380–2387

7. Goldhaber SZ. Contemporary pulmonary embolism thrombolysis. *Chest* 1995;**107**(1suppl):45S–51S

8. McLaughlin VV, Genthner DE, Panella MM, Rich S. Reduction in pulmonary vascular resistance with long-term epoprostenol (prostacyclin) therapy in primary pulmonary hypertension. *N Engl J Med* 1998;**338**:273–277

Reference

Egermayer P, Town GI, Turner JG, Heaton DC, Mee AL, Beard ME. Usefulness of D-dimer, blood gas, and respiratory rate measurements for excluding pulmonary embolism. *Thorax* 1998;**53**:830–834

10

Lung Cancer

Jeremy George

Lung cancer was a rare disease at the beginning of the twentieth century but now accounts for more deaths than any other malignancy in industrialised countries. Tobacco smoking is believed to account for the vast majority (80–90%) of cases and, as the epidemiological studies linking tobacco with lung cancer were first published nearly fifty years ago,[1] it seems remarkable that a fatal but avoidable disease should have become so common.

The annual death rate from lung cancer in England and Wales is in the region of 30 000 and approaches 170 000 in the USA. Although there are signs that the incidence is levelling off in men, it continues to rise in women and is overtaking breast carcinoma as the leading cause of cancer deaths. This is thought to reflect the smoking habits of women, which are now catching up with those of men.

The results of treatment are very poor with overall five-year survival figures in the region of 7–13%. As a consequence, many clinicians have adopted a rather nihilistic attitude to the disease. In the UK, relatively few patients (< 2%) are entered into clinical trials, while the provision of lung cancer services has been criticised as being non-uniform and often sub-optimal. New treatments and management strategies (which may require a major re-organisation of the clinical service) will be needed if we are to improve the outlook for this common and lethal disease.

Classification, Growth Rates and Natural History

Lung cancer is classically divided into four main groups: adenocarcinoma, squamous cell carcinoma, large cell undifferentiated

Table 1.   Classification of malignant lung tumours

Major group (% occurrence)	Subtype
Squamous cell carcinoma (48%)	Spindle cell carcinoma variant
Small cell carcinoma (24%)	Oat cell Intermediate cell type Combined oat cell carcinoma
Adenocarcinoma (13%)	Acinar adenocarcinoma Papillary adenocarcinoma Bronchio-alveolar carcinoma Solid carcinoma with mucus formation
Large cell carcinoma (10%)	Giant cell carcinoma Clear cell carcinoma
Carcinoid tumour (1%)	Classic carcinoid Atypical carcinoid
Adenosquamous carcinoma (1.5%)	
Bronchial gland carcinomas	Adenoid cystic carcinoma Mucoepidermoid carcinoma Others
Others	

Adapted from the WHO classification [2].

carcinoma and small cell carcinoma. These distinctions are based upon the histological differentiation of the tumour when inspected under light microscopy using routine staining techniques. The World Health Organisation classification[2] recognises subgroups of these cell types and includes carcinoid tumours, bronchial gland carcinomas and other rarer groups (Table 1).

Precise categorisation of the four main cell types is seldom required for routine clinical practice and, for practical purposes, it is more useful for the clinician simply to make the distinction between small cell and non-small cell carcinoma. Small cell carcinomas grow very much more rapidly than non-small cell carcinomas and consequently require different approaches to management.

The relevance of growth rates to understanding survival and treatment responses was first highlighted by Geddes in 1979.[3] He

Table 2.   Natural history of untreated lung cancer based on growth rates

| | Years from malignant change to: | | | |
Cell type	Mean volume doubling time (Days)	Earliest diagnosis (1 Cm: 30 volume doublings)	Usual diagnosis (3 Cms: 35–37 volume doublings)	Death (10 Cms: 40 volume doublings)
Squamous cell	88	7.2	8.4	9.6
Adenocarcinoma	161	13.2	15.4	17.6
Large cell undifferentiated	86	7.1	8.2	9.4l
Small cell	29	2.4	2.8	3.2

Adapted from Geddes [3].

argued that the observed survival and poor results of treatment could be explained by an exponential model of tumour growth. He estimated that 30 volume doublings would be required for a tumour to achieve a diameter of 1 cm, when it might just be detectable on a plain chest X-ray, but that only 10 further volume doublings would be required to achieve a size incompatible with life (Table 2). As the average diameter of a tumour at the time of diagnosis is 3 cms (which approximates to 35–37 volume doublings), it can be appreciated that lung cancers are detected only at very late stages in their development when metastatic spread is likely to have occurred.

The model therefore provides an explanation for the disappointing results of surgery in which patients ultimately succumb to metastatic disease and is consistent with observed survival in untreated patients (Table 2). Although the model may be used to argue the nihilist's case, it may also be used constructively to develop more rational approaches to treatment. Firstly, it would seem logical to combine systemic treatments, such as chemotherapy, with local treatments with the intention of eradicating microscopic metastases. Secondly, the knowledge that individuals at risk of lung cancer are likely to be harbouring clinically silent microscopic tumours provides an incentive to develop strategies for detecting and then eradicating lesions at very early stages before they have metastasised.

Table 3.   Additional risk factors for lung cancer in smokers

Large number of cigarettes smoked
Young age when started smoking
Long duration of smoking
Airflow obstruction
Increasing age
Family history of lung cancer
Previous history of other cancers involving the lung, head and neck
Exposure to other carcinogens e.g. asbestos and radon gas

Clinical Features

Early symptoms may easily be overlooked and so it is helpful to adopt a high index of suspicion in individuals who are at particular risk. Our understanding of risk factors has increased considerably in the last 20 years with the result that it is now possible to identify subgroups of smokers who are especially vulnerable to the disease and whose symptoms consequently merit very careful scrutiny (Table 3).

Symptoms and signs in lung cancer are legion and, for convenience, are divided into 3 groups: those related to local disease, extra-thoracic disease and paraneoplastic syndromes (Table 4). Careful evaluation of symptoms and signs is essential as it alerts the clinician to the likely diagnosis while also providing a guide to operability.

Cough, breathlessness and wheeze

60–70% of all bronchogenic carcinomas arise in the large airways and so are likely to cause problems related to large airway obstruction. A combination of cough, breathlessness and wheeze merit investigation if of recent onset and persistent for two weeks or more. It is important to appreciate that the chest X-ray may occasionally appear normal as some centrally situated tumours may be silhouetted by the mediastinum and vertebrae.

The presence of a fixed monophonic wheeze, inspiratory stridor, or a reduction in breath sounds over part or all of one lung are important signs of localised airway obstruction. Tracheal tumours represent 'classic catches' for the clinician as they are rare and are almost always mistaken as asthma or chronic obstructive

Table 4.   Common clinical problems in lung cancer

Local disease	Extra-thoracic disease	Paraneoplastic syndromes
• Cough	• Bone pain	• Finger clubbing
• Breathlessness	• Neurological:	• Hypertrophic pulmonary
• Wheeze	Epilepsy	osteoarthropathy (HPOA)
• Haemoptysis	Headache	• Anorexia
• Dysphagia	Hemianopia	• Cachexia
• Hoarseness	Hemiparesis	• Weight loss
• Chest pain	• Hepatic pain	• Hypercalcaemia
		• Hyponatraemia
		• Peripheral neuropathy
		• Lambert-Eaton syndrome
		• Anaemia
		• Thrombo-embolic disease

pulmonary disease (COPD) at the time of presentation. Empey formulated a simple diagnostic test for tracheal narrowing by expressing the peak expiratory flow (PEF) in relation to the forced expiratory volume in one second (FEV_1).[4] He found that the PEF tended to be disproportionately reduced in patients with tracheal obstruction, such that the ratio of the FEV_1 (expressed in mls/sec) to the PEF (expressed in l/Min) was likely to be greater than 10 (Figure 1). This situation contrasts with both asthma and COPD where there is a proportional reduction in both indices.

It is important to appreciate that breathlessness may be due to conditions other than large airway obstruction. Pleural and pericardial effusions, radiation-induced pneumonitis and fibrosis, pulmonary embolic disease, lymphangitis carcinomatosa and compression of the pulmonary vessels by tumour are important causes. Careful evaluation is therefore required.

Haemoptysis

Haemoptysis occurs in up to 50% of lung cancer patients at presentation and so this symptom should not be dismissed lightly. However, it is also seen in a number of other less sinister conditions and it may not be practicable to submit every patient for comprehensive investigation. Although there are no rigid guidelines, the decision to investigate is usually determined by the severity and persistence of haemoptysis, the patient's age, chest X-ray appear-

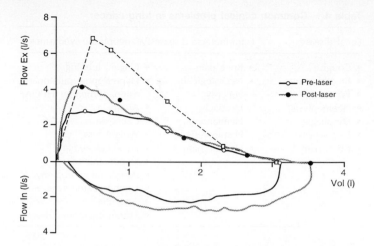

Figure 1. Peak flow, spirometry and flow volume loops are shown for a patient with a squamous cell carcinoma obstructing the lower trachea before and immediately after laser treatment. The ratio of the FEV$_1$ (expressed in ml) to the PEF (expressed in L) was greater than 10 before treatment but returned to a normal after treatment

Lung function	Pre-laser	Post-laser
PEF (L/Min)	167	251
FEV$_1$ (L/sec)	2.09	2.23
FVC (L)	3.08	3.52
Empey index	12.5	8.9

ance and risk factors for lung cancer (Table 3). Patients with abnormal chest X-rays, massive and/or repeated haemoptyses should always be investigated. Similarly, an isolated haemoptysis in a patient at risk of lung cancer should be investigated even if the chest X-ray is normal as there is a significant (approximately 10%) chance of finding an endobronchial tumour.

Diagnosis and Pre-treatment Evaluation

Patients and their families are likely to suffer considerable anxiety and distress while undergoing investigations for lung cancer and

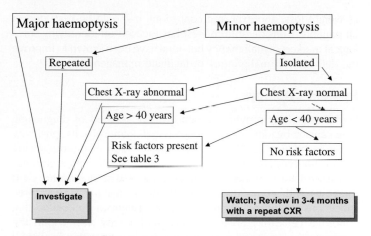

Figure 2. Guide to the management of haemoptysis

so it is essential to conduct investigations with efficiency and sensitivity. Although it is acceptable to make a clinical diagnosis of lung cancer in patients who are clearly unfit or unwilling to undergo any form of definitive treatment, histological and/or cytological confirmation should generally be obtained.

Laboratory investigations

A full blood count and biochemical screen are essential for patient management. Patients frequently become anaemic as part of a paraneoplastic syndrome or as a result of marrow infiltration by secondary tumour. Liver enzymes are likely to be elevated in patients with extensive liver metastases, while the serum albumen tends to be low in patients with advanced disease and is a poor prognostic sign.

Ectopic hormone production occurs commonly in patients with lung cancer and may cause profound metabolic and biochemical disturbances. Patients with small cell lung cancer may develop the syndrome of inappropriate antidiuretic hormone secretion (Table 4) and Cushing's syndrome as a result of ectopic ACTH production, while patients with squamous cell carcinoma may secrete parathyroid hormone-related peptide and become hypercalcaemic. Hypercalcaemia may also occur in association with bone metastases and, as it may produce a number of non-specific symptoms (such as weight loss, anorexia and confusion), it should be excluded in all patients. Considerable interest has focused on identifying serological markers of malignancy but none have been shown to improve the detection of malignancy or facilitate management.

Sputum cytology

Sputum cytology provides a non-invasive method of diagnosing lung cancers by identifying exfoliated malignant cells. Its sensitivity varies in relation to the cell type and location of tumour, being highest for centrally situated squamous and small cell carcinomas and lowest for peripheral adenocarcinoma. The diagnostic yield increases with cumulative samples and so a minimum of three specimens should be obtained. It is important to appreciate that abnormal cells may arise from extra-pulmonary sites within the aero-digestive tract and from pre-invasive lesions within bronchial epithelium which may be difficult to locate with conventional bronchoscopy (see below). As a result of these limitations, the use of sputum cytology is now usually confined to patients who are unwilling or unfit to undergo fibreoptic bronchoscopy. Nevertheless, there is considerable interest in developing and refining techniques for screening individuals at risk of lung cancer (see below).

Fibreoptic bronchoscopy

Fibreoptic bronchoscopy should be regarded as a standard investigation in patients with centrally situated lesions. It is superior to CT scanning in detecting superficial tumours situated within the central airways and is an extremely safe procedure. The combination of bronchial biopsy (3–4 biopsies) with brush cytology optimises the chances of obtaining a diagnosis and is associated with a diagnostic yield of at least 70%.

Although peripheral lesions are usually diagnosed by fine needle aspiration (see below), some centres routinely perform fibreoptic bronchoscopy with transbronchial biopsies and brush cytology under fluoroscopic control. The diagnostic yield is low for small tumours but rises to 60–70% for tumours with a diameter of 2 cms or more.

Bronchoscopy may also provide useful staging information. The location and extent of endobronchial tumour has an important bearing on a patient's suitability for surgery (see below), while the demonstration of a paralysed left vocal cord implies mediastinal invasion and thus inoperability. More direct evidence of mediastinal disease may be obtained by the technique of transbronchial needle aspiration, which allows sampling of subcarinal lymph nodes and which has a sensitivity in the region of 50%.

Percutaneous fine needle aspiration and biopsy

The usual approach to diagnosing peripheral lesions is with fine needle aspiration or biopsy under X-ray, CT or ultrasound guidance. Fine needle aspiration employs a fine diameter needle (20–22G) and provides material for cytology, whereas needle biopsy uses a larger diameter needle (14–18G) to provide a core of tissue for histology. The diagnostic accuracy for malignancy is 80–95%. A negative result does not exclude malignancy and patients may reasonably be referred for surgery if a clinical suspicion of malignancy remains high. The technique may not be adequate for the diagnosis of lymphomas, sarcomas and rare tumours where tissue architecture is required to make a firm diagnosis. Pneumothorax is the most important complication and occurs in up to 30% of procedures, with 5–10% requiring aspiration or drain insertion. Haemorrhage and tumour seeding along the needle track are well recognised but extremely rare complications.

Computed tomography

CT scanning is invaluable for both the diagnosis and staging of lung cancer. It may assist the diagnosis by characterising pulmonary lesions, and thereby provide an assessment of the likelihood of malignancy (see below), while also locating lesions for more invasive diagnostic procedures. CT scanning is not an essential investigation for patients who are clearly unsuitable for surgery or radical radiotherapy but should be performed in all patients who are being considered for curative treatment. The liver and adrenals are frequently involved with metastatic disease and may conveniently be included when imaging the chest. Although cerebral metastases occur in a small proportion of patients at presentation, routine scanning of the brain is not recommended unless there is clinical evidence of metastatic disease.

CT scanning has important limitations. In particular, it provides a relatively poor assessment of mediastinal lymph node involvement, with an estimated sensitivity and specificity of 79% and 78% respectively. Limited mediastinal disease may go undetected while a substantial proportion of enlarged mediastinal nodes (>1 cm diameter) may be benign. Enlarged mediastinal nodes should therefore not necessarily preclude surgery (see below).

CT scanning also provides a relatively poor assessment of chest wall and mediastinal invasion, with estimated sensitivities ranging from 60–75%. Although magnetic resonance imaging (MRI) is believed to be superior to CT in this context (as a result of its multiplanar imaging capability), experience with this technique is limited and it is not widely practised. It may therefore not be possible to decide on the feasibility and extent of surgery until the time of thoracotomy.

Mediastinoscopy and mediastinotomy

Further investigation of the mediastinum is required in patients with enlarged lymph nodes who, in other respects, appear to have operable disease. Cervical mediastinoscopy offers reasonable access to right paratracheal and subcarinal glands, while left sided glands are best approached by mediastinotomy. Multilevel nodal disease and extracapsular spread are usually taken as evidence of inoperability.

Radionuclide bone scanning

Bone metastases are well recognised in lung cancer and may lead to bone pain and pathological fractures. Radionuclide scanning provides a sensitive test for metastatic disease, though false positive results are well recognised. It is therefore not routinely undertaken unless there is a clinical suspicion of metastatic disease. The finding of multiple areas of abnormality on the scan is regarded as strong evidence of metastatic disease, whereas a solitary lesion should be regarded with suspicion and investigated further.

Investigation of pleural effusions

Although pleural effusions in patients who are known to have malignancy are likely to be due to metastatic disease, they may occasionally be due to coincidental benign conditions. Proof of malignancy is therefore advisable. The diagnostic yield of pleural aspiration in malignant effusions is high (65%) but may be increased marginally with the addition of 'blind' pleural biopsy. Ultrasound- and CT-guided pleural biopsies should be obtained if the initial investigation is negative. Thoracoscopy is more invasive but has an

Table 5.   Causes of a solitary pulmonary nodule

Infectious granuloma (Tuberculous/fungal)
Non infectious granuloma (Wegener's Granulomatosis, Rheumatoid nodule)
Bronchial carcinoid
Hamartoma
Metastasis
Primary bronchial carcinoma

even higher diagnostic yield, confirming malignancy in 95% of cases. It also provides an opportunity to proceed directly to a pleurodesis.

The management of the solitary pulmonary nodule

Up to 40% of lung cancers develop beyond the segmental airways and it is not unusual for lung cancers to present as small solitary nodules of 1–2 cms diameter on the chest X-ray. Similarly, with the more frequent use of CT scanning, even smaller lesions of 0.5–1cm diameter may be detected. Resection of lung cancers at such early stages may be curative but not all pulmonary nodules are malignant (Table 5). It is therefore important to differentiate benign from malignant conditions.

Previous chest X-rays or scans should be obtained for comparison as it may be possible to establish that the nodule has formed at the site of previous infection or infarction and is therefore likely to be benign. Alternatively, it may be possible to establish that the nodule has not changed in size. Although growth rates for lung cancer are variable, volume-doubling times are believed to range from 1–18 months. If the lesion has not doubled its volume (equivalent to a 26% increase in diameter) in 18 months, it is most unlikely to be malignant. Alternatively, it may be possible to exclude malignancy if the nodule has increased in size very quickly such that infection or infarction become more likely possibilities.

If old X-rays or scans are not available, the clinician must make a judgement on the probability that the lesion is malignant. This may be based on the patient's known risk factors for lung cancer (Table 3) and on the radiology of the nodule. CT scanning is particularly informative as it allows lesions to be characterised according to their size, shape and patterns of calcification, while also allowing an assessment of tissue invasion. Nodules of 2cm or more in diameter have a higher probability of being malignant than smaller nodules. Lesions that are linear and lack nodularity are more likely to be benign, while nodular lesions with irregular edges are more likely to be malignant, particularly if they are spiculated. Although calcification per se does not exclude malignancy (up to 7% of bronchial carcinomas are calcified when imaged with CT), it is possible to recognise patterns of calcification that are almost always due to benign conditions. These include uniform calcification within the lesion and laminated concentric calcification, which may occur in healed tuberculous or fungal granulomas. Finally, the presence of bone or chest wall erosion by the lesion should be carefully evaluated. Although infections such as tuberculosis and actinomycosis may lead to erosion, malignancy is very much more probable. If these diagnostic criteria are applied to solitary pulmonary nodules, CT scanning has a sensitivity of 70% and specificity of 60%.

Solitary pulmonary nodules may also be assessed by positron emission tomography (PET). PET scanning is usually performed after the administration of 18F-2-deoxy-2-fluoro-D-glucose (FDG), which is a glucose analogue that has been tagged with a positron-emitting isotope. Malignant cells are likely to be more active metabolically than the cells of adjacent normal tissues and take up and accumulate FDG more avidly. False positive scans may occur in inflammatory lesions while false negatives may be seen in slow growing tumours such as carcinoids, well differentiated adenocarcinomas and alveolar cell carcinomas. Although experience with this technique is limited, it is thought to be superior to CT scanning with a sensitivity of 95% and specificity of 70%. It is an expensive technique, which is not widely available in the UK, though it may become the investigation of choice.

Opinions vary as to how to manage the solitary pulmonary nodule in which malignancy cannot be excluded with confidence. Some clinicians opt to observe, with interval chest X-rays or CT scans, and only intervene if there is evidence of growth within an arbitrary 4–6 month period, while others favour an immediate open biopsy, which is both diagnostic and therapeutic. The practical difficulties of adopting a "wait and see" policy are formidable. Inadvertent delays in follow-up may ensure that potentially operable lesions progress to inoperability while some patients may find the suspense and anxiety of waiting quite unbearable. However, the mortality and morbidity associated with thoracotomy are appreciable (see below) and should be considered in each case.

The author's approach is to offer surgery to any patient who is sufficiently fit to undergo surgery if there is an appreciable risk of malignancy based on their individual risks factors for malignancy. If the patient is unwilling or has borderline fitness for surgery, every attempt is made to obtain a tissue diagnosis so that the risk of surgery may be balanced against the risk of taking no action.

Assessment of fitness for surgery

The peri-operative mortality associated with pneumonectomy and lobectomy are 10% and 5% respectively. Careful consideration should therefore be given to each patient's ability to withstand a thoracotomy. In general, the risks of surgery increase with age and with co-existent diseases, particularly those affecting the heart and lungs.

Much importance is attributed to objective measurements of lung function. It is generally accepted that a pneumonectomy will be tolerated if the FEV_1 is greater than 2.0 l/second and that a lobectomy will be tolerated if the FEV_1 is greater than 1.7 l/second, while hypoxaemia ($PO_2 < 60$ mm Hg/7.9 kPa) and hypercapnia ($PCO_2 > 45$ mm Hg/5.9 kPa) are regarded as important contra-indications to surgery.

Baseline measurements of lung function may be misleading when tumour is encroaching onto a major airway or blood vessel, however, as the removal of involved lung tissue is unlikely to impair lung function further. Radionuclide lung scanning may be particularly informative in this situation as it allows a regional assessment of lung function and so enables post-operative lung function to be predicted with a degree of confidence. The post-operative FEV_1 is estimated by multiplying the perfusion value of the residual lung (expressed as a percentage of total lung perfusion) with the pre-operative FEV_1. Patients are usually judged to be fit for pneumonectomy if the estimated post-operative FEV_1 is greater than 1 l/second and fit for lobectomy if the estimated value is greater than 0.8 l/second.

Although these guidelines may provide reassurance on a patient's fitness for surgery, they should be interpreted with some flexibility in patients with borderline fitness. Firstly, it may be possible to obtain small but significant improvements in fitness by commencing inhaled steroids and bronchodilators and by stopping smoking. Secondly, consideration should be given to the patient's overall attitude and approach to surgery. A highly motivated patient with borderline lung function may cope better with post-operative complications and mount a faster recovery than a fitter but less motivated patient. Finally, it may be possible to offer patients with borderline fitness tissue sparing operations involving bronchoplastic procedures or segmental and wedge resections of lung parenchyma. It is therefore important that all potentially operable patients are seen by a surgeon.

Staging and Surgical Management

Staging in lung cancer is important as it provides a guide to treatment and life expectancy. It also facilitates comparisons to be drawn between groups of patients undergoing different treatment protocols.

Small cell carcinoma

Small cell carcinoma has a rapid rate of growth and is almost always too extensive for surgery at the time of diagnosis. As the mainstay of management is systemic treatment with chemotherapy, staging is classified quite simply as either limited or extensive disease. Limited disease refers to disease confined to the ipsilateral hemithorax and supraclavicular group of lymph nodes while extensive disease refers to all other more extensive stages.

Non-small cell carcinoma

Staging in non-small cell carcinoma is more elaborate and is based on a system originally devised by Mountain in 1986[5] and which has subsequently been revised.[6] The current system is now derived from a database of over 5 000 patients treated for primary non-small cell lung cancer from 1975–1988.

The principle of staging is to combine subsets of patients, according to their TNM descriptors (Table 6), into categories or stages that have important bearings on both treatment options and expectations of survival (Table 7). Staging may be either clinical (based on clinical and radiological findings) or surgical (based on definitive pathological findings). The staging system is necessarily detailed and complex. The following account will highlight the important principles and consider areas of controversy.

The first objective is to identify patients with technically operable tumours. Although patients with early stage disease may refuse or be unfit for surgery, it is generally accepted that stages IA, IB,

Table 6. T N M definitions

Primary tumour (T)

TX	Primary tumour cannot be assessed, or tumour proven by presence of malignant cells in sputum or bronchial washings but not visualised by imaging or bronchoscopy
T0	No evidence of primary tumour
Tis	Carcinoma in situ
T1	Tumour 3 cms or less in greatest diameter, surrounded by lung or visceral pleura, without bronchoscopic evidence of invasion of more proximal than lobar bronchus (i e. not in a main bronchus).
T2	Tumour with any of the following features: More than 3cms in greatest diameter Involves main bronchus, 2cms or more distal to main carina Invades visceral pleura Associated with atelectasis or obstructive pneumonia that extends to the hilar region but does not invade the entire lung
T3	Tumour of any size that directly invades any of the following structures: chest wall, diaphragm, mediastinal pleura, or pericardium; tumour in the main bronchus less than 2 cms distal to the main carina but without involvement of the main carina; or associated atelectasis or obstructive pneumonia of the entire lung
T4	Tumour of any size that invades any of the following: mediastinum, heart, great vessels, trachea oesophagus, vertebral body or carina; or tumour with a malignant pleural effusion or pericardial effusion, or satellite nodule(s) within the primary bearing lobe

Lymph node (N)

NX	Regional lymph nodes cannot be assessed
N0	No regional lymph node metastasis
N1	Metastasis in ipsilateral peribronchial and/or ipsilateral hilar lymph nodes, including direct extension
N2	Metastasis in ipsilateral mediastinal and/or subcarinal lymph nodes
N3	Metastasis in contralateral mediastinal, contralateral hilar, ipsilateral or contralateral scalene, or supraclavicular lymph nodes

Distant metastasis (M)

MX	Presence of distant metastasis cannot be assessed
M0	No distant metastasis
M1	Distant metastasis

Table 7. Lung cancer staging and survival

Stage	TNM subset	Per cent surviving 5 years	
		(Clinical staging)	(Surgical staging)
0	Carcinoma in situ		
IA	T1N0M0	61	67
IB	T2N0M0	38	57
IIA	T1N1M0	34	55
IIB	T2N1M0	24	39
	T3N0M0	22	38
IIIA	T3N1M0	9	25
	T1N2M0	13	23
	T2N2M0		
	T3N2M0		
111B	T4N0M0	7	Not applicable
	T4N1M0		
	T4N2M0		
	T1N3M0	3	
	T2N3M0		
	T3N3M0		
	T4N3M0		
IV	Any T, any N, M1	1	NA

Tables 6 and 7 adapted from Mountain [7].

IIA and IIB are operable, while stages IIIB and IV are inoperable. Controversy, however, surrounds the management of stages 0 and IIIA.

Stage 0 disease refers to the unusual situation of carcinoma in situ. It has been assumed that lung cancers develop through a series of pre-invasive stages and that carcinoma in situ progresses ultimately to invasive carcinoma. Some clinicians therefore advocate surgery, or other intervention, with the intention of eradicating local disease. However, as there is no definitive evidence that some or all of these pre-invasive lesions will progress to malignancy, it has been argued that such an approach is unduly invasive and that careful surveillance is more appropriate.

The management of patients with stage IIIA disease is controversial as surgical opinions vary as to the resectability of T3 and N2 disease. T3 tumours, which invade the chest wall, mediastinal pleura and/or pericardium, are technically operable by 'en bloc' dissection of the tumour and adjacent structures. However, the feasibility of such surgery can often only be determined at the time of thoracotomy due to the lack of resolution of pre-operative imaging.

Greater controversy surrounds the management of patients with involvement of the mediastinal lymph nodes. There has been some confusion over the classification of nodal disease and the distinction between mediastinal and hilar nodes. This has recently been clarified such that the mediastinal lymph nodes are now regarded as being located within the mediastinal pleural reflection, while the hilar lymph nodes are regarded as being confined to within the visceral pleura. N1 disease refers to ipsilateral peribronchial and hilar lymph node involvement, while N2 disease refers to ipsilateral mediastinal and subcarinal lymph node involvement.

The surgical management of N2 disease is controversial, as surgical series have produced conflicting reports on long term survival. There is no doubt that the prospects of cure are substantially reduced when there is secondary spread to the mediastinal lymph nodes. However, there are claims of significant 5-year survival in patients undergoing radical surgery with clearance of the mediastinal glands. More careful analysis of the published data, however, suggests that it is only patients with very limited involvement of the mediastinum who are likely to have a prospect of cure. In practice, patients with mediastinal disease, which is apparent on CT scanning or to the naked eye at mediastinoscopy or thoracotomy, are unlikely to have a prospect of cure. However, patients with limited microscopic involvement may be cured. Some surgeons routinely dissect the mediastinal lymph nodes, with frozen section analysis, and only proceed to a lung resection if the lymph nodes are free of metastatic disease. Where there is limited involvement, the surgeon may still proceed with an operation if it is felt that there may be a prospect of clearing the entire disease. In such situations, the question of operability can only be left to the individual judgement of the surgeon on the day. Clearly, a physician cannot make such a decision and so it is important that all borderline cases are discussed with a surgeon. If not, some patients will be denied potentially curative surgery.

Radiotherapy for Non-small Cell Lung Cancer

Radiotherapy represents the mainstay of treatment for the majority of patients with non-small cell lung cancer and may be given with either curative or palliative intent. Radical radiotherapy may be given to patients with small volume tumours, with limited regional lymph node involvement, who refuse or are unsuitable for surgery. Palliative treatment is generally given to relieve symptoms in the large number of patients whose disease is too extensive to be encompassed in a radical field of treatment.

The principle of radical radiotherapy is to deliver a dose that is sufficiently high to kill all tumour cells within the primary site and regional lymph nodes. Control of disease within the primary site is associated with a reduction in systemic metastases and improved survival. The total radiation dose has an important bearing on tumour response, with large volume tumours requiring higher doses. Unfortunately, the doses required to destroy tumour cells approach the radiation tolerance of surrounding normal tissues, the oesophagus, spinal cord and lung parenchyma being particularly vulnerable to radiation damage.

Radiation damage to normal tissues may be ameliorated by fractionation in which the dose of radiation is delivered in small fractions over several weeks. The classical regime is to give daily fractions of 1.8–2 Gy per fraction, 5–6 times per week, for 3–7 weeks up to a total dose of 50–60 Gy. However, the results of treatment have been disappointing with median survival of 8–12 months and 5-year survival in the region of 5–10%. These poor figures have been attributed to poor control of local disease and to extra-thoracic disease arising from outside of the original treatment field.

Poor control of the primary tumour may be due to the proliferation of tumour cells after each fraction of treatment. This problem has been addressed with the development of continuous hyper-fractionated accelerated radiotherapy (CHART) in which fractions of treatment are given at shorter intervals and over a shorter period of time. The intention of treatment is to prevent the re-population of tumour cells between treatments. In a recently published randomised multicentre trial, CHART (36 fractions of 1.5 Gy, 3 times per day in 12 consecutive days up to a total dose of 54 Gy) was compared with conventional radical treatment (30 fractions of 2 Gy up to a total dose of 60 Gy in 6 weeks) in patients with non small cell lung cancer.[7] The results demonstrated a significant survival advantage of 9% at two years for patients receiving CHART, while subgroup analysis suggested that the largest benefit occurred in patients with squamous cell carcinoma where survival was improved by 14%. It has recently been recommended that systems now be established to enable CHART to be offered to patients with early stage inoperable non-small cell lung cancer. This will require radiotherapy to be available at weekends on an in-patient or hotel basis and will incur additional costs. However, a recent cost benefit analysis has shown that the cost for each life year gained compared with conventional radiotherapy is likely to be modest when compared with other anticancer treatments.

The majority of patients with non-small cell lung cancer have disease that is too advanced for curative local treatment and relief of symptoms is all that can be offered. Palliative radiotherapy provides effective relief for common symptoms such as cough and haemoptysis in 80%, breathlessness due to large airway obstruction in 50%, superior vena caval obstruction (SVCO) in 60% and pain due to bone metastases in 50–80%. Symptoms due to brain metastases respond less well, though radiotherapy is thought to be of value in consolidating on any improvement gained with dexamethasone. Ideally, palliative treatment should allow patients to spend as much time as possible at home. With this aim, palliative radiotherapy regimes have been developed in which larger doses are given in fewer fractions (2 fractions of 8.5 Gy one week apart) with results that are claimed to be as effective as standard regimes (30 Gy in 10 fractions over 2 weeks).

Side effects of external radiotherapy are common and dose related. These include fatigue, cough, breathlessness, dysphagia related to oesophagitis, and transient myelopathy. Although most problems are self-limiting, irreversible damage to the lungs and spinal cord may occur. Pneumonitis may develop 2–3 months after radiotherapy and, although it usually responds to oral steroids, it may be followed at about 6 months by radiation fibrosis. This usually presents little diagnostic difficulty as the fibrosis is often demarcated by a straight edge representing the margin of the treatment field. More severe and debilitating problems may arise as a result of damage to the spinal cord which tends to occur as a late complication and may result in permanent paraplegia. Great care must therefore be taken to shield the spinal cord from excessive radiation.

Chemotherapy for Non-small Cell Lung Cancer

Chemotherapy has traditionally been regarded as being inappropriate for non-small cell lung cancer. However, several drugs have now been shown to have significant activity (ifosfamide, cisplatin, mitomycin C and vindesine). Recently, a large meta-analysis involving over 9 000 patients recruited into 52 randomised trials was undertaken which compared surgery, surgery combined with radical radiotherapy, radical radiotherapy and best supportive care with the same treatment plus chemotherapy.[8] In the case of patients receiving cisplatin-based regimes, the study showed a 5-year survival advantage of 5% for the first 3 groups and a median survival advantage of 2 months for patients receiving best supportive care. However, due to the relatively small numbers of patients, the treatment effects could not be estimated with sufficient accuracy.

A large multicentre trial, known as the Big Lung Trial (BLT), has now been established in the UK to assess the value of cisplatin-based chemotherapy. In addition to evaluating the effects of treatment on survival, quality of life measurements (see below) are being undertaken in patients receiving best supportive care. It is hoped that the BLT will answer the important question as to whether the benefits of treatment justify the extra costs.

The possibility of improving survival in non-small cell carcinoma with chemotherapy offers hope that the addition of more recently introduced drugs (such as gemcitabine, vinerelbine, taxanes and the topoisomerase 1 inhibitors) will enhance survival further. Although it is unrealistic to expect dramatic survival advantages with chemotherapy, it should be appreciated that a small percentage improvement in survival translates into a large number of lives saved for a disease as common as lung cancer.

Chemotherapy and Radiotherapy for Small Cell Lung Cancer

Nearly all patients with small cell lung cancer have disease that is too advanced for curative local treatments. Systemic treatment with chemotherapy offers the only real prospect of improving survival for the majority of patients and has now become established as the first-line treatment of choice. In untreated patients, median survival ranges from 4–12 weeks but increases to 6–15 months with appropriate combination chemotherapy.

Several drugs have been shown to be active in small cell lung cancer with the greatest responses being seen with combined treatment. The most frequently used drugs include cyclophosphamide (C), adriamycin (A), vincristine (V), etoposide (E), and cisplatin (P), while the most widely used combinations are CAV and EP. Considerable interest has centred on optimising dosage, treatment intervals and duration of treatment together with evaluations of alternating regimes and combination radiotherapy.

The most fundamental question concerns the duration of treatment. There have been several studies comparing few (4–6) with many (7–12) courses of treatment. The consensus view is that there is no appreciable advantage over 6 courses and this has now become a standard regime. Because of the evolution of chemoresistance in patients undergoing treatment, the possibility of alternating regimes has also been considered though it appears that this does not confer a significant survival advantage over sequential therapy.

It is widely assumed that the response to chemotherapy has a classical "S" shaped dose response curve. Attention has therefore been given to administering drugs at doses as near as possible to the 'plateau' of the dose response relationship. Although more patients exhibited complete and durable responses, it became apparent that most patients relapsed and that the long term results were not improved. Moreover, the toxicity of treatment was considerable with patients requiring autologous bone marrow support.

An alternative approach to high dose treatment has been to administer treatment at shorter intervals of 1 week rather than the usual interval of 3–4 weeks, allowing treatment regimes to be completed within 3–4 months rather than 5–6 months. Although a greater number of complete responders are seen with this more intensive treatment, the toxicity is greater with patients requiring longer periods of hospitalisation.

Treatment toxicity may be ameliorated to some extent with the use of granulocyte colony-stimulating factor (GCSF) which has been introduced within the last decade. Controlled trials have shown that GCSF significantly reduces neutropenia, fever and the requirement for intravenous antibiotics in hospital when administered in relation to the first course of chemotherapy. However, its use is not associated with improved response rates and survival.

Small cell lung cancer is very radiosensitive and there has been some debate as to when radiotherapy should be administered.

Essentially, radiotherapy has been given in 3 situations: to improve the control of the primary tumour and regional nodal disease, to prevent cranial metastases, and to palliate progressive disease. Meta-analyses have shown small but significant improvements in survival when thoracic radiotherapy is combined with chemotherapy in patients with limited disease and there is evidence to suggest that early treatment may significantly reduce the risk of developing brain metastases. However, combined treatment leads to increased toxicity and so must usually be offered to patients with good fitness and performance status.

Brain metastases occur commonly in small cell lung cancer and interest has focused on the value of prophylactic cranial irradiation (PCI) for subclinical disease. Treatment is believed to reduce the risk of developing clinically significant brain metastases but there is evidence to suggest that long-term survivors may be at risk of developing progressive neurological and intellectual disability. Although the precise role of PCI has not yet been established, it is still given to patients who exhibit complete responses to chemotherapy but with precautions that are intended to reduce the risks of long-term toxicity. These precautions include avoiding concurrent chemotherapy and ensuring that the total radiation dose does not exceed 36 Gy and that the daily fraction does not exceed 2.0 Gy.

Disease recurrence following chemotherapy occurs in the majority of patients. Treatment with relapse chemotherapy tends to be disappointing though palliative radiotherapy may be extremely effective. Conditions which respond well to radiotherapy include SVCO, symptomatic brain metastases and large airway obstruction. It should be appreciated, however, that these conditions initially respond well to chemotherapy and that this treatment should always be considered as first line treatment at the time of presentation.

Carcinoid Tumours and Their Management

Carcinoid tumours account for approximately 1% of all lung tumours (see Table 1). Two types of tumour are recognised: classic (well differentiated) and atypical carcinoids (moderately differentiated). Classic carcinoid tumours have a more benign pattern of behaviour such that the regional lymph nodes are involved in about 11% patients as compared with 60% for atypical carcinoids. They resemble small cell carcinoma by showing neuroendocrine differentiation and histological distinction may be difficult when reviewing small bronchial biopsy specimens. However, this distinction is of great importance as their behaviour and management differ very substantially.

Although carcinoid tumours may present as asymptomatic opacities on the chest radiograph, they more commonly arise within the large airways and lead to recurrent chest infections and persistent symptoms of cough, breathlessness, wheeze and haemoptysis. As with other centrally situated tumours, patients with carcinoid tumours are frequently misdiagnosed and may become severely compromised by large airway obstruction. Rapid relief may be obtained with laser resection allowing more definitive surgery to be performed later as an elective procedure (see below). The results of surgery are excellent with 5-year survival figures in the region of 90–100% for classic carcinoids and 60% for atypical carcinoids.

Endobronchial Therapies

See Chapter 3, pages 73, 74.

Large airway obstruction is an important cause of morbidity and mortality in patients with lung cancer. Although chemotherapy and radiotherapy may provide effective palliation, they are limited by their cumulative toxicity and slowness of response. There is often a need for additional treatments which can provide rapid relief from large airway obstruction and which are effective in patients with recurrent disease who have already received full courses of radiotherapy and chemotherapy.

Three types of endobronchial treatment have been developed to meet these needs (Table 8) and should be regarded as being complementary. Tumour debulking methods are appropriate for airways obstructed by intraluminal tumour, airway stents are appropriate for extrinsically compressed airways, while endobronchial radiotherapy may be used to manage combinations of intraluminal tumour and extrinsic compression.

Treatment should only be offered to patients whose main symptoms are due to endobronchial disease. The benefits of treatment vary according to the level of obstruction, being most marked in patients with centrally situated tumours (e.g. trachea, main carina and proximal main bronchi) but diminish with more peripheral obstruction. Patients are likely to benefit from treatment if patent airways supplying viable lung tissue exist beyond the point of obstruction. Careful patient selection is therefore crucial.

Table 8.   Endobronchial therapies for lung cancer

Debulking of intraluminal tumour

Debridement with forceps
Diathermy resection
Cryotherapy
Laser resection
Photodynamic therapy (PDT)

Airway stenting

Silicone rubber tubes
Expandable metal stents

Endobronchial radiotherapy

Low dose
High dose

Tumour debulking

A number of treatments exist for removing intraluminal tumour from the airways (Table 8). The most basic method involves the use of forceps to debride tumour but this may be associated with bleeding which is particularly hazardous in patients with already narrowed airways. Techniques which allow tumours to be heated (diathermy and laser resection) or frozen (cryotherapy) reduce the risk of bleeding considerably and are more widely used.

Comparative studies between these debulking methods have not been conducted though laser resection (usually with a neodymium YAG laser) is now the most widely practised technique. Studies have shown significant improvements in symptoms, lung function and performance status. It has been found to be particularly useful in patients with severe breathlessness due to tracheal obstruction where the improvement is immediate (Figure 3) and enables subsequent management to be offered electively and in greater safety. In some situations, it has been possible to offer curative tracheal resections after laser treatment. It should be appreciated, however, that laser treatment is technically demanding and that it requires a general anaesthetic. The other important limitation is that the response may not be particularly durable, though this may be prolonged with the addition of endobronchial radiotherapy (see below).

More recently, interest has focused on the use of photodynamic therapy (PDT) which allows tumour to be destroyed with some

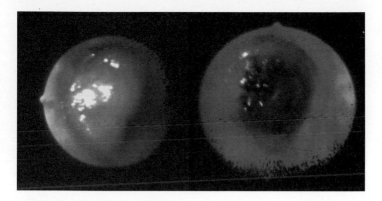

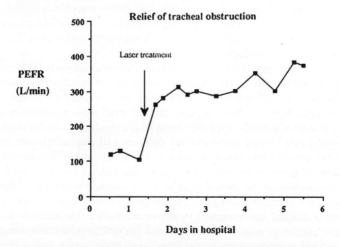

Relief of tracheal obstruction

Laser treatment

PEFR (L/min)

Days in hospital

Figure 3. The bronchoscopic appearances (top) of a tracheal tumour are shown before and immediately after laser treatment. The functional improvement was very rapid and is evident from the patient's peak flow chart (bottom)

selectivity. The principle of treatment is to administer a photosensitising drug which is retained by malignant tissues. Illumination of the involved airway with light of a suitable wavelength (usually emitted by a laser) activates the drug to produce a localised cytotoxic effect mediated via singlet oxygen. Although normal tissues are also affected, damage to collagen is avoided and healing is excellent with the result that the structural integrity of the airway is maintained.

Most clinical experience with PDT has been obtained with the drug, Photofrin, which is a derivative of haematoporphyrin. Preliminary studies comparing Photofrin PDT with YAG laser resection suggest that it may provide more effective and durable palliation. The important advantage of PDT is that it allows tumour destruction to a greater depth. Its important disadvantage, however, is light sensitivity, which requires the avoidance of direct sunlight for several weeks after treatment.

Airway stents

Extrinsically compressed airways are best managed with stents. The first stents were constructed from silicone rubber and, although they were very effective at relieving airway obstruction, their placement was technically difficult while their bulk interfered with mucociliary clearance and predisposed to infection.

More recently, a variety of expandable metal stents have been developed which can be positioned within the airways with greater ease at bronchoscopy. One of the earliest designs was the Gianturco stent, which is constructed from stainless steel wire arranged in a zig-zag configuration into the shape of a cylinder. It can be compressed and loaded into a hollow delivery catheter which can be introduced across extremely narrow strictures within the airway. When aligned in the correct position, the outer catheter is withdrawn to release the stent (Figure 4). The expansile properties of the stent then gradually overcome the compressive effects of the tumour with a gradual improvement in airway diameter. The metal of the stent in contact with the bronchial wall becomes epithelialised and does not interfere with mucociliary clearance, while metal that overlies a lobar orifice is not epithelialised. Unlike their silicone rubber counterparts, they are most unlikely to compromise ventilation when deployed in the more peripheral airways. Their important disadvantage is that they cannot prevent intraluminal tumour encroaching within the airway. However, covered stents are now being developed which may overcome this problem.

Endobronchial radiotherapy

Airway obstruction is frequently due to a combination of intraluminal tumour and extrinsic compression, for which neither laser treatment nor stenting are wholly appropriate. Although many

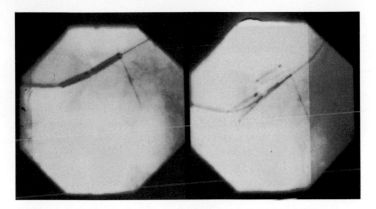

Figure 4. An expandable metal stent, loaded within a delivery catheter, is shown as it is being aligned within a bronchial stricture (left figure). The delivery catheter is then withdrawn and the stent is released into the airway (right figure). The expansile properties of the stent then overcome the compressive effects of the tumour responsible for the bronchial narrowing

patients may have received full courses of external radiotherapy, it may be possible to deliver further radiotherapy with endobronchial radiotherapy (brachytherapy) in which a radioactive source is placed within the involved airway. The dose of radiation falls off steeply with distance, according to the inverse square law, such that very high doses are delivered to the tumour and peribronchial tissues but negligible doses to the lung parenchyma, spinal cord and oesophagus.

A number of techniques for delivering endobronchial radiotherapy have been developed. The most sophisticated involve the use of high activity Iridium-192 sources which are loaded by remote control into afterloading catheters which have been positioned bronchoscopically within the airways. Treatment can be completed within 10–15 minutes under sedation, to deliver doses of up to 15 Gy in a single fraction at 1 cm radius from the source. Treatment has the advantages of being simple and easy to administer and can be offered on a day case basis.

Although endobronchial radiotherapy has been given with curative intent to a small number of patients with limited endobronchial disease with poor medical fitness, the main indication is as palliation. In a recent overview of the American literature involving over

600 patients, bronchoscopic improvement was noted in 80–100% of cases, while lung re-expansion was obtained in 64–88% patients with complete or partial atelectasis. Symptoms of cough, breathlessness and haemoptysis were relieved in 75–100%, though it is clear that cough responds less well than breathlessness and haemoptysis. As with laser treatment, physiological studies have demonstrated significantly improved indices of lung function and performance status. The response to treatment is claimed to be durable with two thirds of patients requiring no further treatment during their lifetime. However, interpretation of the published data is complicated by the heterogeneity of the patients studied, with some patients being offered treatment as a primary palliation and others as salvage treatment.

The most common complication is radiation oedema and bronchitis which occurs in up to a third of patients. This may be hazardous in patients with severe obstruction of a central airway and it may be necessary to protect the airway with prior laser treatment. Radiation strictures may occur as a late complication but are rare. Of more concern are the reports of fistula formation and torrential haemoptysis. However, these events usually occur at a relatively late stage in patients with longer overall survival and it is possible that they are due to recurrent tumour rather to the effects of treatment.

Quality of Life and Treatment Decisions

It is a harsh reality that the majority of lung cancer patients will not be cured and that the mainstay of their treatment will be to relieve their symptoms. The success of treatment should therefore not be judged solely in terms of survival, or a reduction in tumour volume, but should also include a measure of the patient's symptoms and overall wellbeing. Successful anticancer treatments may ensure that patients both live longer and feel better but, until recently, little attention has been given to their quality of life.

Quality of life defies a simple definition but encompasses the physical and psychosocial aspects of a patient's life. Although imperfect and incomplete, methods for measuring quality of life have now been designed and are already beginning to influence treatment decisions. The clinician may have little difficulty in selecting surgery for a patient with an early stage tumour as the long term benefits of cure obviously outweigh the morbidity and mortality associated with the operation. However, the decision to offer chemotherapy to a patient with advanced non-small cell lung cancer is very much more difficult when the perceived benefit is increased survival of only two months. Treatment may be justified, however, if treatment leads to a significantly improved quality of life. Alternatively, quality of life studies may demonstrate that the side effects of treatment outweigh the benefits of improved survival.

Quality of life studies may also be helpful in deciding on the timing of treatment. Traditionally, definitive anticancer treatments are given to patients with newly diagnosed disease while palliative care is offered in the later stages of the disease. However, quality of life studies indicate the benefits of an early palliative care input when the patient is coming to terms with the diagnosis of lung cancer. This subject is covered in more detail in Chapter 29.

Prospects of Early Detection in High Risk Groups

The poor outlook in patients with lung cancer is generally attributed to the late presentation of the disease. An obvious approach has been to develop methods for detecting lung cancers at very much earlier stages when treatment is more likely to be curative. It has been known since the studies of Auerbach and colleagues that changes of metaplasia, dysplasia and carcinoma in situ may occur over wide areas of the tracheobronchial tree and that they are particularly common in individuals who have smoked heavily and/or developed invasive lung cancer.[9] These observations have led to the widely held belief that lung cancers (particularly squamous cell carcinomas) develop through a series of morphological stages from metaplasia to dysplasia, to carcinoma in situ and then to invasive disease.

The possibility of detecting these pre-invasive lesions with sputum cytology was raised by the findings of a longitudinal study of radium workers in whom abnormal epithelial cells were found years before a clinical diagnosis of lung cancer was made.[10] However, a multi-centre trial conducted at the Mayo Clinic,[11] Johns Hopkins,[12] and Memorial Sloane-Kettering[13] Hospitals failed to demonstrate improved long-term survival in patients who had undergone intensive screening with sputum cytology. Although more cases of early stage lung cancers were detected in the screened populations with improved 5-year survivals, this was attributed to lead-time and length-time bias, as the eventual mortality from lung cancer was identical to that of the control groups.

Despite the disappointment of this trial, interest has continued in the development of sputum cytology as a screening tool by utilising immunocytochemical and molecular genetic tumour markers and there is evidence to suggest that its sensitivity may be enhanced significantly. However, the visualisation of early lesions within the tracheo-bronchial tree by conventional bronchoscopy may be technically very difficult, as they may only be a few cell layers thick and a few millimetres in surface diameter.

In order to facilitate the detection of these lesions, bronchoscopic systems are now being developed that exploit differences in the fluorescence properties of normal and abnormal bronchial epithelium. Preliminary experience suggests that fluorescence bronchoscopy may lead to a 6 fold increase in the detection of dysplasia and carcinoma in situ. However, this in turn creates the dilemma as to how these lesions should be managed when there is no absolute certainty that some or all will progress to invasive malignancy. The hope for the future is that markers of tumour progression will enable genuinely pre-malignant lesions to be identified and then eradicated before they progress to invasive disease.

An important limitation of bronchoscopy is its inability to detect lesions within the peripheral airways. CT scanning enables small peripheral lesions to be detected but, until recently, its slow scanning times and excessive radiation exposure have made it unsuitable for screening. However, with the development and refinement of spiral CT, it has become possible to reduce scanning times and radiation exposure significantly. Preliminary experience in screening high-risk populations with this technique has been encouraging such that 80–90% of bronchial carcinomas have been found to be stage 1.

Standards of Care

There is now growing concern that the management of lung cancer in the UK falls short of accepted standards of practice in several important respects. Reviews of unselected groups of patients with lung cancer have recently demonstrated wide variations in management practices, which relate to the age of the patient, place of residence and speciality interest of the hospital clinician to whom the patient has been referred. A substantial number of patients are not referred to chest physicians or specialists with an interest in thoracic oncology and there is evidence to suggest that these patients are less likely to undergo appropriate investigations and less likely to receive active treatments such as surgery, radiotherapy or chemotherapy. As the proportion of patients with lung cancer who undergo surgery in the UK is substantially less than in Europe and North America, concerns have been expressed that some patients with operable tumours are being denied the chance of curative surgery in our present system.

There is also evidence of extreme delays in the management of lung cancer patients. In one recent study,[14] the average interval from first presentation to surgery was found to be 4 months. Although there is no evidence to suggest that management delays of this magnitude adversely affect eventual clinical outcomes, they must inevitably heighten the anxiety and distress suffered by patients and their families. Common sense therefore dictates that we should manage our patients more efficiently.

A number of recommendations have now been drawn up which attempt to address these important deficiencies.[15,16] The most recent come from the British Thoracic Society and cover a range of issues which include management delays, collaboration between different hospital specialists, provision of palliative care and standards of communication between specialist, patient and general practitioner.[16]

In particular, it is recommended that all patients, regardless of age, be referred immediately to a respiratory physician when there is radiological or other evidence of lung cancer. The respiratory physician should see inpatient referrals within two working days and outpatient referrals within 1 week. Unless there are compelling reasons to the contrary, histological and/or cytological evidence of malignancy should be obtained in all patients. All patients who are potential candidates for surgery should have staging computed tomography. There should be no more than 4 weeks' delay between accepting a patient for thoracotomy and proceeding to surgery, while the interval between the first consultation with a respiratory physician and surgery should be no more than 8 weeks.

Although rigid guidelines have not been drawn up on the organisation of individual lung cancer services, a 'team approach' involving a respiratory physician, specialist nurse, oncologist, surgeon, pathologist, radiologist, and palliative medicine physician is strongly recommended. The problems posed by lung cancer are varied, while the range of treatments is increasing to such an extent that it is now no longer feasible for just one specialist to take sole responsibility for the lung cancer patient.

References

1. Doll R, Hill AB. Smoking and carcinoma of the lung. Preliminary report. *Br Med J* 1950;**2**:739

2. WHO Histological Typing of Lung Tumours, 2nd ed. Geneva: World Health Organisation 1981

3. Geddes DM. The natural history of lung cancer: A review based on rates of tumour growth. *Br J Dis Chest* 1979;**73**:1–17

4. Empey DW. Assessment of upper airways obstruction. *Br Med J* 1972;**3**:503

5. Mountain CF. A new international staging system for lung cancer. *Chest* 1986;**89** (suppl):225s–233s

6. Mountain C.F. Revisions in the international system for staging lung cancer. *Chest* 1997;**111**:1710–17

7. Saunders M, Dische S, Barrett A et al. Continuous hyperfractionated accelerated radiotherapy (CHART) versus conventional radiotherapy in non-small cell lung cancer: a randomised multicentre trial. *The Lancet* 1997;**350**:161–165

8. Non-small Cell Lung Cancer Collaborative Group — Chemotherapy in non-small cell lung cancer:a meta-analysis using updated data on individual patients from 52 randomised clinical trials. *Br Med J* 1995;**311**:899–909

9. Auerbach O, Gere JB, Forman JB et al. Changes in the bronchial epithelium in relation to smoking and cancer of the lung. *N Engl J Med* 1957;**256**:97–104

10. Saccommanno G, Archer VE, Auerbach O et al. Development of carcinoma in situ of the lung as reflected in exfoliated cells. *Cancer* 1974;**33**:256–70

11. Fontana RS, Sanderson DR, Taylor WF, Woolner LB et al. Early lung cancer detection: Results of the initial (prevalence) radiological and cytologic screening in the Mayo Clinic study. *Am Rev Resp Dis* 1984;**130**:561–5

12. Frost JK, Ball WC, Levin ML, Tockman MS et al. Early lung cancer detection:Results of the initial (prevalence) radiologic and cytologic screening in the John Hopkins study. *Am Rev Resp Dis* 1984;**130**: 549–54

13. Flehinger BJ, Melamed MR, Zaman MB, Heelan RT et al. Early lung cancer detection: Results of the initial (prevalence) radiologic and cytologic screening in the Memorial Sloane-Kettering study. *Am Rev Resp Dis* 1984;**130**:555–60

14. Billing JS, Wells FC. Delays in the diagnosis and treatment of lung cancer. *Thorax* 1996;51:903–6

15. Standing Medical Advisory Committee. Management of Lung Cancer: Current Clinical Practices. London: Department of Health 1994

16. BTS Recommendations to respiratory physicians for organising the care of patients with lung cancer. *Thorax* 1998;**53** (Suppl 1):S1–8

11

Pleural Diseases and Techniques

Gerrard Phillips

SECTION 1. PLEURAL EFFUSION

Clinical Features

These depend on the underlying cause and rate of formation.

Symptoms

Of the effusion:

- chest pain: implies involvement of the parietal pleura and, if dull, may indicate malignancy
- cough: mechanism unknown
- Dyspnoea

Of the cause:

- neoplasia, TB, connective tissue disease, smoking, asbestos exposure, drugs and foreign travel

Signs

Of the effusion:

- alteration in size of the hemithorax.

If the pleural pressure is increased the hemithorax will be increased in size and the intercostal space concavity lost. If the pleural pressure is reduced, as with obstruction of a major bronchus or a trapped lung, the hemithorax will be smaller and the normal concavity of the intercostal spaces will be exaggerated. In many patients, the hemithoraces are equal in size and the intercostal spaces are normal.

- reduced movement of the ispilateral hemithorax
- reduced tactile vocal fremitus and percussion note
- absent breath sounds
- aegophony and whispering pectroliloquy may be audible at the upper border of the effusion
- if moderate or large, mediastinal displacement away from the side of the effusion. If not, suspect volume loss of the ipsilateral lung eg obstructing carcinoma

Of any underlying cause:

- neoplasia, connective tissue disease.

Imaging

The plain chest radiograph

The PA and/or lateral chest radiograph is usually the first investigation. Normal lung is of lower density than fluid and tends to float on the effusion, whilst maintaining its normal shape. This allows the pleural fluid to accumulate in the most dependent part of the hemithorax, initially in a subpulmonary location. Up to 75 ml of effusion can occupy the subpulmonary space without spillover. At least 75 ml are required to obliterate the posterior costophrenic sulcus on the lateral view, and a minimum of 175 ml to obscure the lateral costophrenic sulcus on the upright PA or AP view. When 1 litre of fluid is present, the effusion usually reaches the level of the fourth anterior rib. The characteristic meniscal shape of the upper border of a pleural effusion is an 'apparent' phenomenon caused by the greater depth of pleural fluid (in A-P extent) that exists laterally.

In moderate/large pleural effusions, the mediastinum should be displaced away from the side of the effusion. If not, disease of the ipsilateral lung should be suspected, such as obstruction of a major bronchus.

A large pleural effusion, particularly on the left, can cause inversion of the diaphragm, paradoxical diaphragmatic movement with respiration, and thereby sudden worsening of breathlessness which can be ameliorated by removal of a relatively small amount of pleural fluid.

Subpulmonary pleural effusions are easily missed. Radiological signs suggesting their presence include (a) elevation of a hemidiaphragm (b) the apex of the apparent hemidiaphragm is more lateral than usual (c) the apparent diaphragm slopes much more sharply toward the lateral costophrenic angle (d) loss of the usually apparent lung markings below the level of the diaphragm (e) on the left side > 2 cm separation between the diaphragm and the gastric air bubble. The posterior costophrenic angle is usually blunted, but may be clear. A lateral decubitus view can confirm the presence of a suspected subpulmonary effusion, by demonstrating the presence of free pleural fluid.

In a supine film it is easy to miss the presence of even moderate pleural effusions. The earliest sign is blunting of the costophrenic angle, followed by increased homogeneous density superimposed over the lung, loss of the diaphragmatic silhouette and decreased visibility of the lower lobe vasculature. Apical capping and accentuation of the minor fissure are other features. The increased density caused by pleural fluid may be distinguished from that attributable to a parenchymal process by (a) preservation of the vascular structures (b) its homogeneous nature and (c) the absence of air bronchograms.

Atypical pleural effusions occur when the underlying lung is diseased. In lower lobe disease, the effusion will collect posteromedially, causing opacification in the posteroanterior (P-A) chest X-ray to be higher on the mediastinal than on the axillary border, its upper border curving downward and laterally toward the lateral costophrenic sulcus, thereby simulating atelectasis and consolidation of the middle and lower lobes.

Fluid located in the fissures may simulate a pulmonary mass lesion when viewed on a P-A chest radiograph. However, on a lateral view, such loculations have a characteristic sharply defined biconvex appearance and blend into the interlobar fissures. Loculations occurring between the lung and the chest wall produce a characteristic D-shaped appearance, the base of the D being against the chest wall and the convexity protruding inward toward the lung.

Ultrasound

This can differentiate pleural thickening from pleural fluid. It can also demonstrate whether the fluid collection is (a) echo free (anechoic), (b) complex septated (fibrin bands in an anechoic effusion), (c) complex non septated (heterogeneous echogenic material), (d) homogeneously echogenic. It can identify loculations and determine the best site for attempted thoracentesis, pleural biopsy or intercostal intubation. It is essential that any procedure is performed as soon as possible after the ultrasound examination (best at the same time) and with the patient in the same position.

Computed tomography

Chest CT is not necessary in all patients with suspected pleural disease and ultrasound is preferred when the issue is to determine whether or not pleural fluid is present. However, CT can detect pleural abnormalities more readily than standard radiographs and can distinguish them from lung parenchymal and extrapleural disease. Pleural processes usually have an obtuse angle with the chest wall in contrast to parenchymal disease. Free pleural fluid produces a sickle-shaped opacity in the most dependent part of the thorax posteriorly. CT is particularly useful in distinguishing empyema from lung abscess. Contrast enhancement can help distinguish pulmonary from pleural processes.

Table 1. Diagnoses that can be established definitively by pleural fluid analysis

Disease	Diagnostic pleural fluid tests
Empyema	pus, putrid odour, culture
Malignancy	cytology
Lupus pleuritis	ANA
Tuberculous pleurisy	positive AFB stain, culture
Oesophageal rupture	high amylase, pleural fluid acidosis
Fungal pleurisy	positive stain, culture
Chylothorax	triglycerides (>1.2 mmol/l), lipoprotein electrophoresis (chylomicrons)
Haemothorax	haematocrit (pleural fluid/blood >0.5)
Urinothorax	creatinine (pleural fluid/serum >1.0)
Peritoneal dialysis	protein (<10g/l), glucose (16–22.5 mmol/L)
Extravascular migration of central venous catheter	milky if lipids were infused, pleural fluid/serum glucose >1.0
Rheumatoid pleurisy	characteristic cytology

Diagnostic Approach to Pleural Effusions

Analysis of the fluid itself is fundamental. At least 30–50 ml should be aspirated but only in approximately 25% of cases can a definite diagnosis be established by pleural aspiration. However, a presumptive diagnosis can be reached in a further 50% of patients when the pleural findings are considered with the clinical context.[1] Diagnoses that can be established with certainty by pleural aspiration are shown in Table 1. Gross observation of the appearance and smell of the aspirated pleural fluid may also suggest the diagnosis. Examples are given in Table 2.

Table 2. Observations of pleural fluid helpful in diagnosis

Colour of fluid	Suggested diagnosis
Pale yellow (straw)	Transudate, some exudates
Red (bloody)	Malignancy, benign asbestos pleural effusion, postcardiac injury syndrome, or pulmonary infarction in absence of trauma.
White (milky)	Chylothorax; pseudochylothorax.
Brown	Long-standing bloody effusion; rupture of amoebic liver abscess.
Black	Aspergillus
Yellow-green	Rheumatoid pleurisy
Colour of Enteral tube feeing	Feeding tube has entered pleural space
Central venous catheter infusate	Extravascular catheter migration.

Character of fluid	Suggested diagnosis
Pus	Empyema
Viscous	Mesothelioma
Debris	Rheumatoid pleurisy
Turbid	Inflammatory exudate or chylothorax.
Anchovy paste	Amoebic liver abscess

Smell of fluid	Suggested diagnosis
Putrid	Anaerobic empyema
Ammonia	Urinothorax

Table 3. Causes of transudative pleural effusions

Effusion always transudative	Comment
Congestive heart failure	Acute diuresis can result in pseudoexudate
Cirrhosis	Rare without clinical ascites
Nephrotic syndrome Acute glomerulonephritis	Usually subpulmonary and bilateral
Peritoneal dialysis	Develops within 48 hours of initiating dialysis
Hypoalbuminaemia	Oedema fluid rarely isolated to pleural space
Urinothorax	Caused by ipsilateral obstructive uropathy
Atelectasis	Caused by increased intrapleural negative pressure
Constrictive pericarditis	Bilateral effusions
Trapped lung	A result of remote or chronic inflammation
Superior vena caval obstruction	May be due to acute systemic venous hypertension or acute blockage of thoracic lymph flow

Classic exudates that can be transudates	Comment
Malignancy	Due to early lymphatic obstruction, obstructive atelectasis, or concomitant disease
Pulmonary embolism	23% incidence; due to atelectasis
Sarcoidosis	Stage II and III disease
Hypothyroidism	From hypothyroid heart disease or hypothyroidism per se

Transudates

These are caused by imbalance between the hydrostatic and oncotic pressures across the pleura, and are most often the result of systemic conditions. They are usually bilateral. Causes are listed in Table 3, but the commonest are cardiac failure, hepatic cirrhosis, the

Table 4.   Commonest causes of pleural effusions

Transudates	Cardiac failure Hepatic cirrhosis Nephrotic syndrome Acute glomerulonephritis
Exudates: Infections	Parapneumonic Tuberculosis Subphrenic abscess.
Malignancy	Bronchial carcinoma Breast carcinoma Metastatic malignancy
Connective Tissue Disease	Rheumatoid arthritis SLE
Other	Pulmonary embolism Subdiaphragmatic (pancreatitis/subphrenic abscess) Trauma (haemothorax) Chylothorax

nephrotic syndrome, acute glomerulonephritis, and any cause of hypoproteinaemia (Table 4).

In cardiac failure the heart should be enlarged. In an autopsy series, 72% with congestive cardiac failure had pleural effusions and in 88% of cases these were bilateral. Only 8% had an isolated right pleural effusion and 4% an isolated left pleural effusion.[2] Therefore unilateral effusions, bilateral effusions with a significant size discrepancy, or bilateral effusions in the absence of cardiomegaly should prompt a search for alternative causes. The presence of pleural effusions in cardiac failure correlates with the degree of pulmonary venous hypertension and not with the degree of systemic venous hypertension. Isolated right heart failure such as cor pulmonale is rarely the cause of a pleural effusion and should also suggest an alternative diagnosis. After treatment of cardiac failure, the protein and LDH may increase to the exudative range.

In liver disease, pleural effusions occur in approximately 6% of cases and usually follow the development of ascites but may precede it. They are common on the right, probably because either diaphragmatic lymphatics are better developed on this side, or there are microscopic diaphragmatic defects.

Pleural effusions in the nephrotic syndrome are usually due to the systemic hypoproteinaemia but, in acute glomerulonephritis, the associated left ventricular failure is probably responsible.

Pleural effusions are rare in superior vena caval obstruction in adults.

Exudates

These usually result from **local** rather than from systemic disease. There are three main causative processes

- capillary protein leak due to pulmonary and/or pleural inflammation
- impaired lymphatic drainage of the pleural space — proteins are absorbed via the lymphatics, chiefly those of the parietal pleura
- movement of fluid from the peritoneal space — acute and chronic pancreatitis, chylous ascites and peritoneal carcinomatosis

Exudates are usually unilateral, although they may be bilateral in lymphoma, metastatic disease, pulmonary embolism and SLE. They usually resolve more slowly than transudates, because resolution depends on protein re-absorption by lymphatics in contrast to the flux of fluid across the normal pleural membrane. They are much more likely to be followed by residual pleural thickening and adhesions. Causes of exudative pleural effusions are shown in Table 5, but the more common causes are listed in Table 4.

Method of distinguishing exudates from transudates

Light and Coworkers[3] were able to correctly separate 99% of pleural effusions based on the following three criteria

- pleural fluid protein/serum protein ratio greater than 0.5
- pleural fluid lactate dehydrogenase (LDH)/serum LDH ratio greater than 0.6
- pleural fluid LDH greater than two thirds the upper limit of normal of the serum LDH.

The presence of one or more of Light's criteria indicates that the effusion is an exudate. The sensitivity and specificity of this

Table 5. Causes of exudative pleural effusions

INFECTIONS
Bacterial pneumonia
Tuberculous pleurisy
Parasites
Fungal disease
Atypical pneumonias
Nocardia, Actinomyces
Subphrenic abscess
Hepatic abscess
Splenic abscess
Hepatitis
Spontaneous oesophageal rupture

IATROGENIC
Drug-induced
Oesophageal perforation
Oesophageal sclerotherapy
Central venous catheter
    misplacement/migration
Enteral feeding tube in pleural space

MALIGNANCY
Carcinoma
Lymphoma
Leukaemia

INCREASED NEGATIVE
INTRAPLEURAL PRESSURE
Atelectasis
Trapped lung
Cholesterol effusion

OTHER INFLAMMATORY DISORDERS
Pancreatitis
Benign asbestos pleural effusion
Pulmonary embolism
Radiation therapy
Uraemic pleurisy
Sarcoidosis
Postcardic injury syndrome
Haemothorax
ARDS
Carcinoma
Chylous ascites
Urinothorax

CONNECTIVE TISSUE DISEASE
Lupus pleurisy
Rheumatoid pleurisy
Mixed connective tissue
    disease
Churg-Strauss syndrome
Wegener's granulomatosis
Familial Mediterranean Fever

ENDOCRINE DYSFUNCTION
Hypothyroidism
Ovarian hyperstimulation
    syndrome

LYMPHATIC ABNORMALITIES
Malignancy
Yellow nail syndrome
Lymphangioleiomyomatosis

MOVEMENT OF FLUID FROM
ABDOMEN TO PLEURAL SPACE
Pancreatitis
Pancreatic pseudocyst
Meig's syndrome
Chylothorax

distinction were 99% and 98% respectively in the original series. These features incorrectly identity some cardiac failure transudates as exudates. This difficulty may be compounded by diuresis, which may elevate pleural fluid protein. Light has suggested that in cardiac failure, if the serum-to-pleural albumin gradient exceeds 12 g/l, the effusion is probably a transudate. More recently, several alternatives to Light's criteria have been suggested, but non have supplanted them. These have included a pleural fluid cholesterol of greater than 1.2 mmol/l, a gradient between the serum and pleural fluid albumin greater than 12 g/l and a pleural to serum bilirubin ratio of greater than 0.6.

Useful diagnostic tests on pleural fluid

Protein

Exudates usually have a pleural fluid protein content of greater than 30 g/l. However, about 10% of transudates have a protein content of above 30 g/l and occasional exudates will have a pleural fluid protein below this level. Tuberculous pleural effusions almost always have total protein concentrations above 40 g/l. When pleural protein concentrations are in the 70–80 g/l range, Waldenstrom's macroglobulinaemia and multiple myeloma should be considered.

Lactate dehydrogenase

Very high pleural fluid LDH levels, exceeding 1000 IU/l, are typically found in empyema, rheumatoid arthritis, paragonimiasis and sometimes in malignancy. High LDH levels are also found in effusions secondary to *pneumocystis carinii* pneumonia. Typically the protein content of such effusions is low. A pleural fluid/serum LDH ratio greater than 1.0 and a pleural fluid/serum protein ratio less than 0.5 are suggestive.

Glucose

All transudates and many exudates have pleural fluid glucose concentrations similar to blood. However, if the pleural fluid glucose level is less than 3.3 mmol/l, or the pleural fluid/serum glucose ratio is less than 0.5 — a number of conditions are suggested

- rheumatoid pleurisy
- complicated parapneumonic effusion/empyema

- malignancy
- tuberculosis
- SLE
- oesophageal rupture

The lowest glucose concentrations are found in rheumatoid arthritis and empyema. In TB, SLE and malignancy levels are usually 1.7–2.8 mmol/l.

pH

The pH of normal pleural fluid is approximately 7.60. Transudates usually have a pH of 7.40–7.55 and exudates of 7.30–7.35. A pleural fluid pH of less than 7.1 suggests that a parapneumonic effusion is 'complicated' and requires drainage. A malignant pleural effusion with a low pH usually has a high positive yield on pleural fluid cytology, responds less well to chemical pleurodesis, and indicates a short patient survival.

Amylase

A raised pleural fluid amylase (> upper limit of normal for serum or a pleural/serum ratio > 1.0) suggests acute or chronic pancreatitis, oesophageal rupture or malignancy.

Nucleated cells

The **total** count is virtually never diagnostic. However, counts above 50,000/μl, are usually found only in complicated parapneumonic effusions and empyema. Exudates due to bacterial pneumonia, acute pancreatitis and lupus pleuritis usually demonstrate cell counts in excess of 10,000/μl, whereas chronic exudates, such as may be found in TB and malignancy, usually have cell counts less than 5000/μl.

The predominant cell type is dependent on the temporal relationship between the acute pleural injury and thoracentesis. The initial cellular response is neutrophilic, but this changes to mononuclear if the pleural injury does not persist. When the lymphocyte count is 85–95% of the total pleural fluid cell count, the cause is likely to be TB, lymphoma, sarcoidosis, chronic rheumatoid pleurisy, yellow nail syndrome or chylothorax. A lymphocyte count constituting 50–70% of the total is found in up to 50% of carcinomatous pleural effusions.

A pleural fluid eosinophilia (more than 10% eosinophils) suggests a benign, self limiting disease and is often associated with the presence of air or blood in the pleural space. There is usually a pleural fluid lymphocytosis too. There is no correlation with the peripheral blood eosinophil count. The differential diagnosis includes: pneumothorax (commonest), haemothorax (peak eosinophil count at 7–14 days), pulmonary infarction, benign asbestos pleural effusion, parasitic disease, fungal disease, drugs. Pleural fluid eosinophilia is uncommon in TB and malignancy.

Mesothelial cells are often found in transudates, but are less common in exudates. Mesothelial cell counts above 5% make TB an unlikely diagnosis.

The Undiagnosed Pleural Effusion

After the clinical assessment and initial pleural aspiration, the cause of a pleural effusion remains unknown in up to 25% of cases.[1] Often, a more thorough clinical evaluation will reveal the cause: a remote history of asbestos exposure, a relevant drug history (nitrofurantoin, amiodarone, drug-induced lupus-like syndromes), or the presence of ascites (patients with hepatic hydrothorax may not have clinical ascites as the ascitic fluid may move quickly into the chest). Undiagnosed pleural effusions are usually *exudates*, since the number of possible diagnoses to be entertained for transudative effusions is more limited. Transudative effusions that can cause diagnostic difficulty include those occurring in constrictive pericarditis, when the effusion although usually transudative can, on occasion, be exudative; and malignancy and pulmonary embolism, when usually exudative effusions may sometimes be transudative — as occurred in one third of the pulmonary embolism pleural effusions in one study.

The undiagnosed exudative pleural effusion is more problematic. A suggested approach is as follows

Repeat the pleural aspiration

Use a heparinised bottle and ensure the sample reaches the laboratory within 1–2 hours and is examined by an experienced cytopathologist. The literature suggests that the diagnostic yield from a single pleural aspirate ranges from 33–70%, but averages 60%.[4] The yield is higher for carcinoma of the breast and lung. The diagnostic yield may be increased by simply repeating the pleural aspiration. In one series the cumulative positive cytology rate rose from 53% to 74% when four separate samples were analysed. Negative cytology does NOT exclude malignancy.

Perform a pleural needle biopsy

This can be undertaken at the same time as the repeat pleural aspiration. The Abram's needle has remained the most popular, although there are others — Cope's needle, the Raja needle and the Tru-cut needle. Pleural biopsy should be undertaken at the lowest **safest** point that fluid can be located, since early metastases occur low in the pleural space. Sampling from two adjacent sites may increase the diagnostic yield, as may ultrasound localisation of any pleural masses. However, the increased diagnostic yield with pleural biopsy is low — only 7% in one series when fluid cytology was negative. Its sensitivity for malignancy averages 50% (range 40–72%).[5] However, most observers report increased sensitivity when pleural aspiration and biopsy are combined.[6] Operator skill is critical, and there have been suggestions for establishing a pleural biopsy service run by a Respiratory Team. Pleural biopsy is particularly important when a diagnosis of TB is being considered, since the sensitivity and specificity of pleural biopsy culture is high.

Consider additional diagnostic procedures

- VQ scanning
- chest CT: this is generally unrewarding but may, on occasion, demonstrate evidence of asbestos exposure, loculation with pleural enhancement in empyema, lymphadenopathy with malignancy
- bronchoscopy: this is rarely helpful in elucidating the cause of a pleural effusion unless the patient has cough, haemoptysis, a parenchymal lesion, a massive effusion or ipsilateral mediastinal shift on the chest radiograph
- thoracoscopy: this has excellent diagnostic yield for malignancy and TB, but is unnecessary in the latter since pleural tissue is often positive
- open pleural biopsy: even this may fail to establish the diagnosis. In one series, 51 patients were reported in whom this eventuality pertained. On follow up, 31 patients did not have a recurrence. Of the remainder, a diagnosis was eventually established in 18 cases, of whom 13 had malignancy ([6]lymphoma and [4]mesothelioma).

Observe the patient

This is a reasonable option if additional diagnostic procedures fail to achieve a diagnosis. In some clinical circumstances, it may be an alternative to option 3 (additional procedures), particularly if the patient is elderly and frail. In younger, fitter patients, however, it is unlikely that simple clinical observation would be acceptable unless additional diagnostic methods had failed. Nevertheless, the time course of a pleural effusion may be extremely informative

- pulmonary embolism: effusions resolve in 5–7 days without infarction and 7–14 days if infarction occurs
- uncomplicated parapneumonic effusions: resolve in 1–2 weeks
- abdominal surgery/post partum: small effusions commonly occur and resolve spontaneously in 1–2 weeks
- post cardiac surgery: effusions may last several weeks
- TB: pleural fluid may take 6 weeks to 4 months to disappear
- benign asbestos disease, rheumatoid arthritis, radiation: effusions may persist for several months
- yellow nail syndrome, trapped lung (eg chronic empyema): may cause effusions that persist for years

Trial of antituberculous therapy

This may be a reasonable option if TB is a likely diagnosis. This is particularly the case in an elderly, frail patient who is deteriorating and in whom there may be a six week wait for the results of pleural tissue culture.

Collagen Vascular Diseases

Rheumatoid arthritis

In one large study of 516 patients with rheumatoid arthritis, 21% had a history of pleurisy and 3.3% of pleural effusion. It is commoner in men, may occasionally antedate the onset of clinical rheumatoid arthritis, but on average occurs 13 years after the onset of disease and lasts a mean of 14 months. Rheumatoid effusions are more common in patients with rheumatoid nodules but are not related to disease activity. The effusion is exudative and may have a green colour due to the presence of cholesterol crystals. Characteristic findings include a low glucose (< 1.5 mmol/l) and pH (< 7.2), reduced C_3 and C_4 components of complement and a positive rheumatoid factor, although the latter is not a specific finding. At thoracoscopy, the parietal pleura has a 'gritty' or frozen appearance due to the presence of multiple small granules which, histologically, consist of small papillae containing capillaries. The visceral pleura looks normal or is only mildly inflamed.

Small effusions require no treatment and may resolve spontaneously leaving pleural thickening. Larger effusions should be aspirated and, if recurrent, pleurodesis considered. Corticosteroids are not proven. Persisting effusions may result in extensive pleural fibrosis requiring pleurectomy. Patients are not at increased risk of empyema. Pulmonary rheumatoid nodules, which typically have a subpleural distribution, may occasionally rupture into the pleural space, causing pneumothorax and bronchopleural fistula.

Systemic lupus erythematosus

In one large study of 105 patients with SLE, 16% had pleural effusions and > 50% gave a history of pleuritic pain. Pleural involvement may occur early in the course of the disease or be a presenting feature. Pleural effusions are often bilateral. Patients present with fever, pleuritic pain and breathlessness. The pleural fluid is exudative. In contrast to rheumatoid effusions, the pH is usually > 7.35, the glucose normal and the LDH < 500 IU/l. There is a high lymphocyte count, although occasionally the leucocyte count is raised. The C_3 and C_4 components of complement are reduced, rheumatoid factor is usually negative and there is often a high titre of antinuclear antibody. Effusions often resolve spontaneously. Pain may be relieved by non-steroidal anti-inflammatory drugs and, in contrast to rheumatoid arthritis, effusions caused by SLE respond well to corticosteroids.

Pleural effusions are occasionally seen in polyarteritis nodosa, scleroderma, dermatomyositis, ankylosing spondylitis, temporal arteritis, Wegener's granulomatosis and Churg-Strauss syndrome.

Pulmonary Embolism

Between 40–50% of patients with pulmonary embolism have a pleural effusion. The effusion is usually maximal at presentation or within 3 days, so that it is very unusual to see increase in size beyond this time unless there is recurrent PE. In 98% of patients there is a history of ipsilateral chest pain. Pleural effusion is almost always associated with pulmonary infarction, though there is radiographic evidence of this in only 55% of cases. The mean effusion size is 15% of the hemithoracic volume and 98% are unilateral. However, bilateral effusions and massive effusions have been described. Pulmonary infarction on X-ray is associated with larger and longer lasting pleural effusions.

Pleural fluid characteristics in PE are variable. In one study, 65% were blood stained and 65% were exudates. Radiographic evidence of pulmonary infarction correlates with blood staining. The white blood cell content is variable. There are often large numbers of neutrophils, and there may be a high proportion of mesothelial cells and eosinophils.

The presence or absence of a pleural effusion does not alter treatment.

Subdiaphragmatic Causes of Pleural Effusion

These include the following:

- pancreatic disease
- abdominal lymphoma
- subphrenic abscess
- intrahepatic infections — amoebic abscess, hydatid cysts
- paragonimiasis

Miscellaneous Causes of Pleural Effusions

Drugs

- lupus-like syndrome
  hydralazine, procainamide, phenytoin, isoniazid, chlorpromazine.
- oculomyocutaneous syndrome
  caused by practolol.
- others
  nitrofurantoin, dantrolene, methysergide, bromocriptine, procarbazine, methotrexate, ergotamine and amiodarone.

Dressler's syndrome

Usually small and bilateral.

Familial mediterrean fever

Pleurisy occurs in 50%.

Radiotherapy

Occasionally associated with pleural effusion.

Sarcoidosis

The prevalence of pleural effusion is 1.9%. They are usually small lymphocyte-rich exudates

Myxoedema

The prevalance rate is 18–50%. Effusions often have borderline transudate/exudate characteristics, may be unilateral or bilateral and are usually < 1/3 the volume of the hemithorax.

Amyloidosis

There are a small number of case reports of pleural involvement.

Yellow nail syndrome

The lymphatic hypoplasia that characterises this syndrome results in lymphocytic exudative effusions which may be large and bilateral. The fluid reaccumulates after aspiration and pleurodesis/pleurectomy may be required.

Uraemia

A fibrinous pleuritis is common and may develop despite dialysis. Pleural effusions are common but other causes, such as volume overload, need to be excluded. True uraemic pleural effusions are exudates and often blood stained. 80% are unilateral. They may be small or large. They usually respond to treatment of the uraemia but may be followed by fibrosis. 20% of patients with the nephrotic syndrome develop a transudative pleural effusion.

Urinothorax

This is rare.

Ascitic effusion

Transdiaphragmatic passage of ascitic fluid via pores or lymphatics in the diaphragm may result in a pleural effusion. This is seen in hepatic cirrhosis, peritoneal dialysis, the ovarian hyperstimulation syndrome (IVF treatment) and Meig's syndrome. The latter has four components: (a) ovarian fibroma (b) ascites (c) pleural effusion (d) resolution of the ascites and pleural effusion with removal of the tumour. Subsequently theca cell, granulosa cell and Brenner tumours of the ovary have been included. The fluid is thought to be produced by 'transudation' from the surface of the usually large tumour. It traverses diaphragmatic defects to reach the chest. It is usually an exudate and may be blood stained. 65% are right sided and 22% bilateral. The main importance is to realise that, in the case of a pelvic tumour, ascites and a pleural effusion may not necessarily indicate metastatic and incurable disease.

Cryptogenic bilateral fibrosing pleuritis

A small series of four patients has been described.

Asbestos exposure

Please see Chapter 17, page 472.

Parapneumonic Effusions and Empyema

Empyema means pus in the pleural space. The commonest cause is pulmonary infection (55%). Other causes include thoracic surgery (21%), trauma (6%), oesophageal perforation (5%), spontaneous pneumothorax and thoracentesis (2% each).[7] A pleural effusion occurs in approximately 40% of cases of pneumonia, and may evolve into an empyema in approximately 15% of these cases via three stages:

1. uncomplicated parapneumonic effusion
   an exudative, predominantly neutrophilic effusion.
2. complicated parapneumonic effusion
   produced by persistent bacterial invasion of the pleural space.

This latter causes an increased number of neutrophils. These, and the bacteria, metabolise glucose anaerobically, resulting in a pleural fluid acidosis and a reduced glucose concentration, whilst

Table 7. Pleural fluid analysis in parapneumonic effusions

	uncomplicated parapneumonic effusion	complicated para parapneumonic effusion	empyema
pH	> 7.30	7.1–7.29	< 7.1
Glucose mmol/l	> 2.2	< 2.2	< 2.2
LDH IU/l	< 1000	may > 1000	usually > 1000

neutrophil lysis raises the concentration of lactate dehydrogenase (LDH). Because patients have often already received antibiotics, and because bacteria are rapidly cleared from the pleural space, complicated parapneumonic effusions are often sterile.

3. empyema

This is characterised by the presence of bacterial organisms seen on gram stain, or a frankly purulent appearance. In the early stages the appearances are fibropurulent; the purulent fluid is accompanied by fibrin clots and membranes in the pleural space which result in loculation. In the later stages, invasion by fibroblasts transforms these fibrin membranes into thick, inelastic fibrous peels.

Distinguishing parapneumonic effusions and empyema

Pleural fluid analysis may help to distinguish the above three stages (Table 7). Pleural fluid pH may be superior to the other two chemical analyses.[8] However, this presupposes that the fluid is collected and transported under strictly anaerobic conditions, and that the pH measurement is undertaken immediately in a calibrated blood gas analyser. The measurement is less useful if there is a systemic acidosis and infection by *proteus* species may induce a local metabolic alkalosis. Recommendations for the pleural fluid pH value indicating intercostal tube drainage have varied. A suggested approach is given below.

Bacteriology

The microbiology of parapneumonic effusions is similar to that of the primary pneumonia. The majority that are culture positive are due to aerobic organisms, principally *Streptococci* (mostly *Strept. pneumoniae*) and *Staphylococci* (mostly *Staph. aureus*) amongst gram positive isolates and *Escherichia coli, Klebsiella Spp, Pseudomonas Spp, and Haemophilus influenzae* amongst gram negative isolates. Anaerobic organisms, however, feature prominently in empyema. Whist 15% are caused exclusively by such organisms, they may be cultured in association with other organisms in 36–76% of empyemas. The most frequent anaerobes are *Bacteroides Spp. and Peptostreptococcus*. Mixed culture results are common.

Clinical features

It is difficult, on purely clinical features to determine the presence of a parapneumonic effusion/empyema unless this is large. Aerobic infections tend to have a shorter more acute time course, whereas anaerobic organisms tend to occur in patients with poor oral hygiene, alcoholism, or aspiration, and are associated with a more subacute/chronic time course.

Imaging

The main finding on plain chest X-ray is an ipsilateral pleural effusion. A decubitus film may aid interpretation. The most typical sign of an empyema is an encapsulated effusion in an unusual position.

Ultrasound is a key investigation but is operator dependent. It is particularly useful for 'targeting' the aspiration/tube drainage of small or loculated effusions. Septated and loculated effusions are more likely to be complicated parapneumonic effusions and dense echogenic patterns are more often associated with empyemas or haemorrhage.

In one series, contrast-enhanced CT showed parietal pleural thickening in all cases of empyema and in 56% of parapneumonic effusions. There may be increased contrast uptake by the thickened parietal pleura and increased density of the adjacent subcostal tissue in empyema. CT may demonstrate parenchymal abnormality, lung abscess or endobronchial obstruction. On MRI scanning complicated parapneumonic effusions and empyemas tend to be associated with alterations of the peripheral fat layer and innermost intercostal muscle layer of the chest wall.

Management

The key to the management of parapneumonic effusions is to first determine whether or not they are complicated. One suggested approach is as follows

- measure the pleural fluid pH except for those that are frankly purulent or have a positive Gram stain, in which immediate tube drainage is recommended irrespective of the pH
- glucose measurements are only of value when there is doubt about the pH measurement
- proceed according to the pH
  - (i)   ≤7.0   tube drainage is usually indicated.
  - (ii) >7.0   the pH should not be the sole criterion to determine drainage. However, effusions with pH 7.0–7.2 should be observed closely and repeat thoracentesis undertaken, as tube drainage may well be necessary. If the pH is >7.2, observation alone should suffice, and if >7.3 a complicated course is very unlikely.

Uncomplicated parapneumonic effusions

These usually respond to antibiotics alone. As is the case for pneumonia, antibiotics should be started immediately specimens have been taken for bacteriology. In patients with community acquired pneumonia a second or third generation cephalosporin, or a beta-lactam/beta-lactamase inhibitor combination, should be used. Metronidazole or clindamycin should be added if anaerobic infection is likely. A macrolide should be included if mycoplasma or *Legionella* is suspected, although such parapneumonic effusions are rarely complicated. In severe nosocomial pneumonia, a third generation cephalosporin or imipenem are good alternative choices. Remember that if Gram-negative infections are suspected aminoglycosides may not be effective in the presence of a purulent, acidotic effusion and a low pO_2.

Complicated parapneumonic effusions

There are no controlled trials to guide selection of therapy. Until these have been done, there will remain a preference for early pleural cavity drainage and to manage such patients as if they have an empyema.

Empyema

Successful management requires achieving three main goals

- adequate systemic antibiotic therapy to sterilize the empyema cavity. Antibiotics alone are often less successful in empyema than other infections. This may be due to depletion of antibodies and complement from the empyema fluid.
- complete drainage of pleural fluid.
- complete obliteration of the empyema cavity; this requires successful re-expansion of the lung.

There are no convincing data to support additional local instillation of antibiotics into the empyema cavity.

There are a variety of methods for draining the pleural space, with no conclusive evidence favouring any one. A number of factors may guide choice: patient fitness, whether the fluid collection is loculated (best determined by ultrasound), and the duration of the empyema. Multiloculated empyemas are difficult to manage successfully with simple drainage techniques, and the inflammatory exudate starts to organize by the end of the third week, adding to this difficulty.

The techniques available for pleural space drainage in empyema are:

Repeated needle thoracentesis and antibiotic instillation

A prospective randomised study is needed.

Intercostal tube drainage

This is usually the preferred method. There are four main decisions to make: (a) whether or not radiological guidance is necessary (b) whether or not more than one tube is necessary (c) whether to use a small bore or large bore tube (d) whether or not to use intrapleural fibrinolysis.

Except in very straight forward circumstances, it is best to take advantage of radiological guidance for optimal tube placement. In complicated multiloculated empyemas, more than one tube may be required, and here ultrasound guidance is probably mandatory. Increasingly, small bore tubes have been demonstrated to be successful provided they are radiologically guided and provided the fluid in the pleural space is not thick pus. They may be particularly effective when combined with intrapleural fibrinolysis.

The idea of introducing a fibrinolytic agent into the pleural space in empyema is based on the supposition that adequate pleural drainage is impeded by the loculation of pleural fluid by fibrin septae and by fibrinous clot which can block drains. The first randomised controlled trial of the use of intrapleural streptokinase was published recently.[9] Twenty-four patients with systemic sepsis and a pleural effusion related to community acquired pneumonia were treated by systemic antibiotics and radiologically guided insertion of a 14 F catheter connected to an underwater drain and flushed with 20 ml of normal saline six hourly. For the first 3 days following catheter insertion twelve patients were randomised to receive a once daily instillation of 250,000 IU streptokinase in one of the 20 ml flushes. After instillation of streptokinase the catheter was clamped for 2 hours and then returned to suction. Three days after initiating streptokinase, the catheters were removed, provided drainage had fallen to < 150 ml per day on two consecutive days. The study determined that the mean volume of pleural fluid drained was significantly greater in the streptokinase group, both over the three days that streptokinase was given (0.39 l vs 0.12 l) and in total (2.56 l vs 1.06 l). Ten of the twelve streptokinase patients achieved > 75% reduction in the volume of their pleural collection, compared with four out of the twelve controls ($p < 0.05$). Three of the controls were referred for surgery, but none in the streptokinase group. There were no adverse events associated with streptokinase.

More evidence is required to show whether or not intrapleural streptokinase truly does affect the need for surgery, morbidity, mortality and length of hospital stay. However, it would seem reasonable to consider its use in patients with a parapneumonic effusion/empyema in whom ultrasound shows fibrinous septation or loculation and in whom the response to pleural drainage alone is incomplete.

Surgical drainage

In an ill patient with uncontrolled sepsis early recourse to surgery may be necessary. Otherwise, if the above methods fail to result in resolution of the parapneumonic effusion/empyema within two weeks, a surgical opinion should be requested. Between three weeks and three months after development of the empyema, the inflammatory adhesions are very vascular and may progress to pleural fibrosis, trapping the lung, preventing it re-expanding properly and obliterating the pleural space. Because the tissue is so vascular during this time, the morbidity of surgery is greater. It is therefore preferable to operate either before three weeks or after three months.

Thoracoscopic lysis of adhesions and debridement may be possible. However, this approach tends to be more successful earlier in the disease and may fail in the case of more extensive pleural adhesions. Its success rate is around 60%. The more standard approach of open thoracotomy and decortication has a success rate of up to 95% but carries with it the risks of major surgery. Early in the course of the empyema, this technique is indicated principally to control infection when other methods have failed, rather than from consideration of eventual lung function outcome, since even thick pleural peels can gradually resolve and lung function return to normal over many months, once the infection has been controlled. Late decortication to correct persisting impairment of lung function is usually only performed after several months. In patients who are unfit for thoracotomy and decortication, the alternative procedure of open thoracostomy may be considered. A vertical incision is made through the chest wall with rib resection to allow open drainage at the inferior border of the empyema cavity via a chest tube. This latter is gradually advanced outward as the track closes, but resolution usually takes 60–90 days.

The unresolving empyema

In this event, a number of possibilities need to be considered

- reassess the microbiology
- consider TB
- exclude a foreign body or carcinoma
- consider the possibility of a bronchopleural fistula
- in empyema secondary to subphrenic abscess, reassess whether the latter has been adequately drained

Empyema may complicate surgery to the chest, possibly with an attendant bronchopleural fistula. In the past these were managed by chronic open thoracostomy. Today, there are a number of techniques to achieve closure of the space including pleural space irrigation with antibiotics, space filling muscle pedicles and surgical closure of bronchopleural fistulae.

Tuberculous Pleural Effusions

In the West, tuberculous pleural effusions account for 5% of all disease due to the organism. However, in sub-Saharan Africa, where 15 million new cases of TB are expected in the next five years, the frequency is approximately 30%, and the frequency of co-existent HIV infection is approximately 60%.

Most tuberculous pleural effusions are associated with primary TB and develop six weeks to six months after infection. However, tuberculous effusions can occur with post primary TB and after reactivation. They are thought to occur after rupture of a subpleural focus of disease into the pleural space, and are in large part due to a delayed hypersensitivity reaction to the presence of mycobacterial antigens, although an infective element is also possible. There is an initial influx of neutrophils, followed by macrophages which predominate until day four. Thereafter, lymphocytes are predominant, particularly memory type helper T-cells (CD4+, CDW29+).

Clinical features

There is usually an acute febrile illness with a dry cough (94%), pleuritic chest pain (78%) and no elevation of the peripheral blood white cell count. When questioned, however, many patients have been unwell for weeks with fevers, night sweats, anorexia and weight loss.

Investigations

Skin tests

A negative tuberculin reaction has been reported in up to 30% of immunocompetent individuals; however, almost all patients become positive when retested 6–8 weeks later.

Radiology

Tuberculous effusions are unilateral in 95% of cases and usually occupy less than one-half of the hemithorax. Associated parenchymal disease is present in up to 50% of patients. In 75% of these there is upper lobe disease suggesting reactivation, with the remainder having lower lobe disease suggestive of primary disease. However, CT scanning reveals parenchymal disease in > 80% of cases. The parenchymal disease is usually ipsilateral to the pleural effusion.

Aspiration

The fluid is characteristically straw coloured and is almost always an exudate with a protein content of > 30 g/l, and > 50 g/l in 50–77% of cases. The LDH is elevated in 75% of cases. A low pH and glucose concentration can occur but are not diagnostically useful findings. The nucleated cell count is usually 1000–6000/mm^3 and there is lymphocyte predominance in 60–90% of cases. Neutrophils may predominate early in the time-course. The mesothelial cell count is usually < 5%; higher counts make TB unlikely. Similarly, an eosinophil count > 10% should lead to consideration of alternative diagnoses.

Organisms are rarely seen on direct staining of pleural fluid smears. The sensitivity of pleural fluid culture is also low, at 10–35%, although this rises to 50% with bedside inoculation for mycobacterial culture. In isolated tuberculous effusions (no parenchymal changes), sputum culture is positive in only 4–11% of cases, but figures are much higher (20–50%) if there is co-existent parenchymal disease.

Pleural biopsy

The histology of the pleural biopsy specimens is positive in 72% of cases on the initial sampling. Although this figure may rise to 80% with additional biopsies at separate procedures, these are not usually necessary if at least one pleural biopsy sample is sent for culture — sensitivity 90%.[10]

Special tests

Whilst some claim that adenosine deaminase levels > 45 U/l are 100% sensitive and 95–97% specific for TB, a recent review suggested a lower specificity of 89%. The place of this test is as yet uncertain. Pleural fluid gamma interferon levels may turn out to be more useful with sensitivity and specificity values > 90% in a recent series. Measurement of pleural fluid tuberculous antigens and antituberculous antibodies, and use of the polymerase chain reaction, perform less well.

Treatment

This is no different from the treatment of pulmonary tuberculosis. Most patients become apyrexial within two weeks and their effusion resolves within six weeks. However, it is by no means uncommon for patients to take up to two months to become apyrexial and four months for their effusion to resolve. Oral corticosteroids may shorten the duration of fever and the time to resolution of the pleural fluid. However, it is less certain that they have any effect on the development of pleural thickening which may occur in 50% of cases. In a recent study, there was no beneficial effect on clinical outcome.[11] For this reason, it may be preferable to drain as much fluid as possible at the start of treatment, by needle thoracentesis. Because of hepatic enzyme induction by rifampicin, a higher dose of prednisolone (60–80 mg daily) than usual may be required, but this can usually be discontinued over 4–6 weeks.

Tuberculous pleural effusion in HIV infection

Pleural fluid culture is positive in 33–91% and pleural biopsy smear in 44–69%, both higher than in HIV negative patients. Treatment is similar to that in non-AIDS patients.

Tuberculous empyema

This is now rare. There is pus containing numerous tubercle bacilli in the pleural space. Like tuberculous bronchopleural fistula, it is usually seen in older patients with reactivation of extensive pleuropulmonary disease. Treatment may be complicated, requiring complex and difficult surgery in addition to standard antituberculous chemotherapy.

Uncommon Pleural Infections

A number of fungal infections can involve the pleural space. *Pneumocystis carinii* is discussed in the section on AIDS. *Aspergillus* species, particularly *A. fumigatus*, usually colonise a residual space. *Coccidiodes immitus* frequently involves the pleura both as a primary infection and following rupture of a pulmonary cavity. *Actinomycosis* and *nocardiosis* may also occur as primary pleural infections. Since they are often destructive, they can simulate tumour. Other fungi, such as *Blastomycosis dermatitides, Histoplasma capsulatum* and *Cryptococcus neoformans* only rarely involve the pleura.

Approximately 20% of viral and *Mycoplasma* pneumonias are associated with a small pleural effusion. *Coxiella burnetii* is also commonly associated with a pleural effusion. Opportunistic myco-bacterial infection occasionally causes a pleural effusion.

Parasitic infections which involve the pleura include *Amoebiasis*, *Paragonimiasis*, *Gnathostomiasis* and *Hydatid.*

Acquired Immune Deficiency Syndrome (AIDS)

Pneumothorax

This occurs predominantly in patients who have, or who have had, *Pneumocystis carinii* infection. The risk is higher if the patient is receiving aerosolized pentamidine, is a smoker, has pneumatocoeles on chest X-ray or has a CD4 count < 100/µl. Approximately 4–5% of patients who have current or past *Pneumocystis carinii* pneumonia (PCP) are affected. This is usually due to predominant upper lobe multiple subpleural lung cavities, due to subpleural necrosis, resulting in emphysematous blebs and multiple cysts. Pneumothorax is particularly prevalent in those receiving aerosolized pentamidine as prophylaxis for PCP, perhaps because the drug doesn't reach the periphery of the upper lobe, allowing chronic low grade infection to persist here.

Approximately 65% develop a recurrence and, in one series, the in-hospital mortality was 50%. The visceral pleura is necrotic, allowing bronchopleural fistulae to develop, and making management very difficult. Conservative treatment with an intercostal tube and a sclerosing agent usually fails. It is usual to attempt this first but, if it is unsuccessful within three days, the choices are either to attach a Heimlich valve to the chest tube or to attempt a video assisted thoracoscopic procedure.

Pleural effusion

This has been observed in 27% of hospitalised patients with AIDS in one large series.[12] Two-thirds of these were due to infectious causes (Table 8). In one series, 31% were due to bacterial pneumonia of which the commonest was due to *Streptococcus pneumoniae*. Other causes include *Haemophilus influenzae*, *Mycoplasma pneumoniae*, *Legionella pneumophila* and *Nocardia asteroides*. It is much less common for them to develop into empyemas (11%), perhaps because of monocyte/macrophage cytokine dysregulation. *Pneumocystis carinii* is an uncommon cause of pleural effusion, accounting for approximately 15%. It may be possible to identify the organism in the pleural fluid.

Table 8. Causes of pleural effusions in AIDS

INFECTIOUS
    Bacterial pneumonia
    Pneumocystis carinii
    Mycobacterium tuberculosis
    Mycobacterium avium-intracellulare
    Nocardia asteroides
    Cryptococcus neoformans
    Septic embolism
    Toxoplasma gondii
    Leishmania species

NON INFECTIOUS
    Hypoalbuminaemia
    Congestive heart failure
    Uraemic pleurisy
    Atelectasis
    Acute respiratory distress syndrome
    Kaposi's sarcoma
    Lymphoma

Mycobacterial infection accounts for approximately 10% of pleural effusions in patients with AIDS. This is usually TB. Effusions due to TB in patients with AIDS are often large.

Cryptococcus neoformans can cause a pleural effusion with or without parenchymal abnormality. Pleural fluid and serum antigen detection and culture allow diagnosis; treatment is with amphotericin B. *Histoplasma capsulatum* and *Toxoplasma gondii* are rare causes of pleural effusions in AIDS.

There are a variety of non-infectious causes of pleural effusions in patients with AIDS. Lymphoma occurs in 5–10% of patients, mostly B-cell non-Hodgkins in type (NHL), although a rarer form is the Kaposi's sarcoma-associated virus (KSHV) lymphoma. Only 6–30% of NHL in AIDS patients demonstrate intrathoracic involvement other than a pleural effusion. Pleural effusions tend to be large and serosanguinous. Prognosis is poor, with a median survival of only 4–6 months.

Kaposi's sarcoma is one of the most common causes of pleural effusions in patients with AIDS. Pleuropulmonary disease occurs in 20%, of whom 60% present with pleural effusions which are predominantly bilateral and often large. Chest X-ray usually shows interstitial or alveolar infiltrates. Chylous effusions may occur. The diagnosis is sometimes difficult to establish, because the parietal pleura is not involved, making pleural biopsy unrewarding. Thoracoscopy or open lung biopsy can be used, but the risks are high. Typical bronchoscopic findings may be useful.

Other causes of pleural effusion in AIDS patients include congestive cardiac failure and hypoalbuminaemia.

Malignant Pleural Effusions

Pleural effusions are a common development in patients with malignancy. Lung cancer is the commonest mitotic lesion to produce a pleural effusion, accounting for 36%.[13] Carcinoma of the breast is the next most frequent (25%) with a pleural effusion occurring in up to 50% of cases, followed by lymphoma (10%), ovarian carcinoma (5%) and gastric carcinoma (2%). The cause of the malignancy is unknown in 7%. The effusion may be caused by

- direct pleural invasion — positive cytology/pleural biopsy
- lymphatic obstruction — negative cytology/pleural biopsy. Some term these 'paramalignant' effusions. Lymphatic obstruction is probably the commonest cause
- local tumour effects — bronchial obstruction causes atelectasis, trapped lung or pneumonia
- systemic tumour effects.

The lymphatic system of the parietal pleura plays a major role in the resorption of pleural fluid and proteins. Stomata, openings between parietal pleural mesothelial cells, lead to lymphatic lacunae just below the pleural surface, which coalesce into lymphatics draining via intercostal trunk vessels principally to the mediastinal lymph nodes. Interruption at any point in this pathway may result in a pleural effusion. Post-mortem studies suggest that impaired drainage from the pleural space is the predominant mechanism, with a strong relationship being observed with mediastinal lymph node involvement and only a weak relationship with direct pleural metastasis. Blood staining may be due to direct blood vessel invasion, occlusion of venules, new vessel growth or increased capillary permeability. Characteristically, malignant effusions are lymphocytic, mainly due to T-cell involvement.

Direct parietal pleural involvement in lung cancer is due either to direct spread from the visceral pleura via adhesions, or via exfoliation into the pleural space. Visceral pleural involvement is probably due to pulmonary artery invasion and embolization, most commonly due to adenocarcinoma. Bilateral pleural involvement in lung cancer is usually due to hepatic involvement with haematogenous spread to the contralateral lung. In breast cancer, there may be chest wall lymphatic invasion or spread from the liver. Primary sites in the abdomen and pelvis involve the pleura via the latter of these two mechanisms. Although other mechanisms may be operative, pleural effusions in Hodgkin's disease are mostly due to impaired lymphatic drainage, whereas in non-Hodgkin's lymphoma direct pleural infiltration predominates.

Clinical features

Breathlessness and cough are commonest. Dyspnoea appears to be multifactorial in origin — reduced chest wall compliance, contralateral mediastinal shift, decreased ipsilateral lung volume and the effects of any coexistent endobronchial obstruction or parenchymal infiltration. The degree of relief from thoracentesis is variable. The increase in TLC is approximately one third of the fluid volume removed, while FVC improves by half this amount. Other symptoms include chest pain and, since malignant pleural involvement usually indicates advanced disease, weight loss and cachexia. In one large series, however, 25% of patients were asymptomatic at the time their pleural effusion was discovered, and in 50% of these it was the first indication of malignancy. Approximately 20% of lymphoma patients have no respiratory symptoms when their effusion is diagnosed. Most patients have effusions > 500 ml and therefore have physical signs.

Radiology

Approximately 75% of patients with malignant/paramalignant effusions have fluid volumes of 0.5–2 l, but in 10% the volume is < 0.5 l and in a further 10% the effusion is massive; 70% of patients with a massive effusion will have a malignancy. Fifty percent of patients with bilateral pleural effusions and normal cardiac size have malignancy, although other causes include hypoalbuminaemia, lupus pleuritis, rheumatoid pleurisy, benign asbestos pleural effusion, constrictive pericarditis and cirrhosis.

The mediastinum should be displaced to the opposite side in the face of a large (> 1.5l) effusion. If this does not occur, malignancy is usually present and the following should be considered:

- carcinoma of the ipsilateral main stem bronchus
- fixed mediastinum due to malignant nodes
- mesothelioma — the X-ray appearances are due largely to pleural disease rather than to fluid
- extensive tumour infiltration of the ipsilateral lung, mimicking a large effusion

Pleural fluid findings

The fluid may be serous, serosanguinous or bloody. It is usually an exudate, but may be a transudate in 5% of cases, particularly early on since it may take weeks for protein to exit from the parietal pleural lymphatics to increase the protein concentration from its usual value of 15 g/l in normal pleural fluid. In a third of patients the pH is low (< 7.3) and so is the glucose (< 3.3 mmol/l). The number of nucleated cells is in the range 1500–4000/μl, comprising lymphocytes, macrophages and mesothelial cells. Lymphocytes predominate (50–70% of cells) in 50% of malignant effusions. The frequency of finding malignant cells varies. The principal points are as follows

- the initial thoracentesis is positive in approximately 60% of malignant effusions. If three separate specimens are taken, this figure increases to 80%, since the third specimen contains more freshly exfoliated cells
- the frequency of positive cytology depends, in part, on the tumour type. It is unusual to obtain positive cytology in squamous carcinoma, since pleural effusions are produced by bronchial obstruction or lymphatic blockade. Adenocarcinomas are more frequently positive than sarcomas. Cytology is more often positive in non-Hodgkin's lymphoma (75%) than in Hodgkin's disease (25%)
- the accuracy of cytological examination of pleural fluid in reaching a histological diagnosis is 40–87%
- some effusions in malignant disease are due to conditions such as cardiac failure, pulmonary embolus, pneumonia, lymphatic obstruction and hypoproteinaemia, and so will have negative cytology

The sample should be taken into a heparinised syringe. Several hundred ml should be removed. This won't improve the initial diagnostic yield but, if negative, may result in a greater number of exfoliated malignant cells several days later when the procedure is repeated. The yield from pleural biopsy in proven malignant effusions is 50–60%. Initial pleural metastases begin near the mediastinum and diaphragm. As the disease progresses, they become more costal and cephalad. Percutaneous pleural biopsy should be reserved for the second thoracentesis if the initial thoracentesis is negative. If the second pleural aspiration and first pleural biopsy are negative, a third aspiration and second biopsy are unlikely to be rewarding.

If malignant pleural effusion is suspected, but the pleural aspiration and biopsy are negative, the main options are:

- observe the patient for a few weeks and then repeat the studies
- thoracoscopy
- open pleural biopsy

Bronchoscopy is rarely helpful unless there are features suggesting an endobronchial lesion, and the role of CT is undefined, although it may, on occasion, reveal additional helpful features. Failure to identify a malignant pleural effusion is rarely a disservice to the patient, who usually will have incurable disease. Exceptions are breast, prostate, thyroid and small cell carcinoma which may be responsive to systemic therapy, germ cell tumours and lymphomas. The prognosis of pleural effusion in carcinoma of the lung, stomach and ovary is a few months only. However, patients with breast cancer may survive several months to years. Survival in lymphoma tends to be intermediate. In the case of lung cancer, a pleural effusion usually indicates inoperability. However, 5% of these may be paramalignant and potentially resectable, so it is important to establish this. For malignant pleural effusions in general, low pH (< 7.30) and glucose (< 3.3 mmol/l) signify a poorer survival (mean two months) than normal values for these parameters (mean 10 months). Reported 30 day mortality rates for malignant effusions are 29–50%.

Treatment

The usual intention in the management of a malignant or paramalignant effusion is palliation. A number of therapeutic options are available and their selection will be determined by consideration of a number of factors

- tumour type
- degree of breathlessness
- whether breathlessness is principally due to the effusion

- rate of reaccumulation of the effusion after initial thoracentesis
- possibly, the pH and glucose content of the pleural fluid, since low values predict a poor response to pleurodesis and poor survival
- patient's general health

The therapeutic options to be considered are as follows.

Observation

Appropriate if the patient is asymptomatic or has very advanced disease with an anticipated very short survival.

Repeated thoracentesis

May be indicated on an outpatient basis for debilitated patients with advanced disease in whom the recurrence rate is slow, especially if they want to avoid hospitalisation. However, most effusions recur in 1–3 days. Problems include repeated protein loss and the potential for infection.

Chemotherapy

This will only be appropriate in a small number of patients, particularly those with small cell lung cancer, lymphoma and some subjects with breast cancer, where a systemic chemotherapeutic/hormonal approach may improve the patient substantially for a time, if successful.

Radiotherapy

May occasionally be useful when mediastinal lymph node involvement predominates, as in some patients with small cell carcinoma of the lung and lymphoma. It may also be effective in lymphomatous chylothorax. Usually, however, the morbidity from radiation pneumonitis far outweighs any potential benefit in most patients.

Chest tube drainage and chemical pleurodesis.

Before considering this, the following should be established

- that the pleural shadowing is predominantly due to fluid
- that symptoms are due to the pleural effusion and relieved by an initial aspiration

- that the effusion is recurrent. Obviously, if the effusion does not recur, or does so only very slowly, pleurodesis may not be indicated. However, malignant/paramalignant effusions usually do recur and often do so moderately rapidly. There is evidence that successful pleurodesis is less likely if the pleural malignancy is advanced, so that some would advocate attempting pleurodesis earlier rather than later.

- pleural pH. This is more used in the USA than in the UK. A pH < 7.3 is associated with not only a poor prognosis but also a poor response to pleurodesis. Successful pleurodesis in one study was achieved in none of the patients with a pleural pH < 7.15, 33% with pH < 7.20 and 90% with pH > 7.30.

- that the lung is re-expandable. Success with a non surgical approach is unlikely if this condition is not met.

- the life expectancy. If anticipated survival is short, an aggressive attempt at controlling the pleural effusion is unlikely to be warranted. Clinical performance status, for instance the Karnofsky index, and pleural pH may be useful here. In 125 patients with metastatic pleural malignancy those with pH < 7.20 had a mean survival of 1.9 months.

Before proceeding with pleurodesis, a number of factors pertinent to the procedure need to be considered by the operator

- the method of pleural drainage. To be successful, the pleural space needs to be as completely drained as possible, in particular to reduce dilution of the selected sclerosant. Recently, the British Thoracic Society undertook a study comparing needle aspiration with intercostal tube drainage prior to attempting tetracycline pleurodesis for cytologically confirmed malignant pleural effusions. Subsequent pleurodesis was successful at 12 weeks in 7 of 33 (21%) in the needle aspiration group and 25 of 32 (78%) in the intercostal tube drainage group, confirming the superiority of intercostal tube drainage.

- the type of sclerosant

A recent review of the literature between 1966 and 1992 determined that, of the 1168 patients included, 752 (64%) had a complete response based on clinical examination and chest X-ray (14). Non-antineoplastic agents were superior, with complete success in 577 of 770 patients (75%) compared with only 175 of 398 (44%) with anti-neoplastic agents. The principal agents and their success rates were: bleomycin 54%: tetracycline 67%: doxy-cycline 72%: *Corynebacterium parvum* 76% (now withdrawn): minocycline 86%: talc 93% (153 of 165 patients).

American authors claim that talc is superior to tetracycline and bleomycin, yet it remains little used in the UK other than by Thoracic Surgeons. It is not produced in sterile form and has to be sterilised by the user. The slurry is produced by mixing talc with normal saline. A suggested dose is 5 g of talc in 50 ml of normal saline. This can be introduced via an intercostal tube, whereas talc poudrage requires thoracoscopy. Complications include fever (up to 70% of patients) and rarely empyema, arrhythmia and the acute respiratory distress syndrome. Severe pain is less frequent than with tetracycline. Although success rates with talc slurry of 91% have been reported, and are comparable with figures for talc poudrage, the studies concerned have been quite small, and some authors therefore favour poudrage.

Tetracycline is favoured in the UK. The usual doses used are 1–1.5 g in 50 ml normal saline. However, based on animal studies comparing low and high dose tetracycline with other agents, some authors have recommended a dose of 3 g. In the USA, production of tetracycline is ceasing. Alternatives include doxycycline (but this often requires repeated doses) and minocycline (but this may provoke vestibular symptoms and haemothorax has been reported in experimental studies).

Thoracoscopy with talc poudrage

This is less easily available, more invasive and requires a greater level of technical skill. The higher morbidity and up to 5% mortality need careful consideration Nevertheless, it is highly effective.

Pleural abrasion and pleurectomy

This is virtually 100% effective in controlling malignant pleural effusions, but the required thoracotomy is a major undertaking in an often ill patient group, with attendant morbidity and mortality. A thoracoscopic approach is obviously less invasive, but tends to be reserved for those who are in good condition and have a reasonably long expected survival or have failed chemical pleurodesis.

Pleuro-peritoneal shunt

This is usually used for patients with intractable symptomatic pleural effusions who have failed chemical pleurodesis and cannot undergo surgery. Palliation may be achieved in 80–90% of properly selected patients. It is particularly useful for chylothorax since it allows chyle to recirculate. The major problem is shunt failure, most commonly due to clot occlusion of the catheter. Concerns about peritoneal seeding don't seem to have materialised; this was seen in only 2 of 40 patients in one study.

Primary Pleural Tumours

These are rare and account for only 2.8 cases per 100 000 registered pleural tumours with only a few case reports of most. They include localised benign and malignant fibrous tumours, localised malignant mesothelioma, primary pleural lymphoma, pleural thymoma and pleural sarcomas

Haemothorax

Causes of blood within the thoracic cavity include:

- trauma
- iatrogenic — insertion of CVP lines
- pulmonary embolism
- pneumothorax — rupture of an adhesion
- malignancy
- ruptured aorta/aortic dissection — usually left sided

Traumatic haemothorax

may occur in the absence of rib fracture. The diagnosis may therefore be missed and may not be made till weeks or months later, when further expansion has been caused by osmotic effects.

- stable patients without active bleeding may be managed conservatively. Blunting of a costophrenic angle indicates the presence of approximately 300 ml of blood. Volumes greater than this may need to be drained by an intercostal tube. This may have to be image guided if the volume is not large. The preferred site is the 5th intercostal space in the mid axillary line. A large bore chest tube should be used. Although a large volume of blood may be drained initially, this usually slows subsequently with lung re-expansion, and up to 85% of patients may be managed without surgery.

- Volumes of 300 ml or less should be followed by daily chest X-ray and drained if they enlarge.
- unstable patients with evidence of active bleeding require surgery. Surgery is indicated for:
  - completely opacified hemithorax
  - > 1l immediate drainage on chest tube insertion
  - ongoing bleeding of > 200 ml/hr for > 3hrs.
  - shock despite volume replacement.
- a clotted haemothorax may occur if management is delayed by 7–10 days. It may be confirmed by pleural aspiration. Treatment is surgical. If management is very delayed, a thickened peel, which may calcify, forms around the clot making thoracotomy for decortication more difficult.

Non traumatic haemothorax

- if small, observation or tube drainage may suffice
- surgery is indicated for the same criteria as above.

Chylothorax and Pseudochylothorax

These two conditions both result in a turbid or milky lipid containing pleural fluid. In the case of chylothorax, the fluid is lymph derived principally from the gut, and the cause is obstruction or disruption of the thoracic duct. The fluid has a high chylomicron triglyceride content, exceeding 0.6 mmol/l and often > 1.2 mmol/l, and a low cholesterol content. By contrast, pseudochylothorax occurs in the setting of a chronic pleural effusion (usually > five yrs) with pleural thickening and is not related to thoracic duct disease. Chylomicrons are absent, the triglyceride content is usually < 1.2 mmol/l and the cholesterol concentration usually exceeds 6.5 mmol/l.

Chylothorax (Table 9)

Typically the lymphatics from the abdomen and lower body drain into a common 'sac' behind the upper abdominal aorta (cisterna chyli) just anterior to the first or second lumbar vertebra and passes through the aortic opening of the diaphragm into the posterior mediastinum (thoracic duct). It runs upward between the azygos vein and the aorta, lying against the right side of the oesophagus. At the level of the third to fifth thoracic vertebra it crosses the

Table 9.   Causes of chylothorax

	Cause	Percent of total
A	**Non Traumatic**	72
	MALIGNANT	45
	Lymphoma	37
	Other	9
	NON MALIGNANT	27
	Idiopathic	14
	Miscellaneous	8
B	**Traumatic**	28
	Surgical	25
	Non surgical	3

midline and continues cephalad behind the aortic arch, adjacent to the left side of the oesophagus. It finally empties into the point of confluence of the left subclavian and internal jugular veins.

The thoracic duct carries chyle, defined as lymphatic fluid of gastrointestinal origin. There is a total flow of 1.5–2.4 l/day.

Any process which obstructs or disrupts the thoracic duct can produce a chylothorax. It is a weak structure and easily damaged, even occasionally by vigorous stretching! This usually results in a right sided fluid collection since the duct lies predominantly on the right. If affected at crossover, bilateral chylothoraces may occur and, in its most cephalad portion, a left chylothorax.

Aetiology

In a recent review of 191 patients with chylothorax, 72% were nontraumatic in origin and, of these, 63% were due to malignancy. Lymphoma, commonly non-Hodgkin's lymphoma, was the single commonest cause, accounting for 50% of nontraumatic cases (Table 9). Of the traumatic causes, surgery was the commonest. Rarely it occurs in sarcoidosis, amyloidosis, tuberculosis, filariasis, thrombosis of the superior vena cava and cardiac failure. However it is worth mentioning a number of specific diseases which affect lymph vessels:

- lymphangioleiomyomatosis (LAM)
- yellow nail syndrome
- haemangiomatosis

For the chest physician, it is worth singling out LAM. In a recent review of this rare condition, 28% of patients developed a chylothorax.

Clinical presentation

Chest pain and fever do not occur because chyle is bacteriostatic and does not evoke an inflammatory response. Traumatic causes may occur as long as 10 days later.

Investigations

Milky fluid is often recovered at aspiration of a pleural effusion. However, in one report less than 50% of chylothoraces were milky, and 12% were serous or serosanguinous. Some were yellow, bloody or even green. A turbid aspirate that clears with centrifugation is unlikely to be a chylothorax; if a cloudy supernatant occurs, the diagnosis is likely but must be distinguished from a pseudochylothorax. The typical biochemical features of chyle have already been discussed.

Once a chylothorax has been confirmed, further investigation will depend on the aetiology

- nontraumatic — CT thorax and upper abdomen, since lymphoma is the commonest cause. CT may also reveal other mediastinal (retrosternal goitre, vascular thrombosis) or pulmonary (lymphangioleiomyomatosis) causes.
- traumatic — if surgical, the site is often suspected. If nonsurgical, CT thorax or even lymphangiography may be required to localise the site of disruption.

If no cause is found thoracoscopic thoracic surgery is often the next step. If the aetiology is not confirmed at operation patients should be followed up closely.

Management

No prospective controlled studies exist. A staged care plan progressing from initial more conservative treatment to later surgical options depending on response, is best. Prolonged drainage of chyle depletes essential nutrients and lymphocytes, resulting in malnourishment and immunosuppression in approximately 14 days.

Nontraumatic chylothorax

Patients with lymphoma or carcinoma

- 55–68% will respond to tumour radiotherapy
- if this fails, intercostal tube drainage and chemical pleurodesis are usually attempted, but may not be successful
- occasionally, pleuroperitoneal shunting

Patients with idiopathic chylothorax

- conservative treatment may be successful in 80% particularly if the chylothorax was caused by unrecognised minor trauma. Such treatment consists of intercostal tube drainage and a low fat diet with supplementation by medium chain triglycerides which enter the portal system directly rather than being absorbed via intestinal lymphatics. If this fails, total parenteral nutrition may be tried. The aim of such options is to reduce production of chyle
- if there is no response to conservative treatment after two to three weeks, surgical options should be considered
- lymphangioleiomyomatosis, SLE, sarcoidosis: in these instances, the chylothorax may respond to appropriate medical treatment

Traumatic chylothorax

Non surgical

Conservative management with intercostal tube drainage and total parenteral nutrition is successful in 50%. If this fails, surgery is indicated by about 14 days since, thereafter, the risk of immuno-suppression increases. Earlier surgical intervention may be appropriate if the patient is becoming malnourished.

Surgical

There is a 50% mortality, particularly since the chylous nature of the fluid may not be immediately recognised, with attendant malnutrition and immunosuppression. Initial conservative treatment is followed by early surgical care in younger fitter patients and in chylothorax after resection of a malignancy such as oesophageal carcinoma. Observation alone, without chest tube insertion is best post pneumonectomy unless there is mediastinal shift, when inter-costal tube drainage followed by surgery is recommended.

Pseudochylothorax

This may occur in the setting of a chronic pleural effusion, usually of greater than 5 years' duration, particularly those encapsulated by a grossly thickened pleura. The fluid is turbid or milky, and has the following features:

- cholesterol crystals — not invariably present
- cholesterol > 6.5 mmol/l, triglycerides < 1.2 mmol/l
- absence of chylomicrons

Predisposing conditions include:

- tuberculosis
- rheumatoid arthritis
- poorly treated empyemas/haemothoraces

Management

This is determined by:

- severity of respiratory symptoms
- ability of the lung to properly re-expand
- the nature of the underlying disease

It should be remembered that active TB should always be excluded and that intervention may do more harm than good.

- asymptomatic patients should be observed.
- in symptomatic patients options include thoracentesis (but beware the risk of introducing infection) and decortication (but if the underlying lung won't expand to obliterate the space, an acceptable situation may be converted into one with a chronic fistula).

SECTION 2. PNEUMOTHORAX

A hospital serving a population of 200 000 may expect to treat 25 cases per year. Normally, intrapleural pressure is 4–5 cm H_2O more negative than intra-alveolar/atmospheric pressure at functional residual capacity, due to recoil of the lung inwards and the chest wall outwards. This negative pressure keeps the lung expanded. When air enters the pleural space, this negative pressure is reduced or ablated and the lung collapses. Air may enter the pleural space following (a) trauma or (b) spontaneously.

In spontaneous pneumothorax, an alveolus spontaneously ruptures, air flows into the pleural space until the pressure equalizes, flow then ceases and the defect closes. If this does not happen, and a physiological 'valve' forms, air may continue to enter the pleural space on inspiration and be unable to escape during expiration. This may lead to a highly positive intrapleural pressure with depression of the diaphragm and mediastinal shift to the opposite side, compressing the normal lung. Cardiopulmonary collapse may ensue. Although this has been attributed to impaired venous return, hypoxaemia and respiratory failure due to shunting are probably more important. This entity is termed a tension pneumothorax.

Spontaneous pneumothoraces may be further subclassified as follows

- primary — no underlying lung disease
- secondary — underlying lung disease present

The commonest underlying disease is COPD. Others include asthma, fibrosing alveolitis, sarcoidosis, pneumoconiosis, cystic fibrosis, bronchial obstruction and staphylococcal pneumonia (especially in children). In the USA, AIDS is rapidly becoming a common predisposing cause in hospitals where large numbers of such patients are treated, largely due to pneumocystis pneumonia. Rarer predisposing conditions include histiocytosis X, lymphangioleiomyomatosis, pulmonary neurofibromatosis, Ehlers-Danlos and Marfan's syndromes and congenital lung cysts.

Primary Spontaneous Pneumothorax (PSP)

In fact, even patients in this group often do have underlying lung disease:

- subpleural blebs and bullae are found in 48–100% of patients on the ipsilateral side, and 79–96% of patients on the contralateral side[15]
- CT based studies have demonstrated blebs and bullae — designated 'emphysema-like changes' (ELCs) — in approximately 80% of PSP patients compared with 0–20% of controls. However, no study has demonstrated that ELCs are the actual cause of PSP
- subpleural blebs and bullae are believed to be caused by inflammation of distal airways resulting in stenosis and a check-valve mechanism producing distention of distal parenchyma. In the majority of cases, smoking is thought to be an important causative factor. 91% from four separate PSP studies were

smokers[7] and smoking increases the risk of PSP 9–fold in women and 22–fold in men. There is a dose-response relationship with the number of cigarettes smoked per day

Clinical presentation

PSP is 2–3 fold commoner in men, with a peak age in the early 20s. A first PSP is rare after age 40. The aetiological factors include smoking (*vide supra*) and height (in tall individuals the apical intrapleural pressure is more negative, perhaps encouraging ELC formation). There are a few reports of familial PSP and of HLA associations. Atmospheric pressure changes > 1 kPa are associated with an increased incidence of PSP.

Surprisingly, PSP usually occurs when the patient is at rest. The typical symptom is sudden pleuritic chest pain. Dyspnoea often occurs, but its degree depends on the size of the pneumothorax and, in SSP, the extent of the underlying lung disease. It often improves, even prior to resolution/treatment, and may in part be due to afferent impulses generated by the rapid change in lung volume. In small PSPs, there may be no abnormal physical signs. In moderate and large PSPs, there may be a tachycardia and slight expansion of the ipsilateral chest wall. The trachea and apex beat may be displaced to the contralateral side. Movement, tactile vocal fremitus and breath sounds are reduced on the affected side but the percussion note is increased. A small left PSP may be associated with a pleuropericardial click (Hamman's sign).

Imaging

On plain chest X-ray, there is usually a white visceral pleural line, separated from the parietal pleura by an avascular collection of air. The line is either straight or convex towards the chest wall. In upright patients, the gas accumulates in an apicolateral location. As little as 50 ml may be visible. The size of the pneumothorax is due to both collapse of the lung and expansion of the chest wall. Hypoxic vasoconstriction of the affected lung preserves its trans-radiancy. A small haemothorax may occur due to the rupture of pleural adhesions. In tension pneumothorax there is flattening or inversion of the ipsilateral diaphragm and contralateral shift of the mediastinum. The size of a PSP is difficult to gauge from a plain chest X-ray. A lateral width of 1 cm corresponds to approximately a 10% pneumothorax. The correlation between size estimated by chest X-ray and by CT, which is much more accurate (r = 0.99 with a pneumothorax model) is only 0.71. However, the clinical status of the patient is much more important than pure radiographic size.

An inspiratory film should be obtained in patients with suspected pneumothorax; two recent studies have not demonstrated any advantage of an expiratory film. There is at present no evidence to support the routine use of CT in PSP in order to identify ELCs and to try to predict the risk of recurrence.

Approximately 500 ml air are needed for a pneumothorax to be certainly visible on a supine chest X-ray. The pleural gas outlines the anterior pleural reflection, costophrenic sulcus ('deep sulcus sign') and the anterolateral border of the mediastinum. A lateral decubitus film is extremely sensitive for the detection of pneumothorax. Rarely, a pneumothorax may form at the site of an atelectatic lobe ('pneumothorax ex vacuo'), particularly the right upper lobe. In this situation, rapid collapse produces an abrupt decrease in intrapleural pressure with subsequent release of nitrogen from pleural capillaries. Bronchoscopy rather than pleural drainage is the treatment.

The condition most likely to mimic a pneumothorax is a large subpleural bulla. However, the visible medial wall of the bulla is usually concave towards the chest wall. If there is doubt, a CT scan should be obtained, since inserting a chest drain into a bulla may lead to a bronchopleural fistula.

Recurrence

The recurrence rate of PSP, whether treated by observation, simple aspiration or intercostal tube drainage (ITD), ranged from 16–52%, with a mean of 30%.[15] In a more recent retrospective British study of 275 episodes of PSP in 153 patients over a four year period, the recurrence rate was 54.2%.[16] Most recurrences occur within 6 months to 2 years.[15] Independent risk factors for recurrence include age, female sex, male height, continued smoking and pulmonary fibrosis.[16]

Management

The aims of treatment are to remove air from the pleural space and to reduce the likelihood of a recurrence. A recent American survey of the practice habits of 409 physicians of whom the majority were chest physicians determined that there was still great variation in the approach to management of PSP and SSP.

Simple observation and oxygen

If the air leak has ceased spontaneously, the air in the pleural space will be slowly re-absorbed at the rate of 1.25% of the volume of the hemithorax per 24 hours. The volume of the collapsed lung and of the hemithorax can be calculated from the PA and lateral chest X-ray, although not very accurately, and the time needed for re-expansion approximately determined. Two reports have suggested that oxygen supplementation can increase this basal rate 3–4 fold, by increasing the pressure gradient favouring re-absorption. Simple observation with or without oxygen is believed to be appropriate only if the pneumothorax is < 15%. There are concerns however. In one study 9 of 40 patients treated by observation required tube thoracostomy.

Aspiration of the pleural space

In the 1980's, two prospective studies in which PSP and SSP were combined, gave success rates of 53% and 58% respectively for simple aspiration. One study determined the technique to be successful in 75% of 48 PSPs and 37% of 30 SSPs.

Subsequently a prospective randomised study organised by the British Thoracic Society (BTS) compared simple aspiration with ITD. In this study, 35 patients were randomised to simple aspiration and 38 patients to ITD. Overall, 28 out of 35 patient randomised to aspiration were successfully treated by this technique, although 5 patients required two aspirations. The remaining seven patients required ITD. There was no difference between the two groups in recurrence rate at one year and none of the aspirated patients required pleurectomy. Their pain scores and length of stay were significantly lower than the ITD group. As a result of this study, the BTS has published guidelines for the management of spontaneous pneumothorax.[17]

Intercostal tube drainage

In the UK, the main indications for ITD are (a) failure of simple aspiration (b) tension pneumothorax. In the American literature, many still favour ITD. Based on the BTS recommendations, guidelines for the insertion and management of chest drains have been developed, by the Wessex Chest Physicians, and are shown in

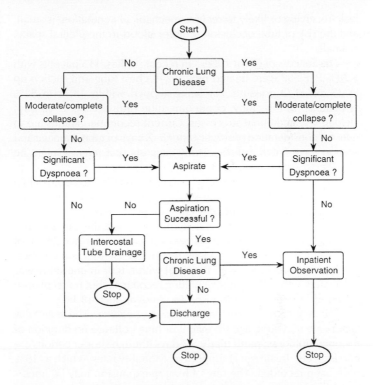

Figure 1.   Pneumothorax guidelines. Initial pneumothorax management

Figure 1. A number of important questions pertaining to the use of chest tubes remain:

The Size of the Tube: In one series of 71 episodes of mixed PSP and SSP managed using either a 5.5 or a 7.0 F tube attached to a Heimlich valve, the success rate (complete/almost complete re-expansion) was 84.5%. However, patients with bronchopleural fistulae can have air leaks of as large as 16 l/mn. Since flow through a chest tube is proportional to the fifth power of its radius, the smallest internal diameter that could accommodate a flow of 15.1 l/mn at –10 cm H_2O suction is 6 mm. Thus a tube < 28 F may not cope with a large flow.

It would seem reasonable, therefore, to use a small bore chest drain when the pneumothorax is not large, the risk of a large air leak (receiving or likely to receive mechanical ventilation) is small, and the risk of tube occlusion (fluid or blood in the pleural space) is small.

The Success of Chest Tubes: In recent studies, 115 patients with > 20% PSP/SSP were treated by 20–24F chest tube and suction up to 25 cm H_2O pressure. Air leaks stopped within 48 hr in 82% of patients. In this study, continuing tube drainage up to 10 days yielded few additional successes. Current recommendations are to refer for consideration of surgery after 5–7 days of tube drainage and suction have failed, but this study suggests that referral might be considered earlier — at 2–3 days.

The Use of Suction: Several studies have failed to demonstrate an advantage of the routine use of suction. It should therefore be used for the management of a continuing air leak.

The Timing of Chest Tube Removal: Once the air leak has ceased, the standard advice is removal after a further 24 hr of observation demonstrates no leak recurrence (see section on chest tube insertion and removal). Removal within 6 hr in one study was associated with a 25% chance of lung recollapse, but no recollapse occurred in patients randomised to removal after 48 hr.

The risk of re-expansion pulmonary oedema: The main risk factors are (a) young age (b) extent of lung collapse (c) duration of the pneumothorax, particularly > 3 days (though shorter periods are not risk-free). Treatment is supportive. Mortality rates as high as 19% have been recorded. The rate of lung re-expansion may be important.

The prevention of recurrence: The use of a chest tube does not prevent later recurrence. The recurrence rate for PSP is 32–34% and for SSP 30–43%.

The use of tetracycline pleurodesis: In contrast to its use in malignant pleural effusions it can be extremely painful. It is the author's opinion that pleurodesis should only be used in PSP when this is being treated surgically. It may, however, have a small role in SSP, principally in patients in whom recurrence would be potentially life-threatening but whose lung function/general health are too poor to allow a surgical pleurodesis.

Video Assisted Thoracoscopy (VAT) and thoracotomy

The main indications for surgery are

- the lung remains unexpanded after 5–7 days
- a bronchopleural fistula persists for 5–7 days

- recurrent pneumothorax. — though not all surgeons will operate after a single recurrence in an otherwise fit patient who tolerates the pneumothorax well and is not at risk through occupation or hobbies
- contralateral pneumothorax
- simultaneous bilateral pneumothoraces
- a first pneumothorax in a patient in a high risk occupation such as diving or flying

In many centres VAT is superseding open thoracotomy. In the VAT technique, bullous disease is treated by electrocautery, laser, suture ligation or stapling, and a pleurodesis is effected by mechanical means, chemical or talc. Because of safety concerns, talc is not used in younger patients with benign disease. In open thoracotomy, recurrence is prevented by mechanical abrasion or pleurectomy. Recurrence rates after these latter two are 2–5% and <1% respectively. The total significant complication rate for thoracotomy is 2.2% (combined series of 642 patients). There has only been one prospective randomised comparison of VAT and thoracotomy. VAT had longer operation times but there was a trend for it to be associated with lower analgesic use and shorter hospitalisations. VAT was felt to be less reliable in SSP.

A median sternotomy can be used for bilateral disease. Authors claim less pain and shorter convalescence. In patients with diseases such as cystic fibrosis, who could be future transplant candidates, more limited pleurodesis is performed, since extensive procedures may make subsequent transplantation more difficult.

Secondary spontaneous pneumothorax

The commonest predisposing condition for SSP is COPD. Several points are worth noting about SSP in COPD:

- patients with more severe COPD are more likely to develop SSP
- a pneumothorax can be confused with an emphysematous bulla, but the two can be distinguished by CT (*vide supra*)
- persistent air leaks are more common
- recurrence rates are higher than for PSP — approximately 50% over 3 y in one study
- simple aspiration is less likely to be successful and some suggest a lower threshold for considering ITD
- in the event of a persisting air leak, earlier referral for surgery should be considered

- a more aggressive approach towards preventing recurrence is indicated, ideally surgical

Other diseases particularly associated with SSP include:

- AIDS: *vide supra*
- cystic fibrosis: 8% develop a pneumothorax overall and, by age 18, 20% will have experienced one. As many patients have poor lung function, they are more likely to be treated by ITD
- TB: patients do badly unless treated by ITD

Pneumothorax and flying

Aircraft are pressurised to 8000 feet at which altitude the inspired oxygen concentration is 15% and trapped air will expand by 38%. There is little experience of pneumothorax and flying, and much will depend on whether the pneumothorax is spontaneous, iatrogenic or traumatic and on whether or not there is underlying lung disease. Past military practice has involved grounding patients for 6 months. The author advises patients not to fly for 6–12 weeks, depending on the clinical situation, and particularly not to board the aircraft if they have any suspicious symptoms.

Catamenial pneumothorax

This occurs within 1–2 days of the start of menstruation, is almost always right sided, and is usually small. It may be recurrent. Since the pneumothorax is often small and resolves spontaneously, it may be missed so that the cause of the patient's pleuritic chest pain remains unknown.

Bronchopleural fistula

This consists of an abnormal communication between any part of the bronchial tree and the pleural space. It is most commonly due to a pneumothorax but in the past TB was a common cause. A 28 F chest drain (or larger) may be required to cope with the large air flows which are sometimes found. Suction may be necessary and may have to be increased to high levels — 50–75 cm H_2O negative pressure. It is important to use a low pressure high flow system. If a low flow system is used, it may not be able to cope with the size of the air leak and will then act as an impedance to drainage. Fistulae from terminal bronchioles often close spontaneously. Those from larger airways rarely do. A surgical opinion should be sought if the fistula persists for 3 days or more.

Subcutaneous emphysema

In the context of a pneumothorax being treated by ITD, subcutaneous emphysema usually means that the drainage is inadequate. Consideration should be given to checking the function of the chest drain or to inserting a larger or an additional drain. Subcutaneous and mediastinal emphysema are not, in themselves, dangerous. However, in the case of mediastinal emphysema, rupture of air into the contralateral pleural space may produce a simultaneous bilateral pneumothorax which could be life threatening.

SECTION 3 PLEURAL TECHNIQUES

Performing a pleural aspiration

- localise the pleural effusion: clinically and X-ray if large; ultrasound if small
- explain the procedure and obtain the patient's consent. Position the patient seated, leaning forward over a table/the bed, with the arms forward. Rotating the patient slightly to the opposite side may splay the ribs a little
- aseptic technique
- if a single needle pass is anticipated, and pleural biopsy is not intended, local anaesthesia may not be necessary. If it is, infiltrate the skin and the tissues down to and including the pleura with 1% lignocaine
- insert a 21–gauge venepuncture needle connected to a 50 ml syringe (± a 3 way tap) perpendicularly to the chest wall immediately above a rib to avoid the neurovascular bundle
- obtain the sample

Performing a pleural biopsy

- proceed as for pleural aspiration points (i)–(iv)
- aspirate a SMALL volume of pleural fluid first to confirm the position is correct. Do NOT proceed if pleural fluid cannot first be obtained
- make a 'stab' incision with a scalpel through the skin and subcutaneous tissues

- ensure that the trocar has been inserted into the inner of the two main 'cylinders' of the Abram's needle and that the biopsy hole is closed
- introduce the Abram's needle through the skin incision. Exert firm but sensible pressure with the dominant hand whilst gripping the needle near it's tip with the other hand which should function as a buffer to prevent sudden forceful insertion. Rotate the needle back and forth with a 'skewer' action so that it SLOWLY advances in a CONTROLLED fashion until the parietal pleural is penetrated
- remove the innermost stillette, leaving the other two 'cylinders' of the needle in place. Place a thumb over the end of the needle to prevent air entering. Connect a 20 ml syringe. Alternatively the stillette can be removed, and the syringe connected, prior to use
- rotate the inner cylinder in an anticlockwise direction to open the biopsy chamber. The small 'bobble' on the hub of the needle indicates the orientation of the chamber
- withdraw the entire assembly slowly a little until the biopsy chamber 'catches' onto the parietal pleura. If biopsying at, for instance, 3 o'clock it is now vital to maintain very firm pressure indeed both in the withdrawal direction **and** in a rightward direction, whilst keeping the biopsy port snagged on the pleura. Keeping the outer needle steady, rotate the inner cylinder clockwise to close the biopsy chamber and cut a biopsy from the pleura. Withdraw the entire assembly. Sometimes a slight tearing sensation is felt as this is done
- rotate the inner cylinder anticlockwise to open the biopsy chamber and extract the biopsy using a sterile needle
- repeat for further biopsy specimens. It is usual to take 4–6 biopsies in total. Three main positions are used — 3,6 and 9 o'clock. The 12 o'clock position should NOT be used to avoid damaging the intercostal neurovascular bundle
- biopsy specimens should be placed in saline for TB culture as well as in formalin for histology
- a single 3–0 silk suture or steristrip may be needed to close the skin wound

Inserting an intercostal chest drain (Figure 2)

- throughout the procedure explain what is happening and reassure the patient. Patients prefer premedication. Consider an opiate

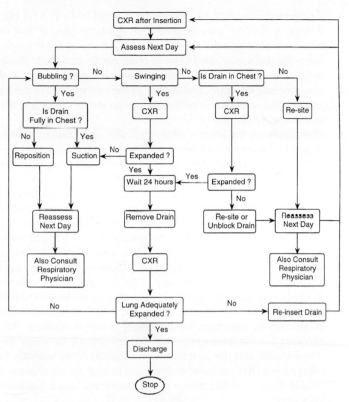

Figure 2. Chest drain management

if there is no evidence of type II respiratory failure. Atropine will prevent vasovagal symptoms

- always double check the correct side for insertion from the chest radiograph just before intubation. The usual site is the 4th or 5th intercostal space in the mid-axillary line. There is no advantage from inserting a 'low' drain, even for fluid, and this can be dangerous. A drain of appropriate size in any position will restore negative pressure, allow lung re-expansion and result in expulsion of air or fluid (unless this is loculated). Position the patient supine with the HEAD OF THE BED ELEVATED 45° (patient 'head up') and the patient's arm behind the head, resting away from the chest wall. Mark the site of insertion with a marker pen

- a pneumothorax may be drained by a small (< 14 F) tube but, if large, a 20–24 F may be preferred. If a large pleural leak or blood are anticipated, a 28 F tube should be used (*vide supra*). Since the drain may need to be in place for several days, sterile technique is essential. Double check by dismantling and reassembling the drain. Ensure that all the connections fit tightly and that the underwater bottle containing sterile water is ready and correctly primed

- after palpating the intercostal space, raise an intradermal bleb of local anaesthetic and then infiltrate the deeper tissues down to the parietal pleura, particularly around the periosteum on the upper surface of the lower rib using at first a blue, and then green, needle. Use either 1% or 0.5% lignocaine (by diluting 1%). Remember that to ensure the track the drain will take is anaesthetized may mean infiltrating more widely and that the maximum recommended dose of lignocaine (3–4.5 mg/kg body weight) can easily be exceeded (toxic serum levels >5 mg/L; toxicity varies with body weight and route of administration). Therefore, 0.5% lignocaine may allow use of a larger volume of solution and be preferable. It may also be preferable to first anaesthetise the skin alone and make the skin incision. The deeper layers can then be infiltrated more accurately, thus allowing for the frequently experienced 'travel' between the skin incision and the deeper layers. Aspirate intermittently to ensure a vein has not been entered and to look for air or pleural fluid in the syringe to confirm when the pleural space has been breached

- when the local anaesthetic has worked, make an incision in the skin and subcutaneous fat; this should be less than 2 cm, to ensure a tight fit of the drain. Then insert one <u>MATTRESS</u> suture, (not a purse string) across the incision, leaving the ends loose for subsequent sealing of the wound on drain removal (complicated circular stitches are unnecessary and leave an unsightly scar). Use No.1 or No.2 silk as this is very strong (ie thicker than 1–0, 2–0). Using <u>BLUNT DISSECTION</u> with forceps, make a wide track through the intercostal muscles down to and <u>THROUGH</u> the parietal pleura

- the sharp metal point of a trocar can be lethal if inserted forcibly and the drain can usually be inserted without it, following adequate, blunt dissection with a pair of metal artery forceps in an apical direction. A finger can be used to aid dissection and to breach the pleura. The artery forceps can then be applied

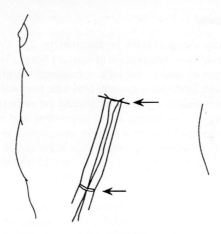

Figure 3. **Diagram of recommended suture to secure a chest drain**
(Respiratory Medicine, 2nd Ed. Brewis RAL, Corrin B, Geddes DM,
Gibson GJ)

to the inside tip of the chest drain, creating a firm blunt tip. If
the trocar is used it should be employed only as a drain 'stiffener'
and not to create a pathway. If ANY resistance is met, the
operator should stop and recreate the track with the blunt
forceps. If using a trocar, it should only JUST enter the chest,
and the drain should be 'fed in' off it. Connect to the underwater
seal

- two throws of the mattress suture, without locking it, will close
  the skin tightly around the drain. Then tie to the drain as
  indicated in diagram (Figure 3). Bind the drain flat against the
  chest wall eg with 'sleek' or, preferably, a transparent dressing.
  Do this yourself and with care, or the drain may become
  dislodged.

- should suction be needed, use either the large volume, low
  pressure Vernon-Tubbs pump or the simpler adapter for wall
  suction (Puritan Bennett Thoracic Drainage Regulator). Start
  with −5 to −10 cm H_2O pressure

- prescribe adequate oral and intramuscular analgesia

- the underwater seal must <u>always</u> be kept below the level of the
  chest. Do <u>NOT</u> clamp the drain unless to avoid reexpansion
  pulmonary oedema. Clamping is unnecessary and potentially
  dangerous

- perform chest X-ray

Tube removal

The respiratory swing should be damped to 2–3 cm H_2O and bubbling should have stopped for at least 24 hours. Test for cessation of air leak by asking the patient to cough lightly. <u>DO NOT</u> clamp the drain. Since some patients find tube removal unpleasant, consider premedication. The drain should be removed with the patient holding his/her breath at full inspiration and performing a valsalva manoeuvre to create a positive intrapleural pressure. That part of the suture securing the drain should be cut as close to the drain as possible. A thick pad of gauzes should be held by the left hand lightly over the drain insertion site, whilst the tube is removed RAPIDLY with the right hand. AT the INSTANT the drain leaves the chest, VERY firm pressure is applied with the gauzes over the wound site and MAINTAINED for a good 5–10 minutes, until the drain track has closed (test by lightly lifting the gauzes for a few seconds). The suture securing the skin can then be calmly tied. A chest X-ray should then be obtained.

Note: it is possible to place an apical chest drain via a posterior intercostal approach to drain a residual apical pneumothorax in particularly needy circumstances. However, the technique is more demanding and will not be described here.

Performing a chemical pleurodesis

Method

- insert either a 20–28 F or a small bore 10–14 F intercostal chest drain and connect to an underwater seal
- ensure that the pleural space has been as completely drained as possible, so that the instilled agent is not diluted and the pleural surfaces are in close contact during the initial inflammatory insult (chest x-ray)
- chemical pleurodesis can be painful, particularly if the pleura is normal. Premedicate the patient with an opiate if there is no contra-indication
- introduce 250 mg lignocaine (25 ml 1% lignocaine), made up to a total volume of 30–50ml with normal saline, into the pleural space via the chest drain. This is best done using a 'bladder' syringe which will make an airtight seal when inserted into the end of the drain. Lignocaine toxicity is unlikely at doses

of < 3 mg/kg body weight. Flush the chest drain with a further 20 ml normal saline. Clamp the drain for 10 minutes

- instill the pleurodesing agent. The author uses 1.5–3.0 g of tetracycline. 5 g of sterile talc in 50 ml normal saline is an alternative (there are concerns about the continuing availability of tetracycline). The tetracycline is made up to a total volume of 50 ml with normal saline and injected slowly using a bladder syringe. The chest drain is then flushed with a further 20 ml normal saline

- clamp the chest drain (but there is evidence that clamping may not be necessary)

- recent studies suggest that patient rotation is not necessary

- the optimum dwell time is unknown but, experimentally, mesothelial cells are sloughed within minutes following intrapleural tetracycline. In the author's opinion, therefore, one hour should suffice

- do not use corticosteroids or nonsteroidal anti-inflammatory drugs to control pain unless really necessary. These will suppress the very inflammation that the operator is trying to induce!

- after one hour, unclamp the drain and reconnect to the underwater seal. Apply suction of –10 to –20 cm H_2O pressure to try to optimise pleural apposition. The first 3 hours is most critical

- in the case of a pleural effusion, remove the drain when drainage is < 100–150 ml fluid per day. This should be within 2–3 days.

- obtain a chest X-ray.

- a possible algorithm for the management of malignant pleural effusions has been produced by the BTS and is given in Figure 4).

References

1. Collins TR, Sahn SA. Thoracentesis: Complications, Patient experience, and diagnostic value. *Chest* 1987;**91**:817

2. Race GA, Scheifly CH, Edwards JE. Hydrothorax in congestive heart failure. *Am J Med* 1957;**22**:83–89

3. Light RW, MacGregor MI, Luchsinger PC, Ball WC. Pleural effusions: The diagnostic separation of transudates and exudates. *Ann Int Med* 1972;**77**:507

4. Sahn SA. The pleura. *Am Rev Respir Dis* 1988;**138**:184–234

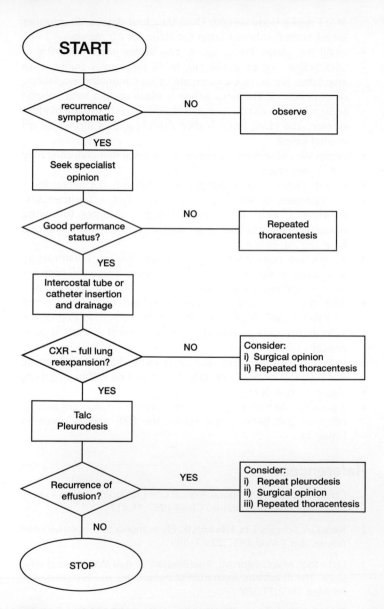

Figure 4. Algorithm for the management of malignant pleural effusions

5. Walshe ASP, Douglas JG, Kerr KM, McKean ME, Gedden DJ. An audit of the clinical investigation of pleural effusion. *Thorax* 1992; **47**:734–737

6. Mungall IPF, Gowen PN, Cooke NT, Roache TC, Cooke NJ. Multiple pleural biopsy with the Abrams needle. *Thorax* 1980;**35**:600–602

7. Light RW. Pleural diseases, 3rd edn. Baltimore: Williams and Wilkins 1995

8. Heffner JE, Brown LK, Barbieri C, De Leo JM. Pleural fluid chemical analysis in parapneumonic effusions — a meta-analysis. *Am Rev Respir Crit Care Med* 1995;**151**:1700–1708

9. Davies RJO, Traill ZC, Gleeson FG. Randomised controlled trial of intrapleural streptokinase in community acquired pleural infection. *Thorax* 1997;**52**:416–421

10. Levine H, Metzger W, Lacera D, Kay L. Diagnosis of tuberculous pleurisy by culture of pleural biopsy specimen. *Arch Int Med* 1970; **126**:269

11. Galarza I, Canete C, Granados A, Estopa R, Manresa F. Randomised trial of corticosteroids in the treatment of tuberculous pleurisy. *Thorax* 1995;**59**:1305–1307

12. Joseph J, Strange C, Sahn SA. Pleural effusions in hospitalised patients with AIDS. *Ann Intern Med* 1993;**118**:856

13. Sahn SA. Pleural diseases related to metastatic malignancies. *Eur Respir J* 1997;**10**:1907–1913

14. Walker-Berard PB, Vaughan LM, Sahn SA. Chemical pleurodesis for the treatment of malignant pleural effusions. *Ann Int Med* 1994; **120**:56

15. Schramel FMNH, Postmus PE, Vanderschueren RGJRA. Current aspects of spontaneous pneumothorax. *Eur Respir J* 1997;**10**:1372–1379

16. Sadikot RT, Greene T, Meadows K, Arnold AG. Recurrence of primary spontaneous pneumothorax. *Thorax* 1997;**52**:805–809

17. Miller AC, Harvey JE. Guidelines for the management of spontaneous pneumothorax. *Brit Med J* 1993;**307**:114–116

Appendix I

Management of spontaneous pneumothorax

Notes accompanying algorithm (Figure 1)

1 Degree of collapse
   Small = small rim of air around lung; Moderate = lung collapsed halfway towards heart border; Complete = airless lung, separate from diaphragm.
   Tension = any pneumothorax with cardiorespiratory collapse. It requires immediate cannulation. It is rare.

2 Significant dyspnoea
   This means an obvious deterioration in usual exercise tolerance. Aspiration may be necessary, whatever the size of the pneumothorax.

3 Chest drain
   If aspiration fails, ie same size or large pneumothorax, then there is a persisting air leak and a chest drain should be inserted — see later.

4 Respiratory physician's opinion
   Consider early advice, or possibly a Respiratory Physician's opinion, at 48 hours. Important considerations in management are
   1 assessing why re-expansion has not been achieved (for example, air leaking around the drain site, tube displaced or blocked, large persistent leak)
   2 the use of suction to re-expand the lung (this can be lengthy, requires appropriate equipment and pressure settings, influences how and where confirmatory radiographs are taken, and involves care from experienced nursing staff)
   3 whether early thoracic surgery would be appropriate (for example, failure of conservative measures, need to prevent recurrence)
   4 consideration of chemical pleurodesis in certain cases
   5 management of surgical emphysema
   6 if this is a recurrence of a pneumothorax.

5 Discharge checklist
   1 Consider patient's proximity to the hospital, transport access, whether he/she lives alone
   2 CXR

3 If chronic lung disease
   (a) bronchodilator +/– inhaled or oral steroids
   (b) spirometry
4 Advice on flying/diving (the latter is contraindicated)
5 Advice for recurrence of pain or breathlessness
6 Return to work
7 Follow up = 7–10 days.

12

Lung Infections

John T Macfarlane

Introduction

Lung infections constitute a significant part of the workload for both general and respiratory physicians. Those specialising in respiratory medicine need a clear idea of the aetiology, investigation and management of both simple and complicated lung infections when confronted with requests for opinions on patients both on the wards and in the outpatient clinic.

The classification of lung infections is shown in Table 1. They are traditionally divided into bronchial infections (acute bronchitis, acute exacerbations of chronic bronchitis, recurrent bronchial infections and bronchiectasis) and pneumonia (community acquired pneumonia, hospital acquired pneumonia, pneumonia in the immuno-compromised host, and pneumonia peculiar to particular geographical areas in the world).

Bronchial Infections

Acute bronchitis

This is generally defined as an acute illness associated with cough and discoloured sputum production in a previously well individual. It is generally thought that the primary infecting insult is usually viral and such patients are rarely seen in hospital unless a complication develops. Numerous studies demonstrate that antibiotics offer little or no benefit for most cases of acute bronchitis; even so, the majority of patients receive them. Complications include secondary bacterial infection (usually *Haemophilus influenzae, Streptococcus pneumoniae* and rarely *Staphylococcus aureus* and *Moraxella catarrhalis*).

Table 1. A practical classification of lung infections

I. BRONCHIAL INFECTIONS
    I.A. ACUTE BRONCHIAL INFECTIONS
        [1] Acute bronchitis
        [2] Acute exacerbation of chronic bronchitis

    I.B. CHRONIC BRONCHIAL INFECTIONS
        [1] Recurrent bronchial infections
        [2] Bronchiectasis

II. PNEUMONIA
    II.A. COMMUNITY ACQUIRED PNEUMONIA (CAP)
        [1] Non severe CAP
            (a) No unusual such factors present.
            (b) Host or environmental risk factors present.
        [2] Severe CAP

    II.B. HOSPITAL ACQUIRED PNEUMONIA (HAP)
        [1] Non severe HAP
            (a) No unusual risk factors present.
            (b) Host or environmental risk factors present.
        [2] Severe HAP
            (a) Early onset.
            (b) Later onset.

    II.C. IMMUNOCOMPROMISED ASSOCIATED PNEUMONIA (IAP)

    II.D. GEOGRAPHICALLY ASSOCIATED PNEUMONIA (GAP)

III OTHER INFECTIONS
    III. A. Lung abscess
    III. B. Empyema
    III. C. Other

Sometimes the cough may persist for several weeks and be a reason for outpatient referral. Although this may represent hyper-reactivity or be a presentation of asthma, often it merely reflects the long natural history of some cases of self limiting, 'post viral' cough.

Acute exacerbations of chronic bronchitis

This is a common reason for acute hospital admission.

Recurrent bronchitis

I use this term to include patients who have had recurring or persisting cough and purulent sputum over a number of weeks or months, but who do not have the features suggestive of established bronchiectasis or chronic bronchitis. Such patients have invariably had several courses of antibiotics before being referred to the outpatient clinic. Causes to consider include persisting bacterial bronchial infection due to ineffective prior antibiotics or beta-lactamase producing strains (usually *Haemophilus influenzae*; rarely *Pseudomonas aeruginosa* or *Moraxella catarrhalis*) It is worth obtaining a good sputum specimen for culture. Another common cause is chronic sinus infection with post nasal drip and recurrent bronchial soiling with aspirated material. Some patients are found to have occult, mild bronchiectasis.

Bronchiectasis

This is discussed in Chapters 7 and 15.

Pneumonia

Pneumonia can be discussed in a number of different ways. The scheme illustrated in Table 1 provides a useful structure from which to consider aetiology and management. As regards aetiology, the concept of 'core' pathogens is helpful. Such pathogens must always be included in any management plan. Additional pathogens become important under special situations where host and environmental factors and other circumstances are present.

Community acquired pneumonia

Community acquired pneumonia (CAP) has an incidence of around four per thousand population per year, this figure being much higher at extremes of age. It occurs twice as often in the winter months, probably because viral respiratory illnesses predispose to bacterial infection of the lower respiratory tract. Some pathogens have a different epidemiological pattern. Legionella pneumonia is much commoner in the summer months, largely related to foreign travel. Q fever (*Coxiella burnetti* pneumonia) occurs particularly in the spring during the lambing and calving season. By contrast *Mycoplasma pneumoniae* occurs in epidemics every three or four years, when it becomes the second commonest cause of CAP, being unusual at other times. Occasionally other epidemiological clues can be helpful to the clinician, such as recent bird contact (psittacosis), exposure to water systems such as showers, jacuzzis and defective air conditioning (legionella infection) or recent foreign travel (e.g. legionella infection, exposure to penicillin resistant pneumococci from Mediterranean countries or geographically restricted infections).

Aetiology

A key factor guiding therapy for CAP is knowledge of the potential pathogens. The spectrum is influenced by host factors (e.g. age, pre-existing disease) disease factors (severity, clinical picture) and epidemiological or circumstantial factors (e.g. season of the year, current epidemic). Geographical variations are also important when faced with a patient from abroad. In adults, 60 to 80% of CAP cases are caused by bacteria, 10 to 20% are 'atypical' and a similar proportion viral. *Strep pneumoniae* is the commonest and should be regarded as the 'core' pathogen, being responsible for up to half of identified cases and probably many of those where no pathogen is identified. Other pathogens vary in importance in relation to host or environmental risk factors (Table 2).

Clinical features

The general symptoms and signs of pneumonia are well known. Comparative studies of groups of patients with pneumonia suggest that clinical features cannot differentiate those with 'typical' bacterial pneumonia from those with 'atypical' infections. However, at the individual patient level, the clinical picture can sometimes be helpful in placing an atypical infection within the differential diagnosis (Table 3). There are several different ways of defining what is meant by an 'atypical' infection. I take this to mean community acquired pathogens including *Mycoplasma pneumoniae, Chlamydia pneumoniae, Chlamydia psittaci, Legionella pneumophilia* and *Coxiella burnetti,* which being intracellular, do not respond to aminopenicillins but do respond to antibiotics such as macrolides, tetracyclines and some quinolones.

Non-respiratory symptoms may be prominent in some patients and mask the diagnosis of pneumonia. Pneumonia may present as confusion, especially in the elderly, their only sign of the true diagnosis being an elevated respiratory rate and localising chest

Table 2.   Likely causes of adult community acquired pneumonia (CAP) with estimates of the overall percentage. (In a third to a half of cases, no pathogens can be identified. Many of these are thought to be pneumococcal in origin)

Non severe cap		% of total
Core pathogens		
Strep pneumoniae		30–50%
Respiratory viruses		15%
(?Chlamydia pneumoniae?)		? 15% ?
Additional pathogens	Additional risk factors	
Haem influenzae	Chronic lung disease	3–10%
Moraxella catarrhalis	Severe chronic lung disease	1%
Staph aureus	Influenza virus. Diabetes. Corticosteroids	2–3%
Legionella pneumophila	Exposure to infected water sprays/mists	3–6%
Mycoplasma pneumoniae	3–4 yearly epidemics	3–15%
Chlamydia psittaci	Bird contact	1–2%
Coxiella burnetti	Animal contact	1%
Influenza Virus	Winter epidemics	10–15%
Herpes varicella	Contact with chicken pox	Rare
Severe cap		% of severe cases
Core pathogens		
Strep pneumoniae		30–50%
Legionella pneumophilia		15% +
Staph aureus		5%
Additional pathogens	As for non severe CAP	Unusual

signs, but is also common in any severe pneumonia. Confusion is a particular feature of legionella pneumonia of any severity.

The differential diagnosis of pneumonia most commonly includes pulmonary infarction and pulmonary oedema and less commonly primary or metastatic lung cancer, eosinophilic pneumonia and acute allergic or cryptogenic alveolitis.

General investigations

Investigations are performed in CAP to confirm the diagnosis, to

Table 3. Clinical features that may sometimes differentiate a 'typical' bacterial pneumonia (usually pneumococcal infection) from an 'atypical' pneumonia (usually mycoplasma infection)

Typical	Atypical
Incidence increases with age	School or working age
Pre-existing disease	Previously well
Abrupt onset	Insidious onset over days
Specific respiratory features (haemoptysis, purulent sputum, pleural pain)	Non specific respiratory features (dry cough, mild dyspnoea, wheeze)
Marked systemic upset (rigors, high fevers, severe malaise, confusion)	Mild/moderate systemic upset
WBC, ESR, CRP high	WBC normal. ESR, CRP mildly raised
Chest radiograph homogeneous shadowing in over 80%	Chest radiograph patchy shadowing in half
Often responds to β lactam antibiotics	No response to β lactam antibiotics

[WBC = white cell count: ESR = erythrocyte sedimentation rate: CRP = C reactive protein]

determine aetiology, to assess severity, to determine the impact of the pneumonia on any underlying condition (such as chronic obstructive pulmonary disease or cardiac failure) and to provide data for epidemiological purposes. The suggested basic requirements for investigation of CAP are shown in Table 4.

Shadowing on a chest radiograph is the requirement to diagnose pneumonia. Most commonly this will be lobar or segmental homogeneous shadowing in bacterial pneumonias and also in over half the cases of atypical infections. Diffuse patchy, nodular or ground glass opacification may point to atypical infection or in severely ill patients, bacteraemic pneumonia.

A full blood count, hepatic and renal biochemical profiles, and a blood sugar should be performed on all hospitalised cases. In most cases of bacterial pneumonia the white blood count (WBC) is elevated over 15×10^9/litre, will usually be mildly raised in legionella infections ($11–15 \times 10^9$/litre) and will be normal in over

Table 4.   Suggested investigations for community acquired pneumonia in hospitalised patients

NON SEVERE CAP

Sputum culture (if available)

Blood culture

Pleural fluid culture (if present). [Essential to exclude empyema]

Full blood count

C reactive protein [bacterial infections usually associated with levels >50 ml/l]

Renal, electrolyte and hepatic biochemistry

Chest X-ray

Oxygen saturation

SEVERE CAP

Sputum Gram stain

Viral/atypical serology

Legionella and pneumococcal antigen detection in urine

Invasive tests

two thirds of viral or atypical infections. Mildly abnormal liver function tests are not uncommon in bacterial pneumonia; raised blood urea, hyponatraemia, hypoalbuminaemia and hypokalaemia can be present in any severe pneumonia. Hyponatraemia is also a feature of legionella infection being seen in half of cases.

Oxygen saturation should be checked and monitored in all the patients hospitalised with pneumonia and arterial blood gases checked if saturations fall below 93%, breathing air.

Specific microbiological investigations

Blood cultures should always be taken in patients ill enough to be hospitalised with CAP. They are positive in less than a fifth of cases but do provide a reliable, specific aetiological diagnosis and bacteraemia is associated with a worse prognosis. Sputum, if available, should be sent for culture but the result is only sometimes of positive value. Any pleural fluid should always be sampled to exclude a developing pleural infection or empyema (see section on parapneumonic effusions and empyema on page 286).

Bacterial antigen detection, if available, can be useful for diagnosis. The detection of legionella antigen in urine can be extremely useful for quick and early diagnosis and before serum antibodies are detectable. The test should be rapidly available to all laboratories. Pneumococcal polysaccharide capsular antigen may be detected in 80% of sputa, a third of urines and a smaller proportion of serum samples from patients with pneumococcal pneumonia but the test has limited availability. New bedside legionella and pneumococcal urine antigen test kits are becoming available.

Although serological methods to test acute and convalescent antibody levels are widely available to diagnose viral, atypical and legionella infections, the results are rarely available in time to influence initial management. Similarly, viral isolation is of little practical value in most cases.

In patients who fail to respond to empirical therapy, who are severely ill or in whom the diagnosis is in doubt, invasive techniques may be indicated to sample lower respiratory secretions or lung tissue (see Chapter XX on bronchoscopic and invasive techniques). These are rarely necessary for patients with CAP.

General management

General management, including appropriate fluid and oxygen replacement is essential. Pain relief should be given for pleural discomfort which may compromise breathing. Physiotherapy in the acute phase is of little benefit unless the patient has underlying chronic bronchial disease with copious amounts of purulent sputum. Monitoring should include regular pulse, respiratory rate, temperature and oxygen saturation recordings.

The early recognition of severe infection is an essential requirement and such patients, when identified, should be monitored closely, preferably on a high dependency (HDU) or intensive therapy unit (ITU). The British Thoracic Society identified four simple criteria, the presence of two or more of them having a high sensitivity, but low specificity for severe life threatening pneumonia. Subsequent studies have supported this simple formula as being of some practical value in detecting severe infections on admission. Other factors have also been identified as being associated with a poor outcome in studies using univariate or multivariate analysis.

Fine and colleagues (see References) have developed and tested prospectively a more complicated prediction rule for pneumonia severity which classifies patients into five risk categories. This has

**Table 5.   Pointers to severe pneumonia and the need for close
monitoring or intensive care unit transfer**

'Core' features identified by the British Thoracic Society study.[2] (presence
of ≥2 associated with 10–20 x increased risk of death).

- New confusion
- Respiratory rate >30/min
- Shock (DBP < 60 mm Hg; SBP < 90 mm Hg)
- Blood urea > 7 mmol/l

Other important adverse features noted in different studies of CAP severity

Age > 60.

Male sex.

Pre-existing disease.

New atrial fibrillation.

Leucopenia or marked leucocytosis.

Hypoxia (PaO_2 < 8kPa)

Multilobe radiographic shadowing.

Bacteraemia.

the practical advantage of not only identifying patients with severe
pneumonia but also grouping patients who have low risk of mortality and hence may be treated either as an outpatient or with oral
antibiotics and short hospital stay. If this risk prediction formula is
validated in the countries, such as the UK, this may form the basis
for more logical management at all levels of illness severity. Pointers
to severity of infection are shown in Table 5, taken both from the
BTS criteria and also those from Fine and colleagues.

The requirement for assisted ventilation for increasing respiratory failure is usually apparent within the first 48 hours of hospital
admission. The survival rate following assisted ventilation for CAP
is over 50%, emphasising the importance and benefit of this type
of therapy. Death most commonly occurs within the first week but
survivors may need ventilation for many days. Anecdotal experience suggests that extra corporeal membrane oxygenation (ECMO)
may has a place for 'buying time' for antibiotics to work in the
presence of early onset, life threatening hypoxia uncorrectable by
mechanical ventilation.

Unplanned transfer from a general ward to the ITU following

'unexpected' cardio-respiratory arrest is far from ideal and is associated with increased mortality.

Specific management — antibiotic therapy

Antibiotic choices vary according to severity of illness, history of pre-existing disease, clinical or epidemiological clues to likely aetiology and the presence of antibiotic hypersensitivity.

Adult non-severe CAP. A proportion of patients with mild or moderate pneumonia can be managed with oral antibiotics. *Strep pneumoniae* is the most common 'core' pathogen in this category. Clinical or epidemiological clues may point to an atypical organism (e.g. mycoplasma, legionella or chlamydia infection). *H influenzae* must be considered in the presence of chronic lung disease. An aminopenicillin such as oral amoxycillin or IV ampicillin is an appropriate initial choice.

If there is no improvement at 48 hours, then the diagnosis should be reviewed.

If an atypical infection is suspected at this stage, a macrolide such as erythromycin can be substituted or added. In the presence of chronic lung disease, resistant bacteria such as betalactamase producing *H influenzae* or *M catarrhalis* may be possible and a quinolone (ofloxacin or ciprofloxacin, but watch for interaction with theophyllines with the latter), co-amoxiclav or a parenteral cephalosporin such as cefuroxime can be substituted. There is little logic in using erythromycin in older patients because of the infrequency of atypical pathogens in this group and poor activity against *H influenzae* (Table 6). Although *C pneumoniae* infection is reported in the elderly, it's role in disease activity is not clear.

Another option is to remove the guess work and prescribe an aminopenicillin and a macrolide as initial therapy for adult non severe CAP. The advantages must be balanced against the increased side effects and cost of combination therapy. Monotherapy using newer macrolides and quinolones may become possible in the future.

Adult severe CAP. Any antibiotic choice must cover all likely pathogens, pending results of microbiological tests. The likely 'core' pathogens include pneumococcal, legionella and staphylococcal infection. Combination antibiotics including an intravenous macrolide (e.g. clarithromycin) and a betalactamase stable antibiotic

Table 6.   Empirical management of non-severe community acquired pneumonia (CAP)

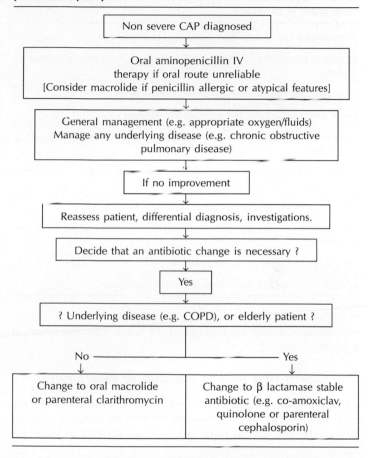

Non severe CAP diagnosed

Oral aminopenicillin IV
therapy if oral route unreliable
[Consider macrolide if penicillin allergic or atypical features]

General management (e.g. appropriate oxygen/fluids)
Manage any underlying disease (e.g. chronic obstructive
pulmonary disease)

If no improvement

Reassess patient, differential diagnosis, investigations.

Decide that an antibiotic change is necessary ?

Yes

? Underlying disease (e.g. COPD), or elderly patient ?

No — Yes

Change to oral macrolide
or parenteral clarithromycin

Change to β lactamase stable
antibiotic (e.g. co-amoxiclav,
quinolone or parenteral
cephalosporin)

(such as a second or third generation cephalosporin or co-amoxiclav) should be used initially. If legionella is thought likely, then rifampicin or ciprofloxacin should be added.

Duration of antibiotics

Duration of antibiotic therapy is dictated by clinical improvement and not by rigid rules. Up to a week of antibiotics is usually adequate for uncomplicated pneumonia. The switch from IV to

Table 7. Factors to consider in patients who fail to improve with initial therapy for community acquired pneumonia (CAP) in approximate order of likelihood

Improvement just slower than usual (e.g. elderly)

Diagnosis of pneumonia incorrect (? Pulmonary infarction or pulmonary oedema).

Less usual pathogen present and not covered by antibiotic.

Usual pathogen present but resistant to antibiotic.

Complicating pre-existing disease (e.g. chronic lung disease, bronchiectasis, lung cancer).

Intra-thoracic complication (e.g. parapneumonic pleural effusion, empyema, lung abscess).

Extra pulmonary complication (e.g. distant sepsis).

Complication of therapy (e.g. cannula related sepsis, antibiotic hypersensitivity).

Patient not receiving or taking antibiotic.

Correct antibiotic but inadequate dose or absorption.

oral therapy should be considered 24 hours after resolution of pyrexia.

The patient who fails to improve, or deteriorates

This should be a reason for a full reappraisal of the patient preferably with advice from a respiratory or infection specialist. Factors to consider and actions to be taken are summarised in Table 7.

Complications

Increasing age and the presence of underlying lung disease are associated with slower recovery. Pointers to the development of complications can be provided by considering the factors mentioned in Table 7. The commonest complication is the development of a parapneumonic effusion. This is often badly managed.

Parapneumonic effusions and empyema. The commonest complication, in around a third of patients with pneumonia, is the development of a parapneumonic pleural effusion. Even if not infected, this can be the cause of persistent fever following resolution of pneumonia and any effusion detected should always be sampled to exclude impending or actual empyema. The characteristics of the fluid aspirated can give a guide to correct management.

Parapneumonic effusions can progress seemlessly from the sterile exudative stage (where the fluid looks clear), through the fibropurulent stage (where the fluid looks cloudy or is frank pus — i.e. an empyema) where bacterial, leukocytes and fibrin accumulate in the pleural space and loculations develop, to the final stage of organisation, where fibroblast produce an inelastic pleural peel surrounding the pleural infection.

Parapneumonic effusions and empyema are examined in Chapter 11.

Lung abscess is a less common local infective complication of pneumonia. Normally lung abscesses will drain spontaneously through the bronchial tree, being associated with sudden increase in purulent sputum production. Consequently percutaneous drainage of lung abscesses are only occasionally needed and run the risk of soiling the pleural space and causing an empyema. Less commonly lung abscesses will discharge into the pleural space, forming a concomitant empyema or pyopneumothorax. The presence of a lung abscess normally requires prolonged appropriate antibiotic therapy for four to six weeks, depending on clinical and radiographic progress.

Occasionally pneumonias may resolve slowly persisting areas of consolidation and collapse consistent with an organising pneumonia and eventually lead onto areas of persistent scarring. In such circumstances the possibility of endobronchial obstruction should be investigated.

Hospital acquired pneumonia

Introduction

Hospital acquired pneumonia (HAP) is defined as pneumonia occurring more than 48 hours after hospital admission, excluding infection incubating at the time of admission. Pneumonia is the third most common hospital acquired infection and is associated with an 'attributable' mortality of up to 50%. The usual pathogenesis is aspiration of bacteria colonising the upper respiratory tract, together with impaired mechanical and immunological host defences.

Haematogeneous spread of infection from a distant focus, and inhalation of pathogens from contaminated respiratory equipment or from the hospital environment (e.g. water system colonised with legionella) are less common mechanisms. With impaired host defences, aspirated bacteria are able to become established and cause pneumonia. The incidence of oropharyngeal colonisation by enteric Gram negative bacteria (EGNB) increases in proportion to the length of hospital stay and the severity of underlying illness. These bacilli arise by the direct contamination of the pharynx from the hospital environment and from the patients upper gastrointestinal tract.

Aetiology of infection

As with CAP, a clear understanding of the likely pathogens causing HAP under different circumstances is essential for logical management. The spectrum of potential pathogens are different from those for CAP.

The most sensible classification of pathogens causing HAP depends on assessing four factors including: [a] the time of onset, [b] severity, [c] the presence of co-morbid disease and, [d] other risk factors for specific pathogens. This allows grouping of likely pathogens and thus guidance for initial empirical antibiotic selection.

The group of 'core' pathogens to be considered in all cases of HAP, include EGNB (*Escherichia coli, Klebsiella species, Proteus species, Enterobacter species* and *Serratia marcescens*), *H. influenzae* and Gram positive organisms such as *Strep pneumoniae* and methicillin sensitive *Staph aureus* (MRSA). Additional pathogens must be considered in certain circumstances including resistant Gram negative organisms such as *Pseudomonas aeruginosa* and *Acinetobacter species*, methicillin resistant *Staph aureus* (MRSA), *Legionella species* and anaerobic bacteria (Table 8).

If HAP occurs within five days of hospitalisation, it is more likely that community pathogens colonising the oropharynx (*Strep pneumoniae, H. influenzae* and *Staph aureus)* cause the infection. EGNB become more common with increasing hospital stay as the oropharynx becomes colonised by 'hospital' pathogens.

Clinical features

The characteristic clinical features of HAP include fever, purulent sputum or tracheobronchial secretions, leucocytosis and new or

Table 8. Aetiology and empirical management for different categories of hospital acquired pneumonia (HAP)

1. (a) Non severe HAP. No unusual risk factors present.

'Core' pathogens likely	Antibiotic choice
Enteric Gram negative bacilli H influenzae Strep pneumoniae Methicillin sensitive Staph aureus	'Core' antibiotic e.g.second or third generation (non pseudomonal) cephalosporin or β lactam/β lactamase inhibitor combination

1. (b) Non severe HAP. Specific risk factors present.

Additional pathogen to consider	RISK FACTORS	Additional antibiotics
Anaerobes	Impaired swallowing. Witnessed aspiration. Dental sepsis. Recent thoraco-abdominal surgery	As dictated by likely additional pathogen e.g. Clindamycin or Metronidazole or Co-amoxiclav.
Staph aureus	Coma. Head injury. Neurosurgery. Diabetes mellitus. Renal failure.	e.g. Flucloxacillin or Vancomycin (if MRSA possible)
Legionella species	High dose steroids. Epidemic in hospital.	e.g. Macrolide ± Rifampicin
Pseudomonas aeruginosa	High dose steroids. Multiple prior antibiotics. Prolonged mechanical ventilation. Underlying bronchiectasis.	As for severe HAP below 2 (b)
Methicillin resistant Staph aureus	MRSA prevalent locally	"

2. (a) Severe HAP. Early onset (within 5 days of hospital admission).		Antibiotic choice

'Core' pathogen likely	'Core' antibiotic

2. (b) Severe HAP. Later onset
Additional pathogens to consider

Pseudomonas aeruginosa Acinetobacter species [MRSA in some hospitals]	Aminoglycoside or quinolone PLUS Antipseudomonal antibiotic e.g. ceftazidime, meropenem or aztreonam [+/- Vancomycin]

persisting infiltrates on the chest radiograph. Unfortunately pre-existing and co-existing illness can cloud the diagnosis. The situation is particularly confusing in the ICU, where patients frequently develop other conditions that can obscure these findings or give rise to a similar picture. Purulent tracheal secretions are invariably present in patients on prolonged mechanical ventilation for a variety of causes apart from pneumonia. In one study less than half of the patients with fever and ventilator associated pneumonia diagnosed on clinical grounds had the diagnosis confirmed microbiologically.

General investigations

The chest radiograph, WBC, C reactive protein (CRP) and oxygenation should be assessed and may be a helpful pointer to infection. Cavitation on the chest radiograph is suggestive of infection particularly by EGNB, anaerobes or fungi, but can also be seen with pulmonary infarction.

Specific microbiological investigations

Blood cultures should always be obtained, but are positive in less than 20% of HAP cases. Sometimes the source of bacteraemia may not be from the lungs. Serological tests for viral and atypical pathogens are rarely of value, unless nosocomial legionella pneumonia is a possibility.

Making a confident microbiological diagnosis from culturing respiratory secretions is often impossible, due to contamination of the specimen with oropharyngeal bacteria. Thus expectorated sputum culture results may be misleading particularly if EGNB are isolated and only a third to a half of sputum cultures provide reliable information when compared with specimens obtained by invasive techniques. Endotracheal aspirates are simple to obtain in patients on mechanical ventilation, have a high sensitivity but a very low specificity.

Much has been published about the value of invasive techniques (both bronchoscopic and percutaneous) for managing HAP. Much of this work has focused on diagnosing VAP. Of these technique the protected specimen brush, broncho alveolar lavage and percutaneous lung needle aspirate (for patients not on mechanical ventilation) appear to provide the best results, in experienced centres. However questions regarding the applicability of published experience to every day clinical situations in hospitals where such clinical and laboratory expertise is not readily available makes the place for the routine use of such invasive procedures unclear. If invasive techniques are to be performed and the results acted upon, institutions should develop protocols agreed by the clinicians and microbiologists which dictate a systematic approach to performing the techniques, handling the specimens in the laboratory and applying the results to management. Little value is likely to accrue from these tests done occasionally, in a non planned way.

General management

Patients with HAP frequently have co-existing disease which may deteriorate as a result and require additional therapy. Sometimes the diagnosis of pneumonia may not be clear and empirical therapy may be given for more than one condition such as HAP and pulmonary oedema, until the situation becomes clearer.

Antibiotic management

Guidelines from North America provide the best basis for the practical, empirical management of HAP, based on the groupings already described. As with CAP, patients with severe infection should be identified early and start combination antibiotic therapy to cover all likely pathogens. Table 8 summarises an approach to antibiotic management.

Immunocompromised associated pneumonia (IAP)

Introduction

Acute respiratory illness is very common in the immuno-compromised population who include patients with lymphoproliferative, myeloproliferative and solid tumour malignancies, those receiving cancer chemotherapy, recipients of organ transplants, patients receiving immuno-suppressive or corticosteroid therapy for non-malignant diseases and patients with congenital or acquired immuno-deficiencies. The latter group are not considered further in this chapter.

Pulmonary infections are only one of the potential causes of acute respiratory illness and radiographic shadowing in this group of patients. Non infectious causes of pulmonary infiltrates which need to be considered in the differential diagnosis include pulmonary oedema, drug induced lung injury, radiation pneumonitis, lung haemorrhage, spread of the underlying neoplastic process and non-specific interstitial pneumonitis. The list of potential infectious causes is also considerable including bacteria, viruses, fungi, mycobacteria and parasitic infections all of which can cause immunocompromised associated pneumonia (IAP).

The picture of IAP is further complicated as many haematology and oncology units employ both chemoprophylaxis to reduce the chance of infection and also aggressive empirical antimicrobial therapy to cover likely bacterial, fungal and viral pathogens at the first sign of lung infection. This empiric approach is justified by the speed of infection, the wide spectrum of potential pathogens (sometimes present in mixed infections) and the difficulty of making a rapid and confident diagnosis of the cause of acute lung shadowing without resorting to invasive techniques in this group of susceptible patients.

Although these patients form a heterogeneous group, it is possible to develop some logic to the aetiology and management of IAP by assessing:

- the type, duration and severity of immunological defect
- the time the pneumonia occurs after the initial insult
- the time course of the acute illness
- the radiographic pattern (Table 9)

Clinical features

Symptoms and signs localising to the respiratory tract may be minimal or absent, especially in the context of severe immunosuppression. Cough and dyspnoea are the most common symptoms but these and fever may also be found in many non-infectious processes.

Clinical features may be helpful for identifying non-infectious causes in the differential diagnosis. Radiation pneumonitis typically develops 4–8 weeks following completion of a course of radiotherapy, earlier in previously irradiated lungs. An obvious time relationship may be apparent between receiving cycles of chemotherapy and developing drug induced pneumonitis. Evidence of tumour progression in other organs may point to neoplastic involvement of the lung. Features may be present of pulmonary oedema or cardiac failure. Pulmonary oedema may be contributed to by large volumes of intravenous fluids given in conjunction with certain chemotherapy regimes or during resuscitation of a septic patient.

Table 9. Factors that are associated with different pathogens for immuno-compromised associated pneumonia

Pathogens	Defect*		Timing after Insult/transplant		Speed of onset			Radiographic shadows		
	T cell	Humoral/ granulocytes	< 1 month	1–6 months	Acute few days	Sub acute 1–2 weeks	Insidious	Focal	Diffuse	Nodular/ cavitations
Bacterial										
Gram positive bacteria		+	+		+			+		
Enteric Gram negative bacilli		+	+		+			+		+ (abscess)
VIRAL										
CMV	+			+	+	+			+	
FUNGAL										
Aspergillus	+	+		+	+	+		+		+
Cryptococcus	+					+		+		
Candida		+								
Nocardia	+						+			+
Mycobacterial	+			+	+	+		+		
Pneumocystis	+			+	+	+	+		+	+

*T Cell defects associated with lymphomas, solid organ transplantation, corticosteroids. Humoral/granulocyte defects associated with myeloma, leukaemias, chemotherapy.

Haemoptysis may point to alveolar haemorrhage, but can also occur with cavitating infections such as aspergillus.

Occasionally, non-pulmonary physical signs can be useful. For instance ecthyma gangrenosum suggesting pseudomonal septicaemia, skin nodules from disseminated cryptococcus or nocardia, yellow white retinal patches with associated haemorrhage in disseminated CMV infection, or necrotising nasal lesions in mucormycosis and sometimes aspergillus. Neurological features may suggest intracranial fungal, tuberculous, neoplastic or other infective causes.

As summarised in Table 9 the timing of onset and the tempo of the illness may also narrow the differential diagnosis. Bacterial infections usually occur early in the course of immunosuppression whereas CMV pneumonia occurs between 1–6 months following organ transplantation typically between 1–2 months. Pneumocystis may develop as corticosteroid therapy is being withdrawn. Bacterial and pneumocystis pneumonias tend to develop rapidly over a few days, CMV, aspergillus and mucormycos over a period of 1–2 weeks whereas tuberculosis, cryptococcosis and nocardiosis follow a more insidious course.

General investigations

The chest radiograph can be particularly helpful (Table 9). Generally pneumocystis and viral pneumonias cause diffuse bilateral (sometimes perihilar) infiltrates as does drug induced lung injury, pulmonary haemorrhage and interstitial pneumonitis. Radiation pneumonitis has sharply demarcated limits, related to radiation fields. Nodular looking infiltrates may point to nocardia or cryptococcus infections both of which can cavitate, as can fungal, mycobacterial and necrotising bacterial infections. Focal, homogeneous consolidation is particularly a feature of bacterial and some fungal infections such as aspergillus.

Aspergillus may show progression of multiple nodules to produce single or multiple areas of homogeneous 'round' consolidation or wedge shaped pleural based lesions mimicking pulmonary infarction (due to vascular invasion and thrombosis).

General and specific microbiological investigations

Non invasive diagnostic techniques including sputum Gram and acid fast stain and culture, and blood culture should be obtained but are rarely diagnostic. Similarly, serology is rarely helpful. In a transplant patient with diffuse lung shadowing, the rise in CMV antibody titres over pre-transplant levels would suggest a diagnosis of CMV pneumonia. Serology for fungal infections appears neither reliable nor widely available. Serology may be helpful for legionella pneumonia; usually only *L. pneumophila* sero group one is detectable by urinary antigen.

Pneumocysts may be found in induced sputum specimens and are diagnostic.

All too often the respiratory specialist is asked to assess a critically ill, immunocompromised patient to consider invasive lung sampling (broncho alveolar lavage, transbronchial lung biopsy or opinion regarding open lung biopsy). Often such patients have already received multiple chemotherapy for bacterial, fungal, viral and pneumocystis infections. In such circumstances, it is unlikely that invasive samples will detect a diagnosis that would radically alter therapy; simplification of therapy often being the most likely benefit.

Management

Most haematology, oncology and transplant units have established protocols for the management of acute febrile episodes and pulmonary shadowing. Respiratory specialists should be involved in developing these guidelines and agreeing on the place of invasive techniques within the protocol, depending on local circumstances and clinical and laboratory expertise. For many the protocols include the early use of broad spectrum antibiotics for acute focal shadowing, adding amphotericin if improvement does not occur quickly. In the presence of diffuse shadowing, early therapy for pneumocystis and CMV is used depending on CMV status and prior use of pneumocystis prophylaxis.

Notes on specific situations

Bone marrow transplantation (BMT). Pulmonary complications may appear in up to 50% of people receiving BMT, an increasingly commonly used technique. Bacterial infections occur within the first two weeks after transplantation and are the most common late infections after six months, often associated with chronic graft versus host disease (GVHT). *CMV* infection is common and may develop into pneumonia, usually 50–60 days after transplantation.

Risk factors include use of sero positive donor products for sero negative recipients, increasing age, total body irradiation and GVHD. Gancyclovir and *CMV* hyperimmunoglobulin have altered the outlook considerably. *Herpes simplex* and *RSV* pneumonitis are occasionally seen.

Marrow transplant recipients are the most susceptible of all transplant patients to invasive pulmonary aspergillosis which often presents insidiously with non-specific symptoms such as fever, dyspnoea and a dry cough. Pleural pain and haemoptysis are pointers to the diagnosis. The radiographic features have already been described. The outcome remains poor. This has encouraged the early use of empirical amphoteracin B therapy. Prophylactic amphoteracin should be used for patients with prior aspergillus disease who require additional courses of chemotherapy. Some recommend the resection of residual lung cavities or nodules to reduce the incidence of further infection or fatal haemoptysis, once the patient is in a stable clinical and more immunocompetent state.

Units have a different incidence of fungal infection, often related to the local environmental contamination with fungal spores. Nearby building work can be associated with a rise in aspergillus infections. An air controlled environment can reduce outbreaks of aspergillus infection.

The incidence of pneumocystis pneumonia has dropped sharply since the introduction of routine prophylaxis with trimethoprim — sulphamethoxazole (TMP-SMX). When it occurs, it is usually around two months after transplantation. Response to treatment is usually good if instituted early.

Kidney transplantation.   *CMV* infection is the most common infectious complication after renal transplantation although the incidence has fallen since the introduction of cyclosporin based immunosuppression and matching of *CMV* antibody negative donors and recipients. Aspergillus pneumonia may sometimes be seen during the treatment of allograph rejection. Pneumocystis pneumonia is uncommon in centres that use TMP-SMX prophylaxis. The use of chemoprophylaxis in at risk individuals also reduces the frequency of mycobacterial infections.

Liver transplantation.   Bacterial or fungal infections that develop after liver transplantation often arise from the liver or biliary system, typically being caused by ENGB or candida. Otherwise the pattern of infection is similar to other solid organ transplant situations with a significant reduction in infection associated with the use of cyclosporin based immunosuppression and chemoprophylaxis.

Heart and lung transplantation. In this situation the lungs are particularly vulnerable to infection due to the initial acute lung injury related to surgery. Bacterial pneumonias are the major early infectious complication; usually due to EGNB and sometimes legionella infection. Other infections are similar to other transplant situations and fungal pneumonias are relatively uncommon.

Geographically restricted pneumonias

Modern and rapid travel means that clinicians may be faced with infections rare in their own environment. In practice, this is an uncommon clinical situation. Examples include parasitic infections of the lung (e.g. paragonimiasis causing lung shadowing and haemoptysis), unusual bacterial infections (melioidosis caused by *Pseudomonas pseudomallei* from South east Asia, pulmonary anthrax, diphtheria, brucellosis pneumonia, *Pasteurella multocida pneumonia,* plague pneumonia due to *Yersinia pestis* and tularaemic pneumonia due to *Francisella tularensis*) and fungal infections endemic in some countries (coccidioidomycosis, common in south western United States, central and south America, *Histoplasma capsulatum* pneumonia common in temperate climates along river valleys in north, central and south America, India and south east Asia and some Caribbean islands).

Conclusions

The correct assessment and management of pulmonary infections is one of the most challenging aspects of respiratory medicine and a frequent cause of referral for specialist respiratory opinion. Clear and logical understanding of the likely aetiology and value of investigations is of primary importance when deciding on appropriate management. Antibiotic choice will frequently be empirical in the first instance. Although there is an increasing complexity in the differential diagnosis of acute lung shadowing as one progresses from CAP, through HAP to IAP, a clear appreciation of the clinical and laboratory information should allow a positive and helpful assessment and opinion to be given.

Further Reading

1. Anonymous. Hospital-acquired pneumonia in adults: diagnosis, assessment of severity, initial antimicrobial therapy, and preventative strategies. A consensus statement, American Thoracic Society, November 1995. *American Journey of Respiratory & Critical Care Medicine* 1996;**153**:1711–1725

2. Anonymous. Guidelines for the management of community-acquired pneumonia in adults admitted to hospital. The British Thoracic Society. *British Journal of Hospital Medicine* 1993;**49**:346–350

3. Fanta CH, Pennington JE. Pneumonia in the Immunocompromised host. In: Pennington JE, ed. Respiratory Infections Diagnosis and Management, 3rd ed, pp 275–294. New York: Raven Press 1994

4. Fine MJ, Auble TE, Yealy DM et al. A prediction rule to identify low risk patients with community acquired pneumonia. *N Eng J Med* 1997;**336**:243–250

5. Macfarlane JT. An overview of community acquired pneumonia with lessons learned from the British Thoracic Society Study. *Seminars in Respiratory Infections* 1994;**9**:153–165

6. Niederman MS. An approach to empiric therapy of nosocomial pneumonia. *Medical Clinics of North America* 1994;**78**:1123–1141

7. Niederman MS, Bass JB Jr, Campbell GD, Feinn AM, Grossman RF, Mandell, et al. Guidelines for the initial management of adults with community-acquired pneumonia: diagnosis, assessment of severity, and initial antimicrobial therapy. American Thoracic Society. Medical Section of the American Lung Association. *Am Rev Respir Dis* 1993;**148**:1418–1426

8. Pennington JE. Hospital-acquired pneumonia. In: Pennington JE, ed. Respiratory Infections Diagnosis and Management, 3rd ed, pp 207–227. New York: Raven Press 1994

9. Pittet D, Harbarth S. What techniques for diagnosis of ventilator associated pneumonia? *Lancet* 1998;**352**:83–4

10. Torres A, Gonzalez J, Ferrer M. Evaluation of the available invasive and non-invasive techniques for diagnosing nosocomial pneumonias in mechanically ventilated patients. *Intensive Care Medicine* 1991;**17**:439–448

13

Tuberculosis

L Peter Ormerod

Introduction

M. tuberculosis is the commonest world-wide infection with 1.7 billion infected and 8 million clinical cases with 3 million deaths per annum, and is rarely spread other than by person to person infection. The incidence of TB had been falling in developed countries throughout this century, but has risen over the last 10 years. In England and Wales cases have risen from a nadir of 5000 cases in 1987 to approximately 6000 per annum. This rise is due to a number of factors which interact.[1] Ethnicity is the biggest single factor. Persons of Indian Subcontinent (ISC) or Black-African ethnic origin have an annual incidence of 120/100000, compared with 5/100000 for the white ethnic group. Over 50% of cases in England and Wales are now in ethnic minority groups, and the increase in most developed countries is largely in such ethnic groups. The highest rates are in the first three years after initial entry, but return visits to countries of high prevalence may also be a risk factor.

In the white ethnic group over half of cases are aged 55 years and over, with an incidence ranging from 1–2/100000 for ages 15–29 to between 10–20/100000 for aged over 75 years. To date TB/HIV co-infection has played only a minor role in the UK. In 1993 only 2.2% of notified TB cases having unlinked anonymised testing were HIV-positive. Allowing for under-notification which is significant in HIV/TB, no more than 5% of TB cases are likely to be HIV-positive. The TB/HIV interaction is higher in some European countries e.g. Spain and Italy, and in the USA. The TB/HIV interaction is most significant in Sub-Saharan Africa where now 70% of TB cases are HIV-positive. The interaction in South-East Asia, including the Indian Subcontinent, is likely to increase rapidly in the next decade.

Social deprivation is also a risk factor. Most of the increase in TB in England and Wales has been in the most deprived 10% of the population. Rates of pulmonary tuberculosis of between 1500–2000/100000 per annum have been reported in the street homeless in London in 1994–5. The incidence of drug resistance is currently low in the white ethnic group, but is higher in ethnic minority groups, in those who are HIV-positive and in those with previous treatment. Multidrug resistant TB (MDR-TB) is increasing globally, and currently accounts for 2% of isolates in England and Wales.

Clinical Features

The initial infection is often symptomless and only a positive tuberculin test shows that it has occurred. Occasionally immunological phenomena such as erythema nodosum or phylectenular conjunctivitis accompany this tuberculin hypersensitivity. In children enlarged mediastinal lymph nodes can cause bronchial obstruction presenting as cough. Dissemination occurs at the time of initial infection but only manifests some time afterwards, often many years. Only some 10–15% of those infected will develop clinical disease over a lifetime. The highest risk is in the first year after infection.

Most clinical disease occurs as post-primary forms in tuberculin sensitised individuals.

General symptoms

Fever particularly nocturnal, accompanied by sweats, is a common feature of pulmonary or disseminated disease. Weight loss also occurs, being most common with pulmonary and abdominal disease and can be considerable (>10kg). Anorexia and a feeling of malaise are also common.

Respiratory symptoms

Cough initially with mucoid then passing to purulent sputum is the commonest symptom. This is often accompanied by streak or more pronounced haemoptysis. Breathlessness tends to occur late when there is either significant parenchymal damage, or if a pleural effusion develops. Chest pain is not common, some patients with mediastinal lymphadenopathy have a dull retrosternal ache. A more localised chest wall pain can occur with parenchymal disease. With long-standing disease there can be loss of volume and tracheal shift towards the most affected side.

Non-respiratory tuberculosis

Lymphadenopathy

Usually involves the neck but can be axillary or less commonly inguinal. The enlargement is relatively painless and not accompanied by much erythema or oedema i.e. a 'cold abscess'. The nodes can be matted together or discrete, often become fluctuant and may discharge leaving a sinus if untreated. In ISC ethnic patients 10% with peripheral TB nodes also have mediastinal lymphadenopathy on chest X-ray.

Bone/joint

The clinical features are of pain and swelling in the appropriate areas. A cold abscess in association with spinal disease occurs in up to 15% of cases. This can cause neurological signs if there is an extradural collection, or spread paraspinally to the psoas muscles and point under the inguinal ligament causing hip flexion, 'psoas spasm'.

Abdominal

Weight loss is frequent. The commonest site of disease is ileocaecal. Some patients present with a short illness simulating appendicitis. Some present with intestinal obstruction, and some with a story of weight loss, fever and more diffuse pain. An abdominal mass, commonly in the right iliac fossa is felt. Ascites is often present, and may dominate the presentation. The 'classical' doughy abdomen is actually very uncommon.

Skin

The symptoms in scrofuloderma — skin involvement from underlying disease are those of the underlying disease e.g. node or bone/joint. Primary skin tuberculosis is very uncommon in white persons. Erythema nodosum may accompany primary infection in children and young adults.

Central nervous system

The symptoms of TB meningitis are non-specific initially with malaise and headache being commonest; fever and/or photophobia and neck stiffness are not invariably present (Stage I disease). As the disease progresses, focal neurological signs e.g. hemiparesis or cranial nerve palsies can develop or concious level becomes clouded (Stage II disease). Coma is a late manifestation (Stage III disease). Choroidal tubercles are rarely seen in developed countries, papilloedema may occur if obstructive hydrocephalus develops. Some 20–30% of classical miliary cases have TB meningitis. Tuberculomas can occur without meningitis — presenting with focal features depending on site. Tuberculomas can occur in association with meningitis or develop during treatment.

Genitourinary

Renal involvement is often insidious. Microscopic haematuria or occasionally frank haematuria can occur. Bladder involvement leads to frequency and nocturia and loss of bladder size. Dysuria and prostatic symptoms can occur. Testicular/epididymal TB causes pain and swelling and can simulate tumour. Endometrial or tubal disease is often 'silent' and may present with primary or secondary infertility or pelvic pain.

Miliary or disseminated TB

Fever and weight loss are the major symptoms. Some 'classical' miliary TB patients have TB meningitis (see above). 'Cryptic' or disseminated TB may have few signs other than fever. TB should be in the differential of a PUO particularly in ethnic minority patients.

HIV-positive patients

HIV-positivity increases by at least 100-fold the chances of clinical disease in a tuberculosis infected person. This tends to involve nodes (intra- and extra-thoracic), or be disseminated, considerably more often than in HIV-negative individuals. Clinical features may be more general and non-specific.

Investigations

Respiratory

The chest X-ray shows the *extent* of disease and can strongly suggest tuberculosis. *Activity* is determined from microscopy and culture of respiratory secretions. Pulmonary TB has a predeliction for the upper lobes, particularly posterior segments, and if in the lower lobes the apical and posterior segments. Parenchymal disease often progresses to cavitation. The pattern is less typical in those HIV-positive with lower zone predominance, lack of cavitation, and increased mediastinal lymphadenopathy reported. In children and in some ethnic minority groups mediastinal lymphadenopathy is a common presentation, when a primary focus may or may not be visible. CT scan of the thorax can be useful in assessing possible bronchostenosis, and shows mediastinal lymphadenopathy well, with the periphery of the gland enhancing with contrast whilst the caseous centre remains non-enhancing.

Bacteriological confirmation is important for confirmation of diagnosis and, in view of rising drug resistance rates, to obtain susceptibility results. Three morning sputum samples should be examined by microscopy and culture for acid-fast bacilli. Those with acid-fast bacilli on direct microscopy should be regarded as infectious if inpatients (see under isolation advice). If TB is strongly suspected but no respiratory secretions are available, fibreoptic bronchoscopy and lavage/trap specimens from the appropriate lobe/ segment is indicated. This procedure may also show unexpected endobronchial involvement. It is also worth sending any post bronchoscopy sputum for analysis. If contamination of endoscopy washers with atypical mycobacteria is a local problem, a parallel sample of washer fluid may need to be examined to exclude false positive microscopy. In children with no respiratory secretions morning gastric washings may be indicated. For pleural effusions pleural biopsy and cytology for culture, protein and cytology (lymphocytes) should be carried out.

The tuberculin test (Heaf: Mantoux) shows if tuberculosis *infection* has occurred, but a positive test does not necessarily mean disease. The tuberculin test is most useful in contact tracing or new immigrant screening (see later). The Heaf test is preferred[2] as being easier to standardise and read (Box 1). There is a poor correlation between a positive tuberculin test and clinical disease in those aged over 35 years. The tuberculin test can also be falsely suppressed e.g. HIV-positivity, extensive disease (miliary or pulmonary).

Box 1   Tuberculin test

Negative	Positive	Strongly Positive
Heaf 0–1	Heaf 2	Heaf 3–4
Mantoux* induration < 4mm	Mantoux induration 5–14mm	Mantoux induration >15mm

* Mantoux 10TU: 0.1ml of 100TU/ml i.e. 1:1000

Heaf grade 0–2 or Mantoux induration under 15mm is consistent with BCG vaccination. In non-BCG vaccinated subjects Heaf 2 or Mantoux 5mm or greater is positive. Heaf is the preferred method of testing as there is less intra- and interobserver error. False negative tests occur in immunocompromised patients e.g. HIV-positive

---

Certain X-ray/clinical situations in ethnic minority groups should be regarded as TB until proved otherwise and investigated accordingly (Box 2). In ISC and other ethnic minority groups isolated mediastinal lymphadenopathy supported by a positive tuberculin test should be regarded as TB and treated accordingly. Mediastinoscopy is only indicated if there is failure to respond in 2–3 months, or if the tuberculin test is negative or only weakly positive. In the white ethnic group this presentation of TB is uncommon, histology should be sought to exclude lymphoma, sarcoidosis and carcinoma.

Box 2   Clinical situations

These situations in ethnic minority groups should be regarded as TB until proved otherwise

1. Mediastinal lymphadenopathy
2. Pleural effusion
3. Persistent peripheral lymphadenopathy (>4 weeks)
4. Monoarthritis

Non-respiratory sites

As with respiratory disease bacteriological confirmation and susceptibility tests are important. Biopsy material (**NOT in preservative**) or pus should be sent for microscopy and culture. Histological diagnosis may be required from biopsies, and the diagnosis is sometimes not suspected until histology is received.

Peripheral lymphadenopathy

Accounts for 50% of extrapulmonary disease is all ethnic groups. In ethnic minority groups peripheral lymphadenopathy persisting for four weeks or longer should be suspected as being TB until proved otherwise. If there is fluctuation needle aspiration shows typical green pus and biopsy is not needed. For non-fluctuant nodes biopsy for histology *AND* culture should be carried out. Surgery does not improve resolution but helps obtain bacteriological confirmation and susceptibilities. In 10% of ISC patients there is associated mediastinal lymphadenopathy.

White children under five years can develop granulomatous and discharging cervical nodes due to non-tuberculous mycobacteria (*M. malmoense* and *M. avium intracellulare*). The nodes often show many AFB on histology, and are accompanied by a weakly positive tuberculin test. Non-tuberculous disease should be suspected in these circumstances. The treatment of such cases is by node excision not by drug treatment.

Bone/joint

The spine is the site of 50% of disease. There are X-ray features of a discitis with loss of disc space and erosion of the adjacent vertebral margins. CT or NMR scanning is indicated if there are neurological signs or evidence of cord compression. A monoarthritis in an ethnic minority patient should be investigated for TB. Arthroscopy or joint aspiration for culture and/or histology may be needed. Bone scans are positive before there is plain X-ray bone erosion.

Gastrointestinal disease

Small bowel disease and peritoneal involvement are the commonest presentations. For TB ascites a peritoneal tap shows a lymphocyte rich exudate. Small bowel barium studies shows stricturing and sometimes multiple lesions which cannot be differentiated from inflammatory bowel disease, or in the colon from carcinoma. Laparoscopy often provides histological (and culture) confirmation.

Genitourinary disease

IVP may show calcification, calyceal clubbing/distortion and ureteric beading/stenosis. Standard urine microscopy shows a sterile pyuria. Three early morning urines for AFB culture should be sent. Renal function may be impaired by parenchymal disease or obstruction. Biopsies from bladder, prostate, epididymis or testis show granulomata. In females TB may present as infertility due to either endometrial disease or tubal involvement. D & C for AFB culture is appropriate if there are granulomata on endometrial biopsy.

Skin disease

Half of skin disease is due to scrofuloderma — skin involvement due to underlying structural disease usually node, bone/joint or genitourinary. Diagnosis is made from biopsy and/or culture. Other forms of skin TB, lupus vulgaris or the tuberculides are diagnosed from clinical appearances supported by a positive tuberculin test and histology. PCR may show mycobacterial DNA in the skin in the tuberculides e.g. erythema induratum (Bazin's disease).

Central nervous system

The CSF in TB meningitis shows a raised white cell count with a lymphocytic or monocytic predominance, reduced glucose and raised protein. AFB may not be visible on microscopy. PCR of CSF may give false negative results because of inhibitors in the CSF. CT scan may show meningeal enhancement, or features of hydrocephalus, and sometimes tuberculomata which can be single or multiple, which enhance with contrast, and can occur without meningitis.

Pericardial disease

Pericardial fluid as with other serous membrane disease shows a lymphocyte rich exudate. Echocardiogram to confirm diagnosis of effusion and guide pericardiocentesis is widely available.

Miliary/disseminated

'Classical' miliary tuberculosis has a typical X-ray appearance with 1–2mm nodules uniformly scattered throughout all zones. 30% of classical cases have associated meningitis and an LP may confirm the diagnosis. Some cases of disseminated or 'cryptic' disease have fever, weight loss but no specific chest X-ray changes. The tuberculin test can be negative. TB should be in the differential of any PUO especially in ethnic minority groups. Liver biopsy has the highest yield of diagnosis in this group (histology +/– culture). A trial of antituberculosis drugs may be needed to make the diagnosis, fever responding usually in 7–14 days.

General

'Routine' blood tests may show normochromic anaemia, raised ESR or CRP/viscosity, raised globulin and reduced albumen, non-specific abnormalities of liver function, and a low sodium (degree of SIADH). None of these are diagnostic of TB in themselves. Consideration should be given to HIV testing TB cases based on an individual risk assessment. Active TB however can cause a moderately reduced CD4 count, which returns to normal in those HIV-negative with treatment.

Differential diagnosis

There can sometimes be difficulty separating tuberculosis and sarcoidosis. Box 3 compares and contrasts the two conditions. The relevance of positive or negative tests for tuberculosis are given in Box 4.

Contact tracing

Screening household contacts of cases yields 1–10% of notifications. Detailed advice on contact tracing has recently been published.[3] Contact tracing is required for respiratory disease to see if contacts have been infected, and for children and those with forms of tuberculosis which usually occur within one year of infection (e.g. eythema nodosum, meningitis) to try to find the source of the infection. The flow diagram (Figure 1) gives advice depending on whether the notified case was sputum smear-positive, and the age, BCG status and tuberculin response. Chemoprophylaxis may be required for some contacts (see under management).

Box 3   Comparison of Tuberculosis and Sarcoidosis

System	Sarcoidosis	Tuberculosis*
Respiratory	predeliction for upper zones mediastinal lymphadenopathy (often BHL) cavitation rare endobronchial disease fairly common Tuberculin test usually weak or negative	predeliction for upper zones mediastinal lymphadenopathy (can be BHL) often cavitation endobronchial disease less common Tuberculin test usually strongly positive +ve microscopy or culture for mycobacteria in respiratory secretions
Peripheral glands	Not uncommon do not discharge granulomas on histology	Common fluctuation and/or discharge in 15–30% Pus may be obtained granulomas on histology
CNS	Lymphocytic meningitis with normal glucose Mononeuritis multiplex	lymphocytic meningitis with reduced glucose
Gastro-intestinal	rarely involved	Ascites — peritoneal nodules Intestinal obstruction — bowel involvement — often ileocaecal
Skin	Lupus pernio over bone lesions Other skin lesions (usually negative or weak tuberculin test)	Scrofuloderma over bone/ gland/urogenital disease Other forms associated with strongly positive tuberculin test
Bone	Cystic changes	Bone destruction e.g. loss of spinal disc space
Liver	may show granulomas	granulomas in up to 75% miliary disease
Genito-urinary	Kidneys occasionally involved involved Urether, epididymis, testis, fallopian tube and endometrium rarely involved	GU involvement sometimes seen Commoner in white patients Epididymis,testis, fallopian tube and endometrium often involved
Other	Conjunctiva and buccal mucosa often asymptomatically involved blind biopsy show granulomata in significant proportions	

(Kveim biopsy positive in 70% acute: 50% chronic)

Box 4   Utility of positive and negative tests for tuberculosis and possible errors

Investigation	Positive test	Negative test	Possible error
Tuberculin test	Infection but not necessarily disease		poor correlation between positive test and disease over age 30
		Can be false negative	negative test can occur in disseminated or extensive disease or in HIV-positive
Ziehl-Nielsen stain	Mycobacterium species on microscopy	Insufficient to detect or negative	Lab reagent or cross-contamination can give false-positive
Auramine stain (better for screening)	as above	as above	as above
PCR test	Identifies mycobacterium and (species)	Suggests not present	Inhibitors e.g. in CSF can give false-negative. Contamination e.g. with environmental mycobacterium can give false positive
BACTEC culture	More rapid culture than conventional		

BCG vaccination[2]

BCG is currently recommended for previously unvaccinated persons at school aged 10–13, where it has been shown to give 70–80% protection which lasts for at least 15 years, and for the following selected groups:

- tuberculin negative new immigrants from high prevalence countries aged under 35
- tuberculin negative household contacts of respiratory disease
- neonates of ethnic minority groups e.g. ISC or Black-African
- tuberculin negative previously unvaccinated Health Care Workers. In those with a definite BCG scar, even if tuberculin negative, there is no evidence to support repeat BCG vaccination

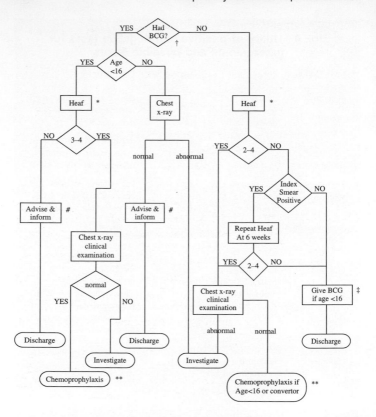

Examination of close contacts of pulmonary tuberculosis.

Contacts of non-pulmonary tuberculosis need not usually be examined (see text). Note: children under two who have not had a BCG vaccination who are close contacts of a smear positive index patient should receive chemoprophylaxis irrespective of tuberculin status (see text).

† Previous BCG cannot be accepted as evidence of immunity in HIV-infected subjects.

* Negative test in immunocompromised subjects does not exclude tuberculous infection.

Advise patient of tuberculosis symptoms, inform GP of contact.

** Persons eligible for, but not given, chemoprophylaxis should have follow up chest x-rays at 3 and 12 months.

‡ See text

Figure 1. Contact tracing algorithm (reproduced with permission from Thorax)[3]

Management

Notification[4]

All clinical cases of TB should be notified to the local Consultant in Communicable Diseases, including those which are non-infectious, so that appropriate contact tracing can be performed. Persons receiving chemoprophylaxis are not notifiable. Denotify if cultures show non-tuberculous mycobacteria.

Pretreatment precautions

Because of the possible but rare toxic effects of ethambutol on the eye it is recommended that visual acuity should be tested by Snellen chart before it is first prescribed. The drug should only be used in patients who have reasonable visual acuity and who are able to appreciate and report visual symptoms or changes in vision. The notes should record that the patient has been told to stop the drug *immediately* if such symptoms occur, and report to the physician. The GP should also be informed of this. In small children and those with language difficulties ethambutol should be used where appropriate, with the above advice given to parents or other family members.

Renal function should be checked before treatment with either streptomycin or ethambutol. These drugs should be avoided in renal failure if possible, but if used should have serum concentrations monitored and substantially reduced dosages given unless dialysis is used. Liver function should be checked pretreatment for clinical cases. Detailed advice on monitoring liver function and the management of hepatotoxicity has recently been published,[5] which is summarised in Boxes 5 and 6.

Infection control

Most patients can be treated and supervised as out-patients and do not need admission to hospital. If a patient with respiratory TB is admitted to hospital for diagnosis or treatment it is safer to admit initially to a single side ward until sputum microscopy results are available. In HIV-negative patients, with positive sputum microscopy segregation for reasons of infectivity is generally only required for two weeks, as such patients become non-infectious within two weeks of treatment containing rifampicin and isoniazid. Different criteria apply in HIV-positive patients and in those with MDR-TB,[6]

Box 5   Liver function pre- and during treatment

Measure pre-treatment liver function, then:

Known chronic liver disease — weekly LFT's for two weeks; then fortnightly for first two months

Normal liver function — repeat (and stop treatment) only if fever, malaise, vomiting, jaundice or unexplained deterioration occur.

↑
less
↑

Abnormal but not known
chronic liver disease – AST less than 2x normal – repeat 2
　　　　　　　　　　　　weeks

↓
more
↓

　　　　　　– AST 2–5x normal – weekly LFT's for
　　　　　　　2 weeks then fortnightly until normal

　　　　　　– AST > 5x normal or bilirubin up –
　　　　　　　stop rifampicin, isoniazid
　　　　　　　pyrazinamide

　　　　　　　(may need alternative treatment until
　　　　　　　LFT's improve
　　　　　　　(depends if infectious form of TB))

See Reference (5) for more detail

in the former because they are more likely be MDR-TB cases and HIV-positive patients acquire infection much more readily, and the latter may remain infectious for many weeks despite treatment.

TB and HIV

- a risk assessment of nosocomial TB transmission should be made for all patient care areas and there should be a TB infection control plan
- suspected or confirmed pulmonary TB cases should be considered as potentially infectious on every admission until proved otherwise, and segregated appropriately from other patients, taking into account their potential infectiousness, any known or suspected drug resistance. and the immune status of other patients on the same ward

Box 6 Drug reintroduction after abnormal LFT's

Measure LFT's daily, plus temperature

Reintroduce under cover of at least 1 drug, usually ethambutol 15mg/kg

Isoniazid 50mg/day for 2–3 days, then 300mg/day for 2–3 days

    if no reaction/LFT's normal

Add rifampicin 75mg/day for 2–3 days, then 300mg/day for 2–3 days
    then 450mg for weight less than 50kg
        or 600mg for weight over 50kg for 2–3 days

    if no reaction/LFT's normal

Add pyrazinamide 250mg/day for 2–3 days, then 1.0gm/day for 2–3 days
    then 1.5gm for weight less than 50kg
        or 2.0gm for weight more than 50kg for 2–3 days

    if no reaction continue standard chemotherapy

    if further reaction – exclude offending drug
                – use suitable alternative regimen
                  (advice from experienced physician needed)

Occasionally may need desensitisation

For more detail Reference (5)

- potentially infectious TB patients should not be seen in the same outpatient clinic as immunocompromised patients (including HIV)
- patients with potentially infectious TB should be isolated from immunocompromised patients by admission to a separate ward or a negative pressure ventilation room
- a nursing system to reduce staff exposure should be employed. If respiratory protection is used a programme with regular audit and education should be in place
- aerosol generating procedures should only be carried out in an

appropriately engineered and ventilated area for all patients on a HIV ward, and for suspected TB in other wards
- TB treatment should be under the management of an appropriately qualified specialist
- TB patients should remain in respiratory isolation until assessed to be non-infectious (see below), or discharged home
- each TB case must be judged on its merits, and the designated TB physician be involved in the decision to end respiratory isolation.

The following criteria that a patient is non-infectious are suggested but it is recognised that exceptions may occur:

Sputum microscopy-positive cases

- the patient has had a minimum of two weeks of appropriate drug therapy AND
- if potentially being moved to accomodation (inpatient or home) with HIV-positive or immunocompromised patients to have a minimum of three negative sputum microscopy smears on separate occassions over at least a 14 day period AND
- demonstrated tolerance to the prescribed treatment and an ability and agreement to adhere to treatment AND EITHER
- a complete resolution of cough OR
- definite clinical improvement to treatment e.g. remaining afebrile for one week

Negative sputum microscopy cases
(three sputums samples on separate days or if no sputum and bacteriology only from bronchoscopy/lavage)

As above except point 2.

Infection control in MDR-TB

- all patients with known or suspected MDR-TB should be admitted to a negative pressure ventilated room. If none are available locally the patient should be transferred to a hospital where the facilities are available
- the same infection control assessments should be made as for HIV/TB
- staff and visitors should wear dust/mist masks meeting HSE (Health and Safety Executive) criteria during patient contact

- the patient should remain in respiratory isolation in a negative pressure room until assessed to be non-infectious. This involves the same criteria as for HIV/TB but may also involve maintaining respiratory isolation until cultures are negative
- the decision to discharge must be discussed with the hospital infection control team, the local microbiologist, and the Consultant in Communicable Disease/Public Health Medicine
- before a discharge from hospital is made, secure arrangements for the supervision and administration of all antituberculosis therapy should have been made, and agreed with the patient and carers
- all treatment as either an inpatient or an outpatient should be fully supervised (DOT) unless there are exceptional circumstances

Treatment regimens[7] (Box 7)

A six-month regimen comprising rifampicin, isoniazid, pyrazinamide and ethambutol for the first two months, followed by rifampicin and isoniazid for a further four months is recommended as standard for all respiratory TB and all forms of non-respiratory TB except CNS disease, for all ages. For CNS disease the continuation phase should be extended to ten months. The fourth drug (ethambutol) can be omitted *only* in patients with a low risk of isoniazid resistance i.e. previously untreated white patients, who are HIV-negative, and who are not a known contact of drug resistant disease. All other patients should be on the four drug combination.

Box 7 Recommended regimens					
	Initial Phase		Continuation Phase		Total
Adults and Children	Drugs	Months	Drugs	Months	Months
Respiratory and non-respiratory	RHZ(E)	2	RH	4	6
Central Nervous system	RHZ(E)	2	RH	10	12
Chemoprophylaxis	H	6			6
	or RH	3			3
for isoniazid resistant organisms	R	6			6

R=Rifampicin H=Isoniazid Z=Pyrazinamide E=Ethambutol

Table 1. Drug dosages

Drug	Daily dosage			Intermittent dosage		
	Children mg/kg	Adults Weight	Adults Dose	Children mg/kg	Adults Weight	Adults Dose
Isoniazid	5	–	300mg	15 3 times weekly	–	15mg/kg 3 times weekly (max 900mg)
Rifampicin	10	<50kg >50kg	450mg 600mg	15 3 times weekly	–	600–900mg 3 times weekly
Pyrazinamide	35	<50kg >50kg	1.5gm 2.0gm	50 3 times weekly 75 2 times weekly	<50kg >50kg <50kg >50kg	2.0gm 2.5gm 3 times weekly 3.0gm 3.5gm 2 times weekly
Ethambutol*	15		15mg/kg	30 3 times weekly 45 2 times weekly		30mg/kg 3 times weekly 45mg/kg 2 times weekly

* Accurate calculation required to reduce the risk of toxicity (reproduced with permission from Thorax)

If pyrazinamide is not prescribed, or not tolerated, the duration of standard treatment should be extended to nine months, and for CNS disease to 18 months, with ethambutol being given for the first two months. In cases where a positive culture of *M. tuberculosis* has been obtained, but susceptibility results are outstanding at two months, treatment including pyrazinamide (and ethambutol) should continue until full susceptibilities is confirmed, even if this is for longer than two months.

Treatment can be given either daily, or intermittently three times weekly (for dosages see Table 1). For daily therapy combination tablets of proven bioavailability should be used. Compliance is the major factor in outcome. Patient compliance should be monitored at least monthly throughout treatment by a TB nurse or Health Visitor using pill counts, prescription checks and urine tests for rifampicin. For patients unlikely to comply with self medication e.g. vagrants, alcoholics and patients who are mentally ill, are best treated with fully supervised regimens (Directly Observed Therapy: DOT). This is easiest using the standard regimen with three times weekly intermittent drug administration, with suitable dosage adjustments (Table 1). If non-compliance is found at any stage during self treatment, this should be switched to fully supervised treatment. Collaboration with treatment should be sought, given directly supervised (DOT) if necessary. Compulsory admission and detention can be sought under Sections 37 and 38 of the Public Health Act (but only for infectious tuberculosis of the respiratory tract), compulsory treatment however is not allowed. Such compulsory admission should be sought only as a matter of last resort. Pyridoxine 10mg/day is not routinely required but should be given to those at higher risk of peripheral neuropathy e.g. diabetics, alcoholics, chronic renal failure, HIV-positive and malnourished. NEVER ADD A SINGLE DRUG TO AN APPARENTLY FAILING REGIMEN: TAKE ADVICE!

Corticosteroids should be given in addition to antituberculosis treatment for pericardial disease, stage II or III meningitis, and for endobronchial disease in children. They may also be indicated in ureteric disease, in pleural effusion, in patients with extensive pulmonary disease and to suppress hypersensitivity reactions to antituberculosis drugs.[7]

Special groups

See Box 8

Box 8   Special groups

Group	Regimen	Comments
Diabetes	Standard	R reduces efficacy of sulphonylureas
Liver Disease	Standard	Monitor LFT's weekly for 2 weeks, then 2 weekly for first 2 months
Pregnancy	Standard	Avoid aminoglycosides, ethion- or prothion-amides: can breast feed normally
Renal disease	RHZ(E)	Reduce dosage of E or S if used: monitor their serum levels
Maintainance Corticosteroids	Standard	Double maintainance steroid dosage R interaction
Unconcious	RHZ(S)	R and H syrup via NG tube or i.v. Z syrup or crushed tablets via NG tube, S i.m. injection
HIV-positive	Standard	4 drug regimen unless MDR-TB suspected (see later).

Drug reactions/interactions

For drug reactions see Table 2 and for drug interactions see Table 3. For detailed advice on management of hepatotoxicity see Boxes 5 and 6 and Reference 5.

Follow up

Should be at least monthly initially and then two-monthly, early follow-up reinforcing patient education. Monitoring of respiratory disease involves serial X-rays including at the end of treatment, and sputum examinations. If progress is unsatisfactory or compliance is in doubt sputum examination should be carried two months before treatment is due to be stopped. Monitoring of extrapulmonary

Table 2. Drug reactions

Drug	Common	Uncommon
Isoniazid	–	Hepatitis Rashes Peripheral neuropathy
Rifampicin	–	Hepatitis Rashes Febrile reactions Thrombocytopenic purpura* 'Flu' syndrome* Shock/renal failure*
Pyrazinamide	Anorexia Nausea Flushing (initial 7–10 days)	Rashes Hepatitis Vomiting Arthralgia
Ethambutol	–	Retrobulbar neuritis

* Much commoner with intermittent as compared with daily therapy
For full list of potential side effects consult appropriate data sheets and reference 7.

disease is largely based on a clinical assessment with X-rays where appropriate.

With the standard recommended therapy and fully susceptible organisms, relapse occurs in 0–3% of cases. If compliance has been good, and there are no residual clinical problems, follow-up is not required but the GP and the patient should be advised to re-refer should symptoms recur. Those with drug resistant organisms (excluding isolated streptomycin resistance), or with continuing clinical problems should be followed up for at least 12 months. Those with MDR-TB, particularly if HIV-positive require long-term follow-up.

Management of drug resistance

Every reasonable effort should be made to obtain positive bacteriological confirmation of the diagnosis, and hence susceptibility testing. The modifications to the standard regimen required for non-MDR-TB resistances are summarised in Table 4.

Table 3. Drug interactions

Anti-TB Drug	Level Increased by	Level Decreased by	Increases Level of	Decreases Level of
Isoniazid	Prednisolone Ethionamide	–	Phenytoin Carbamezepine Warfarin Diazepam	Enflurane Azoles
Pyrazinamide	–	–	Probenecid	–
Ethambutol	–	AlOH	–	–
Rifampicin	–	PAS Ketoconazole	–	Warfarin Other azoles Sulphonylureas Oral contraceptives Glucocorticoids Phenytoin Diazepam Theophyllines Vitamin D Digitoxin Methadone Protease inhibitors Cyclosporin

If rifampicin resistance is shown by a molecular probe; this is 90% likely to be MDR-TB rather than isolated rifampicin resistance, and the patient should be treated as for MDR-TB until the full resistance pattern is known.

Multidrug-resistant TB (MDR-TB) is defined as resistance to rifampicin and isoniazid with or without other drugs. Treatment is complex and demanding for both patient and physician. Treatment should ONLY be carried out by physicians with substantial experience in managing complex resistant cases AND only in hospitals with fully engineered isolation rooms AND in close liason with the PHLS Mycobacteriology service. *The patient should be transferred for treatment unless all the above criteria are met.* The treatment has to be on an individual basis and includes reserve drugs. Close monitoring is required because of likely increased drug toxicity. All such treatment, which cannot be given intermittently, has to be fully

Table 4. Regimens for non-MDR-TB resistances

Resistance	Initial phase	Continuation Phase	
S	RHZ(E) 2	RH 4	(standard regimen unaffected)
H (known pre treatment)	RZES 2	RE 7	(fully supervised)
H (during treatment)	RHZ(E) till results stop H ensure has had RZE 2	then RE 10	
Z (e.g. *M.bovis*)	RHZ(E) till results continue RHE to 2/12 if RHZ only stop Z	RH 7	(if E included initially)
	RHE 2	RH 7	
E	RHZ 2	RH 4	
R*	HZE 2	HE 16	
SH	as for H resistance		but fully supervised
Other combinations	Discuss with PHLS Mycobacterium Reference Unit and highly experienced physician		

* treat as MDR-TB until full resistances/susceptibilities known

Key R = Rifampicin, H = Isoniazid, Z = Pyrazinamide, E = Ethambutol, S = Streptomycin

supervised (DOT) throughout, as both inpatient and outpatient, to prevent the emergence of further resistance. The principles of management of MDR-TB are given in Box 9.

Box 9   General principles for MDR-TB treatment

* Use 5 or more drugs to which the organism is, or is likely to be, susceptible.

* Continue these until culture negative.

* Then continue treatment with at least 3 drugs to which susceptible.

* Continue for a minimum of 9 further months

* Total duration may exceed 24 months depending on in vitro resistance profile, the available drugs, and the patients HIV-status.

* Consideration may have to be given to resection under drug cover.

* Indefinite follow-up after drug treatment has stopped.

Reserve drugs available (7)   Streptomycin, Capreomycin,
                              Amikacin, Kanamycin i.m.
                              Ethionamide/prothionamide
                              Cycloserine
                              Ofloxacin/ciprofloxacin
                              Azithro/clarithromycin
                              Rifabutin
                              Thiacetazone
                              Clofazimine
                              PAS Sodium

Chemoprophylaxis[7]

In tuberculosis *infection*, the tuberculin skin test is positive, the chest X-ray is normal and the patient is asymptomatic. In tuberculosis *disease*, the skin test is usually positive, and there are clinical signs and symptoms or X-ray changes present. Asymptomatic tuberculin positive persons with normal chest X-rays (infection) are usually

Table 5. Chemoprophylaxis

Group	Context	Tuberculin Test	Regimen/Action
Children 0–15yrs	New immigrant from high prevalence country or contact screening	Heaf 2–4 no BCG Heaf 3–4 BCG history	H6 or RH3
Children 0–15 yrs	Schools BCG programme	Heaf 3–4	H6 or RH3
			<u>Give</u> if history of TB contact or residence in high prevalence country in last 2 years. <u>Consider</u> for others
Children 0–2 yrs	Household contact of sputum smear-positive case	Before tuberculin test	H initially
		If initial test result positive as for household contact	as above
		If initial test consistent with BCG history (0–1 no BCG; 0–2 with BCG)	H 6 weeks
		retest at 6 weeks if no change in result if increase in grade	Stop H convert to H6 or RH3

Table 5. Continued

Group	Context	Tuberculin Test	Regimen/Action
Neonates	Mother sputum-smear positive	No initial test	H3
		Retest at 3 months if negative (0–1)	stop
		if positive 2+	convert to H6
Adults	Tuberculin conversion	Conversion with increase of at least 2 Heaf grades	H6 or RH3
MDRTB Contact (any age)	Close contact MDR-TB	Heaf 2–4 no BCG Heaf 3–4	Close clinical monitoring*
HIV-positive	HIV positive individual	May be unreliable	Close clinical monitoring*
		unless contact smear-positive case when H6 or RH3	

* chemoprophylaxis not superior to monitoring

treated (chemoprophylaxis) to kill the small numbers of tubercle bacilli presumed to be in the body, preventing possible progression to disease at a later date. In such situations it is thought that there are very low numbers of viable bacilli and therefore a very small chance of drug resistance, so allowing either single or dual drug therapy to be effective. Recommendations for chemoprophylaxis for various groups/situations are given in Table 5.

Box 10 suggests relevant information for preparing a referral for suspected TB

Box 10   How to prepare a summary referral of suspected TB

Patient details

Age, sex, ethnic group

Risk factors e.g. New immigrant, HIV-positive, recent contact

Clinical reasons for referral
– symptoms
– investigations e.g. Chest X-ray: sputum microscopy
                    other tests – tuberculin test
                                – ultrasound
                                – histology

Referral for a) opinion b) opinion and take over management

References

1. Watson JM, Fern KJ, Porter JDH, Whitmore SE. Notification of tuberculosis in England and Wales 1982–89. *Comm Dis Report* 1991;**1**:R13–16

2. Immunisation against Infectious Disease. *HMSO* 1996;**32**:219–241

3. Joint Tuberculosis Committee of the British Thoracic Society. Control and prevention of tuberculosis in the United Kingdom: Code of Practice. *Thorax* (submitted)

4. Ormerod LP, Watson JM, Pozniak A, Kumar D, McManus T. Notification of tuberculosis: an updated Code of Practice for England and Wales. *J Roy Coll Phys Lond* 1997;**31**:299–303.

5. Ormerod LP, Skinner C, Wales JM. Hepatotoxicity of antituberculosis drugs. *Thorax* 1996;**51**:111–113

6. Interdepartmental Working Group on Tuberculosis. United Kingdom recommendations for the prevention and control of HIV-related tuberculosis and drug resistant, including multiple drug-resistant, tuberculosis. Department of Health 1998 (Sept 1998)

7. Joint Tuberculosis Committee of the British Thoracic Society. Chemotherapy and management of tuberculosis in the United Kingdom: Recommendations 1998. Thorax 1998;**53**:536–548

14

HIV/AIDS

Michael A Beckles, Marc CI Lipman, Margaret A Johnson

Throughout the world HIV infection has become an important cause of death and chronic disease. Respiratory complications occur in up to two-thirds of HIV-infected individuals. *Pneumocystis carinii* pneumonia (PCP) and tuberculosis are the commonest AIDS-defining diagnoses in the developed and developing worlds respectively. Chest physicians will be involved in the routine and emergency care of patients with HIV infection. They will therefore require a working knowledge of this multisystem disease.

This chapter will discuss the general management of HIV disease, and then focus on its respiratory complications in adults.

Background

HIV is a retrovirus, which preferentially enters and replicates within lymphoid cells; the most common of these is the CD4 lymphocyte. There are two strains of HIV, HIV-1 and HIV-2. HIV-1 is the more virulent, and is responsible for the majority of infections. World-wide, in 1998 there were an estimated 30 million adults and children living with HIV/AIDS. The mode of transmission of HIV is outlined in Table 1.

Table 1. Routes of HIV transmission

Sexual Contact	Parenteral Exposure	Vertical Transmission
Unprotected Intercourse:	Injecting drug users	Mother-to-baby:
Homosexual	Blood products	In utero
Heterosexual	Needle-stick injuries	Perinatal
		Breast-feeding

Table 2.   1993 CDC classification system for HIV infection

CD4 T cell categories	Clinical Categories		
	(A) Acute (primary) HIV, asymptomatic or PGL	(B) Symptomatic (not A or C – see explanation)	(C) AIDS Indicator conditions
≥ 500 cells/μl	A1	B1	C1
200–499 cells/μl	A2	B2	C2
< 200 cells/μl	A3	B3	C3

This classification stratifies patients clinically (A to C) and immunologically (1 to 3). Groups A3 and B3 satisfy the immunological but not the clinical criteria for AIDS. Category B consists of symptomatic conditions that are not included in category C but can be either attributed to, or are complicated by, HIV infection. Examples include thrush (oral or persistent vulvovaginal); moderate or severe cervical dysplasia; thrombocytopenia and peripheral neuropathy. PGL = persistent generalised lymphadenopathy.

HIV has profound effects on the immune system. It is thought that a combination of CD4 lymphocyte depletion, changes in cytokine profiles and alterations in the balance of other immune effector cells (such as macrophages) are responsible for the immunosuppression that characterises HIV infection.

Clinical Features of HIV Infection

There are several clinical stages of HIV infection (Table 2).

Prior to the widespread use of effective antiretroviral therapy, the median time from infection with HIV-1 to the development of a major opportunistic infection or tumour (AIDS-defining diagnosis) was 11 years. Current median survival with AIDS is 2–3 years.

HIV infection can involve any organ system. Depending on the level of systemic immunity this can vary from relatively minor skin disease to fatal infections and tumours. Examples of specific conditions are given in Table 3.

Antiretroviral therapy together with specific opportunistic infection prophylactic agents are now improving both the length and quality of life for HIV-infected individuals. However, they can lead to altered patterns of opportunistic disease (eg *Pneumocystis carinii* pneumonia presenting with upper zone rather than hilar and midzone radiographic opacities in patients using nebulised Pentamidine

Table 3.   The systemic manifestations of HIV infection with examples of specific conditions

Organ/System Involved	Manifestations of HIV Infection
Central nervous system and Spinal Cord	Eyes – Cytomegalovirus (CMV) retinitis, toxoplasma chorioretinitis Meningitis- bacterial, tuberculous, and fungal Encephalitis – herpes simplex, CMV Cerebral toxoplasmosis Lymphoma – B cell Non-Hodgkin's lymphoma AIDS dementia complex Depression Peripheral neuropathies (HIV-related, or iatrogenic) Myelopathy
Heart	Cardiomyopathy Pericarditis/Myocarditis Endocarditis Primary pulmonary hypertension
Lung	**See Below**
Gastrointestinal tract	Oral candida Oesophagitis – candida, herpes simplex, CMV Diarrhoea – wasting syndrome (HIV-related), or infectious, eg cryptosporidium, microsporidium, giardia Colitis – CMV, salmonella Lymphoma Kaposi's Sarcoma (KS)
Uro-genital system	HIV-nephropathy Drug-induced acute renal failure Urinary tract infections KS Penile carcinoma Sexually transmitted infections (STIs) Cervical carcinoma

Table 3.   Continued

Organ/System Involved	Manifestations of HIV Infection
Haematological	Lymphopenia (inversion of CD4/CD8 ratio) Pancytopenia Mycobacterium Avium Complex Lymphoma KS
Dermatological	**Infections:** bacterial, viral and fungal. Particularly seborrhoeic dermatitis, molluscum contagiosum, oral hairy leucoplakia **Tumours:** KS, Lymphoma Drug-induced rashes (particularly sulfa-containing drugs).
Endocrine	Panhypopituitarism Adrenal failure Erectile impotence

as prophylactic therapy); and also produce considerable and disabling side effects (eg hyperlipidaemias and lipodystrophy in patients using protease inhibitor anti-retroviral drugs).

HIV Testing

The principles of testing are outlined in Table 4. It should be appreciated that HIV antibody may not be detectable for several months after infection with HIV (the window period). It is important therefore to define the time of last exposure to HIV, as otherwise a negative antibody test may be misinterpreted.

In general the patient's consent must be sought prior to testing, though in certain situations (eg an unconscious patient or occupational exposure), this can be deferred if the diagnosis is felt to have immediate clinical relevance.

Monitoring

Progression of disease is regularly monitored using the following clinical and laboratory features

Table 4.   HIV testing

Reasons for testing:
- **Clinical suspicion:**   The patient may present with one of the illnesses mentioned in Table 3.
- **Patient request:**   The patient may be aware of the risk factors for HIV transmission and request a test.
- **To screen for infection:** Routine on all blood donations (in the UK and US); and in some antenatal clinics.

The test:
Pre-test discussion is necessary. This should cover the potential pros and cons of testing, the treatments available and include some counselling to reduce future HIV risks. Verbal consent is obtained. An HIV antibody test is performed. If there is a positive result confirmatory tests use either immunoperoxidase or Western blot analysis on a second blood sample.

- symptoms and signs
- blood CD4 T lymphocyte count
- plasma HIV(RNA) viral load

A falling or low CD4 count is associated with increasing risk of developing a major opportunistic disease. A high plasma viral load indicates that a patient has a more rapid rate of progression to systemic disease when compared to an individual with an equivalent CD4 count but a lower viral load.

Anti-retroviral Drugs

Several drugs are now used to treat HIV infection. All of them block HIV replication by acting directly on the virus. The current principle is to use combinations of drugs, usually with different mechanisms of action, to reduce HIV viral load, increase blood CD4 count and improve local and systemic immunity. The classes of compounds used in treatment are listed in Table 5. There are a great number of drug interactions with concomitant therapies. Treatment should be managed in conjunction with physicians or pharmacists with specialist knowledge of this field.

There is no clear consensus on when to start therapy though in theory early treatment (when there is less damage to the immune system) would be advantageous. This has to be balanced against the potential short and long-term side effects of taking these drugs.

Table 5.   Anti-retroviral drugs used in the treatment of HIV infection

Nucleoside analogue reverse transcriptase inhibitors	Non-nucleoside analogue reverse transcriptase inhibitors	Protease inhibitors
AZT (zidovudine)	Nevirapine	Saquinavir
ddI (didanosine)	Delavirdine	Ritonavir
ddC (zalcitabine)	Efavirenz	Indinavir
d4T (stavudine)		Nelfinavir
3TC (lamivudine)		Amprenavir
Abacavir		

Antiviral therapies are most effective if drug resistance can be avoided. This is best achieved when the patient adheres rigidly to the prescribing regime. Drug therapies, therefore, should be tailored to the individual patient's needs and lifestyle.

The classification of anti-retroviral drugs is as follows:

- **nucleoside analogue reverse transcriptase inhibitors (NRTI):** These drugs prevent HIV replication by virtue of their structural similarity to the nucleic acid used by the HIV reverse transcriptase enzyme, which transcribes HIV RNA into a DNA copy. HIV is thus unable to integrate with host cell DNA
- **non-nucleoside analogue reverse transcriptase inhibitors:** This is a structurally diverse group, with potent inhibitory activity of the reverse transcriptase enzyme. It has a similar effect to the NRTI's
- **protease inhibitors:** Their mode of action is to inhibit the HIV protease enzyme, which is responsible for producing new infectious particles when HIV leaves the host cell

Pulmonary Complications of HIV Infection

HIV infected individuals with early disease (ie normal or near normal blood CD4 counts) will present with respiratory illnesses that are similar to the general population both in terms of clinical features and underlying aetiology. Thus bacterial pneumonia is the likeliest serious pulmonary infection in patients with CD4 counts above 200 cells/μl. With declining systemic immunity other (opportunistic) diseases become more prevalent. Historically *Pneumocystis carinii* pneumonia (PCP) was the commonest major opportunistic infection, being seen in up to 70% of all AIDS patients. It was also

Table 6.   Features that suggest *Pneumocystis carinii* pneumonia

History of progressive exertional breathlessness

Previous oral thrush, persistent fever of several weeks duration of unknown cause, weight loss > 5kg (or 10%) of unknown cause

Previous PCP

No use of effective PC prophylaxis or poor compliance with therapy

Not currently taking antiretroviral therapy with good compliance

Blood CD4 count < 200 cells/µl

Desaturation of > 4% with exercise (pulse oximetry or blood gases)

the commonest AIDS defining illness (40% of cases). More recently the widespread use of both PCP prophylaxis and also antiretroviral therapy has reduced the incidence of PCP, though it is still seen in subjects not taking effective preventative therapy. PCP should always be considered in the differential diagnosis of HIV related pneumonia. At low blood CD4 counts (< 100 cells/µl) other opportunistic organisms (eg bacteria, protozoa, viruses and fungi) can also cause severe pulmonary disease.

In practice the initial assessment of a patient with a respiratory illness should determine the likelihood that this may be PCP (Table 6). If clinical suspicion is high (ie several of the criteria in Table 6 are satisfied) then specific anti-pneumocystis treatment should be started, and investigations commenced to rule out this diagnosis. If however a patient has a history more compatible with bacterial infection, then it is reasonable to treat with an antibiotic (eg penicillin, macrolide or cephalosporin) and review the diagnosis in the light of the response to therapy and the results of laboratory investigations. It should be remembered that two or more pathogens can be present in up to 20% of cases, leading to apparent partial treatment response, and 'atypical' clinical presentations. The key point, therefore, is that treatment may need to be initiated on an empirical basis, with investigations performed whilst on therapy. Although this may reduce the diagnostic yield for bacterial disease, it will have little effect on that for *Pneumocystis carinii* provided a properly taken sample is obtained within the first two weeks of treatment.

Table 7.   Examples of bacterial organisms responsible for HIV related pneumonia

Organism	Comments
Streptococcus pneumoniae	Common. Associated with increased incidence of bacteraemia in HIV-positive patients. Pneumococcal vaccine recommended for all HIV-positive individuals >2 years old.
Haemophilus influenzae	Need to take into account local antibiotic resistance patterns.
Staphylococcus aureus	Injecting drug users; Falling blood CD4 counts; Nosocomial pneumonias
Klebsiella spp	Falling blood CD4 counts; Nosocomial pneumonias; neutropenic
Moraxella catarrhalis	Nosocomial pneumonias; neutropenic
Pseudomonas spp.	Falling blood CD4 counts; Nosocomial pneumonias; neutropenic
Nocardia spp.	Gram-positive bacillus; apical infiltrates on CXR. Low blood CD4 counts; Seek specialist advice
Rhodococcus equi	Gram-positive bacillus; history of exposure to farm animals, or manure. Low blood CD4 counts; Seek specialist advice

Bacterial pneumonia

These are 3 to 10 times more common in HIV-infected individuals than matched controls. Injecting drug users are particularly susceptible to recurrent bacterial pneumonias. The presentation and radiographic appearance are similar to those found in the non-immunosuppressed population.

The range of causative bacterial organisms expands as systemic immunity (indicated by blood CD4 counts) declines. The commonest pathogen is *Streptococcus pneumoniae* followed by *Haemophilus influenzae*. In more immunosuppressed patients *Staphylococcus aureus* and gram negative infections such as *Pseudomonas* spp also occur (Table 7). It is important to remember that these patients are at risk of non-bacterial pneumonias (eg viruses, protozoa and fungi) which may present also with cough, breathlessness and pulmonary infiltration.

Pneumocystis carinii pneumonia

This opportunistic fungus typically presents with a history of several days to weeks of exertional breathlessness, dry cough and systemic upset. There are often few signs beyond fever, malaise and breathlessness on exercise. Oral thrush may be present, indicating systemic immunosuppression. Auscultation of the chest will reveal at most a few basal crackles.

The chest radiograph typically shows bilateral alveolar midzone and perihilar shadowing. Ten percent of cases will have normal appearances at the time of presentation. More severe pneumonias may produce interstitial shadowing and ultimately confluent areas of consolidation. Other changes associated with pneumocystis are thin walled pneumatoceles, cystic changes, pneumothoraces and upper zone shadowing (the latter occurring in patients using inhaled Pentamidine prophylaxis). Pleural effusions and mediastinal lymphadenopathy are rare in the absence of other respiratory diseases.

Diagnosis

As outlined above a great deal of information can be obtained from the history, CD4 count and chest radiograph. Sputum and blood cultures and arterial oxygen assessment should be performed. This can be by standard arterial blood gas analysis or transcutaneous pulse oximetry.

The advantage of the former is that it provides information on ventilatory status ($PaCO_2$) as well as the alveolar-arterial oxygen gradient, (A-a) DO_2. Alternatively pulse oximetry is less invasive, far better tolerated by the patient and can also be used more easily in an exercise testing protocol (Table 8). If an HIV-infected individual with respiratory symptoms has a fall in oxygen saturation of >4% from a near normal baseline level when exercise tested, then this can be taken as good evidence of an interstitial/alveolar process. In practical terms this should be assumed to be PCP until proven otherwise.

Other non-invasive tests are also employed in the assessment of respiratory disease. These include:

Table 8.   Protocol for pulse oximetry with exercise testing

- Check pulse oximeter is working properly.

- Attach probe to patient ensuring that area of attachment is warm, clean and dry. If subject is wearing nail varnish, remove this or use another site (eg ear probe).

- Ensure that a good pulse wave is present and once machine has stabilised record both oxygen saturations and pulse rate.

- If oxygen saturations are >92% at rest then proceed to exercise testing.

- If oxygen saturations are <92% then discontinue testing.

- If proceeding to exercise testing, ensure that subject is capable of using exercise bicycle and understands what they need to do.

- Start exercise test looking to maintain exercise state (assessed by rise in pulse rate to pre-determined level) for 10 minutes.

- Monitor subject throughout test period.

- Discontinue test either at end of 10 minute period or if there is a sustained fall in oxygen saturations to < 90%.

- If there are concerns about the validity of the test result, consider arterial blood gas analysis (at rest and if necessary on exercise).

- computed tomography (CT) thorax. High resolution CT scanning is probably most helpful when chest radiographs are normal, unchanged or equivocal. It may indicate areas of ground glass attenuation which usually represent active pulmonary disease. This is not specific for a particular pathogen
- lung function testing. Its main use is to exclude PCP. A normal diffusing capacity (D_LCO) is unlikely to be present in a patient whose respiratory symptoms are due to PCP. It should also be noted that a low diffusing capacity is often found in patients with advanced HIV disease and no respiratory infection
- nuclear medicine. Inhaled technetium-99 DTPA clearance studies may reveal the typical biphasic curve of an alveolitis. Again this is not specific for pneumocystis and can also be seen in heavy smokers. However, a normal DTPA scan will exclude active pulmonary disease in subjects with a normal chest radiograph. Gallium-67 citrate scans may help to distinguish infections from tumours such as pulmonary Kaposi's sarcoma. In general,

however, the above tests exclude rather than confirm diagnoses and thus sampling of pulmonary secretions or tissue is required, using either bronchoscopy with bronchoalveolar lavage (BAL) (and sometimes transbronchial biopsies) or sputum induction. The bronchoscopic techniques are described in Chapter 3. It should be noted that sedative drugs can produce life-threatening interactions with antiretroviral agents. Lorazepam is the benzodiazepine of choice for such individuals.

- induced sputum. This technique involves nebulisation of hypertonic saline via a Respirgard Nebuliser. Its diagnostic sensitivity varies from 40–90%, and is dependent upon operator experience. Other potential disadvantages include the risk of transmission of infection (via the aerosol produced from the coughed secretions) and bronchospasm and/or hypoxemia from the procedure. To minimise the risk of infection it should be performed in a negative pressure side room. The BAL or induced sputum sample should be sent for cytological examination (Pneumocystis, viruses, bacteria, mycobacteria and protozoa; as well as abnormal cell populations), viral, bacterial and mycobacterial culture. It should be regarded as infectious, and handled as a biohazard. The diagnostic procedure of choice depends on the particular experience of the centre. One strategy would be to try and induce sputum and if this were non-diagnostic proceed to bronchoscopy and BAL. If no useful information is obtained from this, then consideration should be given to either repeat bronchoscopy and BAL with a transbronchial biopsy, surgical biopsy or empiric treatment for the likeliest organism. Transbronchial biopsy increases the diagnostic yield of bronchoscopy though is associated with a relatively high incidence of pneumothorax and lung haemorrhage. Surgical biopsy is a much bigger undertaking and requires that the patient is fit enough to tolerate the procedure. The disadvantage of empiric pneumocystis therapy is that treatment takes several days to be clinically effective and is not without side-effects. It also requires the patient to be closely monitored as otherwise non-resolution of symptoms may mean either non-response or non-adherence to treatment.

Assessing the severity of PCP

The clinical features that are used to determine severity are listed in Table 9. This is useful as mild disease can be treated as an

Table 9.   Clinical assessment of severity of *Pneumocystis carinii* pneumonia

	Mild	Moderate	Severe
Symptoms and signs	Dyspnoea on exertion	Dyspnoea on minimal exertion	Dyspnoea at rest. +/– cough, fever
Blood gas tensions (kPa) on air	$PaO_2 > 11$	PaO_2 8.1–11	$PaO_2 < 8$
Arterial saturations (SaO_2) at rest	> 94%	90–94%	< 90%
Alveolar – arterial oxygen gradient (kPa)	< 4.7	4.7–6.0	> 6.0
Chest radiograph	Normal, or perihilar shadowing	As mild, or interstitial shadowing	Extensive alveolar shadowing
Treatment mode	Oral	Oral or IV	I.V.

outpatient with oral therapy whilst sicker patients will need a course of intravenous treatment before switching to oral medication when symptoms and signs improve.

Treatment

Agents used in the treatment of PCP are summarised in Table 10. The drug of choice for treatment of PCP is trimethoprim-sulphamethoxazole (TMP-SMX). It acts to inhibit the synthesis of tetrahydrofolic acid in susceptible organisms and is, therefore, a broad spectrum antibiotic.

TMP-SMX is given for a total of twenty one days. The severity of the illness determines whether it is administered intravenously or orally. The commonest adverse effects seen with TMP-SMX are skin rash, nausea and bone marrow toxicity. If these are mild then symptomatic relief is given (eg antihistamines for skin rash) and the treatment course completed. A second line drug (eg Pentamidine or Dapsone Trimethoprim) may be required if the adverse effect is

Table 10. Drug treatment of *Pneumocystis carinii* pneumonia

	Drug	Dose/Route	Comments	Side Effects
First-Line	TMP-SMX	120mg/kg **i.v. or oral** (in divided doses)	Any grade of pneumonia. For severe PCP, add steroids.	Rash; G-I disturbance; Bone marrow toxicity
Second-Line	Pentamidine	4mg/kg/day slow i.v. infusion	Severe PCP; if changing from TMP-SMX, the latter must be continued for at least 48 hours.	Hypotension; hypoglycaemia; pancreatitis; cardiac arrhythmias.
Second-Line	Dapsone-Trimethoprim	Dapsone 100 mg/kg (p.o.) Trimethoprim 20 mg/kg (p.o.)	Mild to moderate PCP. Avoid in G6PD deficiency*. Give 2 hours before ddI.	Bone marrow toxicity; rash; G-I disturbance.
Third-Line	Clindamycin-Primaquine.	Clindamycin 600mg qds. i.v. and then 300–450 mg qds p.o. Primaquine 30 mg/day (p.o.)	Mild to moderate PCP. G6PD.	Maculopapular rash; G-I disturbance; if diarrhoea occurs, send stools for Clostridium difficile toxin.
Third-Line	Trimetrexate + Folinic acid.	Trimetrexate 45 mg/m^2 Folinic acid 20 mg/m^2	Salvage therapy.	Bone marrow toxicity.
Fourth-Line	Atovaquone	750 mg/day p.o.	Mild to moderate PCP.	Absorption increased by fatty food.

* G6PD deficiency = glucose – 6-phosphate dehydrogenase deficiency

more severe or there appears to be no response to TMP-SMX. The response to initial therapy may take up to one week; though if a treatment change is considered therapies should be overlapped for at least 48 hours.

Patients who have evidence of hypoxaemia (ie a $PaO_2 < 9.3$ kPa, alveolar arterial oxygen gradient > 4.7 kPa or oxygen saturations

< 92% at rest on air) should be treated with concurrent corticosteroid therapy. Several regimens have been used though the important point is to start corticosteroids together with specific anti-pneumocystis therapy as soon as possible. A typical protocol would be oral Prednisolone 40mg twice daily for five days then 40mg daily for five days followed by 20mg once a day for a total of twenty one days.

The overall mortality of PCP is now 10%. If a patient requires mechanical ventilation then the outcome is much worse, with survival at best of fifty percent. The decision whether or not to ventilate a patient must be based on the individual's specific circumstances. In general most clinicans would advise that patients who have deteriorated post bronchoscopy, have a first episode of PCP or have presented in respiratory failure should be ventilated. The use of support techniques such as continuous positive airway pressure (CPAP) devices can tide patients over the first few days of treatment when still hypoxic. In many cases this has avoided the need for formal mechanical ventilation.

Prophylaxis

Primary prophylaxis for *Pneumocystis carinii* is indicated in patients with a CD4 count of < 200 cells/μl, or clinical features of progressive immunosuppression at any CD4 count. These include AIDS, recurrent oral thrush, persistent fever or weight loss of > 10% of unknown cause. Secondary prophylaxis (ie after an episode of *Pneumocystis carinii*) is crucial. Details of prophylactic regimes are summarised in Table 11.

Mycobacterial Infection

Tuberculosis (TB)

This is the commonest AIDS-defining diagnosis in Africa. It can occur at any blood CD4 count. With declining systemic immunity extrapulmonary and atypical features are more frequently found. There is an increased incidence in injecting drug users and individuals who come from areas of endemic TB.

Clinical presentation

Respiratory symptoms and systemic upset.

Table 11. **Prophylaxis of *Pneumocystis carinii* pneumonia**

	Drug	Dosage	Side Effects
First Line	TMP-SMX	960 mg/day	Rash, Bone marrow depression, Gastrointestinal disturbance.
Second Line	Dapsone	100 mg/day	Rash, Gastrointestinal disturbance, haemolytic anaemia (G6PD).
Second Line	Dapsone-Trimethoprim.	Dapsone 100 mg/day. Trimethoprim 15 mg/kg/day.	Rash, Gastrointestinal disturbance, haemolytic anaemia (G6PD).
Third Line	Nebulised Pentamidine.	300 mg/month via Respirgard (jet) nebuliser.	Bronchospasm, metallic taste, renal impairment, hypoglycaemia, pancreatitis, risk to staff and other patients.
Fourth Line	Atovaquone.	750 mg bd.	Rash, disturbance of liver function tests.

Chest radiograph

Apical infiltrates, consolidation, hilar lymphadenopathy, pleural effusions.

Diagnosis

Send several sputum samples for microscopy (Ziehl-Nielsen or auramine staining), culture and sensitivity. More immunosuppressed patients have a lower sputum positivity, and bronchoscopy and BAL may need to be performed. It is important to try and obtain a culture-proven diagnosis of tuberculosis as treatment may be prolonged, is often not well- tolerated and the organism may be resistant. Tuberculin skin test reactivity may be unreliable in subjects with advanced HIV disease, and should not be used as a diagnostic tool.

Individuals with suspected TB must be kept in respiratory isolation until shown to be smear negative or non-infectious. All patients with presumed TB must be notified to the appropriate authorities.

Treatment

Quadruple chemotherapy is recommended as first line treatment in HIV-infected individuals. This is given together with Pyridoxine 10mg once daily for the duration of treatment. Further details are given in Chapter 13. The interaction between rifamycins and antiretroviral agents is complex and specialist advice should be sought. In general rifampicin is contraindicated in patients using either protease inhibitors or non-nucleoside reverse transcriptase inhibitors. Rifabutin can be substituted at a reduced dose (150 mg OD) if concurrent therapy is needed, though this can only be used with a small number of antiretroviral agents (eg the protease inhibitor nelfinavir). Thus a sensible strategy may be to treat the tuberculous disease adequately before starting antiretrovirals.

Prophylaxis

Consider this for close contacts of the index case and previously treated subjects at high risk of relapse. The drug of choice is isoniazid (with pyridoxine) for at least 6 months.

Multi-drug resistant tuberculosis

TB which is resistant at least to rifampicin and isoniazid is an increasing problem worldwide. It results in large part from poor compliance with treatment. It requires directly supervised therapy with multiple drugs for a prolonged period of time.

Mycobacterium avium complex

These organisms are a common cause of disease in patients with very low CD4 counts (< 75 cells/μl). Mycobacterium avium complex (MAC) is the commonest pathogen detected.

Clinical presentation

Lone pulmonary disease is relatively rare, and more typically patients will have systemic upset, fevers, weight loss and deranged liver function and haematological indices.

Chest radiograph

This may be normal or show evidence of pulmonary infiltrates, nodules or cavitation.

Diagnosis

This is usually made on culture from a normally sterile site (eg blood or bone marrow). Sputum and bronchial secretion cultures may demonstrate MAC, though it is important to distinguish respiratory colonisation from true clinical disease.

Treatment

Table 12 outlines treatment for Mycobacterium avium complex. This is usually for several years and may need to be life-long. There is a high chance of drug interactions and it is important to seek specialist advice if treatment is contemplated. In vitro sensitivity testing may not accurately predict patient response to treatment.

Prophylaxis

In the UK MAC prophylaxis is not routinely recommended.

Fungal pneumonias

Apart from PCP, pulmonary fungal infections are rare. They are seen in patients with low CD4 counts (ie < 100 cells/µl). The organisms encountered are typically *Candida* spp, *Aspergillus* spp, *Histoplasma capsulatum*, *Cryptococcus neoformans,* and *Coccidioides immitus.*

Clinical presentation

Cough, dyspnoea, haemoptysis and marked systemic upset.

Chest radiograph

Pulmonary infiltrates, mass lesions, occasionally nodules or alveolitis.

Table 12. **Drug treatment of Mycobacterium avium complex**

Drug	Dosage and frequency of administration	Route of administration	Common adverse effects	Monitor
Rifabutin	150–600 mg/day. (150 mg if patient using Indinavir or Nelfinavir protease inhibitor. 300mg if using Clarithromycin or Fluconazole).	P.O.	Uveitis; Arthralgia; turns bodily secretions red/orange; Neutropenia; Induces cytochrome P450.	Visual symptoms; liver function, blood count.
Clarithromycin	500 mg bd/day	P.O. or I.V.	Rash; Gastrointestinal disturbance; Deranged liver function; Possible interactions with cytochrome P450; potentiating the effects of Theophylline, Warfarin, Digoxin, Rifabutin.	
Ethambutol	15 mg/kg/day. Not recommended for children < 5 years old.	P.O.	Optic neuritis; Uricostatic; Gastrointestinal disturbance; Rash.	Visual symptoms

Investigations

BAL, CT or Lung biopsy (seek specialist advice)

Treatment

Intravenous amphotericin (0.5–0.7mg/kg/day) starting at the low dose, and increasing gradually. Renal function must be closely monitored.

Prophylaxis

Depending on the presence of extra-pulmonary fungal infection, antifungal suppressive therapy with either itraconazole, or fluconazole, may be recommended for life as secondary prophylaxis.

Viral pneumonias

These organisms are not common causes of severe HIV-related respiratory disease. They tend to be copathogens or responsible for non-pulmonary disease. Cytomegalovirus is the most frequently isolated respiratory virus. Others such as Herpes simplex, Respiratory Syncytial Virus and adenovirus are much less common. There appears to be no increased incidence of disease due to influenza-like viruses.

Clinical presentation

Symptoms are similar to those of PCP ie breathlessness on exertion, dry cough and fever.

Chest radiograph

May be normal, or show features of an interstitial pneumonitis.

Diagnosis

This relies on detecting the virus in either pulmonary secretions or tissue. For many clinicians the demonstration of invasive viral disease is also one of the diagnostic criteria.

Treatment

If treatment is indicated then antiviral therapy is used at high intravenous doses. In the case of CMV disease, ganciclovir is the drug of choice at a dose of 5mg/kg/twice a day for twenty one days. This drug can cause bone marrow suppression and the blood count should be monitored regularly. Intravenous foscarnet is another option though this drug has associated nephrotoxicity.

Failure to Improve on Therapy

If a patient fails to improve or continues to deteriorate on apparently

Table 13. Causes of treatment failure in HIV pneumonia

Iatrogenic: Fluid overload; narrow-spectrum antibiotic therapy; drug interaction reducing efficacy of antibacterial therapy; neutropenia.

Wrong Diagnosis: either wrong pathogen, or missed copathogen.

Patient factors: Non-compliance; drug hypersensitivity; non-absorbance due to either vomiting or diarrhoea; concomitant illness (renal failure, diabetes mellitus); advanced disease (very low CD4 counts).

optimal therapy then the diagnosis needs to be reconsidered. The timing of this decision depends on the presumed cause of the pneumonia. In general, indicators of a therapeutic response would be expected by the end of the first week. Causes of failure to improve are summarised in Table 13.

Further Investigation

The choice of investigation depends on the clinical condition of the patient and the range of diagnostic tests offered in the institution. Consult with a specialist if you are in doubt as to which investigation to choose.

Bronchoscopy and BAL

If this has not already been performed and the patient's condition allows, then this is the investigation of choice. BAL can identify pneumocysts as well as copathogens. The former persist for several weeks after the start of treatment and the chest radiograph may remain abnormal up to six weeks after completion of therapy. There is no evidence that persistence of pneumocysts is associated with a worse prognosis. If there has been a partial response to PCP therapy and CMV and PCP are both isolated from the BAL, then a trial of Ganciclovir may be indicated.

CT thorax

The enhanced imaging of the lung parenchyma and mediastinum offered by CT scanning may reveal other causes for persistence of symptoms such as abscesses, lymphadenopathy or new infiltration.

Open Lung Biopsy (or transbronchial biopsy)

Patients who are fit enough to undergo general anaesthetic may be considered for an open lung procedure. Transbronchial biopsies may not provide any more information than BAL; though a site-directed technique such as video-assisted thoracoscopy may be the best compromise between obtaining a reasonable specimen and minimising harm to the patient.

Treatment Options

If both iatrogenic and patient factors have been excluded as a cause of failure to improve then it may be necessary to change treatments. Sensitivity testing may be helpful with bacterial pneumonias though currently has no role in the management of PCP. In the latter case second line anti-pneumocystis therapy may need to be instituted (see Table 10). The relevance of any other co-pathogens must be assessed clinically. It should be remembered, however, that most studies indicate PCP and bacterial pneumonias to be the commonest causes of death in patients being treated for HIV-related respiratory disease.

Non-infective Respiratory Manifestations

The incidence of malignancy in the presence of HIV infection is higher than in the general population. The two most important tumours are Kaposi's sarcoma and Non-Hodgkins Lymphoma (NHL). HIV infection does not appear to predispose to an increased incidence of lung cancer. Non infective chronic interstitial pneumonias can mimic opportunistic disease.

Kaposi's sarcoma (KS)

This is the most common non-infectious pulmonary manifestation. The blood CD4 count is often very much higher (ie > 200 cells/µl) than that seen in opportunistic infections.

Clinical presentation

Pulmonary KS is usually associated with cutaneous oral lymph node or visceral disease. The red-purple KS tumours are characteristic. They start as flat lesions that become raised or nodular over time.

The respiratory symptoms may be non-specific and can be difficult to distinguish from those of opportunistic infection. Patients may present with cough, dyspnoea (usually on exertion), and haemoptysis or features of a pleural effusion. In addition there may be 'B' symptoms, such as unexplained fever, weight loss, and night sweats. On examination of the chest, there may be signs of parenchymal or pleural involvement; sometimes chest examination is normal, and the only positive finding is KS at other sites.

Chest radiograph

This may reveal parenchymal infiltrates, nodules, and mediastinal lymphadenopathy. There may also be pleural involvement (effusions or plaques). It is possible to have pleural disease without parenchymal involvement.

Diagnosis

CT thorax, bronchoscopy, and open lung biopsy may confirm the diagnosis. The characteristic CT features (described above) in the presence of visceral KS may be sufficient. Alternatively, identification of the lesions endobronchially (seen in 50% of subjects with pulmonary KS) may be required. Direct biopsy of these lesions or transbronchial biopsy is not recommended as there is a high risk of haemorrhage.

Treatment

Treatment is reserved for those with disseminated disease, and is currently palliative. Several chemotherapeutic regimens have been employed, but the favoured regimen uses single agent liposomal doxorubicin. Care must be exercised with this preparation, as it causes cardiomyopathy.

Lymphoma

Clinical presentation

HIV-related NHL tends to present extra-nodally. The lung is not often involved; more common sites include the central nervous system, liver, bone marrow, and gastrointestinal tract. Pulmonary systems are often non-specific, with 'B' symptoms predominating.

Chest radiograph

May show multiple nodular lesions and diffuse interstitial infiltrates. There may also be large pleural effusions. Hilar lymphadenopathy is uncommon

Diagnosis

Open biopsy is often required to confirm pulmonary involvement.

Treatment

Combination chemotherapy is the preferred mode of therapy. The prognosis for this highly aggressive tumour is poor (weeks to months) though some patients have prolonged disease-free survival. Concurrent therapy should be given for any opportunistic infections identified and PCP prophylaxis continued during chemotherapy.

Chronic interstitial pneumonias

The presentation of both lymphocytic interstitial pneumonitis (LIP) and non-specific interstitial pneumonitis (NSIP) can resemble opportunistic infections. The pathogenesis of these conditions is unclear though they probably reflect chronic immune activation secondary to either HIV or a co-pathogen. Although severe disease in adults is relatively uncommon it is likely that with improving anti-retroviral therapies LIP and NSIP will be seen more frequently.

Clinical presentation

Patients complain of cough, shortness of breath on exercise and fevers. LIP may also have associated systemic features such as weight loss.

Chest radiograph

Bilateral reticular nodular or interstitial shadowing is present.

Diagnosis

This is usually made on tissue biopsy (the categorisation as either LIP or NSIP reflecting the degree of cellular infiltration and fibrosis).

Treatment

Corticosteroid therapy is effective in up to 50% of cases. If therapy is contemplated it is important, therefore, to ensure that an opportunistic infection has not been missed.

References

Feinberg MB. Changing the natural history of HIV disease. *Lancet* 1996;**348**:239–246

BHIVA Writing Committee on behalf of the BHIVA Executive Committee. British HIV Association (BHIVA) Guidelines for the treatment of HIV-infected adults with antiretroviral therapy. *HIV Med* 2000;**1**:76–101

Joint Tuberculosis Committee of the British Thoracic Society. Chemotherapy and management of tuberculosis in the United Kingdom. *Thorax* 1998;**53**:536–48

Lipman MCI, Gluck TA, Johnson MA. An atlas of differential diagnosis in HIV disease. Parthenon Publishing 1995

Mellors JW, Kingsley LA, Rinaldo CR, et al. Quantitation of HIV-1 RNA in plasma predicts outcome after seroconversion. *Annals of Internal Medicine* 1995;**122**:573–579

Phair J, Munoz A, Detels R, et al. The risk of Pneumocystis carinii pneumonia among men infected with human immunodeficiency virus type 1. *New England Journal of Medicine* 1990;**322**:161–165

USPHS/Infectious Disease Society of America. Guidelines for the prevention of opportunistic infections in persons infected with human immunodeficiency virus. *MMRWR* 1997;**46**(RR-12):12–13

Wallace JM, Rao AV, Glassroth J, et al. Respiratory illness in persons with human immunodeficiency virus infection. *Am Rev Respir Dis* 1993;**148**:1523–1529

Zumla A, Johnson MA, Miller RF. AIDS and Respiratory Medicine. Chapman & Hall 1997

15

Cystic Fibrosis and Bronchiectasis

Diana Bilton

Cystic Fibrosis

Cystic fibrosis (CF) is the most common life threatening genetic disorder in Caucasian people. The estimated frequency of occurrence is one in every 2500 live births in the UK. The mode of inheritance is autosomal recessive and the carrier frequency in Caucasian populations is about 1 in 25.

The CF gene sits on the long arm of chromosome 7 and encodes for a protein called the Cystic Fibrosis Transmembrane Conductance Regulator (CFTR). This protein acts as a chloride channel as well as servicing regulatory functions over membrane chloride channels. Thus CF is a disorder characterised by abnormalities of sodium chloride concentrations in secretory epithelia throughout the body. Figure 1 summarises the pathophysiology of CF as a multisystem disorder.

The presentation of CF is usually in early childhood with clinical features of cough, loose stools and failure to thrive. Other presentations in childhood include meconium ileus, prolonged neonatal jaundice and rectal prolapse. In certain regions a neonatal screening policy exists so that the diagnosis can be made at 6–9 weeks. See Table 1 for diagnostic tests.

In adults symptoms and morbidity relate largely to CF related chest disease but it is important to consider the multisystem nature of the disorder. Table 2 summarises the wide spectrum of clinical features and complications, which can occur in CF adults.

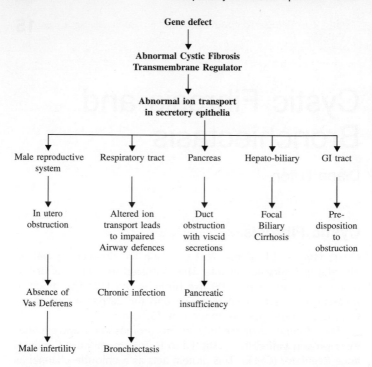

Figure 1.   The pathophysiology of CF as a multisystem disorder

Table 1.   Diagnostic tests for cystic fibrosis

Tests	Technique	Results
Immunoreactive Trypsinogen for neonatal screening	Heel prick Blood specimen	Values raised 2–5 fold in CF neonates
Sweat test	Sweat sodium and chloride concentration of pilocarpine stimulated sweat	Chloride >60–70 mmol/litre Sodium >70 mmol/litre in CF
Nasal potential difference	Measurement of baseline voltage and charge in response to challenge of low chloride solution and isoprenaline	Normal −15 mV to −30 mV CF −35 mV to −60 mV CF no response to low chloride or isoprenaline

Table 2.   Clinical features and complications of cystic fibrosis in adults

Respiratory Tract
> Nasal polyps
> Recurrent sinusitis
> Bronchiectasis
> Haemoptysis
> Allergic bronchopulmonary aspergillosis
> Recurrent pneumothorax

GI Tract
> Distal Intestinal Obstruction Syndrome
> Pancreatic insufficiency
> Malnutrition

Hepatobiliary Disease
> Portal hypertension
> Cirrhosis
> Gallstones

Reproductive Organs
> Male infertility

Metabolic Disorder
> Insulin requiring diabetes – related to pancreatic failure
> Osteoporosis
> Vitamin deficiency
> Salt depletion in hot climates
> Delayed puberty

Musculo-skeletal
> Digital clubbing
> Skin vasculitis
> CF associated arthritis

Simple monitoring in CF adults

At each outpatient attendance spirometry must be recorded. In adult CF patients the FEV_1 declines during a pulmonary exacerbation and should be restored to pre-exacerbation levels with treatment. FEV_1 also guides maintenance therapy against chronic infection in the airways. Damage can occur gradually and if serial recordings are measured, continued decline should trigger a reassessment of

Table 3.   Approaches to management

Sputum clearance	Physiotherapy
	Nebulised rhDNase
Anti-infective	Prophylactic oral anti-staphylococcal agents
	Prophylactic nebulised antibiotics
	IV therapy for exacerbations
Airway therapy	Bronchodilators if reversibility demonstrated
Anti-inflammatory	Steroids
	Ibuprofen

maintenance therapy. In addition, the overall trend of change in FEV_1 over several years allows predictions to be made regarding prognosis.

Weight and body mass indexes are sensitive markers of patient well-being. Weight loss should trigger a check on blood glucose levels, pancreatic supplementation requirements and a dietetic review of intake of calories. If there has been no change in these nutritional factors it is likely that the weight loss relates to an increasing level of lung inflammation and infection and again should lead to further aggressive management of lung disease.

Sputum cultures

Sputum samples must be obtained at regular intervals to assess colonising organisms. In children *Staphylococcus aureus* and *Haemophilus influenzae* predominate. In adults *Pseudomonas aeruginosa* is the pathogen in 80% of patients.

Principles of management

The goal of management is to maintain lung function and quality of life. To young adults with CF, quality of life is paramount and regular treatments need to be negotiated and explained to ensure compliance in the long term. Table 3 summarises the approaches to the management of pulmonary disease in CF. It is crucial that patients carry out daily physiotherapy and that their technique is regularly assessed by the physiotherapist.

Patients need to be regularly assessed and the package of

maintenance therapy reviewed. The use of recombinant DNase to liquefy sputum, has been shown to improve lung function, but the response varies and patients require careful assessment before this is prescribed long term. In similar fashion to asthma guidelines it is always important to assess compliance with basic therapies before adding in anything new.

Treatment of *Pseudomonas aeruginosa*

There is now clear evidence that early aggressive management of the first pseudomonas isolate delays chronic colonisation. This treatment should consist of a combination of oral ciprofloxacin and nebulised Colomycin for at least six weeks. If compliance is an issue or the patient is unwell a two week course of intravenous anti-pseudomonal antibiotics can be given.

Once a patient is colonised with *Pseudomonas aeruginosa* then chronic suppressive therapy is recommended with twice daily nebulised anti-pseudomonal antibiotic. In the UK this is usually colistin (Colomycin) 2 MU twice daily.

There is continued debate regarding the use of intravenous antibiotics. Some centres adopt a policy of prophylactic use of a two-week course of IV anti-pseudomonal antibiotics every three months whereas other centres tend to treat with IV antibiotics on the basis of clinical need. The latter approach in many centres in the UK does in effect mean patients receive IV courses about three times a year because that is the frequency of pulmonary exacerbations requiring IV therapy.

Table 4. Pulmonary exacerbations

Signs and symptoms
Increased cough
Increased sputum production
Change in sputum colour
Fever
Weight loss
New chest signs
Decreased exercise tolerance
Decreased FEV_1
New findings on chest radiograph

Patients are taught early on to recognise the symptoms of an exacerbation and to seek medical advice. Pulmonary function and weight should be measured before starting treatment and a sputum culture obtained. Sputum culture should not delay treatment but is noted after commencement of therapy. The sensitivity of *Pseudomonas aeruginosa* to different antibiotics is reviewed but is not well correlated to clinical response, i.e. patients often get better on an antibiotic to which the pseudomonas is reported as resistant on laboratory testing.

Treatment of a mild exacerbation can be with oral antibiotics. When an exacerbation is more severe intravenous antibiotics are administered. CF patients require high doses of antibiotics for a sufficient period to achieve a clinical response. A two week course is standard but a longer course is required for some patients with more severe disease.

Intravenous antibiotic therapy for *Pseudomonas aeruginosa* should consist of two antibiotics, usually a combination of an aminoglycoside and a β-lactam antibiotic. A standard regimen being ceftazidime 3 g three times daily and tobramycin 10 mg/kg per day in three divided doses (adjusted according to levels). Adoption of aggressive management principles has led to greatly improved survival for patients with this disease. The average age of death is now 29 years. If the trend continues patients born with CF in the 1990s can expect a median survival of over 40 years. In the year 2000 half of the CF patients in the UK will be 'adults'.

These patients are best managed by a multidisciplinary team well trained in cystic fibrosis in centres with facilities designed to cope with these young people.

Management of other organisms

Staphylococcus aureus

Many patients graduate to adult centres on regular flucloxacillin as prophylaxis against *Staph aureus*. There are no good trials to inform us of the best approach in the adult. If *Staph aureus* is absent from sputum samples it seems reasonable to discontinue maintenance flucloxacillin and reinstate if this organism re-occurs.

Burkholderia cepacia

B.cepacia is the organism named after its ability to cause rot in onions. It can colonise previously well CF patients and cause rapid

Table 5.   Team for managing adult CF patients

Consultant Chest Physician
Clinic Nurse Specialist
Specialist Physiotherapist
Dietician
Social Worker
Microbiologist
Psychologist

Other specialists required with knowledge of CF

Diabetologist
Gastroenterologist
Anaesthetist
ENT Surgeon
Obstetrician
Thoracic Surgeon
Rheumatologist
Geneticist

decline and the so called 'cepacia syndrome' characterised by fevers, rapid loss of lung function and rapidly advancing pulmonary shadowing. The outcome of cepacia syndrome is respiratory failure and death. Cepacia syndrome is by no means universal and some patients remain well with little change in lung function following colonisation. *B. cepacia* is transmissible patient to patient. As a result a strict segregation policy has been adopted in CF clinics. A patient colonised by *B. cepacia* must be segregated from other CF patients. For IV treatment a combination of β-lactam and amino-glycosides is recommended. This organism acquires resistance to ceftazidime rapidly and other agents have to be employed. Nebulised colistin has no place in *B.cepacia* patients because of uniform resistance. Oral agents that may be useful for treatment between IV's are minocycline and rifampicin.

Stenotrophomonas maltophilia

With increasing use of broad spectrum antibiotics *Stenotrophomonas maltophilia* has emerged as a colonising organism in CF. It has been associated with increased use of imipenem as it is imipenem resistant. It does not seem to have the devastating effects of *B. cepacia* although some patients are less well and require specific treatment. Septrin can be a useful agent against this particular organism.

Viral Infections

Viral infections are often associated with worsening clinical status and exacerbation of chest disease. Influenza infection can have a catastrophic effect and it is imperative that CF patients receive the flu vaccine each year.

Bronchiectasis

Introduction

Bronchiectasis is the descriptive term given to the condition of chronic dilatation of one or more bronchi. The dilated airway exhibits poor mucus clearance and there is a predisposition to recurrent or chronic bacterial infection.

It is a common misconception that bronchiectasis is no longer a significant problem and has declined in incidence with the advent of improved socio-economic conditions, use of vaccines in childhood and antimicrobial therapy. It is true that the incidence of saccular bronchiectasis, characterised by generalised dilatation associated with severe loss of bronchial wall structure, usually occurring after a severe childhood infection has declined.

More recently with the advent of CT scanning more patients are being recognised with cyclindrical bronchiectasis. The true prevalence of bronchiectasis in the UK remains unknown. Without a high index of suspicion and high resolution CT scan, patients with bronchiectasis are misdiagnosed as asthmatic or bronchitic. In addition published figures have previously been estimated on plain chest radiographs which are insensitive in detecting bronchiectasis.

Clinical features

Bronchiectasis should be suspected when patients present with a history of recurrent chest infections or persistent purulent sputum production particularly in the absence of a history of tobacco smoking. A history of chest pain or haemoptysis complicating exacerbations may also be present. Patients with bronchiectasis may also have true asthma or have wheeze associated with increased sputum production during an infective exacerbation.

In about a third of patients bronchiectasis is associated with upper respiratory tract sepsis ie: chronic purulent sinusitis.

In the pre-antibiotic era, saccular bronchiectasis produced florid clinical signs with patients having gross finger clubbing, malodorous breath, cachectic appearance and coarse crackles. Often today the clinical picture is one of few crackles and absent finger clubbing and a normal chest radiograph. The provisional diagnosis will be made on the basis of a high index of suspicion from the history and then confirmed by a high resolution CT scan.

Investigations

A normal CXR does not exclude bronchiectasis. Studies have shown the plain chest radiograph to detect less than 50% of patients with proven bronchiectasis. High resolution CT has replaced bronchography as the gold standard method of imaging. The sensitivity of CT scanning is dependent on the thinness of sections obtained. High resolution CT scanning is recommended and scans may also be performed in expiration to identify increased transradiency in areas where small airways disease may be present.

It is then extremely important to go beyond the label bronchiectasis and to attempt to define a cause. Bronchiectasis is the end result of a number of pathological pathways and specific causes can be diagnosed in about 40% of cases. The label post infective bronchiectasis can be assigned to patients in whom chronic symptoms follow a severe lower respiratory tract infection with bronchiectasis confined to the affected area. There is debate about the significance of a history of childhood respiratory infection in adult patients who are then symptom free for three or four decades before presenting with recurrent infections and CT evidence of widespread bronchiectasis. In our specialist clinic such patients would not be labelled as post infective.

Underlying causes of bronchiectasis are listed in Table 6 and investigations should be targeted at excluding these underlying causes. The presence of normal total immunoglobulins does not exclude a selective immune deficiency or a specific antibody deficiency and subclass analysis and vaccine responses are useful in classifying patients and identifying those who may benefit from a trial of immunoglobulin therapy.

Table 6.   Causes of bronchiectasis

Type of cause	Important examples
Congenital	Deficiency of bronchial wall, Pulmonary sequestration
Immune deficiency	<u>Primary</u> Panhypogammaglobulinaemia Selective immunoglobulin deficiency <u>Secondary</u> HIV infection, Malignancy (CLL)
Excessive immune response	Allergic bronchopulmonary aspergillosis
Mucociliary clearance defects	Primary ciliary dyskinaesia Cystic fibrosis Young's syndrome
Toxic insult	Aspiration of gastric contents. Inhalation of toxic gases/chemicals
Mechanical obstruction	Intrinsic tumour, foreign body Extrinsic lymph node
Post infective	Whooping cough Tuberculosis

Cystic fibrosis and bronchiectasis overlap

The diagnosis of cystic fibrosis should be considered in any patients with unexplained bronchiectasis, but particularly in the presence of upper lobe bronchiectasis, colonisation with *Staphylococcus aureus* and *Pseudomonas aeruginosa* or male infertility. A normal sweat test no longer excludes a diagnosis of cystic fibrosis as mutations are reported which produce mild disease and a normal sweat test.

If doubt exists a patient can be referred for review at a cystic fibrosis Specialist Centre. Confirming or refuting a cystic fibrosis diagnosis has important implications for family members and offspring.

NB. In a patient where cystic fibrosis is suspected the finding of carriage of a common mutation ie ΔF508 on routine testing should lead to a detailed testing for rare mutations rather than

Table 7. Conditions associated with bronchiectasis

Chronic rhinosinusitis
Rheumatoid arthritis
Ulcerative colitis
Crohn's disease
Coeliac disease
Yellow nail syndrome
Connective tissue disorders

simply assuming the patient is a carrier. There are still a few occasions however when the diagnosis remains in doubt.

Table 8 defines the investigations performed both to delineate the underlying cause as well as to assess the patients current clinical problems. Investigations are obviously tailored appropriately given the history and investigation of each individual.

Management

Management of bronchiectasis can be thought of under five principle headings:

Principles of Management of Bronchiectasis

- Medical treatment of specific conditions
- Mucus clearance   – Physiotherapy
- Antimicrobial chemotherapy – Acute exacerbations
                                             – Chronic suppressive therapy
- Supportive treatment
- Surgical   – Localised resection
                                             – Transplantation

Medical treatment of specific conditions

Identifying patients with panhypogammaglobulinaemia or selective immunoglobulin deficiencies is important as regular intravenous gammaglobulin replacement therapy will dramatically alter the patients clinical course and disease progression. The treatment of acid reflux and aspiration will prevent ongoing acid induced damage to the bronchial tree. Treatment of ABPA with oral steroids may reduce symptoms and prevent further exacerbations.

Table 8.   Investigations of bronchiectasis

Part 1 – To assess underlying cause

CT scan	establishes diagnosis but is not specific for underlying cause. may suggest need for bronchoscopy
Bronchoscopy	if suspicion of bronchial obstruction, tumour or foreign body
Assessment of nasal mucociliary clearance	saccharin test
Nasal brushing/biopsy ± nasal nitric oxide	establish ciliary beat frequency (requires specialist centre)
Measurement seminal analysis	if male infertility present to exclude CF
CF genetics & sweat test	to exclude CF
Immunoglobulins & IgG subclasses vaccine responses to Pneumovax, tetanus & flu	to identify immunodeficiiency ie panhypogammaglobulinaemia subclass deficiency or specific antibody deficiency
Barium swallow ± oesophageal physiology studies	if history suggests aspiration
Measure alpha 1 antitrypsin	to identify alpha 1 antitrypsin deficiency
Autoantibody screen	to identify associated connective tissue disorders or vasculitis

Part 2 – To assess current clinical state

Sputum	standard culture to assess colonisation culture for acid fast bacilli culture for aspergillus
Skin tests	including aspergillus
Lung function test	with assessment of reversibility to β_2 agonists and anticholinergic agents
Blood	differential white count, ESR and CRP, IgE and specific RAST to aspergillus

Mucus clearance

Patients should receive education from a physiotherapist with regard to the best technique of airway clearance for them. Postural drainage can be adjusted according to the affected areas but in general patients should be able to perform the active cycle of breathing techniques combining breathing control, thoracic expansion exercises and the forced expiration technique. Exercise improves mucus clearance and should be encouraged. Physiotherapists should assess patients and recommend appropriate exercise regimens. Assessment of reversible airflow obstruction in the pulmonary function laboratory will allow rational prescription of bronchodilator therapy. It is sensible to advise patients to take their bronchodilator therapy before physiotherapy.

Antimicrobial chemotherapy

The outcome of antibiotic therapy is variable depending on the severity of the bronchiectasis and the colonising organism. In mild bronchiectasis, a single course of the appropriate antibiotic may render the patient well with only small amounts of mucoid sputum. The patient may remain well until a viral infection predisposes to another infective exacerbation. In this situation the patient requires antibiotics only for infective exacerbations associated with muco purulent or purulent sputum, and should be allowed to keep a course of the required antibiotic at home to start as soon as symptoms dictate.

In more severe cases patients may have persistent mucopurulent or purulent sputum production. Every attempt should be made to reduce the sputum volume and shift the sputum towards mucoid appearance. This should be attempted with antibiotics targeted to the organisms and if high dose oral therapy fails then the patient should be admitted for intravenous therapy. In these patients, when 'remission' is achieved if early relapse occurs then chronic 'suppressive' antibiotic therapy orally or via inhalation improves well-being and decreases morbidity.

The choice of antibiotic will be influenced by the colonising organism. The common organisms are non-typeable *Haemophilus influenzae* and *Moraxella catarrhalis*, although in specialist centres there is a higher incidence of *Pseudomonas aeruginosa*. Figure 2 gives a broad guide to the approach to therapy.

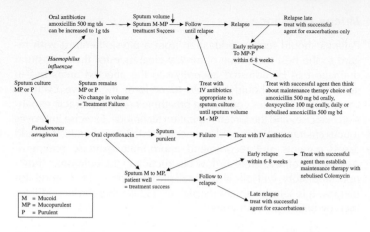

Figure 2.   Guide to therapy for patients with bronchiectasis

Patients often accept a chronic degree of fatigue associated with chronic production of infected sputum and do not expect to get antibiotics until they are very unwell. They are often surprised at how well it is possible to be.

Patients with bronchiectasis require higher doses of antibiotics for longer periods than usually prescribed in COPD. Patients are instructed to take antibiotics until the sputum has cleared and for several days afterwards. This often results in a 14 day course. Each patient may then be given an individual plan regarding mainte- nance therapy and what to do during an exacerbation. Optimum management requires the patient to understand how to manage an exacerbation with early antibiotic therapy. This is best achieved by allowing a patient to have some antibiotics available at home. To make this approach work in practical terms the primary care doctor should be fully informed of the home management plan and his or her agreement obtained. This approach of targeted therapy in suf- ficient dose for the requisite length of time usually leads to less primary care consultations and less courses of antibiotics.

Supportive treatment

Annual influenza vaccination is recommended in these patients. It is important to identify the asthmatic component of the disease in some patients and this should be treated appropriately with inhaled steroids. Recombinant DNase which has been used in cystic fibrosis has not been shown to have any benefit in bronchiectasis.

Surgical treatment

Surgical treatment provides the only curative treatment for bronchiectasis. Surgery is much less commonly used because of the lower incidence of single lobe post infectious bronchiectasis. It is essential that prior to surgical referral it is established that the bronchiectasis is truly confined to a single lobe and that underlying causes which predispose to generalised bronchiectasis are excluded.

Palliative resection can be considered if an area of severe bronchiectasis acts as a sump for infection despite best medical management. In addition if bronchial artery embolisation has failed to prevent recurrent severe haemoptysis then surgery should be recommended. In the context of deteriorating lung function and quality of life despite optimal medical treatment referral for lung transplantation (double lung or heart/lung) should be considered.

Further Reading

Yankaskas JR, Knowles MR, eds. Cystic Fibrosis in Adults. Lippincott: Williams and Wilkins 1999

Hudson ME, Geddes DM, eds. Cystic Fibrosis. Lippincott: Williams and Wilkins 1994

Hill CM. Practical Guidelines for Cystic Fibrosis Care. Churchill Livingstone

16

Diffuse Parenchymal Lung Disease

Athol U Wells

Introduction

Diffuse parenchymal lung disease (DPLD) constitutes an important component of respiratory practice. Whilst these disorders are encountered less frequently than asthma, chronic airflow obstruction and lung cancer, they engender a good deal of diagnostic and therapeutic uncertainty, and their clinical impact is often underestimated. *Optimal management depends primarily on diagnosis*, both in the confident identification of interstitial lung disease (as opposed to infection, pulmonary oedema, diffuse malignancy or alveolar haemorrhage) and in the accurate categorisation of a histospecific diagnosis; a secure diagnosis is a *sine qua non* for prognostic precision and serves as an essential guide to treatment. The therapeutic approach is often critically dependent upon the likelihood of a response to therapy; thus the assessment of 'disease activity' (reversible inflammatory disease) is an integral part of investigation. Precision is also important in the initial staging of disease severity and the monitoring of serial change, both of which have an impact on therapeutic planning. For the most part, general physicians have little experience of interstitial lung disease and lean heavily on respiratory advice, both in the outpatient clinic and for in-patient management. The common clinical presentations can be subdivided into:

- unexplained diffuse interstitial shadowing on chest radiography, with or without associated respiratory symptoms

- disorders known to be complicated by DPLD (usually connective tissue diseases), in which the physician is asked for an opinion on the presence and severity of interstitial disease and the need for treatment
- rapidly progressive DPLD resulting in severe dyspnoea or respiratory failure, requiring urgent in-patient evaluation
- the patient with a secure histospecific diagnosis, in whom a sudden deterioration results in major uncertainties as to the need for investigation or changes in therapy

The greatest barrier to a logical approach to DPLD is the very large number of individual disorders (currently well in excess of 200). The problem has been compounded by opaque terminology which differs between countries, the most notorious being 'cryptogenic fibrosing alveolitis' (CFA)/'idiopathic pulmonary fibrosis' and 'extrinsic allergic alveolitis' (EAA)/'hypersensitivity pneumonitis'. If diagnostic insecurity is to be confronted with the necessary decisiveness, a simple approach to classification is required.

The Classification of DPLD: An Approach to Diagnosis

Does the disease fit a common category?

It is often useful to reach broad diagnostic conclusions before attempting histospecific precision. It is traditional to subdivide interstitial lung disease into the categories encountered most commonly in clinical practice, listed in Table 1. This approach has the major advantage of simplification — most DPLD fall into one of ten groups and the routine use of the classification as a 'check-list' helps to organise thought and prevent major oversights.

Natural history and likelihood of reversibility

An alternative approach is to move directly to conclusions based on perceived natural history (symptom evolution, serial change on chest radiography) and the likelihood of reversible inflammatory disease (previous responsiveness to therapy, a fluctuating course, changes indicative of inflammation on CT). In DPLD such as CFA and EAA, the diagnostic application of clinical criteria defined at a single point in time is a major limitation. The evaluation of *disease behaviour* is integral to diagnosis and often allows the development of a logical therapeutic plan, even when no histospecific diagnosis

Table 1.   Categories of DPLD with diseases encountered most frequently in routine practice in the right hand column

Category of DPLD	Commonly encountered sub-groups
Fibrosing alveolitis (Pulmonary fibrosis)	Cryptogenic fibrosing alveolitis FA in connective tissue disease
Extrinsic allergic alveolitis (Hypersensitivity pneumonitis)	Farmer's lung Bird fancier's lung
Pulmonary sarcoidosis	
Eosinophilic disorders	Eosinophilic pneumonia Churg-Strauss syndrome, other vasculitides Allergic bronchopulmonary aspergillosis
Pneumoconiosis	Asbestosis Silicosis Berylliosis
Cystic lung disease	Langerhans cell histiocytosis Lymphangioleiomyomatosis
Malignant disease	Lymphangitis carcinomatosa
Diffuse alveolar haemorrhage	Systemic vasculitides Idiopathic pulmonary haemosiderosis
Iatrogenic lung disease	Amiodarone lung Nitrofurantoin lung Radiation pneumonitis
Other DPLD	Pulmonary alveolar proteinosis Diffuse bronchiolar disorders

can be achieved. Thus, it is useful to group DPLD into the following scenarios:

- **self-limited inflammatory disease**, including many patients with sarcoidosis, extrinsic allergic alveolitis, and steroid-responsive drug-induced pulmonary disease. Accurate diagnosis and the avoidance of precipitants are the keys to management. Treatment may not be required and seldom needs to be prolonged
- **non-progressive lung fibrosis** that is not extensive or functionally severe, including patients with sarcoidosis, limited chronic EAA, limited fibrosing alveolitis (especially in collagen vascular

disease), pneumoconiosis, and drug-induced pulmonary disease. The documentation of 'benign' behaviour is central to management and may obviate therapy

- **prominent inflammation, with or without fibrosis**. The prognosis may be critically dependent on precision in diagnosis and management. This difficult category includes patients with inflammatory CFA, COP, eosinophilic pneumonitis and a subset of those with sarcoidosis, EAA and drug induced lung disease. Prolonged treatment is often required
- **moderate to rapidly progressive fibrotic disease** with a poor prognosis, as in typical CFA and a subset of patients with chronic EAA and sarcoidosis. Treatment is directed towards preventing or slowing the progression of lung fibrosis. Prognostic precision and accuracy in monitoring changes in disease severity are integral
- **extremely aggressive interstitial processes**, which are rapidly or immediately fatal without prompt intervention, but may sometimes respond well to therapy. These include DPLD (e.g. acute interstitial pneumonitis, a subset of patients with CFA, severe COP), but also disorders simulating DPLD (opportunistic infection, diffuse alveolar haemorrhage syndromes, pulmonary oedema)
- **progressive, non-fibrotic DPLD** for which there is no effective drug treatment. This includes rapidly progressive disease (lymphangitis carcinomatosis) and slowly progressive cystic disease (Langerhans cell histiocytosis (LH), lymphangioleiomyomatosis (LAM)), in which lung transplantation merits careful consideration. Precision in diagnosis and monitoring disease progression are essential
- **unclassifiable DPLD** (i.e. that does not fall clearly into the above categories) and may require prolonged follow-up before declaring itself. These cases present great difficulties, even to experienced respiratory physicians; in the absence of diagnostic and prognostic security, the correct management depends upon constant re-evaluation of changes in disease severity. Tertiary assessment of these complex cases is often fruitful.

History

Useful historical details can be sub-divided into etiological information, the definition of natural history and the symptomatic definition of disease severity.

Aetiological information

Aetiological information is summarised in Table 2.

The definition of natural history

Whenever possible, an attempt should be made to define *disease behaviour* from symptoms and previous chest X-rays. For example a three month history of inexorably increasing dyspnoea is compatible with lymphangitis carcinomatosis, whereas this disorder is highly unlikely in a patient with mild non-progressive dyspnoea and long-standing interstitial abnormalities on chest radiography. A waxing and waning symptomatic course and previous responsiveness to therapy both suggest a significant inflammatory component, as in EAA (with episodic dyspnoea resulting from recurrent antigen exposure). A clear description of natural history often has a major impact on management; for example, progressive DPLD that meets clinical criteria for CFA, looks like CFA on CT and *behaves like CFA* can usually be regarded as CFA for practical therapeutic purposes, without the need for thoracoscopic lung biopsy.

Staging the symptomatic severity of disease

Symptomatic change is an important part of monitoring disease progression and evaluating responsiveness to therapy. Exercise tolerance should be documented carefully at the initial assessment, however the severity of dyspnoea is a much less reliable guide than lung function tests to the intensity of the underlying histopathological process in DPLD. This applies to connective tissue diseases in particular; concurrent systemic disease may worsen exertional dyspnoea, but may also mask respiratory symptoms due to reduced mobility.

Physical Examination

As with the history, physical findings can be sub-divided into diagnostically useful signs, and findings indicative of disease severity (and thus of likely prognosis).

Clinical signs (or their absence) often change the diagnostic balance of probability in DPLD but seldom definitively. *Finger clubbing* is evident in 50–70% of patients with CFA and in some patients with asbestosis, but is not a feature of other DPLD; thus, the presence of definite (but not equivocal) clubbing may bolster

Table 2.   History in diagnosis of DPLD

Age, smoking history	Elderly, smoker – more likely to have CFA or lymphangitis carcinomatosis than EAA or sarcoidosis
Occupational exposures	Pneumoconioses, asbestosis and hard metal exposure may mimic CFA
Exposures relevant to EAA	Even in the chronic fibrotic form of disease, avoidance of antigen exposure may be crucial in preventing further disease progression. A common error in bird fancier's lung is failure to consider antigen exposure outside the home (e.g. in the homes of relatives and friends). If in doubt, any mould or organic dust to which a patient is exposed should be considered as a potential cause of EAA
Drug history	Nitrofurantoin (even intermittent use), sulphasalazine, penicillamine, amiodarone, cytotoxic agents. The list of agents associated with occasional pulmonary complications is expanding. Medline searches are invaluable
Malignancy	Lymphangitis carcinomatosis may simulate CFA radiologically and is found in similar age-groups
Connective tissue disease	Raynaud's phenomenon, arthralgia, myalgia, sicca symptoms, skin symptoms compatible with scleroderma, lupoid butterfly rashes or gastroesophageal regurgitation
Recurrent pneumothoraces	Langerhans cell histocytosis. Lymphangioleiomyomatosis
Other diagnoses (especially if acute or rapidly progressive)	Primary DPLD need to be considered. Opportunistic infection Especially in immunosuppressed patients, and those with connective tissue disease Pulmonary oedema Diffuse alveolar haemorrhage syndromes Alveolar cell cancer Bronchorrhoea

Table 2.   Continued

Pattern of symptoms: cough and wheeze	EAA — (due to the bronchiolitic component of disease) connective tissue disease (in which bronchiectasis may co-exist with interstitial fibrosis). eosinophilic pneumonitis (with associated bronchospasm) Sarcoidosis (in which inflammation is often most severe in a bronchovascular distribution).
Exertional dyspnoea	CFA lymphangitis carcinomatosis pneumoconiosis cystic lung disease (HX, LAM).
Systemic symptoms	sarcoidosis or connective tissue disease and may occur in EAA.

a clinical diagnosis of CFA, but **the absence of clubbing is not diagnostically helpful**. The most useful auscultatory finding is the presence of mid to late **inspiratory crackles** in the lower and mid zones, markedly increasing the likelihood of fibrosing alveolitis or asbestosis, once left ventricular failure has been excluded. The absence of inspiratory crackles should lead the clinician to question a diagnosis of CFA. The **mid-inspiratory squawk** is an under-recognised sign pointing strongly to a bronchiolitic component of DPLD and heard frequently in active (sub-acute) EAA and sometimes in connective tissue disease. **Expiratory wheeze** is a less specific finding, occurring in a subset of DPLD with an airway-centred component, but also in primary acinar diseases such as CFA (in which smoking-related airway disease is often present). In sarcoidosis and LH, respiratory examination is usually normal, even in functionally severe, morphologically extensive disease.

In a small minority of patients, careful systemic examination provides important diagnostic clues, especially in sarcoidosis (**erythema nodosum, lupus pernio, peripheral lymphadenopathy, eye signs, neurological signs, etc**), and in connective tissue disease (**sclerodactyly, proximal scleroderma, telangectasiae, calcinosis, arthropathy, myopathy, etc**). In patients presenting with an acute alveolar filling process, there may be clinical evidence of cardiac disease, especially mitral stenosis.

In irreversible DPLD, clinical evidence of severe functional impairment (***central cyanosis, tachypnoea*** at rest, ***pulmonary hypertension*** with or without ***overt cor pulmonale***) usually denotes a very poor progress. When clinical evidence of severe disease seems disproportionate (i.e. associated with relatively minor disease on chest X-ray or CT), a secondary pulmonary process should be suspected; confounding disorders include emphysema (especially in patients with CFA), primary pulmonary vascular disease (in connective tissue disease), pulmonary thrombo-embolism or occult cardiac disease. A careful clinical evaluation of disease severity is especially important in CFA; in end-stage disease, supervening cardiac disease, unmasked by hypoxia, is the most common cause of death in some series. An awareness of the high likelihood of cardiac disease may lead to a worthwhile reduction in morbidity with the early use of empirical diuretic therapy.

Chest radiography

Sometimes CXR appearances make a major contribution to diagnosis e.g. sarcoidosis. Often, abnormalities are diagnostically inconclusive in themselves, but lead to a more focused definition of the nature of the clinical problem (e.g. unexplained relapsing consolidation, long-standing stable patchy fibrotic change). Key diagnostic considerations are the distribution, extent and pattern of disease, and the nature and rapidity of serial change (the distribution of disease is probably the single most useful observation). The following selected generalisations are sometimes helpful:

- granulomatous disease (sarcoidosis, EAA, TB) is usually associated with upper or upper to mid zone disease on chest X-ray, a degree of reversibility with treatment and a BAL lymphocytosis. Predominantly fibrotic disease (CFA, asbestosis) is often associated with prominent lower zone disease on chest X-ray, irreversible disease and a BAL neutrophilia. However, although a clear zonal distribution on chest X-ray is useful in diagnosis, lack of a clear zonal distribution is a non-specific observation
- multifocal consolidation: migration of infiltrates shown by serial chest X-rays excludes alveolar cell cancer, makes infection unlikely and should focus the clinician on eosinophilic syndromes (especially if the distribution is sub-pleural), vasculitis and cryptogenic organizing pneumonia
- if the chest X-ray is typical of fibrosing alveolitis, evidence from

previous X-rays of long-term stability (e.g. no change for two years) should increase the suspicion of asbestosis or the fibrosing alveolitis of connective tissue disease

- although often present on CT, mediastinal lymphadenopathy on chest X-ray is not a feature of DPLD, apart from sarcoidosis and lymphangitis carcinomatosis. Enlarged mediastinal nodes should heighten the suspicion of tuberculosis or concurrent malignancy (much more prevalent in CFA)

- in fibrosing alveolitis (the DPLD in which the need to define reversibility is greatest), chest X-ray appearances do not discriminate reliably between predominantly inflammatory and predominantly fibrotic lung disease, except in approximately 15% of patients with overt honeycombing (which invariably denotes fibrotic disease)

Pulmonary function tests in diagnosis

The demonstration of functional impairment in a patient with nebulous respiratory symptoms is often the key stimulus of further investigations leading to the detection of occult DPLD. In known but undiagnosed DPLD, it is reassuring when the pattern of functional impairment (the combination of spirometric volumes {FEV_1, FVC, FEV_1/FVC}, plethysmographic volumes {TLC, RV, RV/TLC} and measures of gas transfer {Dlco, Kco} is compatible with the working diagnosis. Of immediate practical value are the designation of the functional defect in an undiagnosed DPLD as **predominantly restrictive, mixed or predominantly obstructive**, based on a combination of estimation of total lung volume (TLC) and measures of airflow obstruction (FEV_1/FVC, RV/TLC); and the **degree of depression of gas transfer**, for a given reduction in lung volumes. While a detailed review of PFT is beyond the scope of this chapter, the following generalisations often have practical value:

- in isolated CFA, asbestosis and chronic fibrotic EAA (without associated emphysema), lung volumes are restrictive but better preserved (as judged by percentage of predicted values) than total gas transfer. A typical pattern of functional impairment (lung restriction or an isolated depression of Dlco) is one of the clinical criteria for a diagnosis of CFA

- fibrotic sarcoidosis may be functionally identical to CFA and chronic EAA, especially in end-stage disease. However, usually Dlco levels are better preserved in sarcoidosis. In otherwise moderate DPLD, severe depression of Dlco markedly reduces the likelihood of sarcoidosis (in the absence of cofounders such as emphysema or pulmonary embolism)

- the demonstration of a mixed functional defect, as shown by relative preservation of lung volumes, a normal FEV_1/FVC ratio, and an elevated RV/TLC ratio (denoting obstruction in the presence of restriction) suggests sarcoidosis, EAA, the DPLD of connective tissue disease and the combination of emphysema and a purely restrictive disease. It is often possible to discriminate between these diseases by integrating PFT and CT findings.

- a severe, predominantly obstructive functional defect (elevated TLC and RV, an overtly obstructive FEV_1/FVC ratio) is occasionally encountered in sarcoidosis or EAA, but should alert the clinician to the possibility of cystic lung disease (LH, LAM).

- measures of total gas transfer (Dlco, Kco) are heavily influenced by the presence of associated emphysema (most commonly in CFA). By contrast, Dlco and Kco levels are relatively little influenced by intrinsic small airways disease (e.g. the bronchiolitic component of EAA or connective tissue disease), provided that the FEV_1 exceeds one litre

- Dlco levels should be corrected for haemoglobin concentration. An anaemia of 10gm/dl results in a fall in gas transfer of approximately 15%

- the interpretation of Kco (Dlco adjusted for VA) is not straightforward, as pulmonary vascular events, interstitial disease and extra-pulmonic restriction all have variable and sometimes conflicting effects: the percentage predicted Kco may be paradoxically normal, despite extensive underlying pathology. Kco values are clinically useful when they are markedly increased (extra-pulmonic restriction, diffuse alveolar haemorrhage) or decreased (emphysema, pulmonary thromboembolism), thus identifying the predominant pathophysiological process; occasionally, when these disorders are suspected, a normal Kco level has an important negative predictive value

- in patients with a severe acute alveolar process, a dramatic elevation in measures of gas transfer (>200% of predicted values), measured by the single breath technique, can be regarded as diagnostic of diffuse alveolar haemorrhage (which may be difficult to diagnose, especially when associated with little or no haemoptysis). However, measures of gas transfer remain strikingly elevated for only 36 hours after haemorrhage has occurred

- arterial gases at rest are helpful diagnostically in a small minority of patients, mainly in a negative sense: in moderate to extensive CFA, hypoxia is the rule and thus preservation of pO_2 argues against the diagnosis. Occasionally, arterial gases may lend support to a diagnosis of extra-pulmonic restriction (i.e. alveolar hypoventilation resulting in hypoxia with a normal alveolar-arterial oxygen gradient)
- exercise testing (the measurement of oxygen desaturation at maximal exercise) has no established utility in discriminating between individual DPLDs, but may be useful in unmasking occult DPLD and thus leading to other diagnostic tests

High resolution computed tomography (CT) in diagnosis and prognostic evaluation

The use of CT in diagnosis is probably the most important clinical advance in the last decade in DPLD. In occult disease, with normal or marginally abnormal lung function indices, CT detects parenchymal abnormalities before chest radiography in a wide variety of DPLD. In established DPLD, CT scanning has substantially increased the accuracy of non-invasive diagnostic evaluation. In CFA, sarcoidosis, lymphangitis carcinomatosis, EAA, LH, LAM and silicosis, CT appearances are often pathognomonic, and when they are not, CT often serves to narrow the realistic differential diagnosis to two possibilities (often readily distinguished clinically). The true impact of CT is understated by formal diagnostic studies in DPLD, as these consist of comparisons in diagnostic sensitivity between CT and chest radiography, which do not take clinical pre-test and post-test probability into account. CT scanning is often pivotal in formulating the best use of ancillary investigations (i.e. those with the highest yield).

In addition, CT has a useful role in predicting the likelihood of a response to therapy, especially in CFA. In general, ***provided that it is the most prominent abnormality***, ground-glass attenuation on CT in DPLD usually denotes responsiveness to therapy. However, ground-glass attenuation often represents fine fibrotic disease when it is admixed with an equally extensive or more extensive reticular pattern. Thus, ***ground-glass attenuation on CT is often but not invariably reversible***, in CFA and in other DPLD. By contrast, a reticular pattern is always irreversible in CFA and treatment is not recommended except where there is progression of disease demonstrated on serial investigations.

Table 3.   Investigations in DPLD

Routine baseline blood tests	Full blood count, biochemical screen
Tests that are central to diagnosis	Plain chest radiography, lung function, computed tomography
Ancillary diagnostic procedures	Bronchoalveolar lavage (BAL), thoracoscopic biopsy (not always necessary but sometimes under-used)
Investigations to identify reversible disease	
Measures of disease severity (including baseline and renal tests)	

Table 4.   Ancillary diagnostic tests

Erythrocyte sedimentation rate	Useful only when markedly elevated (connective tissue disease, vasculitis, infection or malignancy)
Urinary examination	Vasculitis
Auto-antibodies (rheumatoid factor, anti-nuclear antibodies, anti-neutrophil cytoplasmic antibodies)	Connective tissue disorders may present with interstitial lung disease long before the onset of overt systemic manifestations; however, moderately elevated titres are seen in 30% of patients with CFA and should be interpreted with caution. The extractable nuclear anti-DNA topoisomerase antibodies (in systemic sclerosis) and anti-tRNA synthetase antibodies (in polymyositis/dermatomyositis) are associated with more severe lung fibrosis, but have no practical impact on management in established DPLD
Precipitins against fungal antigens (thermophilic actinomycetes, micropolysporium faeni, avian precipitins)	Precipitin positivity is often central to a secure diagnosis of EAA but is not diagnostic in isolation
Immediate skin-prick hypersensitivity to *Aspergillus fumigatus*	A negative result excludes allergic bronchopulmonary aspergillosis

Ancillary diagnostic tests

See Tables 3 and 4.

Radionuclide techniques are of little or no diagnostic value in DPLD (Table 5).

In fibrosing alveolitis and sarcoidosis, the more useful finding is normal DTPA clearance, predictive of non-progression of disease over the next two to three years.

Minimally-invasive diagnostic tests

The role of *bronchoalveolar lavage* (BAL) in DPLD is increasingly open to question. BAL content may occasionally be useful in diagnosis — for example, active EAA is characterised by a striking lymphocytosis. Similarly, there are statistically significant relationships between BAL cellularity and prognosis in individual diseases (e.g. in CFA, a BAL lymphocytosis denotes a good prognosis whereas a neutrophilia and/or is associated with a poor outcome). However, neither diagnostic nor prognostic trends are sufficiently robust to be definitive in individual patients. Furthermore, the use of CT has increased greatly the diagnostic and prognostic information available to the clinician in DPLD: whether BAL adds usefully to CT has yet to be established. Formal assessment of the clinical value of BAL, anchored by a careful definition of pre-test probability, is now long overdue. However, it would be premature to discard BAL

Table 5. Tests which are not useful

Ventilation-perfusion scanning	may add to clinical uncertainty as mismatched defects characteristic of fibrotic lung disease give a spurious impression of thromboembolism
Gallium scanning	adds nothing to diagnosis or the assessment of disease activity in DILD, except in the occasional patient with systemic sarcoidosis
Inhaled ^{99m}Tc-DTPA clearance in current smokers	Results cannot be interpreted
Kveim test in suspected sarcoidosis	No longer permitted, due to BSE precautions

altogether in DPLD, based upon untested speculation. For the moment, the performance of BAL can still be defended, especially when bronchoscopy is warranted for the purposes of transbronchial biopsy.

Most clinicians continue to advocate **transbronchial biopsies** in suspected stage II or stage III pulmonary sarcoidosis (i.e. parenchymal abnormalities on plain chest radiography, with or without hilar lymphadenopathy). Transbronchial biopsies may also be diagnostic in other DPLD including EAA, cryptogenic organising pneumonitis, eosinophilic pneumonitis and lymphangitis carcinomatosis; however, fibrosing alveolitis should not be diagnosed histologically by this means, because useful samples are difficult to obtain and reveal non-specific fibrotic features.

The most difficult investigative decision of all concerns **thoracoscopic biopsy**. A formal lung biopsy is an unsatisfactory 'gold standard'; the test is minimally-invasive, relatively expensive, causes delays in treatment, cannot be performed serially to evaluate change and is impracticable in patients with advanced DPLD. Inter-observer variation in the histological diagnosis of DPLD undoubtedly exists but has never been quantified. For all that, the performance of thoracoscopic biopsy is undeniably crucial in some patients. The unresolved debate concerns the threshold for proceeding to thoracoscopy, which is likely to vary between institutions, depending upon local surgical and pathological expertise.

Currently, it is unclear whether the added diagnostic and prognostic information conferred by CT will reduce the overall need for lung biopsy, or merely refine the indications for histological evaluation. It now appears that in many individual DPLD, a typical clinical presentation in association with typical CT appearances suffices for diagnosis; for example, it is likely that in most patients with CFA, thoracoscopic biopsy adds little to management. However, the added information provided by CT may strengthen the indications for biopsy in a minority of patients, particularly when the CT and clinical features are at odds. The key to rationalising invasive investigation in DPLD is to think of individual diseases in terms of low, intermediate and high pre-test probabilities, and to make an overall re-evaluation with the addition of CT before considering surgery.

Disease Severity

An accurate evaluation of the severity of disease is important because it will influence the immediate therapeutic approach and guide decisions on the frequency of follow-up. Morphologic measures cannot be used routinely for these purposes. Open lung biopsy material is necessarily regional, may not reflect the global severity of disease, and cannot be evaluated serially. CT scanning might, in principle, be used in serial monitoring, but the scoring of disease extent on CT is not a routine radiological skill. Lung function indices are a more reliable guide to the evolution of DPLD than chest radiography or symptoms. It is usual in DPLD to quantify the full range of resting functional indices at first assessment, but the relative accuracy of individual variables in reflecting the morphologic extent of disease is likely to vary between individual disorders. In CFA, total gas transfer (Dlco) best reflects disease extent on CT and at lung biopsy. By contrast, in pulmonary sarcoidosis, the FEV_1 bears the closest relationship to CT findings.

The staging of disease severity in DPLD may be confounded by concurrent pulmonary processes, most commonly emphysema. The coexistence of restrictive disease and emphysema may result in spurious normality of lung volumes associated with devastating depression of gas transfer. In the presence of extensive lung fibrosis, emphysema may be impossible to detect clinically or on plain chest radiography, but is obvious on CT. Thus, in reaching a final evaluation of disease severity, it is useful to consider CT appearances and lung function tests together.

It is conventional, in monitoring DPLD, to focus on alterations in FVC and Dlco. However, the detection of change is often difficult, especially when an increase in symptoms is associated with marginal trends in lung function indices. CT scanning is more sensitive than functional measures in identifying progression or regression of disease, but may detect and over-emphasise trivial change which does not necessarily have therapeutic implications. Currently, clinical consensus continues to favour the central role of lung function tests in routine monitoring, with recourse to repeat CT scanning in selected cases.

Treatment in DPLD

Treatment in DPLD usually consists of oral corticosteroids, with or without immunosuppressive therapy. In instituting treatment, the clinician must have realistic therapeutic goals. It is especially important to discriminate between reversible DPLD, in which a response is expected, and irreversible fibrotic disease, in which case the primary therapeutic goal is the prevention of progression of disease. A balance must be achieved between treating reversible disease optimally and avoiding unnecessary side-effects from an overly aggressive approach to fibrotic disease. Key information in the formulation of a logical therapeutic plan includes:

- evidence of environmental causes
- assessment of the likelihood of significant inflammatory cell infiltration (as judged by CT in most patients and occasionally by thoracoscopic biopsy)
- definition of the 'track-record' of disease, as judged by symptoms, previous chest radiographs and previous responsiveness to treatment
- a confident diagnosis of an individual DPLD

The approach to treatment in CFA can be applied to other DPLD because the range of abnormalities in CFA spans almost the entire DPLD spectrum, from inflammatory to fibrotic appearances on CT and lung biopsy, and from variably indolent to rapidly progressive disease. In a minority of patients with inflammatory disease, early aggressive therapy is warranted, if progression to irreversible fibrosis is to be pre-empted. It is usual to start with high dose corticosteroids (e.g. Prednisolone 60mg daily for three to four weeks), as a therapeutic response will generally become apparent within two to three weeks. The early identification of non-responsiveness in potentially reversible disease is important because the immediate addition of an immunosuppressive agent (usually cyclophosphamide or azathioprine) may be warranted.

Treatment of CFA and the Evidence

More typically, the question confronting the clinician in CFA is whether to treat empirically in the hope of slowing or preventing the progression of disease. This dilemma applies equally to fibrotic sarcoidosis, chronic EAA and other potentially progressive fibrotic DPLD. It is surprising that treatment efficacy in this context has never been studied definitively. In a progressive fibrotic disorder, stability of disease can be regarded as a therapeutic success; however, if deterioration is merely slowed (a more realistic aim in CFA) a placebo-controlled study will be required to demonstrate an unequivocal treatment benefit. Recent therapeutic studies have consisted of comparisons between corticosteroid therapy alone and combinations of corticosteroid and immunosuppressive agents.

Differences in outcome would have lent support to the belief that treatment modulates the natural history of fibrotic CFA. Sadly, all studies have been inconclusive, due in part to small numbers of patients and failure to match precisely for initial disease severity and the degree of inflammation.

In the absence of definitive evidence, the therapeutic approach to fibrotic DPLD has been extremely variable. Many clinicians favour a policy of observation in apparently stable predominantly fibrotic disease and some argue for instituting treatment only when symptoms supervene. However, the latter approach does not take into account the large reserve of the lungs; by the time symptoms develop, major structural damage, which might have been prevented by earlier treatment, is the rule. In the end, each clinician must reach his/her own conclusions on the role of 'civilised' pre-emptive therapy (e.g. Prednisolone 20mg on alternate days) in fibrotic DPLD. However, the following considerations are important when treatment decisions are a close call.

- *a clear 'track-record' of progression of disease* (symptomatically or on review of chest radiographs) is a clear signal that further potentially preventable progression is likely during a period of observation
- even in predominantly fibrotic DPLD, *any hint of associated inflammation* (on CT/biopsy or based on a previous therapeutic response) warrants a trial of therapy. Especially when pulmonary reserve is greatly diminished, minor regression of disease may confer major symptomatic benefits, which may be lost if treatment is delayed
- *definition of an underlying cause* is pivotal because removal of a causative antigen, occupational dust or pharmacological agent may suffice therapeutically, or may allow the early withdrawal of treatment after suppression of an alveolitic component
- *a confident diagnosis of an individual DPLD* may have a major effect on the threshold for intervention, depending upon the expected natural history. Thus, the argument for early treatment in mildly to moderately extensive pulmonary fibrosis is likely to be stronger in CFA than, for example, in EAA, sarcoidosis or fibrosing alveolitis associated with connective tissue disease
- *initial disease severity* is an important consideration. When there is ample reserve, progression of disease may not have catastrophic consequences. However, *when the patient is symptomatic or has moderate functional impairment* (e.g. a

30–40% reduction in lung function indices), further deterioration must be prevented if possible

* *progression of disease during a period of observation* is an obvious indication for treatment. Thus, the meticulous monitoring of untreated patients is essential
* currently, the role of non-invasive tests to identify patients at higher risk of decline remains speculative, although *normal clearance of inhaled ^{99m}Tc-DTPA* may justify deferment of treatment in CFA and sarcoidosis, especially when the decision to intervene is marginal. The role of BAL in identifying poorer prognostic disease requires further study, taking pre-test probability into account
* as discussed in detail below, *patient preferences* are often pivotal. Management decisions should be taken in partnership with the patient. Often, the clinician may believe that refusal of treatment is a mistake, but if the decision is accepted after a civilised discussion, it is often possible to review the decision in the light of subsequent monitoring

Communication with Non-respiratory Medical Colleagues

Because the attainment of a final histospecific diagnosis in DPLD is often a considerable challenge, it is easy to forget that the application of a exact, often arcane, diagnostic label may be of much less interest to a referring non-specialist colleague than a simple statement of prognosis and the formulation of a pragmatic management plan. The most important goals, in communicating with medical colleagues (whether in writing to general practitioners or in assessing in-patient referrals) are:

* **to convey the likely diagnosis, prognosis and responsiveness to treatment.** It is not especially useful to the referring practitioner to provide a lengthy differential diagnosis, although reasonably likely alternative diagnoses which may change management should certainly be mentioned. More importantly, a simple common-sensical integration of the history, CT, biopsy appearances (if any), and lung function findings to provide a summary statement of severity, likely natural history and treated course will usually lay bare the logic of proposed management without the need for further discussion
* **to provide a brief management plan.** It is important to lay down

guidelines for proposed monitoring of disease at first referral, to
ensure that essential baseline investigations have been performed
- **to summarize any discussion with the patient or family.** It is
  usual for the patient (and often the family) to participate in
  decision-making, but some patients choose not to do so but
  prefer to accept medical recommendations without detailed
  discussion. The referring doctor needs to know what information
  has been provided and whether the management plan has been
  significantly modified by choices exercised by the patient
- to summarize major potential toxicities of recommended therapy
  i.e. to recommend tests to monitor drug toxicity, ideally according
  to a locally agreed protocol

Communication with Patients

Interstitial lung disease is particularly threatening to patients because the individual disorders have not been integrated into lay
awareness. There are no novels or films in which CFA or other
DPLDs play a central role, and the rarity of these disorders makes
it highly unlikely that friends or family members will be fellow
sufferers. Few patients have heard of 'pulmonary fibrosis'. Often,
there has been diagnostic confusion before referral, and sometimes
a numbers of alternative diagnoses have been suggested, only to be
discounted. Thus, it is essential to avoid eclectic diagnostic labels
but to speak clearly and concisely in lay language.

This is not always easy. However, in fibrotic disease, most
patients can grasp the concept of a disorder in which 'scar tissue
is laid down' and will then come to terms with the fact that the
cause is unknown (exactly as in many more common disorders).
Inflammation can usually be dealt with by referring to 'swelling of
tissues due to the actions of natural body defences' — most patients
have experienced painful swelling of a finger or toe due to infection.
Patients will then grasp the concepts that scar tissue cannot be
removed, but that inflammation can be treated, and that treating
and suppressing inflammation before it turns into scar tissue may
be vital. The use of treatment in fibrotic disease to try to prevent
further deposition of scar tissue can also be discussed in lay terms.

It is seldom useful to state an 'average prognosis' for an individual DPLD. Even in fibrotic CFA, there is considerable variation
in the rate of progression, and a small proportion of patients survive
for many years. Thus, it is reasonable to leave the patient with the
hope of a good outcome (unless the disease is clearly fibrotic and

pre-terminal). Especially in previously untreated patients, it is often helpful to inform the patient that a much clearer idea of the future will become apparent once it is known whether treatment is associated with improvement, stability or further decline.

A detailed discussion with the patient and family as early as possible is important because in most cases, little or no information has been provided before referral. Even if disease is irreversible, a clear statement of the likely diagnosis is often a great relief. It is usually obvious to the patient, from earlier medical interactions, that DPLD is a difficult area; some uncertainty about outcome is usually accepted readily, especially when the issues are discussed confidently, with an obvious desire to impart information. In this way, a good deal of trust can be engendered with very little effort. The quantity of information to be imparted makes it especially helpful to involve the family in discussion; it is unrealistic to expect the patient to recall all the nuances of communication, especially under considerable stress.

Possible patient phobias should be recognised and confronted. It should be acknowledged frankly that phobias about corticosteroid therapy are not unreasonable. It is often helpful to stress that any therapeutic intervention is a balance of benefit and risk, and that in recommending intervention, the clinician has made the judgement that the risks of toxicity are outweighed by the risks of under-treatment. The aim of reducing corticosteroid dosages to 'civilised' acceptable levels as soon as possible should also be emphasised.

A second under-recognised phobia is that of the radiation dosage associated with CT scans and repeated chest radiographs. If the patient is diffident about undergoing imaging procedures, it is prudent to address the issue of radiation burden immediately. Recently, the high radiation dose associated with contiguous non-high resolution CT scans has been emphasised by the media. By contrast, modern interspaced high resolution protocols (2mm sections at 20mm intervals throughout the lungs) equate with a skin and breast radiation burden of less than 10 chest radiographs, which in turn equate with one or two chest radiographs performed 15 years ago (when radiation dosages were higher). To put this in perspective, the background environmental radiation exposure is equivalent to a (modern) chest radiograph a week; a return flight to the West Coast of the United States results in radiation exposure similar to that associated with CT.

Diagnostic Problems in DPLD

Extensive or 'end-stage' lung disease

'End-stage' lung disease presents a considerable management challenge, especially as a first presentation with severe dyspnoea, devastating functional impairment and widespread shadowing on chest radiography. The key to focused management is the formulation of an accurate diagnosis, but this is not straightforward. Clinical signs, the pattern of functional impairment and chest radiographic appearances are generally non-specific in end-stage DPLD. Bronchoscopy may be contraindicated by severe respiratory compromise; the main potential utility of BAL is to exclude opportunistic impairment. Similarly, thoracoscopic procedures are seldom practicable, and even when a biopsy can be performed, histological appearances are notoriously non-specific in 'end-stage lung'.

In this difficult situation, CT is invaluable. In a large series of 61 patients with 'end-stage lung', (with histological diagnoses made earlier in disease in the majority), an accurate and usually confident first choice CT diagnosis (based upon the pattern and distribution of disease) was made in nearly 90% of cases. The likelihood of reversibility may be suggested by prominence of ground-glass attenuation, as opposed to fibrotic disease. Treatment is usually aggressive with high dose steroids (including pulsed methylprednisolone) and cyclophosphamide.

Diagnostic considerations in fibrosing alveolitis

In CFA, the integration of clinical and CT features usually allows a reasonably secure diagnosis without recourse to thoracoscopic biopsy. However, other DPLDs that may mimic CFA should be kept constantly in mind. These include: *fibrosing alveolitis associated with connective tissue disease*, which appears clinically and radiologically identical to CFA, *asbestosis,* in which the majority of cases have pleural plaques or diffuse pleural thickening evident on CT; *chronic extrinsic allergic alveolitis* which may mimic CFA in all respects, but is rare, especially in the absence of a relevant exposure history; and in any case can be treated as CFA for practical therapeutic purposes. Recently, a new histopathological entity, *non-specific interstitial pneumonitis*, Table 6, has been defined, making up approximately 20% of patients previously diagnosed on lung biopsy as having CFA. This histological picture is associated

Table 6. Classification and features of interstitial pneumonias previously regarded as 'fibrosing alveolitis'

	Usual interstitial pneumonia (UIP)	Desquamative interstitial pneumonia (DIP)	Non specific interstitial pneumonia (NSIP)	Acute interstitial pneumonia (AIP)
Other terminology	CFA, IPF		CFA with some unusual features	'Hamman-Rich'
Clinical features	Insidious progression of pulmonary fibrosis and minimal response to therapy	May progress more explosively than UIP but a good response to treatment is expected	May have similar features to UIP, but more often responsive to therapy, and less progressive when fibrotic	Rapidly progressive disease with onset of respiratory failure within weeks. Response to therapy may be minimal.
Pathological features	Prominent fibroblastic proliferation with honeycomb change. Lesions are at various stages – normal lung may be adjacent to extensive fibrosis. There is minimal alveolar inflammation.	There is diffuse alveolar inflammation with little or no fibroblastic proliferation and no honeycomb change. The degree of interstitial inflammation is variable	Histological appearances homogeneous throughout the biopsy, in both severity and age of lesions. May be fibrotic or inflammatory (interstitial but not alveolar inflammation)	Diffuse interstitial fibrosis, fibroblast proliferation, hyaline membrane formation

In addition respiratory bronchiolitis interstitial pneumonia (RBILD) may occur which is similar to DIP but histological features show interstitial fibrosis is more prominent within the peribronchiolar air spaces and parenchyma. It is associated in the vast majority of cases with cigarette smokers.

with a substantially better prognosis and adds justification to the continued use of thoracoscopic biopsy procedures in suspected CFA when the clinical and CT features are at odds.

Table 6 shows the recently modified classification of interstitial pneumonias associated with a clinical presentation of fibrosing alveolitis.

Unexplained multifocal consolidation

Multifocal consolidation will often have been diagnosed as community acquired pneumonia and has often been treated unsuccessfully with prolonged antibiotic therapy at respiratory referral. The distinction between fixed multi-focal consolidation and changing infiltrates is crucial. Amongst causes of fixed infiltrates, the possibility of *tuberculous or non-bacterial infection*, especially fungal infection, should always be considered. *Alveolar cell carcinoma and lymphoproliferative disease* are often misdiagnosed, sometimes for many months. The differential diagnosis for changing infiltrates is largely immunological and includes *eosinophilic pneumonia, bronchiolitis obliterans organizing pneumonia (cryptogenic organizing pneumonia), allergic bronchopulmonary aspergillosis*, and, occasionally, *acute extrinsic allergic alveolitis* and *sarcoidosis*.

The distinction between fixed and changing multifocal consolidation is straightforward only when serial chest radiographs are available. Moreover, a number of disorders may be partially fixed and partially evanescent. Vasculitic disease, especially *Wegener's granulomatosis*, may presented with consolidation, rather than the classical picture of cavitating nodules. *Pulmonary infarction*, including infarction due to septic or non-septic embolism, may be associated with consolidation. Finally, *recurrent aspiration pneumonitis* due to severe gastroesophageal reflux is often overlooked, especially as reflux symptoms are very common and their significance may be missed.

There is no substitute for considering a wide differential diagnosis when evaluating multi-focal consolidation. In many situations in DPLD, an incorrect diagnosis will not radically alter management. However, missing the diagnoses of Wegener's granulomatosis, widespread opportunistic infection, recurrent aspiration or alveolar cell carcinoma may have devastating consequences, especially if treatment makes the situation worse (e.g. steroid therapy for suspected cryptogenic organizing pneumonitis, when the diagnosis is opportunistic infection). Thus, making a overly rapid diagnosis, based on moderate probability, should be avoided. Bronchoscopic examination is especially important, because culture negativity of BAL and tissue greatly reduces the likelihood of opportunistic infection; moreover, it is often possible to make a definitive diagnosis on transbronchial biopsy (cryptogenic organizing pneumonia, eosinophilic pneumonia, sarcoidosis, alveolar cell carcinoma). It is useful to perform an autoimmune screen (including ANCA titres) at presentation to minimise subsequent diagnostic delays.

Widespread air-space consolidation

Diffuse alveolar filling is often a potentially life-threatening condition. Before respiratory referral, aggressive treatment for *heart failure* has often been undertaken. The possibility of *diffuse alveolar haemorrhage* (DAH) is often overlooked; widespread alveolar haemorrhage is often associated with little or no haemoptysis. Severe *mitral stenosis* may be masked clinically by prominent respiratory signs; urgent echocardiography is occasionally warranted. *Uraemic infiltrates* rarely present a dilemma as the diagnosis is biochemically obvious. *Pneumocystis pneumonia* and other opportunistic infections are an increasing cause of widespread alveolar infiltration. Causes of *adult respiratory distress syndrome* (ARDS) include diffuse pulmonary infection, severe aspiration, toxic inhalation, narcotic overdose, and prolonged hypotension. The differential diagnosis also includes *acute eosinophilic syndromes, desquamative interstitial pneumonitis* and *drug-induced pulmonary infiltration.*

As with multi-focal consolidation, the key to management is to consider a wide differential diagnosis from the outset, and not to overlook possibilities such as mitral stenosis and DAH (especially in patients without haemoptysis). The realistic differential diagnosis often lies between DAH, diffuse infection and ARDS (although causes of ARDS are often readily identifiable). The approach to diagnosis is critically dependent upon the severity of respiratory compromise; early BAL is often useful, both to exclude pneumocystis pneumonia (and other infections) and to diagnose DAH. Other important ancillary clues to suggest DAH include an abnormal urinary sediment, systemic evidence of connective tissue disease (especially SLE), and anaemia (especially a falling haemoglobin concentration). Occasionally, marked elevation of single breath Dlco levels may be diagnostic (although the patient is usually too compromised to undergo formal lung function tests). Whenever DAH is suspected, a full autoimmune screen (including ANCA titres) should be performed. Once a diagnosis of DAH has been confirmed, it is important to identify the underlying cause; an early renal biopsy is often crucial.

Difficulties in the diagnosis of pulmonary vasculitis

The pulmonary vasculitides often pose considerable diagnostic difficulties: it can be argued that the pulmonary vessels (and not the small airways) are the true 'silent zone' of the lung. Vasculitis can

Table 7.   Classification of pulmonary vasculitidies, adapted from 1992 Chapel Hill International Consensus Conference

Primary	Wegener's granulomatosis
	Churg-Strauss syndrome
	Microscopic polyangitis
	Takayasu's arteritis
Secondary	Systemic lupus erythematosis
	Mixed connective tissue disorder
	Systemic sclerosis
	Polymyositis
	Rheumatoid arthritis

usefully be divided into primary and secondary vasculitis. Secondary vasculitis develops as a feature of a well-defined underlying primary disorder such as SLE: the detection of vasculitis is often relatively straightforward, provided the clinician has a high index of suspicion. By contrast, the primary systemic vasculitides are a complex and variable group of disorders. Diagnosis is made more difficult by the absence of overt causative agents and by the similarity in clinical presentation with many non-vasculitic diseases such as endocarditis, other chronic infections and malignancy. A further problem has been the need to update the classification of vasculitis with increasing clinical experience (see Table 7).

It lies beyond the scope of this chapter to describe individual vasculitides in detail. Those commonly involving the lung comprise Wegener's granulomatosis (WG), Churg-Strauss syndrome, microscopic polyangitis and Takayasu's arteritis. Early diagnosis is a realistic goal for clinicians aware of the typical presentations of these rare disorders. However, the great heterogeneity of clinical presentations cannot be over-stated: no two cases of Churg-Strauss syndrome (in particular) are alike. Many patients cannot be readily categorised but have overlap features of two or more vasculitic syndromes. The cardinal histological features of individual disorders may be in evolution or partially suppressed by treatment, leading to non-specific (false negative) biopsy findings. WG apart, serological markers have a low specificity; even in suspected WG, the clinical significance of elevated c-ANCA titres is critically dependent upon the pre-test probability of the disease. False negative c-ANCA levels are seen in at least 10% of WG.

The classification of bronchiolitis

Although airway-centred, the bronchiolitides often have interstitial abnormalities and can be regarded as diffuse lung diseases. The major diagnostic difficulty confronted by clinicians is the procrustean exercise of fitting the clinical picture to the medical literature, which increasingly amounts to a semantic quagmire. The problem is best exemplified by two disorders: 'constrictive obliterative bronchiolitis' (OB) and 'bronchiolitis obliterans organizing pneumonitis' (BOOP). Although these disorders have similar names, their clinical features differ radically (clinically, on chest radiography, on CT, on lung function testing, histologically and in responsiveness to therapy). The reader is referred to a seminal editorial which lays bare what has become a major source of confusion. In essence, 'BOOP' is a true air-space lung disease, presenting with multifocal consolidation (clinically and radiologically), a restrictive defect and usually responding to steroid therapy. OB presents with airflow obstruction and is almost always irreversible. It is difficult to envisage two more dissimilar disorders.

Table 8.   Classification of bronchiolitis

Bronchiolitis	Defining features
Cryptogenic organising pneumonia (COP)*	Multifocal consolidation on CxR and CT, restrictive ventilatory defect, usually regresses with steroid therapy
Obliterative bronchiolitis (OB)	Hyperinflation on CxR, mosaic perfusion on CT, airflow obstruction, irreversible
Follicular bronchiolitis	Reticulonodular abnormalities on CxR, centrilobular nodules and variable ground-glass attenuation on CT, restrictive ventilatory defect or airflow obstruction, regresses with steroid therapy in 50%
Cryptogenic organising pneumonia (COP), bronchiolitis obliterans organising pneumonia (BOOP) and proliferative bronchiolitis are synonymous	

*Bronchiolitis obliterans organising pneumonitis (BOOP).

The resulting confusion might have been minimised by a prompt revision of terminology. Sadly, the issue was not addressed immediately; eventually, separate alternative terminologies were promulgated in Europe and the USA. 'Cryptogenic organizing pneumonia' (COP, the original term used in the first histological description of BOOP) was revived. A dichotomy of 'constrictive obliterative bronchiolitis' and 'proliferative bronchiolitis' (synonymous with BOOP, COP) was proposed and has now entered the medical lexicon. 'Proliferative bronchiolitis' can itself be viewed as a misnomer, as the most proliferative of the true bronchiolitides is 'pan-bronchiolitis', most widely reported in East Asia but increasingly recognised elsewhere. 'Follicular bronchiolitis' is an entirely separate disorder, for which, thankfully, no synonyms exist (at least for the moment).

Occult connective tissue disease: the problem of a disease without a name

A sub-group of patients with DPLD have features suggestive but not diagnostic of collagen vascular disease, and an exact diagnostic label defies definition. Sometimes this takes the form of a mixture of features of defined connective tissue diseases (e.g. SLE, polymyositis, systemic sclerosis) without the satisfaction of rigorous diagnostic criteria for any single disease; these patients are variously characterised as having 'overlap syndromes' or, when features are less well-defined, 'undifferentiated connective tissue disease'. On other occasions, the presentation appears typical of a defined connective tissue disease, but some key diagnostic feature is lacking; the entities of 'lupus sine lupus' (typical clinical presentation but negative serology) and 'systemic sclerosis sine scleroderma' (typical organ involvement without skin manifestations) are increasingly recognised, and it is likely that many other patients verge on these categories. A third variant is the combination of non-specific systemic abnormalities (e.g. raised ESR, Raynauds phenomenon) and a constellation of lung abnormalities suggestive of connective tissue disease (e.g. lung fibrosis associated with bronchiectasis, suggestive of rheumatoid arthritis; lung fibrosis associated with pulmonary hypertension suggestive of scleroderma).

This group of patients, whilst highly academically interesting, causes a good deal of clinical uncertainty. Perhaps the most important principle in formulating a management plan is to accept the uncertainty at face value, and not to try to reach a dogmatic diagnosis. The defined connective tissue disorders were constructed by consensus, in an effort to amalgamate autoimmune phenomena into discrete diseases; textbook descriptions do not capture the full range of disease behaviour to two standard deviations. The reader is referred to a most enlightening and entertaining discussion, written over 30 years ago (see references); as Bywaters implies, diseases such as SLE and systemic sclerosis can be viewed as the mountains and valleys of the autoimmune landscape. However, 'most people live in places which are really neither mountain (nor) valley … but somewhere in between'. In the end, the only safe course for the diagnostician in this situation is to accept uncertainty but to continue to review the diagnosis as the disease evolves.

Diagnosing the complications of advanced DPLD

Fibrotic lung diseases such as CFA do not always progress symptomatically at an even rate but sometimes deteriorate apparently explosively, due either to a sudden increase in disease activity or to a minor worsening which results in a critical reduction in pulmonary reserve. The difficulty for the clinician is that in advanced fibrotic disease, a number of complications may supervene and thus an apparent worsening of lung disease may be spurious. In severe disease, *cardiac complications* commonly arise, triggered by increasing hypoxia; in some large CFA series, cardiac disease is the commonest cause of death. Fibrotic distorted lung tissue may serve as a nidus for *infection*, especially in patients receiving corticosteroid or immunosuppressive therapy. *Pulmonary embolism* is increased in prevalence in CFA (and in other severe DPLD complicated by decreased mobility and cor pulmonale). *Lung carcinoma* is strikingly more prevalent in CFA; bulky symptomatic disease may be masked radiographically by extensive lung fibrosis. Whilst bronchospasm is not, in itself, a complication of fibrotic DPLD, relatively minor *bronchospasm due to smoking-related lung damage* may have a devastating effect when pulmonary reserve is severely compromised. In inexorably worsening, extensive, fibrotic lung disease, the diagnosis and treatment of complications may not greatly alter overall life expectancy, but often substantially alleviates symptoms.

The difficult question for the clinician is how aggressively to investigate a sudden deterioration in a disease like CFA, where progression of disease is the rule. If, as is often the case, decline is primarily due to CFA, intensive investigation is merely a source of added morbidity. In this difficult situation, repetition of CT is often useful. Sometimes, major increases in the extent of lung disease are apparent and further investigation is obviated. A lung carcinoma or focal abnormality compatible with infection may be unmasked. Contrast-enhanced helical CT is increasingly being used for the detection of pulmonary embolism.

Therapeutic Problems in DPLD

The treatment of acute severe DPLD

Overwhelming disease may present acutely in a number of DPLD including CFA, drug-induced lung disease and connective tissue disease (e.g. diffuse alveolar haemorrhage, acute lupus pneumonitis). Due to small numbers at any one centre, optimal treatment has never been defined (other than anecdotally). One important principle is that in aggressive potentially fatal disease, under-treatment tends to be a more serious error than over-treatment. Thus, in patients requiring admission to the intense care unit, in whom a significant inflammatory component of disease is suspected, daily intravenous methylprednisolone (500mg–1000mg) is usually prescribed. Similarly, there is no overall consensus on the indications for immunosuppressive therapy at first presentation, but delay in starting treatment is to be avoided, as several days may be required for an immunosuppressive agent to take effect. However, with the recent development of rapidly acting intravenous cyclophosphamide regimens, this concern is less pressing; in diffuse alveolar haemorrhage syndromes, it is reasonable to use intravenous methylprednisolone initially and to add parenteral cyclophosphamide two to three days later in non-responders.

The treatment of pulmonary sarcoidosis

There are particular difficulties in standardising the indications for treatment in pulmonary sarcoidosis (Table 9). In principle, patients with limited non-progressive inflammation or fibrosis should be observed without therapeutic intervention, and it can be argued that those with overt progressive fibrotic disease ought to be treated in the hope of preventing further deterioration. However, between these extremes, there is a large sub-group with extensive disease consisting of a variable admixture of inflammation and fibrosis, and often the clinical presentation does not discriminate between stable and intrinsically progressive disease. In theory, failure to treat these

Table 9.   Prevalence of clinically overt disease in sarcoidosis

Patterns of disease	Prevalence in all patients
Lung/mediastinal lymph nodes (on chest X-ray or clinically)	90–95%
Non-specific systemic symptoms (fever, fatigue, weight loss, anorexia)	30%
Overt cutaneous disease	25%
Overt ocular disease	10–20%
Symptoms/signs of neurosarcoidosis	5–10%
Overt nasal disease	5–10%
Sicca symptoms (parotid disease)	5%
Overt laryngeal disease	5%
Clinical evidence of myocardial disease	5%
Major liver involvement	<5%
Acute arthritis	<5%
Bone disease	<5%
Chronic arthropathy	<2%
Massive splenomegaly (± hypersplenism)	<2%
Renal failure (due to hypercalcaemia or hypercalcuria)	<2%

patients may result in increasing irreversible fibrosis. In other DPLD, it is generally accepted that patients with extensive inflammation require treatment: spontaneous regression of disease is uncommon, and failure to intervene may have serious consequences, especially if the patient deteriorates rapidly. In sarcoidosis, the situation is less straightforward.

Firstly, a significant percentage of patients with pulmonary sarcoidosis exhibit spontaneous complete or partial regression of disease. When rapid deterioration occurs during a period of observation, a response to treatment is usual and thus the situation can generally be retrieved. Furthermore, although steroid therapy results in short term regression of inflammation, no definitive evidence exists that treatment modulates the long term course of disease in sarcoidosis. Therapeutic decisions are made more difficult by the fact that striking pulmonary involvement on chest radiography is often entirely reversible and may be associated with little or no functional impairment. The justification for intervention is that the potential benefits of treatment should outweigh the risk of side-effects. The problem in sarcoidosis is that the potential benefits of therapy are often uncertain.

Why treat at all in pulmonary sarcoidosis? In the absence of controlled data, clinicians must rely upon personal experience. Those who have treated a large cohort of sarcoidosis patients are convinced that a sub-group benefit greatly from therapy: in sarcoidosis, as in all diseases, lack of evidence of a treatment benefit is not the same as evidence of a lack of treatment benefit. The present consensus favours the long-term suppression of active inflammation once progressive disease has been identified. The difficulty lies in the early identification of those at risk of increasing irreversible disease. Currently, treatment is recommended in patients with *moderate or severe respiratory symptoms* and those with *increasing lung function impairment*. The indications for therapy are more contentious in *asymptomatic patients with persistent pulmonary infiltrates for 1–2 years*: many believe that intervention is warranted in the hope of 'switching off' inflammation and thus modulating the longer term course of disease.

In principle, morphological features on imaging ought to temper decisions on treatment. Stage II sarcoidosis on chest radiography (bilateral hilar adenopathy plus interstitial infiltrates) has a better prognosis, with a higher rate of spontaneous regression than stage III (non-fibrotic interstial infiltrates without hilar adenopathy) or stage IV (fibrocystic ILD) appearances. The threshold for treatment should be highest in stage II disease; by contrast, in overt stage IV disease, there is already evidence of a considerable 'track-record' of progressive fibrosis and thus, symptomatic or lung function decline should stimulate immediate attempts to alter the natural course of disease. Similarly, CT may eventually play an increasing role in identifying the presence of substantial fibrosis when the decision to treat is a close call. Thoracic radiologists have become adept at discriminating between reversible disease and extensive fibrotic disease, in which a response to treatment is unattainable and the cardinal therapeutic goal is the prevention of disease progression.

The prevailing view in the UK and Europe is that high dose corticosteroid therapy is warranted initially (e.g Prednisolone 40–60mg daily for one month), whereas intermediate doses used intermittently, as required, tend to be prescribed in the USA. The rationale for prolonged high dose treatment is the belief that rigorous suppression of inflammation at the outset might down-regulate disease activity and, thus, allow continued control with a 'civilised' maintenance dose (e.g. 20mg of Prednisolone on alternate days). After at least 12 months of treatment, it is usual to try to withdraw steroid therapy (and, in so doing, to establish the minimum steroid requirement to maintain control of disease). In a small minority, in whom continued high doses of corticosteroids are needed, a variety of 'steroid-sparing' agents have been used. These second-line agents, all with their advocates, include methotrexate, azathioprine, cyclophosphamide, hydroxychloroquine and cyclosporin.

The dilemma of whether to increase or decrease immunosuppression

Opportunistic infection is not always easy to diagnose as it sometimes simulates a primary respiratory disease for which the patient is receiving immunosuppressive therapy. Thus, the clinician may be faced with the dilemma of needing to treat a deterioration, knowing that an increase in immunosuppression may be either life-saving or life-threatening. This scenario is probably encountered most frequently in SLE, a disease characterised by a number of defects in immunological defences; patients with SLE are often young and may have a good prognosis if they survive an acute deterioration. Thus, it is important to discriminate between opportunistic infection, lupus pneumonitis and diffuse alveolar haemorrhage in the treated patient presenting with acute severe dyspnoea and pulmonary infiltrates. In this context, the single most important investigation is BAL, even if ventilation is required in order to perform the procedure. The correct management is either to reduce immunosuppression and prescribe appropriate anti-infective agents, based on BAL findings, or to increase immunosuppression (whether the diagnosis is lupus pneumonitis or diffuse alveolar haemorrhage).

Lung transplantation

Single lung transplantation is now the most commonly used transplantation procedure in DPLD. Current experience in DPLD is limited and the indications for transplantation are not well-defined. For example, patients with the limited form of systemic sclerosis (CREST syndrome) and pulmonary hypertension without other major organ involvement are thought to be suitable for transplantation in some centres; however, others have reported poor results. Thus, acceptance of DPLD patients for transplantation is likely to remain highly variable between centres.

A major difficulty in DPLD is to time referral for transplantation appropriately. In slowly but inexorably progressive sarcoidosis, Langerhans cell histiocytosis and lymphangioleiomyomatosis, it is often possible to anticipate when transplantation will become necessary. However, in more unpredictable, potentially explosive disorders (such as CFA), it is easy to miss a brief window of opportunity; a patient may seem to be stable, only to become severely compromised in a matter of months, and the pre-operative period may be prolonged due to the need to reduce the dose of corticosteroid therapy. There is no easy solution to this dilemma, but it is probably preferable to refer patients with CFA when Dlco levels are still 30% of predicted normal or higher.

References

Catzenstein A-LA, Myers JL. Idiopathic pulmonary fibrosis. Clinical relevance of pathological classification. *Am J Respir Crit Care Med* 1998;**157**:1301–1315

Hansell DM, Wells AU. CT evaluation of fibrosing alveolitis — applications and insights. *J Thoracic Imaging* 1996;**11**:231–249

Gay SE, Kazerooni EA, Toews GB et al. Idiopathic pulmonary fibrosis. Predicting response to therapy and survival. *Am J Respir Crit Care Med* 1998;**157**:1063–1072

Geddes DM. BOOP and COP. *Thorax* 1991;**46**(8):545–7

17

Occupational Lung Diseases

Rob Niven and Tony Pickering

Introduction

Occupational lung disease involves interaction between the working environment and some part of the respiratory system from nasal cavity to alveoli. The nature and extent of the exposure to a noxious agent and both the specific physiological and subsequent functional response within the individual will determine the disease presentation. It is almost without exception that occupational lung disease occurs from the inhalation of a dust particle, aerosol, fume or gas. Noxious agents can be presented to the body in a variety of forms:

- dusts   solid aerosols, derived from rocks and minerals
- fumes   solid aerosols (usually metals) formed by condensation from gaseous state
- smokes   solid aerosols derived from combustion
- vapours   gaseous form of substances normally found in liquid or solid state
- mists   liquid aerosol derived from liquid sources in form of droplets
- gases   gaseous form of a substance normally found in that form

Particle inhalation

The type, shape, size distribution and extent of individual exposure in the workplace will be determined by the working practices and this subsequently determines the nature and level of deposition of particles within the respiratory system.

Deposition of particles implies that contact is made between the particle and the alveolar or bronchial wall. Once contact is made, the particle cannot become airborne again. Small particles (< 1 micron) though inhaled, may not come into direct contact with the airway or alveolar surface and are expelled again. Particles of aerodynamic size between 2–5 micron are optimal for deposition in the respiratory tract. Ultra-fine particles 0.5 micron and below have good alveolar penetration and deposition. Particles of greater than 5 micron are most likely to impact in the upper respiratory tract or large airways. In the occupational setting, the nature of the raw material being used and the speed and force of machinery will determine the size of particles and ultimately their deposition within the lung.

Thus factors which may influence the individuals' risk of health effects from exposure in the working environment include:-

- particle size   smaller particles deposit more peripherally
- particle shape   fibres may reach peripherally despite large longitudinal length due to aerodynamic properties
- aggregation   aggregation of particles sometimes achieved intentionally by 'wetting' increases particle size and therefore reduces deposition
- disturbance   disturbance of settled dust or air currents will keep particles in the workers breathing zone for longer increasing exposure
- exercise   physically demanding jobs involve an increase in the minute volume of respiration and lead to mouth breathing, increasing individual exposure.

The resultant physiological response to the occupational exposure will subsequently be determined by:-

- properties of the agent   agent escapes the normal defence mechanisms
toxic local cell damage,
impairment of cell function or of their enzymes
immune mediated response

- clearance

  the effectiveness of the individual natural defence mechanisms will be influenced by smoking habits, pre-existing lung disease, natural variation and exposure to toxic or other irritant gases

- host factors

  including defects either congenital or acquired in the defence mechanisms, immune function and hypersensitivity reactions

- atopic status

  atopic individuals are more likely to react to certain occupational agents

Once exposed and after the agent has exerted a physiological response within the individual, the functional response of the worker will additionally influence the presentation. Epidemiological studies have demonstrated that females report more non-specific symptoms in relation to the working environment than males and Asian workers in the UK report symptoms less frequently than White Caucasians. In practice it is also possible to identify individuals who will withstand or adapt to very severe disabling occupational lung disease, but who fail to report it for fear of job loss or because they think it is expected that they experience their symptoms. Other workers may exaggerate symptoms if compensation is a personal driving force.

Occupational Asthma

Definitions

The terms and definitions used to define obstructive lung disease associated with the work environment are presented below. Unfortunately there is not universal agreement about the usage of these terms and particularly the definition of occupational asthma. The most currently accepted definitions are included.

Occupational asthma
Variable airways obstruction causally related to exposure in the working environment to a dust, fume or vapour.
Hypersensitivity inducer an agent capable of inducing an immunologically mediated airway inflammatory process.
Toxic inducer this may take two forms:

- an agent capable of exacerbating pre-existing airflow obstruction or hyper-reactivity through a non-immunological mechanism (recent attention has focused on the role of passive inhalation of environmental tobacco smoke — the available evidence suggests this only acts as a mild irritant)
- reactive airways dysfunction syndrome — relates to the development of persistent airway reactivity following a single exposure usually to a high level of toxic agent in an individual with no history of pre-existing respiratory disease

Prevalence of occupational asthma

The true prevalence of occupation asthma in the adult asthmatic population is unknown. Various estimates have been made and range between 2 and 15% of total adult asthma cases. Studies within high risk occupational settings have reported prevalences ranging widely: snow-crab processors — 15%; isocyanates — 12%; small mammal workers — 4%. Recent national surveillance schemes may ultimately produce more accurate data, but early estimates of incidence from this scheme suggested 22 cases per million working population per year (with incidence twice as high in men as women).

Aetiological agents

The list of agents accepted as inducers has dramatically increased. In 1989 only 14 agents were compensatable in the UK for occupational asthma. There are currently over 250 chemicals which have been suggested to act as respiratory sensitisers. Compensation from the state is now available for all cases of occupational asthma where there is evidence of exposure to a known respiratory sensitiser in the workplace. The specific regional importance of agents responsible for occupational asthma depends heavily on the local industries. For example in Canada, extensive data is available in wood workers (particularly Western Red Cedar), grain dust and fish/shell fish processing. In the UK, isocyanates, laboratory animals and bakery workers have been extensively studied. More details on aetiological agents can be found from the publications from the national occupational lung disease reporting schemes (SWORD in the UK).

Predisposing factors

Certain factors have been shown to increase the risk of the development of occupational asthma within specific working populations these include:

- **smoking**
  increased risk demonstrated in: tetrachlorophthalic anhydride
  ispaghula
  green coffee bean
  platinum salts
  snow-crab workers
- **atopy** pre-existing atopic status as defined by positive skin prick tests to one or more of a number of common airborne environmental allergens has been shown to be a risk factor for a number of occupational inducers, most notably those with a high molecular weight capable of producing IgE antibodies such as laboratory animals and enzymes (*Bacillus subtilis*) and also for platinum salts.
- **constitutional asthma** while this has been suggested as a risk factor for an increased risk of occupational asthma, good epidemiological data to confirm this is lacking. Problems occur in separating, with certainty, constitutional asthma aggravated by work irritants and respiratory sensitisation. It is however common practice to prevent known asthmatics taking up work exposed to well documented respiratory sensitisers.
- **single peak exposures** it has been suggested anecdotally and supported from predominantly uncontrolled opportunistic studies that single peak exposures to a sensitising agent confers a greater risk of developing occupational asthma than continuous low level exposures.

Clinical features

The symptoms and signs of occupational asthma are as for constitutional asthma. The important feature is the temporal nature of the symptoms in relation to the workplace. They should improve on rest days, but in some cases, particularly after exposure has persisted for months or years after the symptoms first started, many days or weeks of cessation of exposure may be required before symptoms improve. Symptoms are frequently but not invariably recognised as being worse on work days, but because some of the responses are delayed, the symptoms may occur in the evening after work has finished and therefore the relationship to work may not be suspected by the individual. The relationship between first exposure and the onset of disease is highly variable. For most sensitising agents symptoms usually develop within the first two years of exposure though there are exceptions, e.g. bakers for whom a prolonged period of asymptomatic exposure may predate disease.

Diagnosis

The following factors may assist in the diagnosis of occupational asthma. However in complex cases the diagnosis can be difficult and specialist referral is advisable and frequently essential.

Exposure

An accurate occupational history is required to determine the nature of current exposure and to identify the agent which is responsible. There is usually documentable evidence of exposure to a known sensitiser. However difficulties arise in the case of new or previously unidentified potential respiratory sensitisers or in working situations where exposure to more than one respiratory sensitiser coexist.

Clinical history

The presence of work related respiratory symptoms does not make the diagnosis of occupational asthma (respiratory sensitisation). A Canadian study demonstrated that an individual work related symptom had a high sensitivity but low specificity for occupational asthma subsequently diagnosed using occupational peak flow recordings or specific occupational challenge.

Past atopic, smoking and respiratory symptoms should be clearly recorded at initial interview. Potential compensation claims can often alter the perception of individuals with regard to these factors and it is crucial to determine and record their status accurately at the outset. The individual may have already ceased exposure on medical advise or may make a compensation claim retrospectively after finishing work.

Occupational peak flow recordings

If a worker is still working in the implicated industry and their asthma is not severe, occupational peak flow recordings are the primary diagnostic tool. Frequent recordings (usually made two hourly) are taken on work and rest days and preferably during an additional period of absence (holiday of one week or more). It may take some time for the asthma to improve during a period of absence from work and a holiday within the study period will improve the specificity of testing. It should however be remembered that a major proportion of constitutional asthmatics also improve when on holiday. Frequent recordings (two hourly) have also been demonstrated to improve the specificity of the investigation. Inhaled steroids taken during peak flow monitoring reduce the sensitivity of the tool as they modify peak flow variation and the apparent response to occupational exposure. The interpretation of peak flow recordings has traditionally been the responsibility of a specialist opinion following a plot of maximum, mean and minimum peak flow recorded on a day to day basis. Diurnal variation is more sensitive than absolute values, with improvement on rest days compared to working days. Frequent use of reliever medication, may keep maximum recorded peak flow high, but with frequent recording the diurnal variation can be seen to be greater on work days. Figures 1–3 give examples of peak flow charts in occupational asthma. More recently a commercial computer system has been devised to reduce the observer variation in interpretation. OASYS is the one currently available in the UK and gives computer generated graphs and predictions of the diagnosis. Peak flow recordings cannot be used if further exposure is deemed to be an unacceptable risk to the individual for fear of an acute, severe or life threatening attack.

Non-specific bronchial hyper-reactivity
While not diagnostic in any way, the return of normal bronchial reactivity after exposure ceases is a useful monitoring and prognostic tool and can give additional support for the diagnosis if it is in doubt.

Specific occupational agent challenge
Exposure of the individual to the offending agent in controlled hospital conditions is the gold standard diagnostic test. A positive response identified by a 15% early or late fall in FEV_1 after a controlled exposure in excess of any drop occurring following a blinded placebo challenge is the optimum response. A two fold doubling of non-specific hyper-reactivity after exposure compared to pre-challenge can be used as a supportive diagnostic criterion. The practical problem with performing such tests is the determination of an appropriate exposure to imitate a genuine occupational exposure. They should only be performed in centres with experience of the test as too high an exposure could precipitate a life threatening asthma attack.

Immunological investigation

Raised levels of specific IgE (usually using the radio-allergo-absorbent test RAST) are found in cases of occupational asthma to a number of agents and most commonly those with a high molecular weight. These include animal allergens, enzymes, flour and grain workers. IgE to hapten-protein conjugates have been identified in other occupations including anhydrides and reactive dyes. Unfortunately a positive IgE does not diagnose occupational asthma as in a number of industries, raised levels can be seen in currently and prospectively followed employees who remain asymptomatic. In addition IgE antibodies are not commonly found with low-molecular weight chemicals and this limits their usefulness.

Skin prick testing to occupational agents may be performed for example for laboratory animal workers, detergent workers and with platinum salts, but the same limitations exist. In high-risk industries skin testing is used prospectively to identify early sensitisation.

Diagnosis — summary

The diagnostic tools available are limited in their sensitivity and specificity. The diagnosis has such major implications to the health and financial future of the individual that as accurate a diagnosis as possible should be made and it is for this reason that it is frequently advisable to get expert advise before a diagnostic opinion is given to patient or employer.

Management

Pharmacological management of occupational asthma is no different than for constitutional asthma. The major management issue rests with continuing exposure and therefore often with potential individual employment. Many studies have demonstrated that the prognosis of occupational asthma is directly related to the length of time that exposure continues after symptoms develop. Following diagnosis, deterioration of the asthmatic condition should be expected if exposure continues.

Cessation of exposure has to be complete as once sensitised, minimal exposure to the agent concerned may cause marked clinical response. In some cases effected workers may not be able to visit the work site again even to attend Personnel or Occupational Health, without developing symptoms.

Because of the implications to the future employment the advice has to be clear and it is hoped that it is supported by both specialist, general practitioner and occupational health professional where relevant.

Prognosis

Unfortunately, even if work with the offending agent is avoided, it is now known that between 33 and 50% of affected individuals will continue to experience asthmatic symptoms. The prognosis varies with the aetiological agent and may be worse for low molecular weight chemicals. Prognosis is better the earlier exposure ceases after the onset of symptoms.

Compensation

Recent studies have demonstrated profound impact of occupational asthma on earning capacity, long term health status and quality of life. It is not unreasonable that financial compensation is available for individuals with occupational asthma. Two sources currently exist in the UK.

State compensation

A pension is available if a diagnosis of occupational asthma is agreed. The amount of money provided is relatively small and is related to the degree of ongoing disability and will be withdrawn if the asthma remits completely. The process is usually relatively quick and easy but does not preclude a future civil case.

Civil case

The employee may take a civil case against their employer as long as they can prove that the employer did not satisfactorily safe guard their health or were deemed to have acted in a negligent fashion. The amount of compensation is determined by a combination of factors including, the loss of earnings experienced as a result of the ill health and to the 'suffering' experienced. It is important to bear in mind that the diagnosis alone is not sufficient to guarantee success in obtaining compensation if the employer can prove that they acted within best guidelines, gave appropriate information and sufficient occupational health and safety as might have been deemed reasonable for the expected risk. In practice the court rarely finds against the plaintiff unless the diagnosis is in serious doubt.

Reactive airways dysfunction syndrome (RADS)

Reactive airways dysfunction syndrome is the complex of bronchial hyper-reactivity with associated symptoms of cough, wheeze and breathlessness following a significant exposure to an irritant substance. Some of the gases and chemicals that can be responsible are discussed in later sections. The characteristic symptoms are the relatively poor response to treatment with steroids, either inhaled or systemic and the protracted course. The exposures are not always occupational and can follow accidental exposure and domestic or industrial fires. Information on numerous cases can be gained from disasters including the Manchester Air Disaster and London Underground fire. Investigation takes the form of lung function testing, (airways reversibility is variable), non-specific bronchial hyper-reactivity is invariably witnessed, but there is little or no improvement following steroid therapy. Most patients improve slowly over time but many remain permanently effected to some degree.

Occupational bronchitis emphysema or COPD

The terminology for this group of disorders is imprecisely used. A number of occupational exposures have been demonstrated epidemiologically to be associated with an excess of chronic bronchitis or COPD. Many of the studies have defined patients by MRC criteria for chronic bronchitis and lung function. In few of these has the assessment been complete enough to confirm an irreversible process or where studies included an adequate control population. The major methodological problems have revolved around adequate controlling for cigarette smoking. Other studies are inadequate because of lack of exposure measurements to study dose response effects.

Aetiological agents or occupations associated with an excess of either chronic obstructive pulmonary disease, symptomatic chronic bronchitis or emphysema where there is convincing evidence of excess disease in workers after adequate controlling for cigarette smoking and for which a dose response relationship supports the case, include:

- coal workers
- gold miners (predominantly silica exposure)
- cotton textile workers
- cadmium — emphysema specifically

Less convincing but suggestive evidence exists for the following:

- welding
- carbon black workers
- organic dust exposed worker
- asbestos workers

Diagnosis and management

The occupational aetiology is normally only suspected rather than proven in individual cases, but in lifelong non-smokers the suspicion will be much greater. At the current time it is only coal miners with a documented high occupational exposure history who can be compensated for their disease through the state system. Management is as for smoking related COPD, but cessation of exposure should be considered in all but mild disease.

The Pneumoconioses

Pneumoconiosis is a name given to a number of inflammatory lung diseases caused directly by the inhalation of dust aerosols at work. Most of the agents responsible are mineral dusts which have reached the alveolar region. The dust particles have to be retained in sufficient number within the area to cause disease. This may be created by a balance between high or continued exposure and difficulty in clearance.

Basic pathogenesis

Disease occurs in response to inhalation of mineral dusts which cause an inflammatory reaction usually with the formation of collagen. The collagen can form in small nodules and appear as non-specific X-ray appearances, or may form as typical lung fibrosis with extensive collagen formation and progressive disease. With the metal dust diseases, the nodules formed may appear to contain metal components and the opacities may be very dense on X-ray. The density is determined by the atomic number of the mineral. Examples of dusts capable of causing pneumoconioses include:

- dusts heavily laden with silica (>20%) typically cause fibrosis initially in the form of nodules. The nodules are usually up to 5–6mm in size and have a propensity to form in the upper zones
- silica poor dusts. These include coal where silica is not present in high concentrations. The characteristic appearances are of small nodules 5mm in diameter which may later coalesce

- fibrous dusts including asbestos. The lower and posterior parts of the lung are usually affected first. The parenchyma is more diffusely infiltrated than in either of the above causes
- inert dusts (metals). Tin, antimony, barium and oxides of titanium are examples of inert dusts. Their high atomic numbers and reduced clearance give radiological appearances of small very dense opacities. Histologically fibrosis around the dust macules is absent or scanty (Table 1)

Clinical features

Clinical features vary depending on the causative agent and can vary from asymptomatic (simple coal workers pneumoconiosis and some metal diseases such as stannosis), to a severe lung fibrosis (exposure to asbestos or silica). There is contention as to whether the co-existing emphysema in simple coal workers pneumoconiosis is directly caused by the occupational exposure or the frequently co-existent heavy smoking. Recent epidemiological work has suggested that disability in coal miners is caused by obstructive lung disease and not the pneumoconiosis. Symptoms when they occur are usually breathlessness, occasionally accompanied by non-productive cough.

Investigation

Clinical history

Clinical history is relevant to determine the extent of disability based on the impact of the pneumoconioses on the physical capacity of the individual with regard to physical exercise and activities of normal life. However the impact of other diseases on the respiratory state have to be considered and the occupational history is central to this. Assessment of exposure should include nature of the work, hours worked, intensity, duration and use of respiratory protection, which was rarely used prior to the 1980s.

Radiographic appearances

Pneumoconiosis is diagnosed and characterised by the radiological appearances. While there is a poor correlation between the extent of radiological change and respiratory impairment in many cases, the degree of radiological abnormality is probably a better marker of lifetime exposure to dust. To help characterise the radiological changes the ILO (International Labour Organisation) developed a classification schedule based on the presence, size, shape and extent of the radiological appearances on plain X-ray. Clinical pictures are compared to a standard set of films, giving examples of each type of abnormality. The classification is available from the ILO or can be found summarised in the referenced texts.

CT scanning

Computed tomography, especially with high resolution images, demonstrates the overall distribution of nodules, pleural disease and coexistent emphysematous change.

Lung function testing

Pulmonary function can determine the presence and extent of either obstructive (COPD not pneumoconiosis — particularly in coal miners) and restrictive (eg. asbestosis and silicosis) components of disease.

Pathology

It is rarely necessary to perform lung biopsy to make the diagnosis of pneumoconiosis. The exception occurs when a moderate lung infiltrate is associated with what appears to a very minor past exposure.

Management

As with many occupational lung diseases the major management issue relates to further exposure to the offending agent. With silicosis and asbestosis cessation of continued exposure should be mandatory if a firm diagnosis is made as the disease will progress in the presence of continued occupational exposure. Advise is more complex with simple coal workers pneumoconiosis for which the disease does not appear to cause significant physiological impairment although there remains a risk of developing progressive massive fibrosis if exposure continues. For the inert dusts, continued exposure is unlikely to be harmful, but in some cases the radiological appearances will remit when exposure ceases.

Silicosis

Affected Occupations:

- mining — gold, tin, copper, platinum, mica and coal where silica is found in association

- quarrying — granite, sandstone, slate
- tunnelling — seams of rock may contain veins rich in silica
- stone working — involving cutting, sanding or grinding of quarried sandstone
- 'sand-blasting' — abrasive cleaning using sand or salt particles of metals, buildings etc
- glass making — modern technology has reduced exposure and disease now seen only in small industry or workers from developing countries
- foundries — silica sand is used to make the cores and moulds into which the metal is poured
- ceramic industry

Acute silicosis

Acute massive exposures may cause *acute silicosis* which is characterised by fulminant respiratory failure. The exposure has to be high and of small particle size. It may occur in any of the settings above particularly if exposure has been unexpected and with no respiratory protection. Although rare, cases in the UK still occur. Breathlessness is associated with fever, ground glass shadowing on X-ray, and an almost invariable fatal outcome. Treatment with steroids and alveolar lavage has been recommended but without evidence of beneficial effect.

Chronic silicosis

If uncomplicated it is called 'ordinary' silicosis. Features are of breathlessness and cough, although no symptoms may be present at first. Finger clubbing does NOT occur and crackles are not a prominent feature. In the advanced cases respiratory failure may ensue. Radiological appearances vary, but often commence with small nodules in the upper zones. Linear opacities may also be seen. The total dust exposure is well correlated to the extent of radiological change. As the disease progresses, the number and size of nodules increase and the lower lobes may become involved. Nodules may also coalesce to form larger areas of increased density. Hilar lymph node eggshell calcification is seen in some cases and in others the parenchymal nodules appear very dense and may contain microlithiasis. The presence of calcification is not correlated with exposure.

Investigation

Initially lung function tests are normal, but later a restrictive pattern may develop. Positive rheumatoid factors or ANF may suggest the development of suddenly advancing silicosis. ESR is not raised although some reports have suggested serum ACE may be raised in silicosis.

Complications

- tuberculosis — the development of muco purulent sputum or haemoptysis in a patient with silicosis should be considered as suspicious
- pneumothorax
- rheumatoid syndrome (rapid progression with positive rheumatoid factor)
- scleroderma
- cor pulmonale (although this is rare)

A link between silicosis and lung cancer has been the subject of recent topical debate. It appears that if present, it is only in those with historical high exposures with definite fibrosis (not in exposed workers without evidence of established silicosis) and the risk may be no more than that of individuals with cryptogenic fibrosis. The conclusion is, cancer risk is related only indirectly to silicosis once fibrosis has developed.

Simple coal workers pneumoconiosis (SCWP)

Prevalence

The number of coal workers who develop pneumoconiosis is determined predominantly by the level of cumulative exposure to coal dust. On the basis of radiological evidence it rises from 2% at 160 000 hmg/m^3 to 10% at 360 000 hmg/m^3.

Features

Radiological changes are as described in the ILO classification. The nodules are caused by discreet fibrotic nodules with normal lung intervening. Symptoms and signs are usually absent and pulmonary physiology unchanged in the absence of complications or associated emphysema.

Diagnosis

Diagnosis is purely by radiological changes. Rheumatoid factor may be positive in Caplan's syndrome

Complications

- progressive massive fibrosis are areas of dense fibrosis seen in the upper lobes. They contain an excess of black dust and can be distinguished from the areas of coalescence of silicotic nodules on the basis of the absence of the characteristic whorled pattern seen in silicosis. PMF occurs more predominantly if the coal has a high quartz content. Unlike SCWP, PMF is associated with pulmonary impairment, reduced gas transfer and subsequently breathlessness
- tuberculosis is more common in individuals with PMF and may not respond to therapy
- rheumatoid nodules may cavitate and may occur in the presence of a positive rheumatoid factor (Caplan's syndrome) frequently in the absence of simple pneumoconiosis.

There is no evidence that SCWP causes pulmonary heart disease, nor is there a link with cancer of the lung

Pneumoconiosis of inert dusts

The terminology 'inert' is probably inappropriate as any dust may be able to exert a biological effect purely by its presence. However, this title still remains in common usage and relates to pneumoconiosis resulting from a number of dust exposures where the outcome is thought to cause no physiological effect in terms of lung function or symptomatic impairment.

The agents causing these 'benign' pneumoconiosis range from metal fumes to inorganic compounds for which fibrosis and collagen formation are not a feature.

Table 1 gives a summary of some of the agents which fall into this category.

Asbestos Related Diseases

Asbestos is a term used to describe a group of mineral fibres of silicate origin. It is the fibrous nature of the mineral which is the characteristic of asbestos and which is responsible for its pathogenicity. However the physical properties of the fibre, are also

Table 1. Pneumoconiosis of inert dusts

Agent	Specific name	Occupation	X-ray	Specific features
Iron	Siderosis	Mining Steel rolling mills Grinding, fettling Welding (electric and oxyacetylene) Boiler scaling	Profuse small (0.5–2mm) rounded opacities high density	Reddish coloured sputum Pleura, marbled and rust coloured Parenchyma – grey rust coloured nodules Microscopy – aggregates of iron particles
Tin	Stannosis	Milling and grinding of ore Smelting, plating and grinding of tin	Moderate size (2–4mm) Very dense numerous nodules	Macroscopically grey/black nodules Tin containing macrophages
Antimony	Antimony pneumoconiosis	Mining or crusing ore Smelting & alloy workers Manufacture of pigments, glass enamels	Numerous small opacities Denser hilar regions Dust laden macrophages	Orange staining to teeth suggests exposure Rhinitis, nasal septal ulceration/skin rash
Titanium	(Titanosis/titanocosis)	Mining of rock containing ilemlite Pigment manufacture	Small roundish opacities	Carbon like aggregates – peribronchiolar
Barium	Baritosis	Mining Glass manufacture	Extremely dense irregular opacities, clearing after exposure ceases	Pulmonary & pleural grey macules
Low density dusts – marble – cement/concrete – limestone – gypsum – silicon carbide		quarrying construction/demolition quarrying/milling mining, milling carborundum manufacture & abrasives	Normal radiographs	Associated radiographic abnormalities, lung function abnormality and symptoms thought to be due to associated exposure to silica which frequently coexists with these minerals

responsible for its usefulness (fire resistance, non-conductive, resistance to acids, alkalis, physical strength and its ability to be turned into yarn). It is found naturally in Canada, Russia, parts of South America and South Africa, southern Asia and parts of Europe.

Classification of asbestos

Amphiboles	Crocidolite (blue asbestos)
	Amosite (brown asbestos)
	Tremolite
	Anthophyllite
	Actinolite
Serpentine	Chrysotile (white asbestos)

Crocidolite has been particularly associated with the malignant consequences of asbestos exposure. The long straight fibres allow its penetration to the periphery of the lung and are more difficult for the body to remove than chrysotile fibres. A voluntary ban on the use of crocidolite was initiated in 1969, but its' use has been completely banned since 1986 (along with amosite). The fibres of tremolite while straight are shorter and more brittle than crocidolite, with resulting reduced pathogenicity. Tremolite however can contaminate chrysotile at low levels and can be found naturally in soils. It has been postulated that it is the contamination of chrysotile with tremolite rather than chrysotile itself which is responsible for the mesothelioma risk associated with chrysotile mining.

The fibres of chrysotile are smaller and are curved giving them an effective greater aerodynamic size than the amphiboles. Their use outside UK and USA has remained extensive.

Uses and some occupational exposure situations are summarised in Table 2.

Asbestos bodies

These commence as fibres usually greater than 10 micron in length. They are usually incompletely engulfed by a macrophage which breaks down leaving a coating on the fibre. This is initially colourless, but turns brown over time. Thickening tends to occur at each end, giving it a dumb-bell appearance. It is thought that some of these bodies remain in the lung indefinitely, though it is more likely a proportion of them breakdown into smaller fragments and are therefore eventually engulfed and digested. Most of these bodies in

Table 2. Sources and nature of exposure to asbestos

Source	Asbestos type	Uses	Nature of exposure
Mining and milling	chrysotile amphibole	source source	Open cast mining, exposure moderate Underground mining – traditional mining techniques. High exposure risk, reduced by wetting rock to aggregate particles
Asbestos cement	crocidolite & chrysotile	Cladding Roofing Sheeting	Often mixed on site but made into slurry Highest exposed worker – mixing raw asbestos with liquid base Low exposure to vicinity workers
Lagging	crocidolite (historically) chrysotile	Insulation fire protection	Traditionally mixed on site as above – mixing worker high exposed Slurry applied by hand or sprayed on (wet therefore low/moderate exposure) Low exposure to vicinity workers
Textiles	mixed	fire protective fibres/materials	Traditionally spun and woven dry with high exposure to all workers Wetting of process reduces exposure where it is still performed (rare)
Dismantling	mixed	–	Breaking ships, locomotives with heavy asbestos content – high exposure risk Uncontrolled until recently, drilling, sawing, etc, producing high concentration dry asbestos fibres

Table 2. Continued

Source	Asbestos type	Uses	Nature of exposure
Dock workers	mixed	Importing	Traditionally asbestos imported in dry fragile sacking, with resultant moderate exposure Leak-proof sealed bagging reduces risk
Break linings	chrysotile	transport	Low level asbestos exposure
Furnace/kiln workers	mixed	fire insulation	Workers had heavy exposure intermittently when the kilns or furnaces were stripped and reset.
Vicinity workers	mixed	–	Workers in the vicinity and down stream from direct asbestos exposure include electricians and pipe fitters Wives of exposed workers who maintained their clothing may have had similar low level exposure
Environmental exposure	mixed		Low level environmental exposure will occur from asbestos parts used in buildings, naturally occurring asbestos, brake linings etc. No epidemiological risk can be currently attributed to this exposure

environmentally exposed people will be amphiboles, identifying their lung persistence over chrysotile fibres. In individuals heavily exposed to chrysotile, many bodies can be found derived from chrysotile fibres, indicating that they do have a capacity (though less so than amphiboles) to avoid degradation by macrophages.

Estimating lung burden

Pulmonary fibrosis, lung cancer and mesothelioma can all occur with or without asbestos exposure. Attributing the disease to possible asbestos exposure can in part be determined from an occupational history. The presence of high levels of asbestos bodies within lung tissue will support a significant past exposure and therefore an aetiological role. Interpretation of findings will depend on the laboratory techniques used and a large variation occurs. Specimens used, whether alveolar lavage, wet or dried lung preparations and light or electron microscopy for counting all influence the results.

Asbestosis is associated with a high fibre burden (usually >10^6 fibres per g of dried lung), while mesothelioma occurs with lower levels. Levels of asbestos bodies in apparently unexposed workers can range widely, presumably related to environmental or hidden occupational sources or different patterns of removal of fibres within individuals.

Asbestos related disease

The following conditions may occur following significant asbestos exposure:

- asbestosis
- mesothelioma
- lung cancer
- benign pleural plaques
- diffuse pleural thickening
- benign pleural effusion

They will be considered for their prevalence, clinical features, diagnosis and prognosis independently.

Asbestosis

The prevalence of the disease in exposed workers is directly related to the degree of exposure, with a clear dose-response effect. A no effect level of 25 fibres/ml years has been suggested, below which, clinically significant asbestosis will not develop. The latent period between exposure and the development of disease is now, on average, at least 20 years. The signs and symptoms are as for any form of pulmonary fibrosis. Clubbing occurs in about 1/3 of cases. Radiologically, the changes appear first in the lower zones, with fine linear opacities which may cross each other. The linear opacities may become thicker and mimic 'Kerley B' lines. As the disease progresses the linear and irregular opacities become more coarse and extensive with the costo-phrenic and cardio-phrenic angles worst affected. It has been suggested that the CT appearances are more specific for asbestosis with peripheral changes appearing first, but these are not always diagnostic. Lung function shows typical features of a restrictive defect with reduced gas transfer. Broncho-alveolar lavage shows a small increase in neutrophils and lymphocytes. The former may help to differentiate asbestosis from extrinsic allergic alveolitis.

The diagnosis is made in the presence of typical features and a suitable occupational history. The presence of other features of asbestos related disease such as pleural disease will strongly support the diagnosis. Corticosteroids are unhelpful in therapy. Cessation of exposure is obviously mandatory.

The prognosis with regard to the fibrosis after cessation of exposure is usually relatively good. The extent of radiographic change appears to predict the progression which is worse in more advanced disease at diagnosis and in those with a higher historical exposure. Overall prognosis is affected by the high incidence of lung cancer in individuals who develop asbestosis, especially in those who also smoke cigarettes. Lung cancer is the commonest cause of death in individuals with asbestosis (approximately 34%).

Mesothelioma

Mesothelioma is a malignant tumour of the mesothelial membrane of the pleura or peritoneum. The incidence of mesothelioma has been increasing, predominantly in men since the mid 60s and recent estimates suggest we have not reached the peak. Death rates for mesothelioma were 20 per million in men and 3 per million in women in 1984. The vast majority are pleural in origin with a ratio to peritoneal tumour of approximately 10:1. The incidence of disease is much higher in asbestos workers than non-exposed workers and is higher for crocidolite compared to chrysotile exposed workers. There is some suggestion that workers exposed to pure chrysotile have a very low incidence of mesothelioma. The difference between the two fibre types relates to the fibre shape and the persistence of the fibre within the lung as discussed above.

The latent period from exposure to development of mesothelioma is very long (usually 30 years or more) and on this basis it is predicted that in the next 10 years the number of cases will continue to increase.

Unlike asbestosis, a strong dose response relationship is not evident. Most studies have shown that those exposed to high levels of amphiboles and particularly crocidolite are most at risk. About 8% of workers who have asbestosis as a marker of their high exposure go on to develop mesothelioma. However it also develops in individuals with trivial past exposure including down stream workers (including wives of asbestos workers from exposure from contaminated clothing) and this has fuelled the suggestion that small quantities of exposure are sufficient to develop mesothelioma in those predisposed.

The tumour is highly malignant but has a low propensity to disseminate, spreading invasively locally and frequently encircling the lung. It may invade the chest wall, frequently through the tracks of investigation sites (biopsy scars, needle biopsy and needle aspiration).

There are a number of histological variants which have different patterns of progression and a new staging system has been proposed. These are summarised in Table 3.

Clinical features

The presenting feature may be breathlessness where an associated pleural effusion develops. Severe localised chest pain may develop and is usually a later feature. Breathlessness may also occur if the mesothelioma is advanced and compressing or encircling the lung. Signs if present are those of a pleural effusion or thickening.

The radiological features are of a pleural usually lobulated tumour, which may extend around the costal margin or of a pleural effusion. If the tumour is suspected radiologically it is preferable to limit the number of investigation tracks through the chest wall because of the possibility of tumour invasion, which can be an unpleasant and a poorly treatment responsive complication. Large biopsy specimens are preferable to needle biopsies because the histological diagnosis and differentiation from adenocarcinoma is

Table 3.   Histological classification, TNM and Stage group grading classification for mesothelioma

Histological Sub-types
Epithelioid, Sarcomatoid, Desmoplastic, Biphasic, (Other)

TNM staging

Tx	Tumour cannot be assessed
To	No tumour
T1	Limited to ipsilateral parietal and/or visceral pleura
T2	Invasion of any of: ipsilateral lung, endothoracic fascia, diaphragm, pericardium.
T3	Invasion of any of: chest wall, ribs, mediastinal organ or tissue
T4	Invasion of any of: contralateral pleura or lung, perotoneum, intra-abdominal organs, cervical tissues
Nx	Nodes cannot be assessed
No	No node involvement
N1	Ipsilateral, peribronchial or hilar nodes (including direct extension).
N2	Metastases in: ipsilateral mediastinal and/or sub-carinal nodes
N3	Metastases in: contralateral mediastinal or hilar nodes or isplateral or contralateral scalene or supraclavicular nodes
Mx	Distant metastases cannot be assessed
Mo	No distant metastases
M1	Distant metastases at any site

Stage grading

Stage I	T1	No	Mo
	T2	No	Mo
Stage II	T1	N1	Mo
	T2	N1	Mo
Stage III	T1	N2	Mo
	T2	N2	Mo
	T3	No,1,2	Mo
Stage IV	Any T	N3	Mo
	T4	Any N	Mo
	Any T	Any N	M1

difficult and mis-diagnoses are not uncommon. As a result, thoracoscopy or open biopsy may be preferable, depending on local service availability.

Treatment is often conservative although modern chemotherapy has been associated with tumour response in a minority of cases. In a small number of cases with localised disease, radical surgery has been attempted in some centres. The surgery is disfiguring with major chest wall repair being required and evidence of benefit is restricted to a few highly selected patients. Otherwise supportive care, pain control and local radiotherapy for chest wall invasion is recommended for the majority of cases.

The prognosis is poor almost without exception, with a mean actuarial survival of between 12 and 18 months but varying with cell type.

Asbestos and lung cancer

As with mesothelioma and asbestosis, amphibole asbestos offers a greater risk than serpentine (chrysotile) asbestos. For lung cancer however there is a clear dose response relationship between cumulative exposure and cancer risk. There is also epidemiological evidence of a level of exposure below which, lung cancer risk is not increased. As with asbestosis, it is considered that the level is associated with the capacity of the macrophages to maintain a balance of cytokines and once this level has been surpassed, the risk develops. Cigarette smoking and asbestos have at least additive (and probably multiplicative) risk towards lung cancer, suggesting that they act synergistically. There remains a problem with the attribution of lung cancer to asbestos exposure in ex-workers, when the exposure history is unclear and in the absence of asbestosis. At present the state system will only allow compensation for lung cancer in those individuals with asbestosis or other markers of high exposure (diffuse pleural disease).

The diagnosis, management and prognosis of asbestos induced lung cancer is similar to that of non-asbestos cases except that the threshold of suspicion should be higher and the possibility for radical surgery lower if asbestosis is present.

Benign pleural disease and asbestos

Plaques develop from the parietal pleura. They consist of circumscribed areas of hyaline fibrosis which may be partially calcified and in themselves cause no functional impairment. Diffuse pleural thickening emanates from the visceral pleura and if extensive can cause a restrictive ventilatory defect. The prevalence of plaques and diffuse thickening is dependent on the nature of occupational exposure and the method of reporting (radiological, pathological etc.). In one study only 15% of plaques found at autopsy had been documented prior to death. A dose response relationship exists between exposure and risk of plaque formation, but recent studies have suggested that this is not with total cumulative dose but only with time since first occupational exposure (a pattern more akin to mesothelioma than to asbestosis and lung cancer). Approximately 20% of heavily exposed individuals may be expected to develop diffuse pleural thickening or pleural plaques.

Plaques are symptomless and can affect the costal, diaphragmatic or mediastinal/pericardial pleura.

Pleural thickening can occasionally cause non-specific chest pain. Radiology varies depending on the site. Seen tangentially, a sharp medial edge is apparent but when seen face-on, a simple blurred shadow with no sharp borders occurs. The costo-phrenic angle is frequently obliterated. CT is a more sensitive method of detection than plain X-ray.

Both plaques and diffuse thickening may be seen to progress over time even after exposure has ceased. Epidemiologically, neither appears to be a marker of increased mesothelioma or cancer risk, but are markers of significant asbestos exposure. Specific treatment is not usually indicated.

Benign pleural effusions have been demonstrated as being more common than expected in asbestos workers, but proving the aetiological role of asbestos in individuals is more a process of exclusion. Most cases are symptom free and resolve spontaneously.

Compensation for asbestos related disease

State compensation is now available in the UK for asbestosis, diffuse pleural thickening, mesothelioma, primary carcinoma of the lung where there is accompanying evidence of asbestosis and/or diffuse pleural thickening. Claim forms specifically for asbestos related diseases are available from the DSS. Pension for asbestosis is based on degree of disability. Mesothelioma because of its poor prognosis usually attracts 100% disability awards.

Civil cases can be taken against the former employers if they can be identified although problems can occur with bankrupt companies who carried their own insurance. Under the laws of limitation a plaintiff has to lodge his claim within three years of the date on which he was first aware he had developed any asbestos related disease, this includes the presence of pleural plaques. The amount awarded, is calculated by total loss of earnings, actual as well as predicted future earnings over a fifteen year period and for pain and suffering.

The Occupational Alveolitides (Hypersensitivity Pneumonia)

Extrinsic allergic alveolitis

The clinical features, radiological findings and management of allergic alveolitis has been discussed in Chapter 16 on interstitial lung disease. Only the occupational features of the diseases will be discussed in this section.

The sources of antigenic material are derived from two main sources:

- microbial spores
- animal proteins (principally avian).

Acute allergic alveolitis

The acute disease is characterised by cough, breathlessness, malaise, fever and joint aches occuring 4–8 hours after a heavy occupational exposure. Haemoptysis may occur rarely, but chest pain is not a feature. In the absence of continued exposure the symptoms settle after 48–72 hours, although rarely they may take several days–weeks to settle completely. Clinical examination may reveal the febrile response, fine to medium crackles predominantly in the lower halves of the lung and occasionally a characteristic 'squawk' may be heard.

The history of a heavy exposure is important in the diagnosis. The cause of the heavier than usual exposure depends on the industry. For farmers, hay making is the classical example. Cleaning cages for bird fanciers and certain phases of the mushroom cycle in mushroom workers are also relevant.

Reduced gas transfer and a low-grade restrictive pulmonary function impairment may be demonstrated in the acute stage. X-ray shows a fine nodular infiltrate in the lower zones.

Chronic disease

The chronic disease may be preceded by a history of recurrent acute attacks, but the classical symptom of breathlessness on exertion may develop without clear preceding acute disease. The dyspnoea will be progressive if exposure continues.

Crackles are not always present. Clubbing is reported but are and these clinical features may help to differentiate it from idiopathic pulmonary fibrosis, although the occupational history is usually sufficient.

The typical physiological findings are of reduced gas transfer and a restrictive pattern. Radiologically, predominantly linear fibrosis occurs with a tendency to favour the upper lobes.

Investigations

The occupational history is central to the diagnosis and should not be missed. Pulmonary function and radiological changes are as discussed above. Serology shows precipitins positive in 90% of acute cases, but may be less consistent in chronic disease. Bronchoscopy and lavage in both acute and chronic disease demonstrates a lymphocytic alveolitis. Biopsy if performed, shows non-caseating granulomas.

Table 4 summarises the common occupational causes of allergic alveolitis. In addition rarer causes include sequiosis (mouldy sawdust from sequioa tree), cheese workers lung, dry rot lung (domestic exposure), wheat weevil lung, fish meal workers lung, diisocyanate alveolitis, snuff takers lung, wine growers lung, fertiliser workers lung, potato riddlers lung.

Management, prevention and prognosis

Acute disease usually settles spontaneously without sequelae. Once diagnosed appropriate advice to limit exposure is required. Farmers, because of their self-employed nature, may be the most difficult to resolve. Respiratory protective equipment and adequate ventilation during barn procedures may be sufficient to prevent the acute disease.

In chronic disease, cessation of further exposure is required to prevent progression. The disease is usually steroid responsive in its development, but once fibrosis has been established supportive treatment is all that can be offered.

Modern techniques have prevented the disease in many occupational settings, including bagassosis, malt workers and partially in mushroom workers. Because of the economic pressures, exposure continues in farmers (although technological advance has reduced its incidence). Pigeon breeders, by clinical experience, seem unlikely to avoid future exposure but may use respiratory protective equipment.

Table 4. The occupational allergic alveolitides

Title	Agent	Occupational source	Specific features
Farmers lung	Thermophilic actinomycetes (Faeniae rectivigula) (Thermoactinomyces vulgaris) (Saccharomonospora viridis)	Turning stored or mouldy hay Bale opening for feediong livestock Threshing mouldy grain	The disease rarely occurs during April–September (stored hay not used for feeding) Respirators worn during barn operations significantly reduces risk Other fungi may be important in the aetiology
Bird fanciers lung	Avian protein	Cleaning out lofts and cages – high Bird keeping – chronic low exposure Poultry and aviary attenders	Acute disease is associated with high exposure occupational or para-occupational sources Chronic disease occurs in owners of domestic birds
Bagassosis	T. sacchari	Bagasse (sugar cane) handling	Modern processing eliminates actinomycete exposure
Mushroom workers lung	Thermophilic actinomycetes	Mushroom spawning (placing mushroom into agitated compost) Mushroom picking – specific species	Many other allergic and toxic agents may also be present during mushroom cultivation, including many allergenic fungi NO_2, and spores.

Table 4. Continued

Title	Agent	Occupational source	Specific features
Malt workers lung	Predominantly *Aspergillus clavatus*	Spreading barley manually to floors in traditionally malt processes	Aspergillus found in sputum of all exposed workers
Suberosis	*Penicillium frequentans*	Processing and sorting bark for cork manufacture	Cork particles may add to effects of immune response to penicillium
Maple bark strippers disease	Spores (cryptostroma)	Stripping bark from maple trees, paper mills	
Air conditioner lung disease	Thermophilic actinomycetes	Working in offices with contaminated humidification in air conditioning	Extrinsic allergic alveolitis reported from such sources

Organic dust toxic syndrome

The symptoms of this disease are similar to those of allergic alveolitis, with cough and febrile illness predominating. Other signs and symptoms do not occur and precipitins are absent. The cause of the disease is probably due to either inhaled bacterial endotoxin or fungal toxins (or both in combination). The episode is self-limiting lasting up to 72 hours. Blood and alveolar lavage will demonstrate a neutrophil leukocytosis again differentiating it from allergic alveolitis. The condition is benign and a chronic disease does not occur.

Miscellaneous Conditions

A number of difficult to classify respiratory conditions occur in association with specific dust or metal exposure. These conditions are summarised for their occupational and clinical features in Tables 5–7.

Table 5 contains a summary of specific named diseases, while Tables 6 and 7 reports the symptoms associated with metal, dust and toxic gas exposure.

Occupational Respiratory Infections

A number of respiratory infections of bacterial, viral or parasitic nature may have an occupational aetiology and the occupational factors are briefly summarised.

Legionnaires disease

The exposure to *Legionnella pneumophila*, is usually from a contaminated water system such as cooling tower. Epidemics have been associated with occupational exposure in hospitals from contaminated cooling towers and ducting and in domestic housing located alongside contaminated cooling towers as examples. Adequate maintenance of the cooling system should prevent the disease and high risk is associated with a water system which has remained dormant for some time allowing the organisms to proliferate. The exposure risk occurs if an aerosol of contaminated material is released into the environment.

Table 5.   Miscellaneous conditions of dust exposure

Disease	Occupational Setting	Clinical Features	Diagnosis	Prognosis
Berylliosis	Metal and alloy production Electronics (transistors etc) Laboratory process of beryllium Ceramic manufacture Rocket parts, fuel production (historically) fluorescent lights	*Acute berylliosis* Eye and nasal irritation including epistaxis Cough, haemoptysis, chest tightness and breathlessness (SOB). Fever, skin irritation	Crackles, fever Radiologically-pulmonary oedema Histology – haemorrhagic exudates/pneumonitis	Full recovery can occur, steroids and hyperbaric oxygen may assist survival
		Chronic berylliosis Insidious onset of SOB, cough weakness, malaise and arthralgia (may occur after resolved acute disease)	Clubbing, crackles and 'squawks' Pleural rub, hepatomegally Radiologically: like sarcoidosis Histologically; granulomas Beryllium containing cell inclusions	Steroid responsive in early phases Remission following cessation of exposure may be followed by late relapse
Byssinosis	Cotton, flax hemp textile spinning	*Chronic byssinosis* (traditional) Chest tightness and SOB occurring on first working day after rest days Occurs after 10–20 years exposure	No signs Diagnosed by clinical history Accompanying restrictive defect in advanced disease	Impaired lung function and symptomatic chronic bronchitis can occur
		Acute byssinosis Cross shift change in lung function With or without symptoms of wheeze/SOB	Pulmonary function change Usually no signs	Usually full recovery on cessation of exposure. Effect of continued exposure unknown.
Mill fever	Textile industry	Fever, SOB on first occupational exposure	Crackles and radiological infiltrate	Resolves completely
Humidifier fever	Printing industry and other occupations with humidification	Fever, cough, SOB, malaise & arthralgia. First working day periodicity	Crackles, precipitins to humidifier extracts	Usually benign, but persistent
Metal fume fever	Metal industry (Zn, Al, Cu Mg) Welding, galvanising	Fever, SOB	Crackles and radiological infiltrate restrictive impairment and leukocytosis	Resolves completely

Tuberculosis

Occupations at risk include health care workers, mortuary attendants and those with occupational silicosis. In the UK, health care workers should be protected by mandatory BCG vaccination of all high risk workers, but it is evident that occupational cases are still occurring, because of omission of or unsuccessful vaccination.

Chlamydia

Psittacosis may occur in aviary attendants or pet shop workers. Although parrots are the most common source other birds can carry or transmit the infection. Indeed, mammals may also be source of chlamydial infection including sheep. Chlamydia pneumonia, may occur in epidemics in situations of close communities such as university students and army barracks.

The avian related disease should be controllable by appropriate quarantining of imported birds.

It is advised that pregnant women should avoid sheep especially during lambing. Treating effected animals with tetracycline and appropriate segregation should reduce the incidence of the disease.

Q fever

Pneumonia caused by *Coxiella burnetti* was first diagnosed in abattoir workers. Many animals and birds can act as hosts and exposure can occur by indirect means, such as clearing sheds used by animals and straw handling, but in a number of cases the aetiological origin may be unclear. Vaccination may become more widely available in the future for high risk occupations, and serological screening of these workers is used in some situations.

Other occupational sources of respiratory infection include:

- brucellosis   animal source of *Brucella abortus* or *Brucella melitensis*.
  affects abattoir workers, cattle breeders, dairy farmers
- anthrax   inhaled anthrax spores from animal source occupational sources include tanning and skinning of hides, gelatine and fertiliser

Table 6. Summary table of diseases associated with metal exposure

Metal	Occupation	Asthma	Carcinogen	Pulmonary fibrosis	Features
Aluminium	Ore refining, smelting, abrasives	Yes (pot room)	No	Yes (complicated by pneumothorax)	In addition an acute condition similar to acute silicosis is reported
Cadmium	Welding alloys, batteries, pigments Pesticides, atomic reactors, refining	No	No	Acute disease	Haemorrhagic pneumonitis after acute exposure, high mortality chronic exposure → emphysema, renal damage
Chromium	Electroplating, leather tanning	Yes	Yes	No	Possible long term lung function impairment
Cobalt	Electronics, medical prosthetics tungsten carbide (hard metal)	Yes	No	Yes (Hard metal disease)	Hard metal disease = interstitial fibrosis with honeycombing and cyst formation. Hard metal crystals in lung and show on CT (not X-ray)
Copper	Anti-mildew spray	No	Probable	No	Rounded opacities on X-ray, lymphocytic infiltrate
Manganese	Electric batteries, chemical, alloys	No	No	No	Haemorrhagic necrosis, metal fume fever. Increased risk of pneumonia.

Table 6. Continued

Metal	Occupation	Asthma	Carcinogen	Pulmonary fibrosis	Features
Mercury	Electrical – lamps/batteries pharmaceuticals, fungicides dentistry	No	No	DIPF pattern Often after acute illness	Acute tracheo-bronchitis with high fatality Acutely responsive to steroids if diagnosed Raised blood mercury levels
Nickel	Alloys, electroplating, welding	Yes	Yes	?	Acute chemical pneumonia
Titanium	Dyes	No	No	No	Intense irritant → pulmonary oedema
Selenium exposure	Electrical industry	No	No	No	Irritant → Pulmonary oedema if high
Vanadium	Steel manufacture, catalyst	Yes	No	? one study suggested it since refuted	Acute – bronchitis/pneumonia
Zinc (chloride)	batteries, galvanising, oil refining	No	No	DIPF pattern after acute	Acute – pulmonary oedema and pneumonia

Table 7. Summary of occupational exposure to non-metal toxic gases vapours and mists

Agent	Occupation	Features
Ammonia	Pharmaceutical, chemical and fertilizers	Chemical burns, mucosal irritation, pulmonary and bronchial oedema Haemorrhagic sputum, stridor
Chlorine	Chemicals, plastics and pharmaceuticals	Mucosal irritation, chest pain, cough → pulmonary oedema in severe cases Persistent bronchial reactivity or lung function impairment has been suggested.
Hydrogen sulphide	Chemicals, dyes and rubber manufacture	Central respiratory paralysis + mucosal irritation → haemorrhagic pulmonary oedema
Oxides of nitrogen	Silos, pertroleum industry, blasting (mines) Fire-fighters at chemical fires	No immediate effect (therefore exposure may be prolonged) 3–24 hours later →paroxymal cough, wheeze, blood stained sputum, fever Crackles and polymorpholeucocytosis. Second relapse may occur at 2–6 weeks – with associated bronchiolitis obliterans
Phosgene	Chlorinating agent in chemical industry Fire-fighting with chlorinated hydrocarbons	Delayed pulmonary oedema Survivors → complete recovery
Sulphur dioxide	Chemical and paper industries	Acute severe pulmonary oedema → persistent lung function impairment in survivors

• histoplasmosis

manufacture from bones and animal hooves, dock workers, horse and sheep hair handling inhalation of fungus *Histoplasma capsulatum* farm workers, poultry keepers, construction/ demolition workers in effected regions of Eastern and Central USA, Central and South America, South and West Africa

References

Occupational Lung Disorders, 3rd edition. In: Parkes WR, ed. Butterworth Heinemann 1995

Travis WD, Colby TV, Corrin B, Shimosato Y, Brambilla E. Histological typing of lung and pleural tumours, 3rd edition. World Health Organisation 1999

Venables KM, Chan-Yeung M. Occupational asthma. *Lancet* 1997;**349**: 1465–69

Ross DJ, Keynes HL, McDonald JC. SWORD'97: Surveillance of work-related respiratory disease in the UK. *Occup Med* 1998;**48**:481–5

18

Radiotherapy and the Lung

J Paul Dilworth

The lung may be affected by radiation given for treatment of a range of neoplastic diseases including lung, breast, oesophagus, lymphoma, spine and thymus or occasionally as part of total body irradiation for bone marrow transplantation preparation. Radiation damage to the lung is either **acute (1–6 months) or late (>6 months)**.[1] The early, acute pneumonitis only occurs in the irradiated volume and usually resolves but may progress to regional fibrosis.

The delay in onset of radiation damage of months is due to cell turnover times. The initial response is disruption of endothelial cells after a few weeks with capillary occlusion and inflammation followed by epithelial and endothelial repair in the first two months. Intra-alveolar septa may be replaced by collagen and dense fibrosis occurs after six to nine months.

Sub-clinical disease is common with abnormalities in lung function and radiology but severe symptoms are rare. There is a strong correlation between severity of lung disease and dose of radiation and the volume irradiated[2] but much individual variation in susceptibility. Clinically significant pulmonary effects are unusual with less than 3000cGy but usual with greater than 4000cGy. Fractionation of the total dose diminishes pulmonary side-effects whereas concomitant chemotherapy, steroid withdrawal or tobacco smoking increase risk. The risk factors for both acute and late pulmonary side-effects are the same. A principal risk for later development of fibrosis is the presence, timing and severity of the previous subacute pneumonitis.

Clinical Features

The acute radiation pneumonitis presents between 1 and 6 months (median 2 months) after treatment with a non-productive often paroxysmal cough, breathlessness and low grade fever with occasional chest pain. This generally resolves but progressive irreversible breathlessness may occur due to pulmonary fibrosis. The onset is at 3 to 9 months generally peaking and plateauing at 12–24 months. Signs are initially sparse but crepitiaitons over the site of fibrosis with occasional rubs or signs of consolidation occur. There is little correlation between the severity of post-radiation skin changes and the severity of pulmonary involvement.

Less common effects of radiation are pleural thickening, pneumothorax, rib fractures, pericardial effusions and an ARDS type picture. Haemoptysis from airway telangiectasis may rarely be fatal especially as a complication of brachytherapy.

Investigations

On a plain chest radiograph or thoracic CT there is initially a ground glass appearance progressing to an alveolar or interstitial infiltration with nodularity or consolidation in some cases. The principal differentials are recurrence of the underlying neoplasia (eg; lymphangitis or lymphadenopathy) or infection but these are not generally confined to the area of irradiation with a characteristic 'straight-edge effect'. Transient pleural effusions may occur. If fibrosis develops there will be volume loss with elevation of the diaphragm and pleural thickening and occasionally bronchiectatic or cystic changes[1].

Pulmonary function measured by either FEV_1 or gas transfer is frequently impaired after radiation. This initially peaks during episodes of pneumonitis, subsequently partially or completely resolves then may deteriorate again if fibrosis occurs. The fall in TLCO correlates with the area irradiated. If an endobronchial obstruction is relieved there may be an improvement in lung function. Bronchial hyper-reactivity may be enhanced. Some degree of hypoxia is common.[2] Other investigations have a limited role though the ESR and blood neutrophil count are usually elevated.

Treatment

Most patients with sub-clinical abnormalities of pulmonary function or asymptomatic radiographic change require no therapy. If symptomatic pneumonitis occurs corticosteroids (eg, prednisolone 60mg a day for 2 weeks then taper) are helpful along with supportive use of oxygen, cough suppressants and bronchodilators as required. After 6 months steroid therapy is generally ineffective.

References

1. Libshitz HI. Radiation changes in the lung. *Seminars in Roentgenology* 1993;**28**:303-321

2. Marks LB. The pulmonary effects of thoracic irradiation. *Oncology* 1994;**8**:89-100

19

Drug-induced Respiratory Disease (DRD)

Simon CO Taggart and J Paul Dilworth

DRD may be induced by numerous agents and produces a wide spectrum of syndromes. A few are not uncommon, most are rare but the total number of cases is significant. Patients may complain of fever, malaise, cough, chest tightness, breathlessness or pain, and examination may reveal wheeze, crepitations, fluid, pleural rub or bronchial breathing. Chest X-ray findings are equally non-specific e.g. interstitial infiltration, pleural thickening, pleural effusion, pulmonary oedema or consolidation but any combination is possible and none is pathognomonic of any particular drug reaction. In some clinical situations such as diffuse radiological shadowing or bronchospasm the possibility of DRD should always be amongst the differential diagnosis and in some specialities it is a common problem including oncology/haematology, cardiology and rheumatology. The incidence of respiratory disease is high enough with a small number of agents for vigilance to be essential in their use (eg, bleomycin, amiodarone and nitrofurantoin). Other agents known to cause DRD, however, do so only occasionally and the physician should always consider medication as the aetiology of any respiratory symptom and having taken a detailed history consider consulting one of the references of known drug reactions[1]. DRD is under-reported but important.

Table 1. Common causes of drug induced interstitial disease

Bleomycin	Amiodarone
Busulphan	Nitrofurantoin
Chlorambucil	Sulphasalazine
Cyclophosphamide	
Methotrexate	

Interstitial Lung Disease

DRD may often present as pulmonary infiltrates on the chest radiograph. The underlying pathology may be an interstitial pneumonitis (Table 1), fibrosis, pulmonary eosinophilia or bronchiolitis obliterans with organising pneumonia. DRD usually occurs after a delay of weeks or months but may occur years after therapy commenced (eg, nitrosureas).

Presentation is commonly with breathlessness and cough. Fever is common. Liver function tests are frequently abnormal. Several drugs (especially antibiotics) produce an eosinophilia (Table 2).

Pre-disposing factors for the development of DRD include increasing age, a combination of potentially pneumotoxic drugs (eg, oxygen or GCSF with bleomycin) and radiotherapy at a similar time. Most will resolve when the agent is withdrawn but irreversible fibrosis occurs with prolonged treatment with some agents.

Investigation often requires bronchoscopy and lavage to confirm the presence of a lymphocytosis and to exclude infective or malignant disease. Pulmonary function tests generally indicate a restrictive defect with a low gas transfer. High resolution CT scanning may be helpful but is unlikely to suggest a specific aetiology and gallium scanning often shows bilateral increased uptake. Trans-bronchial biopsies are generally non-specific and occasionally an open or thoracoscopic biopsy is required.

Table 2. Common causes of pulmonary eosinophilia

Aspirin
Amiodarone
Isoniasid
Methotrxate
Nitrofurantoin
Penicillin
Sulphonamides

Treatment with corticosteroids is indicated if there is extensive radiographic change or markedly reduced lung function but cessation of the offending agent is often sufficient.

Chemotherapy agents

32% of published reports of DRD are related to chemotherapeutic agents. The commonest five are bleomycin, methotrexate, cyclophosphamide, busulphan and the nitrosureas. Pulmonary disease in these patients frequently results in a diagnostic challenge with the differentials including radiotherapy pneumonitis, infection and recurrence of the underlying disease.

Interstitial lung disease is common with bleomycin occuring in up to 5% of patients treated and fatal reactions occur. Bleomycin induced pneumonitis is thought to be mediated by release of free radicals which damage the pulmonary vascular endothelium and stimulate both the influx of inflammatory cells and cytokine induced fibroblastic recruitment and activity. It is related both to cumulative dose and to the combined administration of other pneumotoxic agents (including radiation) and oxygen. Cases either present acutely with fever, dry cough, dyspnoea and pulmonary infiltrates or chronically with progressive fibrosis sometimes after a period of latency. A nodular appearance may mimic metastatic disease.

Methotrexate induced acute pneumonitis occurs in 1–2% of patients over a 3–4 year period but is generally reversible. It has no specific features but tends to occur in the first few months of treatment and typically presents with cough, dyspnoea, malaise and fever. The systemic symptoms may precede the respiratory symptoms by a few weeks. Other presentations include hypersensivity, eosinophilia and pleural effusions. In rheumatoid arthritis it is associated with older age, diabetes mellitus, rheumatoid pulmonary involvement, previous rheumatoid modifying drugs and low albumin.

Busulphan induced pneumonitis may progress after the drug is withdrawn and the pneumonitis of nitrosureas may occur up to a year after treatment. The pneumonitis induced by cyclophosphamide varies from rapidly progressive to insidious and delayed.

Amiodarone

Amiodarone pulmonary toxicity is one of the commonest forms of drug induced pulmonary disease.[2] Amiodarone may also have a direct cytotoxic effects but evidence also suggests that its metabolites may in some way stimulate the activity of natural killer cells targeted at the constituents of the lung parenchyma. It occurs mainly in men and is uncommon when taking less than 200mg per day or with less than two months treatment. A cumulative dose of greater than 150g is generally required to produce pulmonary toxicity and the likelihood of toxicity correlates with the daily dose. Occasionally symptoms may commence a few weeks after stopping treatment. Pre-existing respiratory disease may increase risk further.

The presentation is generally fibrotic but includes bronchiolitis obliterans organising pneumonia and adult respiratory distress syndrome (ARDS). Histologically there are foamy lipid laden macrophages which may progress to irreversible fibrosis. Occasionally there will be rapid, acute onset but most are insidious. Commonly there is fever, malaise and weight loss with exertional breathlessness, crackles and a high ESR. There may be wheeze and cough with pleuritic chest pain and a pleural friction rub. There are reports of ARDS developing post-surgery and post-angiography in patients on amiodarone.

The chest radiograph most commonly shows bilateral asymmetrical interstitial or alveolar opacities of relatively high density (due to iodinated compounds). Less commonly the abnormalities may be unilateral, migratory, bi-basal, mass lesions or areas of consolidation. A pleural effusion may occasionally occur in conjunction but is rarely the sole abnormality.

The differential diagnosis includes left ventricular failure (LVF), pulmonary embolism or infection. In LVF the ESR is less likely to be elevated and a gallium scan normal whereas the echocardiogram and pulmonary capillary wedge pressure may be abnormal. Foamy macrophages on broncho-alveolar lavage or biopsy are usually present but can be present in patients on amiodarone without other evidence of pulmonary toxicity. Pulmonary function is impaired with a restrictive deficit and reduced gas transfer but does not help to distinguish LVF from amiodarone pneumonitis.

If arrhythmias can be controlled by an alternative strategy the amiodarone should be discontinued. This is, however, often impossible and reduction in dose with concomitant use of corticosteroids is useful in many patients. 80% will improve but 10–20% will progress to respiratory failure and death.

Bronchospasm

Drug induced bronchospasm is usually an exacerbation of pre-existing asthma but may be new. Beta-blockers, including ophthalmic preparations, and cholinergics (e.g. pyridostigmine and pilocarpine eye drops) act physiologically to produce bronchoconstriction.

Up to 5% of asthmatics give a history of NSAID induced bronchospasm on direct questioning and up to 20% on challenge testing. They block the cyclooxygenase (COX-1) and shift arachidonic acid metabolism down the 5 lipooxygenase pathway leading to the production of cysteinyl-leukotrienes which mediate inflammation and cause bronchoconstriction. The classical ASA triad (aspirin sensitive asthma with nasal polyps) is not always seen. Those affected usually have adult onset asthma and may experience life-threatening exacerbations with upper airway oedema. Controlled challenge tests may rarely be necessary to confirm the diagnosis. Leukotriene modifiers have been shown to be helpful but if ineffective desensitisation may be attempted.

Angiotensin-converting Enzyme (ACE) Inhibitors

Up to 20% of patients experience a non-productive cough often worse at night. It is thought to be caused by a build up of bradykinin which is normally metabolised in the lungs by ACE. In about 2% there will be hoarseness and sore throats. This occurs with all ACE inhibitors with a weak relationship to dose. Symptoms usually occur within one month of commencing treatment and resolve within one month of stopping therapy. Of those who experience cough about 25% require a change in treatment. The differential diagnosis includes pulmonary oedema and asthma and a chest radiograph and home peak expiratory flow recordings may be helpful in excluding other causes. Where treatment is essential a non-steroidal anti-inflammatory agent may be tried.

Key Points

- take a thorough drug history
- assess likelihood of a drug reaction by consulting references/ texts
- exclude other conditions thoroughly, especially infection

- consider bronchoscopy ± biopsy
- stop drug if possible
- consider corticosteroids if severe
- reconsider diagnosis if patient fails to respond

References

Foucher P, Biour M, Blayac JP, Godard P, Sgro C, Kuhn M, Vergnon JM et al. Drugs that may injure the respiratory system. *Eur Respir J* 1997;**10**:265–279

Fraire AE, Guntupalli KK, Greenberg D, Cartwright J, Chasen MH. Amiodaone Pulmonary Toxicity: A multidisciplinary Review of Current Status. *Southern Medical J* 1993;**86**:67–77

20

Intensive Care

Brendan Madden

Introduction

Intensive care is an increasingly important speciality which involves a multidisciplinary approach to patient management. Indeed lack of familiarity with the complex monitoring and support systems found in intensive care frequently inspires lack of confidence among physicians, particularly those in training. Although perhaps not at first appreciated, specialist knowledge in respiratory medicine, physiology and infection is a tremendous advantage in this field. The aim of this chapter is to outline the major aspects of support and therapeutic interventions available in the management of patients in the intensive care unit. It is hoped that this information will provide a solid foundation which will not only help familiarise the physician with the basic aspects of intensive care management and emphasise the importance of not looking at single organ systems in isolation but also provide impetus for further learning in this fascinating area of medicine.

Mechanical Ventilatory Support

Principles

Respiratory support forms a major part of intensive care treatment. It is rarely required in isolation from other problems which may have their own adverse effects on respiratory function. The classic indication for ventilatory support is reversible acute respiratory failure. Some patients with acute lung disease however can be successfully treated without tracheal intubation and mechanical ventilatory support using continuous positive airway pressure

Table 1. **Guidelines for introduction of mechanical ventilation**

A General Indications

Inadequate Ventilation as indicated by :

a) Apnoea, upper airway obstruction, unprotected airway

b) Respiratory rate > 35 breaths/minute (normal range 10–20)

c) Tidal volume < 5 ml/kg (normal range 5–7)

d) Vital capacity < 15 ml/kg (normal range 65–75)

e) $PaCO_2$ > 8 kPa (60 mmHg) (normal range 4.7–6.3 kPa; 35–47 mmHg)

f) Negative inspiratory force < 25 cmH$_2$O) (normal range 75–100)

g) V_D/V_T ratio > 0.6 (normal range < 0.3)
(Dead space/Tidal volume ratio)

B Inadequate gas exchange oxygenation as indicated by :

a) Alveolar – arterial oxygen gradient (A-a) DO$_2$ on FiO$_2$ of 1.0 > 47 kPa (350 mmHg) (normal range 3.3–8.7 kPa; 25–65 mmHg)

b) PaO_2 < 8 kPa (60 mmHg) on FiO$_2$ > 0.6

(CPAP) or non-invasive ventilation (NIV) via a tight fitting facemask. Other accepted terms for mechanical ventilation include artificial, controlled, assisted and intermittent positive pressure ventilation (IPPV) and continuous mechanical ventilation (CMV).

In general, the indications for mechanical ventilation fall into two broad categories

• inadequate alveolar ventilation with increasing $PaCO_2$ and
• inadequate gas exchange with increasing alveolar-arterial oxygen gradient and arterial hypoxaemia

Guidelines for mechanical ventilation in acute respiratory failure are shown in Table 1. Clinical judgement must always be exerted in interpreting these guidelines and problems should be anticipated before they arise. For example, it is quite possible that a patient with a respiratory rate in excess of 35 breaths per minute requires ventilatory support. However, if a patient has a respiratory rate of 30 breaths per minute and is clearly becoming fatigued, early elective intubation is preferred to an emergency procedure when the patient has deteriorated to the extent that a cardiorespiratory arrest is present or imminent. Likewise a progressive fall in vital capacity in a patient with myasthenia gravis on full medical support may indicate a need for early ventilation although the critical value of less than 15ml per kilogram has not been reached.

In most cases endotracheal intubation is the preferred technique of airway access. Orotracheal intubation and nasotracheal intubation are other avenues available. Whatever technique is employed, intubation should be performed in a safe and controlled manner by an experienced clinician e.g. an anaesthetist or trained specialist in intensive care. The appropriate endotracheal tube size for most adult males is eight to nine millimetre internal diameter and for women seven to eight millimetre internal diameter. For children a rough calculation can be made using the child's age in years divided by four plus four to provide an approximate internal diameter. It is essential that the endotracheal tube be securely anchored with a tie and the cuff inflation pressure restricted to less than 30 centimetres H_2O, higher cuff pressures do not improve airway protection against aspiration but only increase the risk of damage to the tracheal mucosa and subsequent stenosis.

Tracheostomy is indicated for specific reasons. These include helping to wean patients from ventilatory support following failed attempts at extubation, facilitation of oral nutrition or the need for chronic or permanent ventilation. The same principles of cuff pressure management apply to tracheostomy tubes. This procedure is associated with fewer complications than endotracheal intubation, however, these complications tend to be more serious and include tube displacement, pneumothorax, haemorrhage and infection.

Features of a mechanical ventilator

Most adult patients are supported on volume/time cycled, pressure limited ventilators (Volume Ventilator or Flow Generator). These ventilators deliver pre-set tidal volumes regardless of changes in lung compliance or impedance. Unfortunately, however, inflation pressures must rise to overcome the mechanical load and therefore to protect the patient against inadvertently high pressures a pressure limit must be set. When this limit is reached, the ventilator terminates inspiration regardless of the volume delivered and triggers an alarm. Neonates and infants may be satisfactorily ventilated using

Table 2.   Ventilator parameters

1.   Respiratory Rate

2.   Tidal Volume

3.   Flow Waveform

4. FiO_2 (0.21–1.0)

5.   Inspiratory/expiratory (1:E) ratio

6.   Pressure limit

7.   Positive end – expiratory pressure/continuous positive airway pressure
     (0 to 20 cmH_2O)

time cycled pressure limited devices (Pressure Ventilator or Pressure
Generator). Although these devices are simple and offer reliable
ventilation the delivered tidal volume is difficult to measure. Ventilator parameters are listed in Table 2.

Drive mechanisms propel the air/oxygen gas mixture into the
patient. Some systems deliver the gas to the patient directly (Single
Circuit) and others indirectly though a dual circuit. Several types of
drive mechanisms are available that determine the flexibility,
ventilatory modes and ability to deliver particular tidal volumes in
the presence of abnormal lung mechanics. A variety of control and
monitoring systems are available which cycle the ventilator from
inspiration to expiration. The majority of modern ventilators use
sophisticated electronic cycles with significant improvement in
safety and efficiency. When a clinician has established that a patient
needs to be mechanically ventilated, the mode of ventilation,
ventilatory parameters and ventilatory alarms must be selected. The
most common ventilatory modes employed include control mechanical ventilation, assist control (Triggered Ventilation), intermittent
mandatory ventilation (IMV or SIMV) and pressure support.

Control mechanical ventilation is suitable for paralysed or heavily sedated patients. It provides time and volume cycled, pressure
limited breaths at pre-set rates but does not allow the patient to
breathe spontaneously. Assist control is better tolerated and the
patient requires less sedation. This mode synchronises the ventilator
to the patient's own respiratory rhythm, delivering a volume pre-set,
pressure limited tidal volume. It is necessary to select a trigger
sensitivity (usually minus 0.5 to minus 2.0 cm H_2O) by which the
patient can initiate volume pre-set breaths above the set rates.

Patients have a tendency to hyperventilate on assist control. Intermittent mandatory ventilation enables the patient to breathe spontaneously and supplement positive pressure minute ventilation. In this standard mode there is theoretical risk of stacking a ventilator breath on top of a spontaneous breath. This is not a significant problem usually, however, if an appropriately set pressure limit is selected to prevent inadvertent over-inflation of the lungs. Modern ventilators use triggering or assist facility to synchronise the machine breaths with the patient's own spontaneous breathing pattern (Synchronised Intermittent Mandatory Ventilation, SIMV). This technique is intended as partial ventilatory support. If the patient is taking spontaneous breaths it is better tolerated than control mechanical ventilation, results in lower mean airway pressures and has less effect on the cardiovascular system. It allows the patient to regulate their own $PaCO_2$ to some degree, although rising HCO_3 and alkalosis can be a problem.

Pressure support uses a triggering facility to deliver a pressure limited breath (and not a volume pre-set breath as in assist control). It can be used alone or in conjunction with SIMV when it assists spontaneous breaths. It provides an efficient maintenance and weaning mode that is usually well tolerated. Other modes of ventilation include high frequency (Jet) ventilation which has been used with success in the management of patients with bronchopleural fistula who require re-intubation following pneumonectomy, for those with adult respiratory distress syndrome (ARDS) or following single lung transplantation in patients with emphysema. Reverse I:E ratio (ranging from 1.2 to 1.4) may be employed in a variety of clinical situations which includes ARDS.

Once a ventilation mode has been selected, ventilatory parameters are set before attaching the patient to the ventilator. These parameters are listed in Table 2. Not infrequently tidal volumes of 5ml per kilogram of body weight are all that is required although some patients may have higher requirements. There is little evidence to favour one inspiratory waveform over another, although square waveforms deliver the tidal volume in the least time and with high peak pressures. A decelerating flow pattern results in lower peak pressures, longer inspiratory intervals and lower I:E ratios. The inspired oxygen concentration (FiO_2) should be constantly adjusted to maintain adequate arterial oxygenation without subjecting the patient to the risks of too high oxygen delivery which, if above 0.6, can cause lung toxicity. Setting a pressure limit of approximately 10 cm H_2O above the peak pressure reached during each ventilator cycle, protects the patients against excessive pressures which may be experienced during coughing or straining. Positive end expiratory pressure is used to correct lung volumes in situations such as adult respiratory distress syndrome or cardiogenic pulmonary oedema where lung volumes are typically reduced. Usually starting pressures are in the region of 5 cm H_2O and these are gradually increased to facilitate satisfactory oxygenation with an FiO_2 less than 0.6. It is rarely necessary to exceed levels of 20 cm H_2O.

Weaning from ventilatory support

While patients are being mechanically ventilated, monitoring may be performed by serial arterial blood gas analyses, pulse oximetry, continuous monitoring of end tidal expired CO_2 using a CO_2 analyser, lung function tests (A-aDO_2 and V_D:V_T ratio) and serial chest radiographs. The aim however, is to wean the patient off mechanical ventilatory support as soon as practical. In general, weaning will not be successful if there is an accompanying major organ failure, sepsis or if the patient still requires a high FiO_2 to maintain adequate oxygenation. Weaning is traditionally accomplished with a T piece system using adequate humidification and oxygen concentration. The use of positive end expiratory pressure can subsequently be replaced with CPAP using an appropriate CPAP valve and circuit. There must be no residual effects of sedatives or muscle relaxants and vital signs, arterial blood gas analysis and respiratory variables should be monitored closely during the weaning process. Periods of spontaneous ventilation are gradually lengthened until mechanical ventilatory support is required only at night. The patient is then taken off the ventilator at night after at least two consecutive days of spontaneous breathing. Removal of a tracheostomy tube may be carried out after a further two to three days provided the patient does not require oxygen therapy or ongoing suction. The use of IMV and/or pressure support in weaning avoids the drastic change from CMV to spontaneous breathing via a T piece. Ventilator delivered breathing is progressively reduced as the patient's respiratory function improves. The patient is then weaned to spontaneous breathing by a T piece or CPAP when IMV ventilator breaths are as low as three to four per minute or pressure support required is less than 3 cm H_2O. IMV and or pressure support may be useful in patients who are difficult to wean off CMV e.g. chronic bronchitics and those who require prolonged ventilatory support.

Table 3.   Monitoring the cardiovascular system

A	Non invasive	Heart rate
		Blood pressure
		ECG
		Level of consciousness
		Urine output
		Skin perfusion
		Arterial oxygen saturation
B	Invasive	Arterial blood pressure
		Central venous pressure
		Pulmonary artery flotation catheter measurements
		Transoesophageal echo and doppler measurements

Haemodynamic monitoring and support

Resuscitation of pre or post operative critically ill or haemodynami-
cally unstable patients should take place in a high dependency
area or intensive care unit where it is possible to continuously
monitor the cardiovascular system. There are a variety of non-
invasive and invasive means of assessing a patient's haemodynamics
and these are listed in Table 3. Non-invasive methods should not
be forgotten in an intensive care unit when often emphasis may be
on complex monitoring systems. They are particularly useful when
taken in conjunction with invasive measurements or monitored in
a serial fashion when they may herald the onset of haemodynamic
compromise.

Although arterial blood pressure can be measured indirectly,
critically ill patients require continuous monitoring of blood pressure and frequent analysis of arterial blood. Therefore peripheral
arterial canulation is required. The display of the arterial pressure
waveform is a visual representation of contractility and can add
additional information. One should remember that the blood pressure is the product of cardiac output and peripheral resistance and
therefore does not equate with tissue blood flow. The usual artery
which is canulated is the radial artery but brachial, femoral and
dorsalis pedis arteries can also be used. The central venous pressure
(CVP) represents the pressure in the right atrium and great veins and
therefore equates to right ventricular end diastolic pressure. As this
measurement is a measure of pre load, CVP provides a guide to the
volume of fluid replacement therapy required. There is a wide

Table 4.   Pulmonary artery flotation catheters

Uses	Measurement of pulmonary capillary wedge pressure, vascular resistance, mixed venous oxygen saturation and cardiac output
	Can derive oxygen consumption and delivery and shunt fractions
Indications	Cardiogenic and septic shock
	Adult respiratory distress syndrome
Complications	Mortality up to 2%
	Pulmonary infarction/haemorrhage
	Catheter knotting
	Arrhythmias
	Infection

normal range from 1 to 12 cm H_2O or 0 to 10 mmHg. It is important that the measurement is taken at the appropriate reference level which is usually the mid axillary line in a supine patient.

Pulmonary artery flotation catheters

The mean pulmonary capillary wedge pressure (PCWP) can be measured by a catheter floated into a branch of the pulmonary artery. This measurement (normally 6 ± 2 mmHg) is a useful estimate of left ventricular end diastolic pressure (or pre-load of the left ventricle). It is particularly helpful when the functional behaviour of the left and right ventricles is different and right-sided pressures become an unreliable guide to left ventricular function. Further information regarding these catheters is outlined in Table 4. The catheters are directed by means of a small balloon inflated at the tip. Using the Seldinger technique, a sheath is inserted into a major central vein e.g. internal jugular or subclavian vein. As the catheter is advanced towards the heart, the balloon is inflated and blood flow directs the catheter across the tricuspid valve into the right ventricle and thence through the pulmonary valve into the main pulmonary arterial trunk and from there into the left or right (usually right) main pulmonary artery. The catheter is advanced further until it wedges in a small branch of the pulmonary artery and isolates the catheter tip distal to the balloon from the normal pulmonary artery pressure changes. The catheter tip will measure the PCWP, which equilibrates with the left atrial pressure. Under physiological conditions with a normal mitral valve, at the end of diastole there should be no flow and a continuous column of blood between the catheter tip and the left ventricle. Therefore the PCWP is indirectly a measurement of left ventricular end diastolic pressure. It is usually possible to site the catheter without fluoroscopy by observing pressure traces. One first recognises the central venous pressure waveform and then ventricular, pulmonary arterial and wedge pressure waveforms. In addition to measuring PCWP, measurements of cardiac output, using the Fick principle of indicator dilution, can be made. Mixed venous oxygen saturation can be measured from the distal lumen of the catheter. The pulmonary vascular resistance (PVR) is calculated by an adaptation of Ohm's law of electrical resistance. It is defined as the mean pulmonary artery pressure minus mean PCWP divided by cardiac output and is measured in Wood units. Normally the mean pulmonary artery pressure is 12 ± 6 mmHg and cardiac output is 5l/minute. The pressure drop across the pulmonary vasculature is 6 ± 2 mmHg and normal pulmonary vascular resistance < 1.5 Wood units (120 dynes sec cm^{-5}). In patients with pulmonary hypertension PVR is an important measurement as a favourable response to vasodilator therapy is defined as a greater than 30% reduction in PVR, with a corresponding increase in cardiac output. The conversion from Wood units to dynes second centimetre minus five is multiplication by a factor of 79.9. The systemic vascular resistance is derived from the formula mean systemic arterial blood pressure minus right atrial pressure divided by cardiac output. This measurement is particularly useful if one is considering the use of noradrenaline in managing patients with septic shock or if one wishes to reduce left ventricular afterload in patients with impaired cardiac function.

Further information in the intensive care unit regarding cardiac function can be obtained by transoesophageal echocardiography. This investigation provides information on valve structure and function and estimates of cardiac structure and systolic and diastolic function. Oesophageal Doppler probes can provide useful information on cardiac output.

Shock

In general, shock can be defined as being a high systemic vascular resistance or a low systemic vascular resistance state. Examples of

Table 5.   Shock

Definition	Inadequate tissue perfusion
Consequences	1. Lactic acidosis

	2. ↓ Blood pressure
	        Impaired cardiac contractility
	        Vasodilatation

	3. Specific organ failure from ↓ Perfusion
	        ↓ Consciousness
	        Renal failure
	        Gut permeability altered
	        ARDS

Types	A. High systemic vascular resistance shock
	        e.g. cardiogenic, hypovolemic
	        → ↓ Cardiac output

	B. Low systemic vascular resistance shock
	        e.g. septic, anaphylactic
	        → ↑ Cardiac output

the former include cardiogenic and hypovolemic shock, while septic and anaphylactic shock are typical examples of low systemic vascular resistance shock. In this latter group the systemic vascular resistance remains typically low despite a marked increase in heart rate and cardiac output (Table 5).

Inadequate tissue perfusion leads to lactic acidosis. Initially this can result in breathlessness as a consequence of respiratory compensation. If uncorrected, however, progressive acidosis leads to negative inotropism and fall in blood pressure. This will exacerbate the problem in a downward spiral. Further end organ damage and failure then occurs and patients may develop acute renal failure from acute tubular necrosis, altered levels of consciousness and loss of consciousness from poor cerebral perfusion, impaired hepatic function and altered gut perfusion leading to bacterial translocation. All these factors will exacerbate the initial insult and lead to further deterioration in clinical condition.

Inotropic support

A variety of agents are prescribed, often concomitantly to support the circulation of a patient in the intensive care unit (Table 6).

Table 6.   Measures to improve cardiovascular function in patients with shock

1.   Identify and treat cause
     a)   Optimise fluid balance
     b)   Treat infection
     c)   Reverse anaphylaxis (adrenaline, hydrocortisone)
     d)   Control arrhythmias (drugs, DC cardioversion or pacing)

2.   High systemic vascular resistance shock
     In addition consider   inotropes e.g. adrenaline, dobutamine
                                    phosphodiesterase inhibitors e.g.
                                    enoximone, milrinone
                                    intra aortic balloon counterpulsation
                                    mechanical assist device
                                    surgical intervention e.g. bypass or valve
                                    surgery or transplantation

3.   Low systemic vascular resistance
     In addition consider   nor adrenaline

4.   Support other organ systems

Drugs should be prescribed with careful consideration given to the patient's clinical history and examination and haemodynamic measurements. A clear plan should be made from the onset and regular revision made in conjunction with the nursing and intensive care medical staff. It is usual for inotropic agents to be given via a central venous line, as tissuing from peripheral veins can lead to extravasation of inotropes into the subcutaneous tissues and produce vasoconstriction and ulceration. Typical inotropic drugs are adrenaline and dobutamine. The latter agent also causes reduction in left ventricular afterload by arteriolar vasodilatation. Isoprenaline may be employed to increase heart rate. Noradrenaline preferentially increases systemic vascular resistance by causing arteriolar vasoconstriction. Dopamine is an inotrope, although is frequently used in intensive care units to protect against or to improve renal function in patients with renal impairment. This area is controversial although some believe that dopamine at 3.5mcgs per kilogram per minute is beneficial. Phosphodiesterase inhibitors are inotropic agents (acting via a different pathway to adrenaline) although their major beneficial effect is to produce arteriolar vasodilation and so

Table 7. Causes of acute renal failure

Pre-Renal Failure	Underperfusion due to hypotension resulting from: hypovolemia due to dehydration or bleeding cardiac shock sepsis
Intrinsic Renal Failure	Acute Tubular Necrosis due to renal ischaemia or nephrotoxins, glomerulonephritides Vascular lesions or infection

Post Renal Failure	Obstruction to flow of urine along the urinary tract
	Pelvi-Calyceal
	Ureteric
	  stones or clot
	Extrinsic compression
	  tumour, haematoma,
	  retroperitoneal fibrosis
	Bladder outflow obstruction

reduce afterload on the left ventricle. Examples of these latter agents include enoximone and milrinone. Milrinone may also improve pulmonary blood flow.

Atrial systole contributes up to 20% of ventricular filling and efforts to restore sinus rhythm should be made. Other measures to improve cardiac function in patients with cardiogenic shock include intra-aortic balloon counterpulsation and mechanical assist devices. The intra-aortic balloon pump is usually inserted via the femoral artery and its two major purposes are to improve diastolic perfusion of the coronary arteries and to reduce left ventricular afterload. It is primarily used as a bridge procedure (e.g. following cardiac surgery or as a bridge to cardiac surgery or transplantation). Mechanical assist devices can support the left (LVAD) or right (RVAD) side of the circulation or indeed support both sides (BiVAD). These procedures are also used as a bridge to support patients following cardiac surgery or those who are awaiting cardiac transplantation. Selected patients with cardiogenic shock will require conventional cardiac surgery (e.g. coronary artery bypass grafting, valve surgery, repair of ventricular septal rupture etc) or cardiac transplantation.

Renal Support

Acute renal failure can occur in the intensive care unit for a variety

Table 8. Distinction between pre-renal failure and ATN

Urinary Index	Pre-Renal Failure	ATN
Sediment	Normal	Granular, cell and tubular casts
Sodium	Low, < 20mmol/l	High, > 40mmol/l
Specific Gravity	High, 1.020	Typically fixed 1.010–1.012
U : P Urea ratio	High, 20	Low, 10
U : P Creatinine ratio	High, 40	Low, 10
U : P Osmolality ratio	High, 2.0	Low, 1.2

U = Urine
P = Plasma

of pre-renal, renal and post-renal reasons as outlined in Table 7. Acute renal failure carries a mortality of 8% and describes a condition in which renal function is inadequate to maintain the volume and composition of the patient's internal environment. Anuria refers to the absence of urine output while oliguria describes a urine output of less than 400mls per day. In non oliguric renal failure there is persistent rise in serum creatinine to greater than 200umols/litre despite absence (or correction) of haemodynamic and mechanical causes of renal dysfunction. It occurs more frequently than oliguric renal failure. It should be remembered that the mortality of acute renal failure rises to approximately 70% when associated with one other organ system failure and to 95% when associated with two or more other organ system failures. Table 8 lists ways to reliably delineate between pre-renal failure and established acute tubular necrosis (ATN). The typical manifestations of ATN are oliguria, isothenuria (isosmotic urine) and progressive azotemia. Clinically ATN can be considered under three distinct phases named onset, oliguric and diuretic.

The onset phase follows a renal insult and urine output falls below 400mls per day or anuria develops. At this stage every effort should be made to diagnose and correct the underlying condition which is leading to ATN. The pathogenesis of the oliguric phase is probably multifactorial. Important factors which may be synergistic include:

Table 9.　Complications of ATN

Metabolic Acidosis
Uraemia
Hyperkalaemia
Pulmonary oedema
Infection
Hypocalcaemia (crush injuries)
Bleeding from intestinal tract
Disseminated intravascular coagulation
Multiple organ failure

- interstitial oedema with retrograde diffusion of filtrate which may be resorbed into the circulation
- decreased glomerular capillary permeability leading to a reduction in glomerular filtration rate
- tubular obstruction from cellular casts or afferent arterial vasoconstriction causing cortical ischaemia

After a variable period the diuretic phase occurs and this is typified by polyuria. It does not end all the problems of renal failure. Death may still occur during this phase, usually on account of infection or fluid and electrolyte imbalance. Despite the increase in urine output, renal function remains poor. Blood urea may rise and uraemic symptoms persist or worsen and excessive fluid and electrolytes e.g. K^+ are major hazards. The urine concentrating defect may remain for months. The duration of oliguria does not correlate with the extent of functional recovery. Complications of ATN are listed in Table 9.

Renal function can be assessed by means of clinical signs (presence or absence of features of uremia), blood urea, creatinine and electrolytes, urine output and urine microscopy and biochemistry. One should also remember that impaired renal function can lead to impairment of other organ systems e.g. negative inotropic effect on the heart, adverse effects on liver function and increased susceptibility to infection and bleeding. It is essential therefore that one is aware of these potential complications and that patients are closely monitored. In general the indications for renal replacement therapy are:

- intractable fluid overload
- intractable hyperkalaemia
- intractable acidosis
- signs and symptoms of uraemia

Renal function can be supported using dialysis (i.e. exchange across an osmotic gradient) of the blood (haemodialysis) or using the peritoneal membrane (peritoneal dialysis) with specific volumes of fluid at a known concentration regularly instilled into the abdominal cavity via an indwelling catheter. Alternatively, haemofiltration (or haemodiafiltration) where plasma water is separated from plasma proteins and blood, may be employed. This process has an effective creatinine clearance of approximately 15mls per minute and is not usually associated with the haemodynamic consequences which often accompany haemodialysis. It is therefore often better tolerated by critically ill patients in an intensive care unit. One should also remember to appropriately reduce doses of drugs which are normally metabolized or excreted by the kidneys for patients in renal failure and to monitor drug levels carefully. Careful attention must also be given to nutritional support for these patients.

Nutritional Support

Much has been written about nutritional support for critically ill patients. General consensus exists regarding the main principles of dietetic support. In general, it is agreed that patients should be fed preferably via the gastro intestinal route and that a period of starvation for up to one or two weeks has probably less chance of inducing complications than the early instigation of total parenteral nutrition. The timing of nutritional intervention, particularly total parenteral nutrition (TPN) in patients who are unsuitable for enteral feeding is a cause of much debate. Some believe that post-operative TPN should be considered only when oral or enteral feeding is not anticipated within seven to ten days in previously well nourished patients and five to seven days in those who are malnourished. In patients who are septic, the benefit of early feeding is less clear and indeed the role of TPN has been questioned. Unfortunately, efforts to reduce catabolism in septic patients have been disappointing. TPN regimes with a high proportion of the calories derived from glucose seem to increase catabolism although the ideal constitution of regimes for septic patients remains to be clarified. Any guidelines for the timing of the instigations of various interventions for TPN in

Table 10. Contra-indications for enteral feeding

1.	Complete intestinal obstruction
2.	Gastro intestinal perforation
3.	Recent upper gastro intestinal surgery (in general an intact anastomosis should be demonstrated before NG feeding is started. If a jejunostomy is sited, it should be used according to surgical guidance).
4.	Ileus (persistent)
5.	Inability to pass NG/OG tube or site enterostomy

general and particularly in the case of sepsis are by and large arbitrary.

Specific types of patients may benefit from particular feed constituents. Therapeutic feeds have been categorized as:

- those that are modified which improve uptake of constituents of the feed or reduce diarrhoea (elemental, added fibre etc)
- those which reduce the patient's intake of substances which may be poorly eliminated, result in the accumulation of by products of metabolism or increase the requirement for carbon dioxide removal (low sodium, low protein, high fat etc)
- those which contain specific substances which may modulate the septic response (specific amino acids, fatty acids, RNA etc)

Routine non diabetic post-operative patients do not require specific nutritional support (other than close attention to fluid balance) so long as they are expected to be extubated within 24 hours. For diabetic patients, continuous insulin infusion and calorie intake is required. Post-operative patients who are likely to be ventilated for longer than 24 hours will require a large bore nasogastric tube passed as soon as it is practicable following surgery. Feeding should be commenced after position of the tube has been confirmed. Contra-indications for enteral feeding are listed in Table 10.

Normally when patients are fed enterally they receive feed continuously for 20 hours and are rested for four hours. Feeding sets should be disconnected at the beginning of the rest period and the tube flushed with 20mls of water. Enteral feeding not only provides patients with calories but is an important source of nutrition for the bowel mucosa. Integrity of the intestinal mucosa resists bacterial translocation, which in itself may fuel multiple organ failure. This is particularly important if patients are also being prescribed inotropic agents which can produce gut ischaemia (particularly nor adrenaline). The rest period allows the gastric pH to fall. Gastric acidity is an important host barrier to infection. Failure to allow the gastric pH to return towards its normal acidity may facilitate bacterial and fungal overgrowth.

Diarrhoea is common and not always due to feed intolerance. In the first instance feed should not be stopped and a stool specimen should be sent for microbiological examination, in particular for *Clostridium difficile*. Specific therapy may be indicated (e.g met ronidazole or vancomycin orally for Clostridium infection). As the enteral feed volume increases, the hourly IV maintenance fluid should be concomitantly decreased. When flushing the enteral feeding tube a 50ml syringe should be used to avoid high pressures. 20 to 30mls of water should be flushed down the tube after aspiration and drug administration. Even if the patient is not absorbing, 10mls per hour of feed should be administered, as this may be beneficial to gut mucosa.

Ensure™ is the standard feed used in many intensive care units and all patients (even those that are hypernatraemic) should be started on this as the sodium content is 35mmol per litre. Normally feed is started at 40mls per hour and the nasogastric tube is aspirated after four hours. If a volume in excess of 200mls is returned, 200mls of fluid is replaced and the feed continues at the rate of 40mls per hour. Four hours later further aspiration is performed and if the volume still exceeds 200mls the process above is repeated. One can consider use of a prokinetic agent e.g. Erythromycin 250mg six hourly IV or orally but remember potential drug interactions. Aspirate once again four hours later. If the volume persists above 200mls decrease the rate to 10 to 20mls per hour and review. If however, at any stage the volume returned is less than 200mls, replace the aspirate and increase the feeding rate by 20 to 25mls per hour. Aspirate four hourly and replace up to 200ml of aspirate. If four hourly aspirates continue to be less than 200mls, increase rate by 20 to 25mls per hour every four hours until the prescribed rate is achieved. If the aspirate is greater than 200mls at any one time maintain the rate and consider a prokinetic agent. If two consecutive aspirates in excess of 200mls are obtained reduced the feeding rate by 50% but aim for a minimum rate of at least 10mls per hour.

Total parenteral nutrition is indicated for specific circumstances. It is usually given via a central line and strict asepsis needs to be observed. Routine monitoring for TPN includes one to two hourly blood glucose, daily sodium, potassium, urea, creatinine, haemoglobin and white cell count and thrice weekly magnesium and phosphate. If patients are requiring long-term TPN they will require monitoring of trace elements e.g. zinc, copper and lipids, together with biochemical markers of liver function.

Sepsis

Patients in intensive care units are at risk of developing hospital acquired (nosocomial) infections. This concept is not new and was well described by the Viennese in the 1840s as childbirth fever. Streptococci remained the predominant pathogens in hospitals until the 1950s when they were partly replaced by Staphylococci, which led to major epidemics in hospitals, particularly among the very young and the elderly. More recently epidemics of methicillin resistant *Staphylococcus aureus* (MRSA) have been associated with morbidity and mortality. There have recently been reports of vancomycin resistant *Staphylococcus aureus* in Japan and vancomycin resistant enterococcus is being more frequently encountered in intensive care units in this country. Since the 1960s, Gram-negative bacilli have become increasingly important causes of nosocomial infection. They are particularly associated with cross infection in indwelling urinary catheters and intensive care equipment (e.g. ventilators and humidifiers) and as causes of surgical infection. Patients are at risk of infection in the intensive care unit for a variety of reasons (Table 11), which include the presence of central lines, chest and abdominal drains, urinary catheters and endotracheal intubation with mechanical ventilatory support. They may have failure of one or more organ systems and are frequently on antibiotic therapy, which in itself may facilitate the emergence of resistant microorganisms. Infection in its severest form, i.e. septic shock, is associated with a mortality of 40 to 70% inspite of the best treatment available.

Definitions

Sepsis has been defined as the systemic response to infection, which is characterized by two or more of the following conditions resulting from that infection:

Table 11. Predisposing factors in developing sepsis

A **Impaired General Body Defence Mechanisms**

1. Reticulo-endothelial system e.g. shock, major trauma, burns

2. Cell mediated immunity e.g. immunosuppressive drugs, malignancy, malnutrition

3. Humoral immunity e.g. post-splenectomy

B **Impaired Local Organ Defences**

1. Respiratory system
    e.g. impaired cough, mucociliary clearance, laryngeal dysfunction

2. Alimentary tract
    e.g. alteration in mouth flora, gastric colonisation if pH exceeds 4.0, antibiotics causing bacterial or fungal overgrowth, gut ischaemia

3. Genito-urinary tract e.g. urinary catheterisation

4. Eyes e.g. impaired blinking, loss of irrigation and anti-bacterial properties of tears

5. Skin e.g. lines, drains or catheters

- temperature greater than 38°C or less than 36°C
- heart rate greater than 90 beats per minute
- respiratory rate greater that 20 breaths per minute or $PaCO_2$ less than 32mmHg
- white cell count greater than 12000 per mm^3 or less than 4000 per mm^3 or greater than 10% immature (band) forms

When evidence of organ dysfunction such as altered mental state, lactic acidosis or oliguria is added to the clinical picture of sepsis, the term **severe sepsis** is appropriate. The diagnosis of **septic shock** is restricted to those patients who, in addition to being severely septic, remain hypotensive despite fluid resuscitation. It should also be stressed that the systemic inflammatory response can also be provoked by an number of non infectious stimuli including trauma, pancreatitis, vasculitis and anaphylaxis. This has been termed the **systemic inflammatory response syndrome** (SIRS). This response reflects immune activation with the production of a variety of inflammatory mediators including cytokines. For example, pyrexia

Table 12. Clinical features of septicaemia

1. Inadequate tissue oxygen delivery

2. Reduced systemic vascular resistance

3. Myocardial dysfunction

4. Increased capillary permeability

5. Increased venous capacitance from relative hypovolemia

6. Rise in pulmonary vascular resistance

is mediated by the action of endogenous pyrogen compounds on specific hypothalamic receptors. These, via the action of compounds such as prostaglandins, activate the thermo-regulatory centre. Endogenous pyrogen is primarily released by the effects of exogenous bacterial pyrogens on polymorphonuclear leucocytes (endogenous leucocyte pyrogen) and also by their effects on macrophages. The antipyretic effects of agents such as aspirin relate directly and proportionally to their ability to inhibit prostaglandin synthesis. Corticosteroids inhibit endogenous leucocyte pyrogen released by stimulated macrophages and this explains their ability to abolish or mask pyrexia.

If sepsis is suspected in a patient it is important to perform a careful history and physical examination. Blood, urine and sputum specimens should be sent for microbiological culture, ideally prior to commencing antibiotic therapy. There is no doubt that the appropriate doses of appropriate microbial agents at the right time saves lives. A number of studies have shown improved outcome in the management of patients with pneumonia and septic shock by the early introduction of appropriate antibiotic therapy with satisfactory peak blood levels. In addition, one should always remember the vital role of early surgical intervention in appropriate circumstances e.g. to drain pus and to excise necrotic tissue.

The haemodynamic changes that characterize septic shock (Table 12) are not determined by the nature of the infecting organism but rather by the response of the host to that organism. Gram-negative and positive infection can produce a high output low peripheral vascular resistance state. Such patients typically have low mean

Table 13.   Complications of septicaemia

1.   Metabolic acidosis – usually lactic acidaemia due to anaerobic metabolism

2.   Hyperglycaemia

3.   Coagulopathy including disseminated intravascular coagulation

4.   Gastro intestinal bleeding

5.   Multiple organ failure

6.   Hypercatabolic state – accelerated muscle wasting and negative nitrogen balance

arterial and central venous pressure with increased cardiac output and heart rate in the presence of a low systemic vascular resistance. There is frequently also impaired peripheral oxygen utilization, which is often as a consequence of shunting at a microcirculatory level or to anaerobic tissue metabolism. The net result is reduced arteriovenous oxygen content difference and frequently a lactic acidosis. Although splanchnic blood flow is increased in septic patients, the coexisting increase in oxygen consumption of the gut and liver may result in relative ischaemia of these organs. This may be compounded by inotropic agents e.g. nor adrenaline. It follows therefore that gut ischaemia may facilitate bacterial translocation from the gut into the circulation and lead to the development of multiple organ failure. Complications of septicaemia are listed in Table 13.

Conventional haemodynamic support for patients with septic shock consists of optimising intravascular volume often with the aid of a pulmonary flotation catheter and restoring normal mean arterial pressure, frequently with the use of inotropic support. Antimicrobial therapy consists of a third generation cephalosporin in combination with an aminoglycoside and a penicillin. If anaerobic infection is suspected metronidazole is added. Flucloxacillin, vancomycin or teicoplanin are prescribed for infection due to *Staphylococcus aureus*. Vancomycin and teicoplanin are indicated for methicillin resistant *Staphylococcus aureus* and for enterococcal infections. Prompt surgical eradication is indicated if a septic focus is present.

Pneumonia in the intensive care unit

Pneumonia can occur as a consequence of septicaemia or can lead to the development of septicaemia. One should always remember that septicemia can lead to the development of multiple organ failure.

Although pneumonia can be caused by Gram-positive and Gram-negative organisms, primary Gram-negative pneumonia is uncommon in the normal host. Features which facilitate the development of pneumonia include deficiencies in respiratory defense mechanisms e.g. impaired coughing as a consequence of pain or level of consciousness, impaired mucociliary clearance as a result of opiates, high inspired oxygen or excessive suctioning, impairment of alveolar phagocytic function as a result of smoking or uraemia, laryngeal dysfunction and immunodeficiency states e.g. Acquired Immune Deficiency Syndrome, immunosuppressive therapy for transplant recipients (Table 11).

Nosocomial pneumonia is defined as infection occurring in patients who have been in hospital for more than 72 hours.

References

1. OH TE Intensive Care Manual, Third Edition. Sydney: Butterworths Pty Ltd 1990

2. Intensive Care Reader (Core Module 4). The Royal College Of Surgeons Of England MRCS Distance Learning Course 1996

3. Duke GJ, Bersten AD. Dopamine and renal salvage in the critically ill patient. *Anaesthesia And Intensive Care* 1992;**20**(3):277–302

4. Moore FA, Moore EE, Haenel JB. Clinical benefits of early post-injury enteral feeding. *Clinical Intensive Care* 1995;**6**:21–27

5. McLuckie A, Bihari D. Sepsis in the intensive care unit. *Care Of The Critically Ill* 1994;**10**(6):276–279

21

Acute Respiratory Distress Syndrome

Brendan Madden

Definition

The acute respiratory distress syndrome (ARDS) as defined by the European American Consensus conference, describes a condition of impaired oxygenation defined as a ratio of the partial pressure of arterial oxygen (PaO_2, measured in mmHg) to the fraction of inspired oxygen (FiO_2) that is less than or equal to 200 irregardless of the level of positive end-expiratory pressure (PEEP) employed to increase lung volume and to keep alveoli open (e.g. a patient with a PaO_2 of 100mmHg with an FiO_2 of 1.0 has a ratio of 100). When this occurs in the presence of bilateral pulmonary infiltrates on chest radiograph and a pulmonary capillary wedge (or occlusion) pressure less than or equal to 18mmHg (or there is no clinical evidence of left ventricular failure), the condition is known as ARDS (Table 1).

In ARDS injury to the alveolar-capillary membrane disrupts the endothelial barrier giving rise to the development of non-cardiogenic pulmonary oedema through increased vascular permeability. As the air spaces fill with fluid the pulmonary compliance and capacity for gas exchange deteriorates giving rise to the clinical entity of ARDS.

Many aetiological factors can give rise to ARDS (Table 2) and they can be divided into those that directly damage the lung and those that cause ARDS by the systemic release of circulating mediators. The associated risk factors or clinical conditions and co-existing organ failures are major determinants of survival. Risk

Table 1.   Criteria for diagnosing acute respiratory distress syndrome

1. Clinical Setting
    Initiating insult
    a) Pulmonary
    b) Non-pulmonary

2. Chest radiograph
    Bilateral pulmonary infiltrates

3. Physiological parameters
    a) Impaired oxygenation

    $$\frac{PaO_2}{FiO_2} < 200$$

    b) Pulmonary capillary wedge pressure < 18 mmHg
    c) Decreased lung compliance
    d) Increased shunt fraction and deadspace ventilation

4. Pathological Phases
    a) Exudative
    b) Proliferative
    c) Fibrotic

factor analysis suggests that most early deaths are the result of complications of the underlying illness, whereas late mortality (>72 hours after onset) is a consequence of sepsis. Hepatic failure in association with ARDS has an almost 100% mortality rate and any combination of three organ failures for more than seven days carries a 98% mortality rate. Estimates of mortality rate from all causes of ARDS have ranged from 40–75%. It has recently been shown however that mechanical ventilation with a lower tidal volume than is traditionally used results in decreased mortality.

Pathology

The pathological features of the lung in ARDS result from disruption of the alveolar-capillary unit. The morphological appearances which are termed diffuse alveolar damage can be divided into three phases which overlap, and which correlate with clinical evolution.

Table 2.   Clinical conditions associated with ARDS

RESPIRATORY

Aspiration of gastric contents

Pneumonia

Lung contusion

Smoke and toxin inhalation

Oxygen toxicity

Goodpastures syndrome

Thoracic radiation

Near drowning

Reperfusion injury

NON-RESPIRATORY

Sepsis

Major trauma

Severe burns

Pancreatitis

Multiple transfusions

Disseminated intravascular coagulation

Fat embolism

Systemic hypotension

Pregnancy related
  aspiration
  amniotic fluid embolism
  pre-eclampsia

Head injury/increased intracranial pressure

Drug reaction/abuse

Tumour lysis syndrome

Cardiopulmonary bypass

Exudative phase

This occupies approximately the first week following the onset of respiratory failure. On macroscopic examination the lungs appear rigid, dull red and with increased weight (up to 1 kg each). Unlike classic pulmonary oedema the cut surface of the lung does not exude fluid. This is because the high protein content of the alveolar exudate leads to coagulation. Eosinophilic hyaline membranes which are most prominent in the alveolar ducts are the distinctive feature of early ARDS. They are composed of condensed plasma proteins mixed with cell debris. Immunoglobulin, fibrinogen and complement are also present. The alveolar septa are widened markedly by interstitial oedema, fibrin and extravasated red cells.

The Proliferative phase

This is characterised by the organisation of intra-alveolar and interstitial exudates. Epithelial regeneration is manifest as rows of cuboidal cells which extend along alveolar walls and cover basement membrane that was previously denuded. Many of these cells are type II respiratory cells. Within the alveolar wall there is proliferation of fibroblasts and myofibroblasts which migrate through defects in the alveolar basement membrane into the fibrinous intra alveolar exudate. The exudate is subsequently converted to cellular granulation tissue and finally to dense fibrous tissue. There is also fibrocellular intimal proliferation in small muscular arteries, veins and lymphatics.

Fibrotic phase

This phase begins as early as the tenth day after onset. Macroscopic examination shows the pleural surface to have a coarse and cobble stoned appearance. There may be evidence of healed abscesses and chronic interstitial emphysema. There is extensive remodelling of the pulmonary vascular bed which contributes to irreversible pulmonary hypertension in patients who develop marked pulmonary fibrosis.

Pathogenesis, Cellular Mechanisms and Mediators

ARDS can be caused by agents that directly damage the lung and by those in which a remote disease process is complicated by ARDS presumably as a result of the action of humoral inflammatory mediators. Similar factors can presumably damage the alveolar capillary membrane when released locally, eg, as a consequence of gastric acid aspiration. Sepsis is a systemic insult which leads to global endothelial damage, cardiovascular depression, and multiple organ failure including ARDS (in approximately 25% of cases). The systemic effects of sepsis are associated with the activation, release and synthesis of a variety of inflammatory mediators. These have been extensively studied as have putative interactions with these factors and the cellular and humoral arms of the immune system and coagulation mechanisms. The mediators studied include endotoxin (lipopolysaccharide), a variety of cytokines (which mediate toxic effects of lipopolysaccharide), lipid mediators (formed after the activation of membrane phospholipase A2) and peptide mediators which are formed following activation of the proteolytic cascades of complement and the coagulation systems. How these agents contribute to the development of ARDS is not clear and similarly the interplay between these factors and neutrophils, macrophages, lymphocytes and platelets remains to be clarified.

Pathophysiology

The normal alveolar epithelium is composed of two types of cells. Flat type I cells account for 90% of the alveolar surface area and are easily injured. Cuboidal type II cells make up the remaining 10%. They are more resistant to injury. Their functions include surfactant production, ion transport and proliferation and differentiation to type I cells after injury.

Following the precipitating lung injury in ARDS there is damage to the alveolar capillary membrane, abnormal surfactant metabolism and injury to type II pneumocytes. As a consequence increased vascular permeability ensues giving rise to pulmonary oedema in the presence of surfactant dysfunction and depletion. This can lead to the development of alveolar oedema and atelectasis. The endothelial dysfunction which complicates injury to the alveolar capillary membrane leads to impaired hypoxic pulmonary vasoconstriction exacerbating ventilation perfusion inequality and increasing shunting. Lung compliance and functional residual capacity falls progressively as alveolar oedema and atelectasis involves more of the pulmonary parenchyma.

Diagnosis

The diagnosis of ARDS is made on the basis of historical and clinical presentation, chest radiography, arterial blood gas analysis, haemodynamic parameters and computed tomography of the chest.

Chest Radiography

Initially chest radiography may be normal following the precipitating event but full progression to the typical presentation of diffuse bilateral alveolar infiltrates is usually present within 24 hours following the initial insult. In the early stages of the disease, chest radiography is useful in assisting the diagnosis of conditions such as pneumonia, lung contusion and gastric aspiration. As disease progression occurs, air space shadowing with prominent air bronchograms appear with features of multi-focal consolidation. Exudative pleural effusions may also be present. Subsequently, areas of consolidation may be replaced by interstitial or 'ground glass' patterns. Cyst formation may complicate pulmonary infarction. It can be impossible to delineate cardiogenic from non-cardiogenic pulmonary oedema on the basis of chest radiography alone. Features which favour ARDS include patchy peripheral shadowing, normal heart size and decreased frequency of septal lines. As the underlying process extends to involve more of the pulmonary parenchyma the radiological picture can progress to a 'white-out' of both lung fields. It should be remembered that therapeutic intervention can significantly alter radiographic appearances in patients with ARDS. Excess fluid administration may exacerbate alveolar oedema whereas diuretic therapy may lessen it. Mechanical ventilatory techniques (particularly with PEEP) which increase mean airway pressure can reduce regional lung density by increasing lung inflation which may artificially suggest improvement. Chest radiography is an insensitive guide to disease progression in ARDS. Daily chest radiographs are essential to detect complications such as pneumothorax, pneumomediastinum (from barotrauma) and complications of flotation catheter or endotracheal tube placement.

Arterial blood gas analysis

Initially arterial blood gas analysis demonstrates respiratory alkalosis with varying degrees of hypoxemia. The hypoxemia is usually relatively resistant to supplemental oxygen via nasal prongs or face mask. As alveolar oedema progresses the pulmonary shunt fraction increases, arterial hypoxemia worsens, pulmonary compliance falls and the work of respiration increases. At this stage mechanical ventilatory support is necessary.

It should be remembered that the shunt equation gives an estimate of the proportion of blood being shunted past poorly ventilated alveoli (Q_s) relative to total blood flow (Q_T)

$$\frac{Q_s}{Q_T} = \frac{C_cO_2 - C_aO_2}{C_cO_2 - C_vO_2}$$

Where C_cO_2 = end capillary O_2 content (calculated from PAO_2), CaO_2 = arterial O_2 content (calculated from PaO_2), C_vO_2 = mixed venous O_2 content (either calculated from mixed venous PO_2 measured from a pulmonary artery catheter or assumed to be 50ml/l less than arterial O_2 content. Alveolar PO_2 (PAO_2) is derived from the alveolar gas equation:

$$PAO_2 = \text{Inspired } PO_2 - \frac{PaCO_2}{\text{Respiratory Quotient}}$$

Respiratory quotient normally approximates 0.8. $Q_s : Q_T$ is normally 3 to 5% of cardiac output.

Haemodynamic monitoring

The role of pulmonary arterial flotation (Swan Ganz) catheters in intensive care management is controversial. Nevertheless in the context of ARDS, Swan Ganz catheterisation provides important information regarding the pulmonary capillary wedge pressure, cardiac output, cardiac index, systemic vascular resistance and pulmonary arterial oxygen saturation (SVO_2).

In addition to confirming that the patient has non-cardiogenic pulmonary oedema, fluid balance can be optimised and inotropic support prescribed if indicated (eg, noradrenalin may be indicated for patients with low systemic vascular resistance as a consequence of bacterial septicaemia). The systemic vascular resistance (SVR) is calculated by the equation:

$$\frac{\text{Mean Arterial BP} - \text{Right Atrial Pressure}}{\text{Cardiac Output}}$$

To convert to dynes sec cm^{-5} one multiplies by 79.9. The normal SVR is 770–1500 dyne sec cm^{-5}. It can be as low as 300 in patients with septic shock.

Computed thoracic tomography

Thoracic CT scanning may provide additional information that is not apparent on chest radiography. It can help to assess the degree of pulmonary involvement in the process which in itself can be correlated with pulmonary compliance and efficiency of gas exchange. Furthermore evidence of barotrauma or localised infection, eg, pneumothorax, empyema or lung abscess not evident on plain chest radiography may be obtained. It may also be possible to ascertain potential steroid responsiveness if scanning reveals parenchymal ground glass shadowing. The role of steroid therapy in ARDS is controversial. However, there is some evidence from uncontrolled studies that sustained courses of high dose steroids given to uninfected patients in the later (fibroproliferative) stage may shorten the clinical course, with few steroid-related complications.

Broncho-alveolar lavage

This can be performed safely in patients with ARDS and provides a useful diagnostic tool for diagnosing nosocomial or opportunistic respiratory infection. Ideally a combination of protected specimen brushing and bronchoalveolar lavage should be performed if pneumonia is suspected as this combination has a sensitivity and specificity > 85% in the diagnosis of nosocomial pneumonia. It is common for increased concentration of polymorphonuclear leukocytes to be present in broncho-alveolar lavage fluid in patients with ARDS. Occasionally eosinophilia may be present (eg, when ARDS is drug related) and this may suggest steroid responsiveness.

Assessment of Lung Injury in ARDS

Efforts to assess acute lung injury have been made by measuring the protein content of alveolar fluid or the flux of radio labelled proteins from blood to lung parenchyma.

Unfortunately these tests are at best supportive rather than diagnostic. Measurement of extra vascular water can be performed and is often three to eight times the upper limit of normal. Interpretation of these measurements however is difficult. Usually lung injury in ARDS is assessed using scoring systems based on the extent of pulmonary infiltrate on chest radiography, the degree of arterial hypoxemia and a measurement of pulmonary compliance. Unfortunately such a scoring system has not been correlated with outcome. Scoring systems such as the Acute Physiology And Chronic Health Evaluation (APACHE) III system or the Mortality Prediction Model are commonly used in clinical trials but their usefulness in patients with ARDS is not clear.

Management

Clinical management is by and large supportive and treatment is therefore aimed at optimising gas exchange, critical organ perfusion and aerobic metabolism during which time the acute lung injury will hopefully resolve. As there are a paucity of controlled clinical trials to justify a variety of therapeutic interventions currently employed in the management of patients with ARDS many of these treatment strategies are controversial. Aspects of care in the management of a patient with ARDS include mechanical ventilation, haemodynamic support and fluid balance, nutritional support, early diagnosis and treatment of infection and other complications, eg, pneumothorax, empyema. A variety of pharmacological agents have been tried with limited success although the literature is lacking in case controlled clinical trials supporting their use.

Ventilation

Ventilatory support is adjusted to maintain acceptable gas exchange with minimal complications. Different units may define acceptable gas exchange differently but one frequently aims for PaO_2 in the region of 8–10kPa, with $PaCO_2$ of 4–6.5kPa and arterial oxygen saturation greater than or equal to 90%. The lowest FiO_2 is employed to attain these goals with tidal volume in the region of 6mls per kilogramme body weight and PEEP (initially less than or equal to 5cm of water). There has been a shift to maintain tidal volumes below earlier recommendations as large tidal volumes (i.e. 10–15mls per kilogramme of body weight) and high peak airway pressures can cause direct injury to the alveolar capillary membrane and hence exacerbate ARDS. Furthermore excessive distention or "stretch" of the aerated lung may cause release of inflammatory mediators which can increase lung injury and also damage other organs. PEEP is applied in order to increase lung volume and keep alveoli open. It should be remembered that 'prophylactic' PEEP does not prevent ARDS in patients at risk of developing this condition although routine use of low levels of PEEP may limit the development of atelectasis. PEEP can be increased in small increments to a maximum of 15cm of water in order to attain arterial oxygen saturation greater than or equal 90% while maintaining non-toxic FiO_2 values (less than or equal to 0.6) with acceptable peak airway pressures (less than 40cm of water). This is because elevated peak airway pressures, and high FiO_2 values can cause lung damage and impede repair mechanisms that normally occur in the presence of lung injury. One should also remember that PEEP can adversely affect haemodynamics.

In inverse ratio ventilation the inspiratory time is prolonged. This increases mean airway pressures while keeping peak airway pressures acceptable. Inverse ratio ventilation can be volume controlled or pressure controlled. Pressure controlled inverse ratio ventilation is gaining increasing popularity in the management of patients with ARDS. Those in favour of this ventilatory modality quote the fact that the pulmonary infiltrates are not distributed homogeneously in the lungs of patients with ARDS and that sustained inspiratory pressures may have their greatest incremental effect on non-functional areas of the lung. The maximum benefit of this type of ventilation can take several hours to achieve which may support the hypothesis that sustained inspiratory pressure is one beneficial mechanism with its use. Further experience and clinical trials with this type of ventilatory support are however necessary. High frequency (jet) ventilation has been used in patients with ARDS who have no primary lung infection, and who have multiple areas of atelectasis. The use of this type of ventilatory support in patients with ARDS is controversial. High frequency jet ventilation delivers dry gas under a high pressure (approximately 345kPa) at rates of 2–10Hz by means of fluidic selenoid, or rotating valve flow controllers. Driving pressure, frequency and I:E ratio are usually adjustable. Gas entrainment in the proximal airway is common but not invariable. Expiration is passive and PEEP may be added. Humidification depends on entrainment of additional humidified gas through a side arm, placing a humidifier before or after the cycling device, or a saline drip into the circuit immediately in front of the jet nozzle. The optimal position of the jet nozzle in the trachea is unknown. Gas exchange occurs by convective gas transport and tidal volumes are small at 1 to 2.5ml/kg. Peak airway pressure is reduced. This type of ventilation has been successfully used in patients with bronchopleural fistula and in patients who have had subsequent reintubation and ventilation following pneumonectomy. A prospective randomised trial of high frequency jet ventilation versus conventional ventilation showed no significant difference in mortality in patients with ARDS. The ventilators employed used frequencies of approximately 5Hz, the resonant frequency of the lung, and maximised alveolar recruitment while maintaining alveolar volume at lower peak inspiratory pressures than would be achievable using conventional methods. Prospective randomised studies are in progress.

Extracorporial membrane oxygenation (ECMO) has been used successfully in children and with some success in adults with ARDS. Venoarterial or venovenous extra corporeal membrane oxygenation may be employed in acute lung injury. The prime objective of ECMO is oxygenation and the transfer of carbon dioxide across the membrane occurs as a secondary effect. Complications such as haemorrhage, bleeding disorders and sepsis have been diminished by advances such as heparin bonded circuits and percutaneous cannulation techniques. Nonetheless these complications still represent a major cause of morbidity and mortality.

If patients have arterial hypoxemia unresponsive to maximal medical therapy, repositioning (in the lateral decubitus or prone position) may be helpful. Management of patients in the prone position requires experience and careful monitoring.

Haemodynamic support, fluid balance and monitoring

Because of the increased capillary permeability in patients with ARDS efforts are made to keep the pulmonary capillary wedge pressure as low as possible while at the same time maintaining adequate perfusion to vital organs. Colloid (eg, blood, human albumin solution) is sometimes necessary to increase (albeit temporarily) plasma oncotic pressure. Inotropic support is prescribed if clinically indicated and is adjusted with respect to haemodynamic measurements (eg, cardiac output, cardiac index, SVO_2, systemic vascular resistance) obtained at Swan Ganz catheterisation. Agents which are inotropes and which increase cardiac index include adrenaline and dopamine, whereas noradrenalin is used to increase SVR (e.g. in patients with septic shock). It should be remembered that PEEP artificially elevates central venous filling pressure.

Every effort is made to preserve renal function. Mortality from acute renal failure alone is approximately 8%. If acute renal failure occurs in association with failure of another organ system, mortality rises to 70%. If there is coexistent renal and two other organ system failure mortality is in the region of 95%. The use of dopamine to improve renal perfusion is controversial and not proved in clinical trials. Furthermore, dopamine (even at so called renal doses of less than 5mcgs per kg per minute) may cause gut ischaemia as a consequence of poor splanchnic perfusion. As a consequence bacterial translocation can occur in the bowel giving rise to bacteraemia, toxaemia or septicaemia. Dopexamine may be a suitable alternative to dopamine with respect to renal function and this agent does not reduce splanchnic blood flow. Should patients develop acute renal failure, renal replacement therapy should be considered early. The standard indications for initiating renal replacement therapy are:

- uncontrollable acidosis
- intractable hyperkalaemia
- fluid overload
- signs and symptoms of uraemia

Feeding

It is important that feeding is commenced early in patients with ARDS. Enteral feeding is preferred and is also important in maintaining gut mucosal integrity. Patients who are intolerant of enteral feeding are given total parenteral nutrition using standard protein, carbohydrate and lipid preparations supplemented with vitamins and trace elements. It is important that haematological and biochemical indices are monitored regularly and trace elements measured at least weekly together with C reactive protein.

Infection

Patients with ARDS are at risk of infection for a variety of reasons. Firstly the nature of the initiating injury, eg, aspiration, trauma or septicaemia may lead directly to lung infection. The patients will have mechanical ventilatory support which increases susceptibility to infection as does the presence of central lines, arterial lines, chest drains and urinary catheters. It is essential therefore that infection surveillance is regular and thorough. One should have a high index of suspicion for infection and sputum, blood, drainage fluid and urine specimens should be sent for microbiological culture if sepsis is suspected. It should also be remembered that the systemic response to infection may be atypical and is often manifest by two or more of the following:

- temperature less than 36° centigrade or greater than 38° centigrade.
- heart rate greater than 90 beats per minute.
- respiratory rate greater than 20 breaths per minute or $PaCO_2$ less than 32mmHg.
- white blood cell count greater than 12 000 or less than 4 000 per cubic millimetre or greater than 10% band forms

As previously mentioned thoracic CT scan may demonstrate lung abscess or empyema not readily visualised on chest radiograph which will require drainage and appropriate antimicrobial therapy. Fibre-optic bronchoscopy with broncho-alveolar lavage is important in the diagnosis of nosocomial or opportunistic lung infection. Broncho-alveolar lavage sputum, and blood can be sent for microbiological analysis. High airway pressures and PEEP together with underlying lung injury can predispose to the development of pneumothorax which requires early diagnosis and, if necessary, intercostal drainage. If persistent air leak necessitates prolonged intercostal drainage, infection in the pleural space may occur.

Pharmacological Therapies

Unfortunately, there is no specific pulmonary arterial vasodilator. However, on account of its short half-life, nitric oxide can act in a selective way on the pulmonary circulation when inspired at concentrations of 5-80 parts per million. Similarly, intravenous or nebulised prostacyclin can cause pulmonary arteriolar vasodilatation. These agents are particularly useful in patients with ARDS who have pulmonary arterial hypertension and right ventricular failure. It should be remembered that in patients with ARDS local reflex mechanisms may reduce perfusion to areas of lung parenchyma which are not being ventilated in an attempt to reduce ventilation perfusion mismatch. It follows therefore that the use of a non-specific pulmonary vaso-dilating agent may increase perfusion to these non-ventilated areas and therefore make the shunt faction (and hence arterial hypoxemia) worse. There is no convincing evidence that either administration of nitric oxide or prostacyclin improves survival in patients with ARDS although both should be considered in selected patients with pulmonary hypertension and right ventricular failure. Further controlled studies are necessary.

A favourable response to vaso-dilating agents is defined as a greater than 30% reduction in pulmonary vascular resistance with a corresponding increase in cardiac output. Corticosteroids are not routinely given to patients with ARDS. They may be considered in those patients with eosinophilia in broncho-alveolar lavage fluid (eg, if ARDS is drug related) or in those patients who have ground glass shadowing on thoracic CT scanning who do not have co-existent infection.

Instillation of surfactant improves survival in infant respiratory distress syndrome. Unfortunately studies have yet to support the use of surfactant in ARDS and indeed it is not known which of the many types of surfactant will confer most benefit. The role of anti-oxidants eg, acetylcysteine (an oxygen free radical scavenger and precursor of glutathione) or ketoconazole (a potent inhibitor of thromboxane and leukotrine synthesis) are unclear.

Pentoxifylline is a phosphodiesterase inhibitor that inhibits the chemotaxis and activation of neutrophils in animal models of ARDS and sepsis. Its role in the management of ARDS in humans remains unclear. Similarly the role for anti-endotoxin and anti-cytokine therapy in the management of ARDS (particularly if due to sepsis) have yet to be established.

Management During the Recovery Phase

Most patients who die of ARDS do so within the first two weeks of their illness. For those who survive, the recovery period is variable and can occur over several months. Generally the majority of the alveolar edema resolves after seven to ten days and new infiltrates visible on the chest radiograph after this time may represent infective or non-infective inflammatory change or the onset of pulmonary fibrosis.

As the alveolar edema resolves, oxygenation improves, although minute ventilatory demands remain high. It is not uncommon for satisfactory arterial oxygenation to be achieved with an FiO_2 of 0.4 to 0.6 and a PEEP of 5–8cm of water. One should be careful in not reducing the airway pressures provided by mechanical ventilatory support (particularly by PEEP) too quickly, as terminal airways remain quite unstable and rapid deterioration in oxygenation may occur. Many authors now recommend that PEEP be decreased slowly by 2-3cm of water every 12 hours. As the majority of patients with ARDS require ventilatory support for at least 10 to 14 days, the question of tracheostomy is frequently addressed. In general the

Table 3. Complications of tracheostomy

During the Procedure

1. Haemorrhage
2. Injury to adjacent structures (pneumothorax, oesophageal damage)
3. Air embolism
4. Anoxia

After Tracheostomy Established

Early	Obstructed tube
	Displaced tube
	Subcutaneous or mediastinal emphysema
	Infection of trachea site
	Respiratory infection
	Haemorrhage (e.g. erosion of innominate artery)
	Tracheo — oesophageal fistula
	Apnoea and severe hypotension (sudden fall of $PaCO_2$)
Late	Tracheal stenosis
	Difficult decanulation
	Tracheocutaneous fistula
	Keloid and granulation tissue formation

indications for tracheostomy include:

- prolonged weaning from mechanical ventilatory support anticipated
- patient unable to tolerate the endotracheal tube without sedation
- failed trial of extubation
- underlying chronic respiratory disease

Clearly the timing will vary depending on circumstances but patients are usually more comfortable with a tracheostomy. Progress with weaning is usually more rapid as sedation can be discontinued and the patient sat out of bed. Tracheostomy can be performed via a formal surgical approach in theatre or percutaneously using a guidewire and dilator technique. Complications of tracheostomy are listed in Table 3.

Pulmonary Function in Survivors

It would appear that recovery of lung function is most rapid in the first six months and reaches a plateau one year after the onset of

ARDS. It is common for survivors to report one or more respiratory symptoms such as dyspnoea and a reduced carbon monoxide diffusing capacity is the most common abnormality of lung function. Such reductions in diffusing capacity are often still apparent even when corrected for alveolar volume, suggesting that the most important defect is a loss of pulmonary capillary surface area. Some patients may develop airflow obstruction and others may develop complications attendant on tracheostomy tube insertion (e.g. tracheal stenosis). Unfortunately, it is not possible to predict which patients will develop significant impairment in respiratory function following ARDS and many centres will follow these patients on a regular basis with serial estimates of lung function. No therapeutic interventions, however, have been shown to improve outcome in this group. Lung transplantation is not considered appropriate in the acute phase of ARDS, largely because of sepsis and attendant other end organ impairment which render mortality of transplantation excessive. It may, however, be an option in selected patients who have chronically impaired lung function following the initial insult, assuming that no other contra-indications to transplantation are present.

Conclusion

ARDS may represent a final common pathway in the lung to a variety of injuries. Treatment is by and large supportive although current research suggests that a variety of vaso-dilating drugs, anti-inflammatory agents and immuno-modulators may have a role to play in the future. Survival appears to be related to the aetiological factor and there is evidence that, in spite of the multi-factorial aetiology, survival in patients with ARDS is improving beyond 50%. It has recently been shown that mechanical ventilatory support using lower tidal volumes (e.g. 6 mls/kg) reduces mortality significantly and increases the number of days without ventilator use. It is hoped that multi-disciplinary clinical collaboration and research will further improve our understanding of the pathophysiology of ARDS and hence lead to improved therapeutic strategies and survival for patients with this syndrome.

References

1.   Petty TL, Ashbaugh DG. The adult respiratory distress syndrome —
      Clinical features, factors influencing prognosis and principles of
      Management. *Chest* 1971;**60**:233

2. Meduri GU, Belenchia JM, Estes RJ, Wundering RG, El Torky M, Leeper V. Fibroproliferative phase of ARDS. Clinical findings and effect of corticosteroids. *Chest* 1991;**100**:943

3. Chastre JC, Fagon JY, Lamer C et al. Procedures for the diagnosis of pneumonia in ICU patients. *Intensive Care Med* 1992;**118**:S10

4. Sprung CL, Rackow EC, Fein IA, Jacob Al, Isikoff SK. The spectrum of pulmonary edema: differentiation of cardiogenic, intermediate, and new cardiogenic forms of pulmonary edema. *Am Rev Respir Dis* 1981;**124**:718

5. Drake RE, Laine GA. Pulmonary microvascular permeability to fluid and macromolecules. *J Appl Physiol* 1988;**64**:487

6. Leatherman JW, Lari RL, Iber C, Ney Al. Tidal volume reduction in ARDS-effect on cardiac output and arterial oxygenation. *Chest* 1991;**99**:1227

7. Kollef M, Schuster D. The acute respiratory distress syndrome. *N Engl J Med* 1995;**332**:27

8. Griffiths M, Evans T. Adult respiratory distress syndrome in respiratory medicine, 2nd Edition, p 605. In: Brewis, Corrin, Geddes, Gibson, eds. London: WB Saunders & Co Ltd 1995

9. Keogh BF, Heard S, Calkins J et al. Ultra high frequency ventilation in severe ARDS: preliminary results from multicentre study. *Eur Respir J* 1991;**4**(Suppl 14):176

10. Rossaint R, Falke KJ, Lopez F, Slama K, Pison U, Zapol WM. Inhaled nitric oxide for the adult respiratory distress syndrome. *N Engl J Med* 1993;**328**:399

11. Lewis JF, Jobe AH. Surfactant and adult respiratory distress syndrome. *Am Rev Respir Dis* 1993;**147**:218

12. Peters JI, Bell RC, Prihoda TJ et al. Clinical determinants of abnormalities in pulmonary function in survivors of the adult respiratory distress syndrome. *Am Rev Respir Dis* 1989;**139**:1163

13. The acute respiratory distress syndrome network. Ventilation with lower tidal volumes as compared with traditional tidal volumes for acute lung injury and the acute respiratory distress syndrome. *N Engl J Med* 2000;**342**:1301–1308

22

Lung Transplantation and Thoracic Surgery

Brendan Madden

Introduction

Lung transplantation has an established role in the management of a variety of pulmonary, vascular and parenchymal lung diseases leading to end stage respiratory failure. The first successful human heart–lung transplant was reported in 1982. Initially this procedure was limited to patients with pulmonary vascular disease although it has been subsequently successfully extended to patients with end stage parenchymal lung disease including cystic fibrosis. More recently single-lung transplantation, double-lung transplantation and bilateral sequential lung transplantation have been successfully employed for patients with end stage respiratory failure.

Indications and Contra-indications to Lung Transplantation

The main indications for lung transplantation are:

- severe respiratory failure despite maximal medical therapy
- severely impaired quality of life
- patient positively wants a transplant

Only patients who have deteriorating, chronic, respiratory failure should be accepted on to the transplant waiting list. In practice the forced respiratory volume in one-second (FEV_1) is usually less than 30% of the predicted value. Careful psychological assessment is necessary to exclude patients with intractable psychosocial insta-

Table 1. Contrindications to lung transplantation

Absolute Contra-indications

1. Non-compliance with treatment.
2. Malignant disease within five years.
3. Hepatitis B surface antigen and Hepatitis C seropositivity.
4. Active aspergillus or mycobacterial infection.
5. Infection with Human Immunodeficiency Virus I & II.
6. Bacterial species in sputum with no *in-vitro* antibiotic sensitivities.
7. Gross malnutrition.
8. Other end organ failure.
9. Prednisolone therapy > 10 mg/d
10. Age > 60 years.

Risk Factors

1. Chemical pleurodesis.
2. Previous thoracic surgery (pleurectomy, abrasion pleurodesis).
3. Pre-operative ventilation.
4. Severe liver disease necessitating combined heart–lung and liver transplantation.

bility that may interfere with their ability to cope with the operation and to comply with the strict post-operative follow-up and immunosuppressive regimens. In most centres the upper age limit is 60 years for single lung transplantation and 50 years for heart–lung, double lung and bilateral lung transplantation.

Contra-indications to lung transplantation are listed in Table 1. Non-compliance with treatment is an absolute contra-indication as it is essential that patients take life-long immunosuppressive therapy and attend the transplant clinic for regular post-operative follow-up. Patients with a history of malignancy can be accepted on the transplant waiting list provided their disease has been successfully treated and the patient has been in remission for at least five years prior to acceptance on to the transplant waiting list. The presence of hepatitis B surface antigen, hepatitis C sero-positivity and human inmmuno-deficiency virus type I and II prelude transplantation as does active infection with aspergillus or mycobacteria. There would be concern about progressive or disseminated infection from these infectious agents in an immuno-compromised patient post lung transplant. Sometimes one encounters pseudomonas or

Burkholderia cepacia species in the sputum of patients with cystic fibrosis to which no *in vitro* antibiotic sensitivities are available. This is uncommon although in theory it would preclude acceptance on to the transplant waiting list. Gross malnutrition has to be vigorously addressed prior to transplantation and this may necessitate insertion of gastrostomy or jejunostomy feeding tubes. Other end organ failure precludes transplantation unless this is also amenable to transplantation, eg, combined heart–lung and liver transplantation in patients with cystic fibrosis who have end stage respiratory failure with portal hypertension. Patients with cushingoid features are excluded until these changes subside with reduction in steroid therapy. There is concern that long term steroid therapy may adversely affect tissue healing (and particularly healing of the major airway anastomoses) after transplantation. Most transplant units do not accept patients over the age of 60 years.

Risk factors which significantly increase early mortality are also listed in Table 1. Chemical pleurodesis and previous thoracic surgical procedures are associated with adhesion formation which may give rise to major bleeding at the time of pneumonectomy. Patients who are pre-operatively intubated and ventilated immediately prior to transplantation may have colonisation of their sputum with resistant bacteria and may develop post-operative infection. Combined heart–lung and liver transplantation has been performed in small numbers of cystic fibrosis patients with respiratory failure and portal hypertension and this procedure is associated with increased early mortality.

Choice of Surgical Procedure

The current indications for heart–lung transplantation (HLT), bilateral lung transplantation (BLT), double-lung transplantation (DLT) and single-lung transplantation (SLT) are summarised in Table 2.

Heart–lung transplantation

HLT can be used in a variety of patients with pulmonary vascular and parenchymal lung disease. It is performed by a median sternotomy incision with cardio-pulmonary bypass. Right atrial, aortic and tracheal anastomoses are made and the coronary-bronchial collateral circulation (which provides an important blood supply to the trachea) remains intact; ischaemic complications of the large airways are therefore uncommon.

Table 2.   Current indications for heart–lung, double-lung and single-lung transplantation

Pulmonary vascular disease

	Primary indication	Alternative Options
Eisenmenger's syndrome	HLT	DLT or SLT with repair of defect
Primary pulmonary hypertension	DLT	HLT, SLT[1]
Complex pulmonary atresia	HLT	
Thromboembolic pulmonary hypertension	DLT	HLT, SLT[1]
Pulmonary veno-occlusive disease	HLT[2]	

Parenchymal lung disease

Cystic Fibrosis	BLT, HLT	DLT
Bronchiectasis	BLT, HLT	DLT
Emphysema	BLT, DLT	SLT
Sarcoidosis	SLT	DLT, BLT
Cryptogenic Fibrosing Alveolitis	SLT	
Occupational Lung Disease	SLT	
Obliterative Bronchiolitis	SLT	
Lymphangioleiomyomatosis	SLT	DLT, BLT
Eosinophilic Granuloma	DLT, BLT	
Adult Respiratory Distress Syndrome	SLT[3]	

HLT, heart–lung transplantation; DLT, double-lung transplantation; SLT, single-lung transplantation; BLT, bilateral lung transplantation.

1. Reperfusion pulmonary oedema in the early post-operative period is a serious risk.
2. Experience limited.
3. Results of transplantation in the acute phase of the illness are poor.

Another cited advantage of HLT is domino cardiac transplantation. In this procedure the heart from a patient who receives HLT for conditions other than Eisenmenger's syndrome can, if healthy, be successfully transplanted into a patient requiring cardiac transplantation alone, so long as there is no severe irreversible elevation in pulmonary vascular resistance. The results of this procedure are very encouraging and, in addition, it offers advantages of short organ ischaemic time and non-exposure of the donor heart to the effects of brainstem death. Psychologically domino transplant recipients respond well in the knowledge that a donor did not die to give them a chance of life and the HLT recipient receives consolation from the knowledge that they were able to help someone else.

With increasing numbers of centres performing cardiac transplantation, the number of heart–lung blocs available for HLT (and therefore, the number of HLTs being performed) are declining significantly. Consequently the primary indications for HLT are being redefined. It is likely that as more and more patients are successfully transplanted with DLT and BLT the only primary indication for HLT will be Eisenmenger's syndrome with a surgically incorrectable cardiac defect.

Bilateral lung transplantation

This procedure allows the patient to retain his own heart but healing of the airway anastomoses may be jeopardised as a result of ischaemia secondary to interruption of the coronary–bronchial collateral circulation.

DLT is performed via a median sternotomy on cardio-pulmonary bypass. The procedure involves anastomoses of the trachea, pulmonary artery and pulmonary veins (to the left atrium). The initial results of DLT were poor principally because of tracheal and anastomotic dehiscence, but recent reports are more encouraging. BLT is performed more frequently worldwide than DLT and HLT. When it is indicated the procedure is usually performed via bilateral thoracotomy incisions or a thoracosternotomy (clam shell) incision. The lungs are inserted in a sequential fashion and bi-bronchial anastomoses are fashioned in addition to pulmonary arterial and venous anastomoses. Airway healing is less impaired than following DLT because the bronchus is supplied with blood partly from the neighbouring hilum. The procedure can also often be undertaken without cardio-pulmonary bypass and thus avoids attendant complications such as bleeding, complement activation and neurological defects.

Single-Lung Transplantation

This is performed through a postero-lateral thoracotomy. Anastomoses are made at the level of the main bronchus, pulmonary artery and pulmonary veins (with a cuff of donor atrium to recipient left atrium). Before 1983, no long term clinical success was achieved with SLT. The majority of early mortality was related to infection, rejection and ischaemic complications of the bronchial anastomosis. However, with increasing experience, the advent of cyclosporin A and careful selection of donor and recipient, encouraging results are now being reported.

The primary indication for SLT is restrictive lung disease, eg, pulmonary fibrosis. The increase in elastic recoil and vascular resistance of the remaining fibrotic lung in these patients ensures a progressive shift of alveolar ventilation and lung perfusion from the native to the transplanted side. Ventilation perfusion mismatching is therefore uncommon. Emphysema is a possible indication for SLT but hyper-expansion of the remaining native lung and the tendency of the allograft to receive a disproportionate amount of air relative to blood makes the outcome unpredictable. BLT may be a better alternative. Patients with primary pulmonary hypertension may be treated successfully with SLT but the development of pulmonary oedema in the transplanted lung in the early post-operative period is associated with a high mortality. As a consequence of this risk many centres advocate BLT or HLT for primary pulmonary hypertension. Pre-existing sepsis, eg, in cystic fibrosis or bronchiectasis, usually precludes SLT because there is a high risk of the transplanted lung becoming infected by sputum overspill from the remaining native lung. SLT and pneumonectomy is not considered appropriate for suppurative lung diseases because of the high risk of breakdown of the bronchial stump and empyema formation in an immunocompromised host.

Lobar transplantation

Living related lobar transplantation has been applied successfully to patients with cystic fibrosis. Intermediate term results are comparable to cadaveric lung transplantation with respect to survival, function and incidence of complications. Following bilateral pneu-

Table 3.   Donor selection

1. No significant cardiac or pulmonary injury.
2. Non-smoker.
3. Age < 50 years.
4. Clear lung fields on chest radiograph.
5. Normal gas exchange (PaO_2 > 15 kPa with an FiO_2 of 35%)
6. No systemic infection.
7. No past history of pulmonary, cardiac or malignant disease.
8. Normal ECG.

monectomy the recipient receives a bilateral sequential transplant of a lower lobe from each of two living donors. There must be detailed independent, clinical and psychological assessment to ensure that the donors and recipient are fully aware of the risks attendant on lobectomy and on transplantation. It is essential that undue pressure is not being brought to bear on the donors or healthy siblings of the cystic fibrosis patient to become donors. It should also be remembered that cystic fibrosis can run in families and therefore more than one child can be affected. As parents can theoretically only donate one lobe each, they should not be put in a position of having to chose between children. Recent work with cadaveric lobar transplantation whereby an adult cadaveric single lung is divided into two lobes, for a smaller bilateral lung recipient, suggests that this may be an encouraging option for selected paediatric candidates.

Donor Selection

Guidelines to determine organ suitability are listed in Table 3. Good donor cardiac and respiratory function are essential to optimise success of cardiac and pulmonary transplantation. The commonest cause of brain death in donors is trauma with brain injury and cerebral vascular events. It is appreciated that with increasing demand and scarcity of suitable donor organs the criteria listed in Table 3 may change.

Donor and Recipient Matching

Matching criteria are based on ABO blood group compatibility, size of thoracic cage and cytomegalovirus (CMV) antibody status.

Potential recipients are also screened for pre-formed antibodies against a panel of HLA antigens. Ideally the donor lung should be slightly smaller than the recipient chest cavity as organs which are too big may predispose to atelectasis and uneven ventilation due to compression. On the other hand, lungs which are too small may fail to obliterate the pleural space with the potential risks of air leak, pleural effusion or empyema formation. CMV infection is a major cause of morbidity and mortality following lung transplantation. Infection can be transmitted by donor organs or blood products. Whenever possible therefore CMV negative recipients should receive CMV negative donor organs and blood products in an effort to minimise post-operative infection as CMV negative antibody recipients of a CMV positive donor organ have a higher incidence of primary CMV pneumonitis.

Pre-transplant Assessment

Patients are admitted to hospital for a period of about one week which enables them to get to know the staff, visit the surgical centre and meet some patients who have already been transplanted. While in hospital a full history and physical examination (which includes height, weight and chest measurements) is performed and assessment of the patient's quality of life and psycho-social suitability is undertaken. There will be a detailed dental and ear, nose and throat examination as chronically infected sinuses of teeth may become potential sources of post-operative infection. Measurments of lung function include FEV$_1$, forced vital capacity (FVC) and arterial blood gas analysis at rest and on exertion. Typically when patients are accepted on to the transplant waiting list their FEV$_1$ and FVC are about 30% predicted and oxygen saturation at rest is between 80% and 90% with marked desaturation on exertion. In addition to chest radiography a CT scan of the thorax is undertaken to assess the state of the patient's pleura as many patients, eg, cystic fibrosis patients often have extensive pleural thickening and adhesions which are essential to document prior to surgery.

Cardiac assessment involves clinical evaluation, electrocardiography, transthoracic two dimensional echocardiography and 24 hour holter monitoring. After careful counselling permission is sought from patients who are being accepted for HLT to become a cardiac donor for the domino procedure. When HLT is performed for conditions other than Eisenmenger's syndrome the patient's heart may be suitable for transplantation into another patient requiring cardiac transplantation alone. In order for a heart to be considered suitable for domino transplantation, valves and left ventricular function must be normal. Mild to moderate tricuspid regurgitation and right ventricular dysfunction are however acceptable. Patients who are being accepted for BLT or SLT will routinely undergo coronary angiography (if there is a potential risk of underlying coronary artery disease) and measurement of pulmonary vascular resistance. The presence of coronary artery disease may necessitate bypass grafting at the time of transplantation or may be an indication for supportive cardiopulmonary bypass. If patients have a mean pulmonary artery pressure in excess of 50mmHg SLT is contraindicated and BLT is considered.

Blood group and routine haematological and biochemical parameters are measured and abnormalities in hepatic and renal function addressed. With regard to lung transplantation liver disease may be associated with coagulation disorders and hence perioperative bleeding or may be a contra-indication to post-operative administration of azathioprine. Serological investigations for infection include those for CMV, Epstein–Barr virus, Australia antigen, toxoplasmosis, human immuno-deficiency virus I and II and herpes simplex. Microbiological examination of the sputum is undertaken for pathogenic organisms, acid-fast bacilli and fungi.

Patient Preparation

It is essential that patients and their family are fully prepared for the events which may ensue following acceptance on to the transplant waiting list. It should be stressed that unfortunately there are more patients requiring transplantation than suitable donor organs and therefore that being accepted on to the transplant waiting list does not guarantee that a suitable donor organ will be found for the patient. Indeed up to 40% of patients die on the transplant waiting list. The patient should also be advised of the risks of transplantation and what to expect in the intensive care unit and during the early post-operative period. They should also understand that following transplantation they will need to take life-long daily immuno-suppresive therapy and will require careful post-operative supervision. It is also important to point out that obliterative bronchiolitis is a potential long-term complication following successful transplantation. The majority of patients and their families realise that without transplantation the chance of survival is minimal. However, with transplantation there is a good chance that they may obtain

Table 4.   Indications for bronchoscopy in lung transplant recipients

1. Reduction in lung function.
2. Reduction in exercise capacity.
3. Abnormality on chest radiograph.
4. Unexplained cough.
5. Unexplained pyrexia.

a substantial improvement in their quality of life. Thus even when fully informed most patients wish to go ahead and have their name placed on the transplant waiting list. Once on the waiting list patients face an uncertain time. It is essential that they can be found at all times and some patients benefit from having an aircall bleep or a portable telephone. During this time transplant support groups are particularly helpful.

Post-operative Management

Routine post-operative immunosuppression compromises azathio-prine and cyclosporin A with intravenous methyl prednisolone for acute rejection episodes. Acute allograft rejection is diagnosed by a combination of clinical and radiological findings, together with respiratory function tests and histopathological examination of transbronchial lung biopsy specimens obtained at fibre-optic bronchoscopy.

Fibre-optic bronchoscopy is performed routinely immediately post transplantation and at the end of the first post-operative week. Thereafter it is only performed if there are clinical indications as listed in Table 4. At bronchoscopy, the anastomosis is inspected and broncho-alveolar lavage fluid specimens are taken for culture and sensitivity, opportunistic pathogen screen and immunocyto-chemistry. Transbronchial lung biopsy specimens are sent for histopathological examination and culture. Diagnosis of infection is made by clinical, serological, pathological and radiological find-ings. Patients are treated with appropriate antimicrobial agents. Complications of lung transplantation are listed in Table 5. It can be appreciated that the specialist nature of the majority of these problems necessitate management in the transplant centre.

Table 5.   Complications of lung transplantation

General

1. Infection.
2. Acute rejection.
3. Airway complications.
4. Bleeding.
5. Multiple organ failure.
6. Complications of immunosuppression.
7. Lympho-proliferative disorders.
8. Obliterative bronchiolitis.

Specific Cystic Fibrosis Related Problems

1. Malnutrition.
2. Liver disease.
3. Salt loss.
4. Diabetes Mellitus.
5. Persisting infection in upper respiratory tract.
6. Meconium ileus equivalent.
7. Malabsorption of cyclosporin A.

Obliterative Bronchiolitis

This is the most serious late complication affecting up to 40% of adult patients within three years of surgery. The incidence is higher in children who receive transplantation under the age of ten years. The diagnosis is made clinically in patients who develop progressive airflow obstruction often in the presence of infection. Common presenting features include reduced exercise capacity, cough and progressive deterioration in lung function. Chest radiography may be normal or hyper expanded lung fields secondary to air trapping may be observed.

Transbronchial lung biopsies do not usually confirm the diagnosis because the affected bronchioles are randomly distributed throughout the lung and are peripheral in location and thus are not routinely sampled at biopsy. The diagnosis may be confirmed by DTPA lung scan or high resolution thoracic CT scan. DTPA scanning may show patchy uptake and deposition of the radioisotope in larger airways. A mosaic appearance due to air trapping may be observed in expiratory CT scans.

The aetiology of obliterative bronchiolitis is unclear but it may reflect a form of chronic allograft rejection. Obliterative bronchiolitis may be a final common pathway for a variety of pulmonary injuries which include rejection and bacterial and viral infection. Other factors including pulmonary denervation and ischaemia may be important. Once the diagnosis of obliterative bronchiolitis is made immunosuppression is augmented with either high doses of oral prednisolone, tracrolimus or total lymphoid irradiation. Unfortunately, most patients will not regain lost lung function and will either stabilise at lower levels of lung function or deteriorate to end stage respiratory failure when the only remaining treatment option is re-transplantation.

Results

One and two year actuarial survival following both HLT and BLT is of the order of 70% and 60% respectively with corresponding figures of 80% and 70% respectively following SLT. Most survivors show a marked improvement in quality of life. Pulmonary function improves rapidly following surgery and FEV_1 and FVC are usually in excess of 70% predicted following HLT and BLT by the end of the third post-operative month. Results of re-transplantation for obliterative bronchiolitis are poor with one year actuarial survival of 30%. These results together with the current shortage of donor organs has led many centres to abandon re-transplantation programmes.

Programme of Long-term Care

Following discharge from hospital patients are managed by the Transplant Unit in collaboration with the referring centre. Each patient receives a home microspirometer on discharge and measures FEV_1 and FVC on a daily basis. Should they experience a greater than 15% reduction in lung function on home testing or develop a cough, pyrexia in excess of 37.5°C or reduction in exercise tolerance they are advised to contact the Transplant Centre. Patients are initially required to attend outpatient clinics on a weekly basis during the first month after hospital discharge but thereafter the frequency of outpatient appointments become less and eventually the majority of patients attend the transplant centre for review every six months. In between they attend their local hospital for routine haematological and biochemical investigations together with cyclosporin A level and lung function testing. The results are faxed to the Transplant Centre and any changes in immunosuppression are made as appropriate.

The referring centre is encouraged to play an active role in the management of the lung transplant recipient and indeed should patients develop problems the majority will present to their local centre. In such situations early communication and, if necessary, prompt referral to the transplant centre is essential.

If a transplant patient presents unwell to an Accident and Emergency Department the following approach may be useful:

- take a full history including details of home spirometry record and perform a physical examination
- treat any acute medical emergency
- check FBC, U+E, LFT's, CXR, arterial blood gas analysis
- discuss the clinical presentation and above results with the transplant centre before deciding on further management

The Future

The major challenges facing lung transplant programmes are shortage of suitable donor organs and the development of obliterative bronchiolitis. The timing of surgery is also vital. It should not be too early because about 30% of patients will die during the first postoperative year, but if it is too late, suitable donor organs may not be found in time and the patient may become too unwell for successful transplantation. It is hoped that the development of new immunosuppressive agents (eg. tacrolimus, mycophenolate mofetil, total lymphoid irradiation), together with improved diagnosis and treatment of rejection and pulmonary infection will reduce the incidence of obliterative bronchiolitis. Major immunological issues and concerns over possible transmission of infection have to be overcome before the use of animal organs (xenografting) can be successfully applied to human lung transplantation.

Lung Volume Reduction Surgery for Emphysema

There has recently been a resurgence of interest in lung volume reduction surgery for severe emphysema. However the concept is not new and was originally proposed in 1957 by Brantigan.

Lung volume reduction reduces total thoracic volume and improves chest wall mechanics in patients with severe emphysema.

Table 6.   Lung volume reduction surgery

Inclusion Criteria

1.   Diagnosis of emphysema defined by imaging and lung function.
2.   Disease not eligible for established surgical procedures such as bullectomy or lobectomy.
3.   Non-smoker.

Exclusion Criteria

1.   Estimated life expectancy < two years.
2.   Age > 75 years.
3.   Using oxygen for > 18 hours/day
4. FEV_1 < 0.5l, TLCO < 30% (in homogeneous disease), RV < 180%.
5. $PaCO_2$ > 6kPa.
6.   Maintenance prednisolone therapy > 10 mg/d
7.   Previous thoracic surgery.
8.   Cardiac failure.
9.   Significant coronary artery disease.
10. Asthma.
11. Kyphoscoliosis.
12. Other major medical disease.

The operation can be performed via a median sternotomy or thoracoscopically and comprises non-anatomical usually unilateral resection of multiple pieces of bullous and non-bullous lungs using a stapling device. The ideal candidate for lung volume reduction surgery has a hyper-expanded rib cage with increased anterior and posterior diameter and a flattened diaphragm. Inclusion and exclusion criteria are listed in Table 6. Many patients referred for lung volume reduction have failed to meet the criteria for lung transplantation.

In centrilobular emphysema, the disease usually affects predominantly the upper zones and apical portions of the lower zones; patients with more severe disease in both upper zones, ie, a heterogeneous pattern (demonstrated by a combination of chest radiography, ventilation perfusion and thoracic CT scanning) may benefit from volume reduction surgery of both upper lobes. In alpha 1 antitripsin deficiency however the disease typically affects the lower zones; these patients tend to be younger and are usually referred for lung transplantation as results of lung volume reduction surgery for this condition are poor.

Table 7.   Indications for thoracoscopic surgery

1. Lung resection.
2. Pleurectomy.
3. Resection of bullae.
4. Spontaneous pneumothorax.
5. Pericardial window; pericardectomy operations for recurrent malignant/ benign pericardial effusions.
6. Other possible applications include sympathectomy and resection of mediastinal tumours.

Mortality after lung volume reduction surgery is in the region of 4%. Patients have noted an improvement in quality of life after surgery and up to 75% are able to discontinue the use of oxygen by the sixth post-operative month. Prospective studies randomising patients between surgery and medical treatment/rehabilitation are in progress. It follows, therefore, that at present although surgery would appear to benefit selected patients significantly in terms of improvement in quality of life and in exercise capacity, this remains to be proven.

Thoracoscopic Techniques

Thoracoscopy was introduced for the surgical management of tuberculosis in the pre-chemotherapy era. In the ensuing years its use declined and was restricted by and large to diagnosis. More recently thoracoscopy has been revisited and shown to have considerable potential for palliation of pleural tumours and in the management of pneumothorax and emphysematous bulla in patients who would not easily tolerate thoracotomy. The recent development of video assisted thoracoscopy (VAT; working through more than one incision simultaneously), has greatly enhanced the range of minimally invasive techniques currently possible through the thoracoscope. This is because it allows the surgeon to use instruments with both hands while maintaining a comprehensive view inside the thorax. Lasers have also successfully been employed in thoracoscopic surgery. Thoracoscopic surgery can be applied to a variety of conditions as listed in Table 7.

Lung resection can be successfully performed via the thoracoscope. It is particularly useful in the management of patients with a pulmonary nodule. Encouraging results of sub-total lobectomy with minimal blood loss using the contact NdYag laser and endoscopic stapler have been reported.

Thoracoscopy is useful in the diagnosis and management of recurrent pleural effusions. Good visualisation of the pleural surfaces can be achieved and pleural biopsies taken. Thoracoscopy can also be used to facilitate chemical pleurodesis. Under direct vision pleural adhesions are freed and talcum powder (or other agent) may be insufflated. When these methods fail, surgical intervention — thoracotomy and pleurectomy — is indicated. Although surgical pleurectomy has a high success rate, patients with neoplastic pleural effusions may be too ill to have such a major procedure. As an alternative thoracoscopic laser pleurectomy was developed to remove the parietal and visceral pleura followed by vapourisation of the remaining malignant tumour on both the parietal and visceral pleura using the free beam NdYag laser. This laser can also be used via the thoracoscope to induce pleurodesis. There are a variety of alternative instruments which can be used via the thoracoscope for blunt dissection and pleurectomy. Lung volume reduction surgery and resection of bullae can also be performed thoracoscopically using a stapling device and pericardial (usually bovine) patches. Spontaneous pneumothorax can be treated very effectively by thoracoscopy. Once again the laser is effective in this circumstance as are stapling and suturing techniques.

There are a variety of causes of pericardial effusions. If repeated pericardiocentesis fails to prevent recurrence and if patients are symptomatic, a permanent measure to decompress the pericardial space is required. Surgery through the thoracoscope to create a pericardial window is a useful alternative to traditional surgical approaches (anterior left thoracotomy, right lateral thoracotomy, sub-xyphoid approach). Laser therapy has a role to play in this procedure because, unlike electrocautery it does not stimulate the phrenic nerve and/or induce ventricular fibrillation even in a patient who has had a permanent pacemaker inserted. Pericardectomy for malignant pericardial effusions has also been achieved thoracoscopically. Other possible applications for thoracoscopic surgery include thoracic sympathectomy and excision of mediastinal tumours, eg, thymectomy for myasthenia gravis. It should be appreciated however that should major bleeding occur sternotomy may be required.

Pneumonectomy, Lobectomy and Segmental Resection

Pneumonectomy

The first successful one stage pneumonectomy was performed in 1933 for a patient with bronchogenic carcinoma. By the 1940s the standard operation for resectable lung cancer was pneumonectomy. It is currently generally accepted that with careful selection and staging, pneumonectomy is the correct treatment for lung cancer that cannot be treated by lobectomy. With advances in modern day respiratory medicine and the advent of potent antibiotics, physiotherapy techniques and bronchomodulatory therapy, pneumonectomy for inflammatory lung disease, bronchiectasis, tuberculosis and other non-malignant conditions is uncommon.

The most frequently employed incision for pneumonectomy is the postero-lateral thoracotomy with access to the pleural cavity via the fifth intercostal space. Careful intra-operative monitoring of blood pressure using an arterial line, of arterial blood gases, of end tidal carbon dioxide and if necessary of pulmonary arterial pressures using a Swan Ganz catheter is necessary. The patient will also routinely have measurements of urine output and pulse oximetry. Single-lung anaesthesia is best provided with the use of a double lumen endotracheal tube. Once thoracotomy has been performed the hilum is dissected to identify the pulmonary artery and the two (superior and inferior) pulmonary veins. Dissection of the bronchus, proximal to the resection margin is kept to a minimum in order to preserve as much as possible of its blood supply intact. The main stem bronchus is divided as proximally as possible in order to avoid the problem of a long bronchial stump.

Indications

The major indication for pneumonectomy is lung cancer that cannot be treated by lobectomy. As a general guideline most surgeons would not accept patients for pneumonectomy who have an FEV1 less than 1.5l. Otherwise the standard anaesthetic fitness for surgery guidelines apply.

Post operative course following pnemonectomy:

- following closure of the thoracotomy wound, air is aspirated from the pneumonectomy space to bring the mediastinum across.

A chest drain is not routinely inserted unless bleeding is anticipated. Some surgeons leave a chest drain in the hemithorax following pneumonectomy to achieve balancing of the mediastinum and to promptly announce significant bleeding. If employed no more than 5 cm H_2O suction should be given as additional suction may have disastrous consequences

- chest X-rays are performed daily to monitor the rising fluid level within the pneumonectomy space and to ensure optimum position of the mediastinum which normally deviates towards the side of surgery). If rapid accumulation of the fluid occurs the mediastinum may be pushed away from the side of the operation and the fluid and air must be aspirated to bring the mediastinum back towards the side of surgery

- bloody fluid accumulates over the following six weeks and air is progressively absorbed from the space. This leads to full opacification of the hemithorax with loss of the fluid level

- over the next few months fibroblastic proliferation occurs within the pneumonectomy fluid. Although this may sometimes proceed to complete fibrous obliteration of the space, fluid usually remains often as a single large collection surrounded by a thick fibrous capsule

- the pneumonectomy space contracts progressively with narrowing of the intercostal spaces and progressive elevation of the diaphragm and further mediastinal shift to the side of surgery. It should be remembered that, as long as fluid remains (which is usually the life span of the patient) it may be colonised by bacterial infection causing an empyema

Following lesser pulmonary resections an alveolar air leak occurs from the raw lung surface and chest drains are necessary until the air leak has stopped. If the remaining lung tissue fails to expand to fill the hemithorax a persistant air leak develops which can lead to prolonged intercostal drainage and thus intrapleural sepsis.

Post operative complications

The post operative complications which may occur following pneumonectomy are listed in Table 8. As the majority of patients have smoking related lung disease, sputum clearance requires intensive physiotherapy assisted by optimal pain control. Pneumonia developing following pneumonectomy is a major complication with a high mortality. It almost always follows inadequate management of

Table 8.   Post operative complication following pneumonectomy

1. Sputum retention
2. Pneumonia.
3. Supraventricular dysrhythmias.
4. Wound infection.
5. Bleeding.
6. Empyema.
7. Bronchopleural fistula.
8. Pulmonary embolism.

sputum problems. Early aggressive antibiotic therapy Is indicated. Should patients require subsequent re-intubation, jet ventilation may be of benefit. Mortality however, in this situation approaches 100%. Supraventricular dysrhythmias, particularly atrial fibrillation, is common in the elderly patient and usually occurs within two to five days following surgery. Treatment is usually successful with digoxin. Up to 10% of patients develop wound infection post surgery and troublesome post operative bleeding occurs in 1 to 2% of patients. Empyema is a potential complication at any time following pneumonectomy although it may present within a few weeks post operatively if related to intraoperative contamination or a bronchopleural fistula. Features of empyema may be insidious and often recurrence of malignancy is suspected. Although aspiration of the pneumonectomy space should be undertaken, cultures may prove negative in up to 30% of patients inspite of clear evidence of infection within the space and turbid fluid on aspiration. Treatment includes surgical drainage, closure of bronchopleural fistula and antibiotic therapy. *Staphylococcus aureus* is the commonest organism encountered although other respiratory pathogens may be isolated. If a mixed growth of upper gut organisms is obtained an oesophago pleural fistula needs to be excluded. A bronchopleural fistula developing in the early post operative period is related to technical deficiencies in closure of the bronchial stump. The patient may expectorate bloody fluid from the pneumonectomy space which can flood the remaining lung, causing immediate death or pneumonitis. Immediate insertion of an intercostal drain may be life saving in this circumstance. If the diagnosis is in doubt, a chest X-ray may demonstrate a drop in the fluid level and increased translucency in the space. Immediate surgical closure of the stump is necessary although mortality is in the region of 50%. If small bronchopleural fistulae occur following pneumonectomy, they may be diagnosed by the development of empyema or by the failure of the pneumonectomy space to become completely opaque on serial chest radiographs. Usually such fistulae close spontaneously following drainage of the space and antibiotic therapy but occasionally re-operation is necessary. Pulmonary embolism is rarely encountered, largely on account of early post operative mobilisation and prophylactic heparin. In hospital mortality for pneumonectomy is between 5 and 8% and for lobectomy is between 1 and 2%.

Lobectomy

The first proper dissection lobectomy was performed in 1912. It was not until the report of long-term survival following lobectomy for peripheral lung cancer in the early 1950s that this procedure became acceptable in the management of lung neoplasia. Before this, lobectomy had been reserved for inflammatory disease such as tuberculosis and bronchiectasis.

Lobectomy remains the preferred method for the surgical therapy of peripheral lung cancer. Pnemonectomy is reserved for the more centrally placed tumours and resections less extensive than lobectomy are carried out in patients with compromised pulmonary function or, very rarely, electively in those with small peripheral tumours. The indications for lobectomy in benign pulmonary diseases includes tuberculosis, chronic lung abscess, bronchiectasis, benign tumours, fungal infections and congenital abnormalities.

The usual approach for lobectomy is via a postero-lateral incision and entry into the pleural space is gained through the fifth intercostal space or through the periosteal bed of the fifth rib when an upper or middle lobectomy is contemplated and through the sixth intercostal space or the bed of the sixth rib when a lower lobectomy is planned.

Segmental resection

Anatomical segmental resection is the excision of one or more bronchopulmonary segments of the lobe with individual ligation and division of the corresponding bronchovascular structures. It was originally developed for the surgical management of tuberculosis and bronchiectasis. More recently it has been applied to the surgical therapy of primary or metastic lung cancer.

References

1. Madden BP, Hodson ME, Tsang V et al. Intermediate term results of heart–lung transplantation for cystic fibrosis. *Lancet* 1992;**339**: 1583–7

2. Madden BP, Radley-Smith R, Hodson M et al. Medium term results of heart and lung transplantation. *J Heart Lung Transplant* 1992;**11**: S241–3

3. Madden BP, Geddes D. Which patients should receive lung transplants? *Monaldi Archives for Chest Disease* 1993;**48**:**4**:346–352

4. Starnes VA, Barr M, Cohen R et al. Living donor lobar lung transplantation experience: Intermediate results. *J Thorac Cardiovasc Surg* 1996;**112**:1284–1291

5. Pomerance A, Madden BP, Burke M, Yacoub M. Transbronchial biopsy in heart and lung transplantation: Clinicopathologic correlations. *J Heart Lung Transplant* 1995;**14**:761–73

6. Madden BP, Kamalvand K, Chan CM et al. The medical management of patients with cystic fibrosis following heart and lung transplantation. *Eur Respir J* 1993;**6**:965–70

7. Hutter JA, Wreghitt T, Scott JP et al. The importance of cytomegalovirus in heart transplant recipiemts. *Chest* 1989;**95**:627–31

8. Griffith BP, Paradis IL, Zeevi et al. Immunology mediated disease of the airways after pulmonary transplantation. *Ann Surg* 1988; **208**:371–9

9. Squier HC, Ries AL, Kaplan RM et al. Quality of well-being predicts survival in transplantation candidates. *Am J Respir Crit Care Med* 1995;**152**:2032–36

10. Brantigan OC, Mueller E. Surgical treatment of pulmonary emphysema. *Ann Surg* 1957;**23**:789–804

11. Wakabayashi A. Thoracoscopic Techniques. In: Hetzel MR, ed. Minimally Invasive Techniques in Thoracic Medicine and Surgery, p 267–286. London: Chapman and Hall 1995

12. The New Airds Companion in Surgical Studies, p 739–742. In: Burnand KG, Young AE, eds. Edinburgh: Churchill Livingstone 1992

23

Chest Trauma and Respiratory Emergencies

W Ellis Morgan and David R Baldwin

This section provides some guidance in the management of acute respiratory emergencies and aspects of chest trauma. It is recognised that trauma is more often the realm of the thoracic or trauma surgeon, but physicians may be called upon to advise on medical sequelae or concomitant conditions. Therefore it is useful to have a working knowledge of the management of trauma victims and emergency treatment of life threatening injuries.

Chest Trauma

In developed countries blunt trauma from road traffic accidents (RTA) is the commonest cause of chest injury. Twenty-five percent of RTA deaths are due primarily to chest injury alone and in a further 25% the chest injury is a major contributing factor. Penetrating injury due to a bullet or a knife is most commonly seen in areas of conflict, in developing countries and in poor urban populations; the majority of victims who survive to reach hospital are salvageable with prompt treatment. Age has an important influence on the likely nature of injuries: The elastic rib cage of young children and the brittle bones of old age render these two groups more susceptible to severe visceral damage from blunt trauma. The mortality rate from trauma increases with advancing years and frailty.

Table 1. Life threatening chest injuries

Airway	may be obstructed and/or disrupted
Breathing	pneumothorax; open, tension or bilateral haemothorax severe lung contusion severe chest wall flail and/or ruptured diaphragm
Circulation	haemorrhage tamponade severe cardiac dysfunction
Dysfunction of the nervous system	head injury drugs metabolic disturbance stroke

Emergency assessment

In the emergency assessment of a trauma victim it is necessary to make a rapid methodical assessment. The primary survey concentrates on the vital functions: A – airway; B – breathing; C – circulation; D – dysfunction of central nervous system (Table 1). Any life threatening problem is immediately treated. During this assessment some history may be available, but it is essential to obtain more history from the secondary survey after the patient has been stabilised. At this stage important history includes that of previous illness, particularly cardiac and respiratory disease and enquiry about any acute medical condition either causing the accident (e.g. epilepsy, diabetes, myocardial infarction) or precipitated by the injury (eg. myocardial infarction). A drug history should be obtained; particularly important are anticonvulsants, steroids, cardiac and respiratory drugs and anticoagulants. Alcohol and drug abuse are not uncommon in trauma victims and may complicate both the acute management and the convalescent period. As soon as practical obtain a chest X-ray and blood gas estimation in patients with significant chest trauma. In the heat of the moment it is all too easy to be diverted by the more obvious injuries such as compound limb fractures and miss a more immediate threat to life, for example, a developing tension pneumothorax.

In comatose trauma victims where the level of consciousness does not correlate with the degree of head injury, other causes of

Table 2.   Indications for emergency thoracotomy

life threatening haemorrhage

tamponade

aortic rupture

massive air leak

large chest wall defects.

large diaphragmatic tears.

all penetrating injuries that are precordial, transmediastinal, transdiaphragmatic or into root of neck.

all unstable patients not responding to resuscitation without obvious cause.

coma should be sought eg. alcohol, drugs, hypoglycaemia, diabetic ketoacidosis, hypothermia, epilepsy, stroke, psychiatric disturbance. After assessment only 15% of chest trauma victims need emergency thoracotomy. The indications for emergency exploration are shown in Table 2.

Chest wall trauma

Soft tissue injury

The site and severity of bruising and haematoma correlate well with damage to the underlying rib cage and viscera. Large boggy haematomas commonly overlie multiple fractures and may obscure flail segments. Large or increasing haematomas at the root of the neck raise the suspicion of bleeding from major vessels. Severe seat belt bruising is associated with sternal fractures and possible myocardial contusion. Injuries over the costal margin are indications for careful examination of the abdomen as well as the chest.

Subcutaneous emphysema at the site of a rib fracture is a common finding and X-ray may reveal an underlying pneumothorax. Subcutaneous air limited to the neck alerts one to the possibility of a major airway tear. Massive subcutaneous emphysema can be dramatic and especially with positive pressure ventilation can cause an alarming inflation of the patient! Such cases always have a large air-leak from the underlying lung or major airway and need the insertion of a large intercostal drain. Often the pneumothorax on X-ray is obscured by the subcutaneous air; if so, insert an intercostal drain (ICD) on the side of trauma.

Penetrating injuries

The site and direction of penetrating wounds indicates which viscera are at risk, although bullets may take a very unexpected path. Urgent exploration is indicated in all unstable patients, wounds overlying the precordium, those that cross the mediastinum, and very high or low injuries which may involve neck or abdominal organs. Lateral and posterior stab wounds are indications for ICD and intravenous infusion, but many do not require thoracotomy, the bleeding and air leak usually resolving with conservative management.

Bony injuries

The bony chest cage offers protection to the thoracic and upper abdominal viscera; it is not designed to withstand the traumas of modern high-speed living. Not surprisingly the severity and extent of rib fractures correlate with the degree of underlying visceral trauma, the exception being young children, whose elastic rib cage may not fracture on impact.

Simple rib fractures are painful! This obvious statement bears emphasising — analgesia must enable the patient to breathe deeply and cough effectively. Patients with chronic lung disease, especially those with a productive cough, are especially at risk and need admission, vigorous physiotherapy and close monitoring, but above all, effective analgesia. A distressed tachypnoeic patient, unable to co-operate with the physiotherapist, developing sputum retention and atelectasis, can be transformed with good analgesia. Paracetamol, non-steroidal anti-inflammatories and opiates are commonly employed but local nerve blocks are woefully underused. In patients with just a few fractured ribs local infiltration with long-acting agents e.g. bupivicaine is useful, but with more extensive injuries a wider area of analgesia can be achieved using intercostal blocks or paravertebral or epidural infusions.

Progressively severe degrees of rib fractures increase the likelihood of pneumothorax, haemothorax (approximately 150 ml of blood per rib fractured) and visceral contusion. Fractures of the first rib have a strong association with injury to the underlying major vessels and multiple fractures of the lower chest wall with injuries to the diaphragm, liver and spleen. The most severe bony injuries result in flail segments which move paradoxically with respiration. The common patterns are postero-lateral flail segments from side impact or anterior flail from steering wheel injuries. Many patients with severe flail segments require immediate intubation and ventilation because of the severity of underlying thoracic visceral damage or severe extrathoracic injuries. Patients with lesser degrees of injury can often be managed conservatively but aggressively with analgesia, physiotherapy, insertion of ICDs, appropriate intravenous fluid replacement, sputum clearance and repeated monitoring of respiratory function, especially blood gases. The need for ventilation is usually dependent on the extent of lung contusion and is indicated by a falling PO_2, a rising respiratory rate and rising PCO_2.

Sternal fractures raise the suspicion of cardiac injury especially contusion. Seat belt sternal fractures sustained at low speeds (less than 30mph) carry a low risk of significant cardiac injury, in contrast to high speed injuries, especially where there is displacement of the sternal fracture or an associated anterior flail segment.

Pleura

In open pneumothorax (sucking chest wound), a full thickness defect of the chest wall allows free passage of air into the pleural cavity. The underlying lung collapses completely and the contralateral lung does not ventilate, the respiratory effort merely causing a paradoxical flapping of the mediastinum. With large defects the patient rapidly develops extreme respiratory distress for which the first aid treatment is to pack the wound rendering it airtight. In moribund patients commence artificial ventilation but leave the wound unsealed. When practical, insert an ICD and proceed to wound toilet and repair. Note that in the presence of dense pleural adhesions (10 to 15% of the population) the normal mechanisms of ventilation will be preserved.

In tension pneumothorax, trauma to the lung or airway results in a one way flow of air into the pleural cavity. The lung collapses, there is a marked mediastinal shift and a build up of intrapleural pressure which eventually exceeds central venous pressure. The patient dies of an obstructed circulation and respiratory distress, with signs of extreme agitation, tachypnoea, raised jugular venous pressure, mediastinal shift away from a resonant non-ventilating hemithorax and a disappearing pulse. In these circumstances, the correct management is to insert a large bore needle into the pleura immediately. The resulting hiss of air should be followed by a returning cardiac output and improved colour. When available insert an ICD.

Note that positive pressure ventilation may rapidly cause a simple pneumothorax to tension; all such patients, even with a small pneumothorax, should have a drain inserted prior to ventilation.

Simple traumatic pneumothorax usually results from air leaks from tear(s) in the lung. Less commonly it arises from a major airway, a chest wall defect, the upper gastrointestinal tract or from iatrogenic causes. Simple pneumothorax can become an emergency if bilateral and in patients with pre-existing severe lung disease. Traumatic pneumothorax is treated by inserting a large ICD (28-32F gauge) which usually achieves rapid and complete lung expansion, allows estimation of blood loss and air leak and obviates the risk of a tension pneumothorax should ventilation be necessary. If the lung fails to expand check the position and patency of the drain, and consider bronchial rupture if the air leak is vigorous or bronchial obstruction if the leak is minimal (either possibility is an indication for bronchoscopy). Positive pressure ventilation can exacerbate air leaks but providing the lungs remain fully expanded continue with intercostal drainage; often the air leak persists until the patient is weaned off the ventilator.

Haemothorax

Massive life threatening haemorrhage within the chest presents with hypovolaemic shock, respiratory distress and a total 'whiteout' on chest X-ray. Salvage depends on rapid intravenous infusion via at least two large cannulae, chest drain insertion and thoracotomy. On opening the chest, bleeding from the heart, lung hilum or great vessels can be torrential especially in crush injuries; with stab wounds it is usually easier to control the bleeding.

Indications for thoracotomy include:

- an unstable patient
- complete opacification of one lung field on chest X-ray
- initial blood loss greater than 1 litre
- continuing blood loss over 200mls/hr for 3 hours
- severe bleeding into the bronchial tree

If a chest drain becomes blocked by clotted blood, this is also an indication of significant bleeding; do not hesitate to insert a second drain and monitor closely.

Initial drainage of several hundred millilitres of blood is not unusual on inserting an intercostal drain after which the drainage usually diminishes. These patients do not usually require thoracotomy, but do need effective drainage to ensure complete lung expansion and to minimise the risk of clotted haemothorax, fibrothorax or empyema. Ultrasound and/or CT scans can be useful in localising and draining pleural blood.

Lung trauma

Localised haemorrhage can present as a discrete lung mass; such haematomas usually resolve over four to six weeks. Traumatic lung cysts can develop from lacerations contained within the lung parenchyma or by cavitation of a haematoma. They usually resolve over a few months, but a few become infected and require drainage or resection

Pulmonary lacerations

Major tears involving the lung hilum can produce massive haemorrhage and air leaks requiring emergency surgery. Peripheral tears usually present with varying degrees of haemo/pneumothorax; the majority can be managed with drainage and volume replacement, but thoracotomy is indicated if the bleeding or air leak is excessive. Haemorrhage into the bronchial tree can threaten to drown the patient in blood and necessitates urgent intubation with a double lumen endotracheal tube and thoracotomy.

Pulmonary contusion

This is the commonest type of lung injury seen with blunt trauma and results in haemorrhage and oedema in the walls and spaces of the alveoli and small airways. Minor degrees of lung contusion show up as localised soft patchy infiltrates on X-ray which resolve in the course of a few days. At the other extreme, as seen in severe blast injuries, there is a widespread and coalescing pattern of consolidation associated with rapidly deteriorating gas exchange and eventual hypoxic death. In practice most patient suffer a combination of lung tears and contusion especially in blunt trauma where there is a strong association with overlying chest wall injuries and significant extrathoracic trauma eg. head injury.

Lung response to injury

Oedema

Increased permeability of the pulmonary capillary endothelium occurs within hours of trauma and results in oedema of the pulmonary tissues. This response is initially most marked in the area of traumatised lung but within several hours there is a generalised effect on the entire pulmonary capillary bed. This picture of leaky lungs or Acute Lung Injury (ALI) is not confined to thoracic trauma but can be triggered by extrathoracic injuries, burns, sepsis etc. The mechanism of damage to the capillary endothelium has been the subject of intense research with a long list of cellular and chemical mediators. In these patients the infusion of large volumes of intravenous fluids, colloid or crystalloid, can result in the accumulation of litres of excess pulmonary tissue fluid leading to rapid respiratory failure. There is a fine line between under and over transfusion in these patients and careful monitoring of venous pressures and cardiac output should ensure that minimum essential volumes are infused. Pulmonary oedema may also result from cardiac injuries (left ventricular failure or mitral incompetence) or previous cardiac disease and in severe head injuries.

Aspiration

Aspirated blood causes an acute pneumonitis. Aspiration of gastric juice provokes an intense chemical inflammatory response in the airways and alveoli together with the risk of pneumonia.

Atelectasis

Loss of surfactant is associated with trauma and predisposes to alveolar collapse. Small and large airways can be obstructed by oedema, blood and secretions resulting in minor or major degrees of atelectasis. Patients with a history of chronic obstructive airways disease or asthma are particularly at risk from major airway plugging with copious or viscid bronchial secretions.

Emboli

The pulmonary capillary bed acts like a biological vascular filter entrapping a cocktail of emboli: fat emboli from fractures; blood clots from deep veins; and air, platelet aggregates and plastic polymers from intravenous infusions. All produce not merely a mechanical obstruction to the vascular bed but can exacerbate endothelial and airway problems.

Management

The combination of the initial lung injury and subsequent response often results in a deteriorating pattern of increasing alveolar/arterial gradient, increasing pulmonary vascular resistance and decreasing lung compliance. Vigorous treatment may avoid the need for ventilation. This includes effective analgesia, intensive physiotherapy, restriction of fluid to essential volumes, intravenous diuretics, minitracheostomy or bronchoscopy for sputum retention, antibiotics for proven infection, and oxygen administration if necessary via CPAP mask. Previous medication especially bronchodilators, steroids and diuretics needs to be continued, if necessary in increased doses.

Ventilation is indicated for respiratory failure and also in comatose patients. Unfortunately, prolonged positive pressure ventilation causes further lung damage from barotrauma, oxygen toxicity and infection. The label Acute Respiratory Distress Syndrome (ARDS) is usually applied to this severe degree of acute diffuse alveolar damage but suffers from an imprecise definition (see ref 5 or page 528). Such patients have a 50% mortality; death usually results from hypoxia or sepsis and multiple organ failure. ECMO (extracorporeal membrane oxygenation) is applicable to patients with severe but rapidly reversible lung injury. In the context of trauma this includes severe inhalational burns and selected cases of ARDS. Haemofiltration is an effective method of offloading excess fluid from waterlogged lungs. Clinical trials have provided no support for the use of steroids in ARDS, but there is increasing interest in nitric oxide and prostaglandin therapy.

Airway

The airway may be obstructed and/or disrupted. Obstruction can occur anywhere between mouth and bronchus with blood, secretions, oedema, vomitus, teeth, foreign bodies or a loss of muscle tone. Particularly at risk are comatose patients and those with severe facial trauma or inhalational burns. Disruption of the upper airway can be extreme in faciomaxillary injuries. Less commonly the cervical airway can be disrupted; more distally tracheobronchial rupture may complicate blunt chest trauma.

Securing the airway is most important. The majority of early post-trauma deaths are airway related. Assume an unstable cervical spine injury until proven otherwise and immobilise the neck with a hard collar or sandbags. Clear the mouth and pharynx with finger and suction, elevate the tongue and jaw and administer 100% oxygen. If no gag reflex is present insert an oral airway. If there is no improvement proceed to orotracheal or nasotracheal intubation, the choice being dependant on the operators experience. For intubation the patient must be unconcious or anaesthetised and the cervical spine kept immobile. Endotracheal intubation may be impossible in facial trauma or burns, necessitating tracheostomy or cricothyroidotomy (not in young children). Problems distal to the larynx require bronchoscopy, ideally with a rigid bronchoscope.

Cervical airway

Blunt trauma to the neck (karate chop and clothes line injury) may completely disrupt the larynx or trachea. The combination of severe airway obstruction and cervical subcutaneous emphysema is an indication for open exploration and intubation of the distal airway. Cut-throat victims may survive the initial injury but present struggling to breathe through a bloody frothing wound and need urgent intubation of the distal airway through the incision provided.

Thoracic airway

Rupture of the thoracic trachea and major bronchi usually result from high speed impacts and crush injuries to the chest. Most tears occur within a few inches of the carina and vary from minor partial thickness injuries to full rupture and disconnection. In severe cases the patient rapidly develops airway obstruction, bleeding into the airway and a major air leak. The air may track into the mediastinum and neck and/or into the pleural cavity. The resulting complete pneumothorax fails to expand on insertion of an ICD which bubbles vigorously. An attempt at tracheal intubation is a lottery which may precipitate a massive air leak and a failure to ventilate. Rigid bronchoscopy is necessary to achieve rapid clearance of the airway, to accurately assess the injury and to facilitate safe intubation prior to surgical repair.

Suprisingly some patients with complete bronchial rupture present no immediate airway problem but develop bronchial obstruction and atelectasis, either in the early weeks from granulation tissue or later from fibrosis. Local resection of the obstruction and airway repair should be possible without resorting to a major lung resection.

Cardiac trauma

Blunt trauma

Most deaths at the scene of high speed accidents are due to cardiac and/or great vessel rupture. In survivors myocardial contusion is often undetected, although in one large study 25% of RTA victims admitted to hospital had sustained a significant cardiac injury. Suspicion of myocardial trauma should be raised if there is severe injury to the anterior chest wall eg. anterior flail, fractured sternum, seat belt bruising. The right ventricle is the most vulnerable chamber but left venticle, septum, great vessels, atria, valves and conducting system are all at risk. The diagnosis of myocardial contusion should be suspected if there are electrocardiographic changes such as ischaemia or arrythmias and elevation of cardiac enzymes. It is diagnosed and monitored by echocardiagraphy. Complications of blunt cardiac trauma include tachy- and brady-arrhythmias, pump failure, cardiac rupture, valvular incompetence and septal defects.

Surgery is indicated for patients with a significant septal defect, valve incompetence and incipient rupture (ventricular aneurysm). Such complications can occur up to one month after trauma, therefore patients with documented cardiac trauma should be rested and monitored during this period.

Penetrating trauma

Most knife and bullet wounds to the heart are rapidly fatal, but of those who survive to reach hospital 50-80% can be saved. Death occurs from exsanguination, tamponade and arrhythmias; salvage depends on rapid intravenous volume replacement and immediate surgery to relieve the tamponade and control bleeding (if need be in the emergency room). The classical signs of tamponade are a raised venous pressure, low cardiac output with a paradoxus pulse, soft heart sounds and a globular heart on chest X-ray. In practice tamponade should be suspected in all precordial and transmediastinal wounds if the neck veins are full despite obvious blood loss and there are signs of a low cardiac output. Pericardiocentesis is traditionally employed to relieve tamponade prior to surgery, but there is ample evidence that in inexperienced hands it causes more harm than good; it is better to concentrate on intravenous infusion and rapid operation. At operation the right ventricle is most commonly involved, followed by the left ventricle, the right atrium and the great vessels. Control of bleeding and repair of the cardiac wound is usually possible by direct suturing without the need for bypass. Injury to the coronary vessels may result in acute infarction and if a major coronary artery is involved direct repair or grafting should be attempted. Less commonly penetrating injuries may result in significant valvular incompetence, septal defect, ventricular aneurysm or coronary fistula, all of which require surgical correction on bypass.

Aortic tears

Over 80% of patients with aortic ruptures die at the scene of trauma and of those that survive to admission the majority suffer a sudden fatal haemorrhage within hours or days. The aorta tears just beyond the origin of the left subclavian artery as a result of a high speed impact. Initially the haemorrhage is contained by the adventitia, mediastinal tissues and pleura and may be recognised on a chest X-ray (erect postero-anterior film if practical). Appearances which suggest aortic rupture include a wide mediastinum (over 8 cm), apical pleural capping, distortion of the aortic knuckle, displacement of the trachea or a nasogastric tube to the right and downward displacement of the left main bronchus. Many radiologists advocate CT scans to diagnose rupture but aortography is the gold standard and is mandatory prior to repair. If aortic rupture is suspected control the blood pressure and pulse rate as for an acute dissection and transfer to a cardiothoracic centre for aortography and repair. A small number of patients survive with undetected tears which stabilise as chronic pseudoaneurysms, these require surgical repair.

Diaphragm rupture

Major disruption of the diaphragm is usually associated with severe crush injuries to the lower rib cage, lung contusion and haemorrhage from the liver and spleen. If the resulting tear is large a mass herniation of the abdominal viscera into the chest can cause severe respiratory embarrassment. Such major injuries are usually obvious on X-ray and need urgent resuscitation and surgery. Most lacerated diaphragms are diagnosed on the left side; the bulk of the liver is said to protect or mask injuries to the right side. Lesser degrees of diaphragmatic trauma are easily missed and may present late (even decades later) with visceral herniation and strangulation e.g. colon, stomach, small bowel.

Oesophageal trauma

Most oesophageal trauma is iatrogenic; less commonly perforation is related to a foreign body or induced by vomiting (Boerhaave syndrome); it rarely results from penetrating or blunt chest trauma. Air may track into the mediastinum, neck or pleura and diagnosis is confirmed by contrast studies. If diagnosed within 24 hours direct repair is possible but many cases are detected late when management is difficult and mortality is high.

Thoracic duct

Trauma to the thoracic duct is uncommon and results in a chylothorax which is diagnosed on insertion of a chest drain. If the daily drainage of chyle exceeds 1 litre for several days (despite a fat free diet) then exploration and ligation of the duct is indicated.

Iatrogenic trauma

Iatrogenic injuries are unfortunately common. Trauma to all the thoracic (and upper abdominal) viscera has been reported, but it is the lung and heart that seem to be the main targets. Trauma to the lung is especially common resulting in haemorrhage into the pleura or lung parenchyma and pneumothorax and may complicate the insertion of a chest drain, transcutaneous lung biopsy (FNA or Trucut), CVP line insertion, transbronchial lung biopsy, aspiration of pleural effusion, pleural biopsy and CPR. Management includes correct insertion of a chest drain, replacement of blood volume if loss is significant and administration of oxygen. The majority of such cases settle on supportive care and do not require thoracotomy. Cardiac trauma may complicate cardiac catheterisation, pacemaker insertion, pericardiocentesis and intracardiac injections. Bleeding is fortunately minor in most cases but urgent exploration is necessary if tamponade or hypovolaemia develop.

Cardiopulmonary resuscitation if vigorous not uncommonly causes fractures of the anterior chest wall especially in the very young and the very old. In extreme cases anterior flail chest and severe contusion to heart, lungs and liver result; a chest X-ray should be routinely performed after successful resuscitation.

Long term sequelae of chest trauma

Pain

Prolonged pain is not uncommon following fractures of the ribs and sternum and thoracotomy incisions. Intercostal neuralgia follows the distribution of the dermatomes and can prove intractable.

Pulmonary function

Loss of volume follows lung resection, chest wall deformity (stove in chest) and paralysed or fixed diaphragm. Reduced mobility of the chest wall will result from severe multiple rib fractures especially if cross union occurs and from fibrothorax complicating empyemas or clotted haemothorax. Wasting of the muscles of respiration is a major factor in patients suffering prolonged ITU and inpatient care; restoration of the respiratory muscle pump will take many months of intensive exercises.

Obstructive defects

Tracheal stenosis may complicate ET intubation or tracheostomy and bronchial stenosis may present late following brochial rupture. Such large airway stenosis presents with stridor or a fixed ronchus and a typical flow/volume loop curve and is amenable to dilation or resection.

Parenchymal damage

Some patients demonstrate continued reduced alveolar gas exchange and microscopic evidence of diffuse alveolar wall thickening, and fibrosis around small vessels and airways. These changes reduce lung compliance, thus increasing the work of breathing and creating a sensation of dyspnoea.

Cardiac injury

Ventricular failure may follow severe myocardial contusion or infarction. Aneurysm and pseudoaneurysm of the ventricle can present late and require surgical repair as may VSD, valve incompetence and arterial fistulae. Pericardial constriction is uncommon following trauma and usually develops as a complication of sepsis.

Herniation

Herniation of abdominal viscera through tears in the diaphragm can occur years or decades after trauma; because of the dangers of obstruction and strangulation such cases should be repaired. Lung herniation is a rare complication of chest wall injuries especially those with large defects; herniated lung is tender and reconstructive surgery is necessary.

Deformity

Crush injuries of the chest wall may result in pectus deformity or stove-in chest. Surgical correction is indicated for cosmetic reasons, or in dyspnoeic patients with a large restrictive defect to restore lost lung volume.

Respiratory Emergencies

Massive haemoptysis

Haemorrhage from the lower respiratory tract of >200 mls per hour is termed massive haemoptysis. The management depends on the severity and on the cause. If the bleed is very severe it may be that the patient suffers severe respiratory embarrassment. Whilst attempts should be made to clear the airway, administration of a strong intravenous sedative such as diamorphine should be considered.

    In less severe cases, if the side from which the bleeding is coming from is known, the patient should be positioned on the same side. This is thought to compress the dependent lung and reduce aspiration of blood into the other lung. The algorithm (Figure 1) indicates how the knowledge of the pathology governs management. Embolisation and surgical resection are only realistic if the bleed is from a discrete area and investigations are directed to define the pathology. Bronchoscopy may be very difficult but can define which lung is bleeding. Rarely, a bleeding area is seen at bronchoscopy and successfully coagulated. If available, rigid bronchoscopy allows better clearance of the airway and control of bleeding. A decision needs to be made whether there is time for transfer to a unit offering rigid bronchoscopy. Pulmonary angiogram may be followed immediately by embolisation as part of the same procedure. In less severe cases, where <200 mls blood per hour is

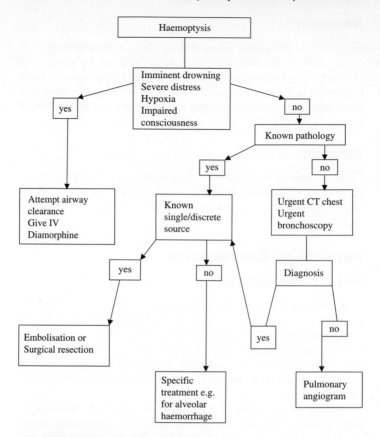

Figure 1. Algorithm for the management of massive haemoptysis

expectorated, procoagulants such as ethamsylate may be used. In all cases clotting disorders should be corrected and agents promoting haemoptysis discontinued e.g. nebulised acetylcysteine.

Tension pneumothorax

Non-traumatic tension pneumothorax is recognised by the presence of unilateral hyper-resonance, absent or reduced breath sounds, tracheal displacement and mediastinal shift. As the tension increases, cardiac output falls resulting in hypotension and collapse. Tension pneumothoraces commonly develop if a pneumothorax occurs during positive pressure ventilation but otherwise they are rare.

If hypotension has developed, a large gauge needle should be inserted which will be sufficient to restore venous return and correct cardiovascular collapse. This should be followed by insertion of an ICD.

Acute upper airway obstruction

Acute stridor is an uncommon emergency presenting to the respiratory physician. A clue to the aetiology can be obtained in the history. Slowly progressive dyspnoea and 'wheeze' suggests tracheal or carinal involvement with tumour whereas a history of constitutional symptoms of infection (fever, malaise) might indicate epiglottitis. The management is directed towards visualising the obstruction and securing the airway, whilst instituting specific therapy. Table 3 shows the more common causes of acute upper airway obstruction.

In all but epiglottitis, it is acceptable to examine the upper airway for foreign body, and then proceed to fibreoptic examination of the airway. If epiglottitis is suspected, there is a danger (particularly in children) of complete occlusion of the airway being precipitated by attempts to examine the oropharynx. Children with this now rare condition adopt the 'sniffing the morning air' posture, are very pale and make a gurgling sound. As a general rule, if the patient has critical airway narrowing as evidenced by respiratory distress at rest, an anaesthetist and an otorhinolaryngologist should

Table 3.   Aetiology of acute upper airway obstruction

Aetiology	Specific treatment (all may require intubation)
Tracheal and carinal tumours	Stenting, endobronchial debridement
Tracheal web	Surgery/laser therapy
Laryngeal tumour	Surgery/radiotherapy
Acute epiglotitis	Antimicrobial therapy
Acute laryngotracheobronchitis	Nebulised adrenaline may be tried
Severe subcutaneous and laryngeal emphysema	Intercostal drain; possible skin incisions
Foreign body	Removal

be present with equipment ready for intubation and tracheostomy. Other respiratory emergencies include acute ventilatory failure due to asthma, COPD, pulmonary embolism and pneumonia are reviewed in Chapters 4, 6, 7, 9 and 12.

Acute lung injury due to inhaled agents

Table 4 shows the agents commonly responsible for acute inhalation toxicity. The main effects are due to non-specific inflammation and the main threat to life is failure of gas exchange.

Thus management is directed towards monitoring clinical status, blood gases and radiographic changes. Supplementary oxygen must be given, if needed but high concentrations may augment the toxicity of some agents. The trachea and larynx may be oedematous leading to stridor and may necessitate either intubation or tracheotomy. Both obstructive and restrictive ventilatory abnormalities may develop and may also necessitate assisted ventilation.

In general, systemic corticosteroids should be given to moderate the inflammation. This is controversial in some circumstances (mineral oil aspiration) but in others (nitrogen dioxide) recommended for six to eight weeks. Antibiotics may be given prophylactically or withheld and the patient monitored for signs of infection. Some agents require specific antidotes (Table 4). A suggested algorithm for management is shown in Figure 2.

Near drowning

Near drowning may occur in the context of other circumstances which may be important in treatment e.g. cardiovascular disease, injury (particularly cervical spinal injury), impaired central nervous system function (alcohol) and hypothermia.

In near drowning there is usually little water inhaled in the early stages because laryngeal and bronchial spasm prevent further water entering. In one study, 22ml/kg body weight were inhaled. Even small amounts of inhaled fresh water cause loss of surfactant. Water is rapidly absorbed leaving atelectetic segments. Sea water is less rapidly absorbed and can block small alveoli. Both result in accelerated hypoxia due to intrapulmonary stunting. Water may be contaminated with bacteria, but severe infections following near drowning are unusual. If submersion continues, hypoxia results in unconsciousness but later hypercapnoea stimulates powerful inspirations which results in aspiration, swallowing and vomiting of large

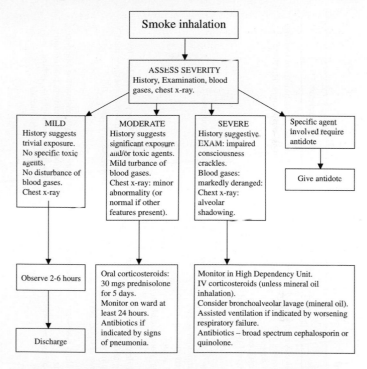

Figure 2.   Algorithm for the management of smoke inhalation

volumes of water. Respiratory arrest occurs before circulatory collapse and this may be useful by removing some products of metabolism from the brain and aiding cooling.

Management

Prolonged resuscitation on site is always appropriate and especially if the water is cold. Several reviews of near drowning have shown favourable outcomes. The cervical spine should be protected if there is any possibility of damage. There is little benefit from trying to empty the lungs — most fluid obtained comes from the stomach. The airway should be established and 4 or 5 respirations given (in the water, if necessary). If the circulation is not restored, full CPR should be maintained continuously once the patient is on a solid surface. Oxygen should be used as soon as available.

Table 4. Acute toxic lung injury due to inhalation

Agent	Where encountered	Clinical effect	Specific antidote	Chronic effects/sequelae
Ammonia	Raw material for chemical industry (fertilisers, explosives, plastics)	Acute inflammation in airways and parenchyma. Large exposures may cause death in minutes due to airways inflammation. Risk in lesser exposures is related more to parenchymal disease and secondary infection	None	Bronchiectasis, bronchiolitis obliterans, fixed airway obstruction described
Aldehydes (acetaldehyde acrylic aldehyde formaldehyde)	Chemical & plastics industry. Products of diesel & petrol combustion. Health care industry	Usually cause immediate & marked irritation to mucous membranes & therefore exposure limited, but can cause pulmonary oedema and acute pneumonitis. Skin rashes, rhinitis, asthma	None	Asthma may continue
Chlorine	Chemical industry paper (pulp) manufacture	Large exposures – rapid death due to asphyxia & acute airway and parenchymal toxicity. Pulmonary oedema may occur – may be several hours later	None	Parenchymal fully recovers low level, chronic exposure may produce mild airways obstruction
Drugs of abuse – cocaine, marijuana.	Cocaine used as an alkaloid base(less common), pneumothorax, pneumomediastinum, pulmonary oedema, pulmonary haemorrhage		None	Chronic airways obstruction Marijuana, cocaine (hypersensitivity pneumonitis, pulmonary eosinophilia, asthma, obliterative bronchiolitis

Table 4. Continued

Agent	Where encountered	Clinical effect	Specific antidote	Chronic effects/sequelae
Metals (elemented oxides salts)	Various industries	Acute mucosa irritation, pneumonitis, pulmonary oedema if inhaled as a fume	Ethylene diamine tetra-acetic acid for cadmium toxicity	Cobalt, chromium, nickel, vanadium – asthma. Nickel – Loeffler's syndrome. Chromium – malignancy. Pneumoconiosis with less reactive metals. Cobalt – 'hard metal disease' (a fibrosis alveolitis). Zinc – as for cobalt. Beryllium – sarcoidosis like all ?[a]
Methyl isocyanate	Chemical industry	Acute pulmonary oedema/pneumonitis (major release in 1984, Bhopal, India)	None	Not known
Minerals oils/petroleum	Acute – shipwreck – firefighters – siphoning petrol	Intense pneumonitis. Diffuse haemorrhagic pneumonia (especially if aspirated)	None	Pneumonitis, fibrosis or asthma
Nitrogen dioxide	Chemical industry mining (explosives). Fires. Combustion of nitrocellulose in radiographic films. Diesel fumes. Welding. Silos	Silos – fillers lung. Following exposure (not immediate effect on mucous membranes) toxic pneumonitis/pulmonary oedema (may recur 2-8 weeks after first episode)	Prophylactic corticosteroids for late pulmonary oedema. Methylene blue for methaemo-globinaemia	Bronchiolitis obliterans

Table 4. Continued

Agent	Where encountered	Clinical effect	Specific antidote	Chronic effects/sequelae
Organic dust syndrome (may be confused with nitrogen dioxide toxicity and acute Farmer's lung)	Unloading silos	Mycotoxicosis: (toxicity from fungal contamination). Inhalation of mucous membranes. Pneumonitis	Does not respond to steroids	
Manure		Liquid manure: Hydrogen sulphide. Main agent causing loss of consciousness, pulmonary oedema. Aspiration leads to infection with multiple organisms		
Phosgene	Clorination in chemical industry welding	Pneumonitis pulmonary oedema		
Sulphur dioxide	Fumigation. Paper industry (bleaching)	Acute effect in mucous membranes warns of exposure & lung damage therefore uncommon. High levels cause death within minutes – haemorrhagic pneumonitis		Progressive airway obstruction.

Table 4. Continued

Agent	Where encountered	Clinical effect	Specific antidote	Chronic effects/sequelae
Welding fumes.	Variety of toxic agents	Metal fume fever: acute influenza-like illness beginning hours after exposure & resolves after 24 hours. Acute pneumonitis induced by nitrogen oxide & other compounds		Asthma (chronium). Bronchitis
Smoke inhalation.	Variable toxicity depending on compounds & extent of combustion (incomplete can be worse)	Hypoxaemia – worse if carbon monoxide or hydrogen cyanide inhaled. High blood levels of either require action. Skin burns may exacerbate risk of pulmonary oedema, infections and ARDS. Risk of morbidity & need for intensive care predicted by chest X-ray, arterial gas tensions & clinical features (black sputum, fire in enclosed space, perioral burn, altered consciousness, altered voice and symptoms & signs of respiratory distress)	If hydrogen cyanide inhaled give amyl nitrate (inhaled) followed by IV sodium nitrate and sodium thiosulphate	Asthma (rare). Bronchostenosis (rare). Bronchiectasis (rare)

If resuscitation is successful ARDS may develop and therefore patients should be monitored in hospital for at least the first 24 hours. There are no indications for corticosteroids. Sputum should be obtained for culture, if present and antibiotics only started if there is evidence of infection. β_2 agonists should be used as indicated for bronchospasm. If raised intracranial pressure occurs this may be treated with mild hyperventilation and other measures.

References

1. ABC of Major Trauma, edited by Skinner, Driscoll and Earlam. British Medical Journal 1991

2. Thoracic Trauma, edited by Hood, Boyd and Culliford. WB Saunders 1989

3. Symbas PN. Cardiothoracic Trauma. WB Saunders 1989

4. Pittet JF et al. Biological markers of acute lung injury: prognostic and pathogenetic significance. *Am J Resp Crit Care Med* 1997;**155**: 1187–1205

5. Shuster DP. Identifying patients with ARDS, time for a different approach. *Intensive Care Medicine* December 1997;**23**(12):1197–1203

6. Modill JH. Serum electrolyte changes in near drowning victims (editorial). *JAMA* 1985;**252**:257

24

Chronic Cough

Ian D Pavord

Introduction

Troublesome cough is a common reason for patients to consult their General Practitioners. Surveys in the USA suggest that it is the fifth commonest symptom based cause for visits to the family doctor. The vast majority of cases are due to viral or bacterial infections of the upper and lower respiratory tract, are easily identified and are self limiting. Other causes such as chronic bronchitis, bronchiectasis, lung cancer and interstitial lung disease usually become obvious after a careful clinical assessment and a chest X-ray. A small proportion will have a persistent cough that defies diagnosis and will be referred for a specialist opinion. A chronic persistent cough is often arbitrarily defined as one lasting for more than three weeks although the majority will have a cough of many weeks duration by the time of referral. In most cases the cough will be dry or productive of scanty sputum. Chronic persistent cough is responsible for between 5 and 10% of respiratory outpatients referrals.

Chronic persistent cough is often wrongly regarded as a relatively trivial problem and accurate diagnosis and management is not afforded a high priority. However many patients experience considerable associated physical and psychological morbidity. Musculoskeletal chest pains, syncope, incontinence, disturbed sleep and social embarrassment are particularly common. Another common error is to regard the diagnosis and management of patients with chronic persistent cough as difficult and unrewarding. A systematic approach based on the so called 'anatomic diagnostic protocol' described by Irwin et al does seem to be successful and various series have reported a high rate of treatment success even in tertiary referral populations.

The anatomic diagnostic approach to chronic cough is based on a more complete understanding of the distribution of cough receptors and the physiology of the cough reflex, and particularly on the realisation that most cases are due to disease of the upper respiratory tract where cough receptors are most plentiful. Irwin has shown that up to 90% of cases are due to rhinitis, asthma and gastro-oesophageal reflux or a combination of these. Many of these conditions can be recognised clinically and successful diagnosis and management is often possible without recourse to expensive or invasive investigations.

Anatomy and Physiology of the Cough Reflex

Cough receptors are present in the larynx, trachea and carina and they extend distally as far as the sub segmental bronchi. Receptors are most plentiful in the upper airway suggesting this is the most functionally important area. There are a number of cough receptors but bronchial C fibres and irritant receptors are probably the most important. Stimulation of these receptors results in an involuntary forced expiratory manoeuvre against a closed glottis followed by glottal opening and a high velocity expiration. Afferent nerve fibres pass to a central cough receptor in the medulla. Factors influencing activity of the central cough receptor are poorly understood but opiates probably exert their anti-tussive effects here.

Box 1.   Protocol for capsaicin cough challenge testing

- prepare doubling dilutions of capsaicin (0.5 to 500 μM) in normal saline from a stock solution (10 mM in absolute alcohol diluted to 1 mM in 30% alcohol solution)

- subjects inhale a single breath of normal saline from functional residual capacity followed by doubling concentrations of capsaicin via a breath actuated dosimeter (output 5–7 μl; mass median diameter 4 μm). Breaths of normal saline can be alternated at random with capsaicin to minimise conditioned responses

- record number of coughs for one minute after each inhalation.

- discontinue when five or more coughs elicited or the highest concentration inhaled. Calculate the lowest concentration of capsaicin causing two (C2) and five (C5) coughs

Table 1.   Approximate incidence of the commoner causes of chronic persistent cough

Diagnosis	Approximate incidence (%)
Rhinitis	25–30
Asthma/eosinophilic bronchitis	20–25
Gastrooesophageal reflux	15–20
ACE inhibitor	5–10
Post viral	5–10
Chronic bronchitis/bronchiectasis	5–10
Unexplained	5–10

The cough reflex can be evaluated by challenge testing using known tussive agents such as the pepper extract capsaicin, citric acid and low chloride content solutions. These agents probably act through different mechanisms although the selectivity of different tussive stimuli in man is incompletely understood. A common protocol for cough challenge testing using capsaicin is illustrated in Box 1. Most cases of chronic persistent cough are associated with a heightened cough reflex, particularly if the cough is dry. This may reflect sensitisation of cough receptor by inflammatory mediators as has been shown to occur in experimental animals and man after administration of various inflammatory mediators including prostaglandins. Successful treatment of the underlying cause of the cough usually results in reduction in cough sensitivity.

Important Causes of Chronic Persistent Cough

Table 1 lists the common causes of chronic persistent cough in patients referred for a specialist opinion and their approximate incidence. The clinical features and treatment of the commoner causes are summarised in Table 2.

Rhinitis

Rhinitis, often associated with sinusitis and post-nasal drip, is probably the commonest cause of chronic cough. The exact mechanism is unknown but may involve extension of nasal inflammation into

Table 2.   Clinical features and suggested investigation and treatment of commoner causes of chronic persistent cough (BDP = beclomethasone diprionate)

Diagnosis	History	Examination	Investigations	Treatment
Rhinitis	Rhinorrhoea, nasal obstruction, sinus pain, sneezing, nasal itch, post nasal drip	Nasal secretions, nasal or pharyngeal mucosal inflammation	Sinus X-ray/CT showing mucosal thickening and/or fluid level	Topical budesonide/BDP 100 μg twice daily. In selected cases: topical ipratropium bromide 40 mg twice daily, oral antihistamine
Eosinophilic bronchitis	No wheeze, dyspnoea.	No signs of airflow obstruction	FEV_1 >80% predicted. FEV_1/FVC >75%. Max within day PEF variability over 2 weeks <20%. PC_{20} >8mg/ml. Sputum eosinophil count >5%	Inhaled budesonide/BDP 400 mg twice daily with prednisolone 30 mg daily for 14 days in selected cases
ACE cough	Cough onset temporarily related to starting ACE inhibitor			Drug withdrawal. Substitution of alternative if appropriate.
Gastrooesophageal reflux	Heartburn, flatulence, waterbrash		Barium swallow, endoscopy and 24 hr oesophageal manometry and pH in selected cases	Weight reduction, elevation of head of bed, avoid eating within 2 hours of bedtime, acid supression. Pro-kinetic agent in selected cases

Table 2. Continued

Diagnosis	History	Examination	Investigations	Treatment
Asthma	Episodic wheeze, dyspnoea and/or chest tightness	Polyphonic expiratory wheeze	One or more of the following: >15% increase in FEV_1 after inhaled salbutamol 200 μg, Max within day PEF variability over 2 weeks >20%, PC_{20} <8 mg/ml*	Inhaled budesonide/BDP 400 μg twice daily with prednisolone 30 mg daily for 14 days in selected cases. As required inhaled $beta_2$ agonist
Post viral	Onset following viral upper respiratory tract infection			Observation
Chronic bronchitis	Productive morning cough >3 months/year for more than 1 year. Smoking history	Coarse crackles		Stop smoking

* PC_{20} to methacholine

the upper airway and larynx with sensitisation of pharyngeal and laryngeal cough receptors. The cough is usually dry and patients may complain of an irritation in the upper airway and a need to frequently clear their throat. They often report nasal obstruction, discharge or frequent sinus headaches and may be aware of post nasal drip. Examination may reveal a nasal quality to the voice, sinus tenderness and inflammation of the posterior pharyngeal wall with evidence of draining secretions. Sinus X-rays or preferably CT scans often show mucosal thickening and the presence of fluid levels. Radiographic abnormalities can be the only evidence of upper airway disease.

Topical corticosteroids are the mainstay of treatment. Where nasal obstruction is prominent, initial additional treatment with topical decongestant sprays may be necessary and antibiotics should be considered if infection is suspected. Topical ipratropium bromide is often helpful when serous nasal discharge is prominent. Surgical treatment may be necessary in some cases, particularly where there are obvious anatomical abnormalities.

Asthma

Chronic cough can be the only presenting feature of asthma. Cough variant asthma is particularly well recognised in children. Paroxysms of coughing at night, after exercise, or in response to allergen exposure should particularly arouse suspicion. The cough is often dry but some patients complain of a morning cough productive of small amounts of tenacious mucopurulent sputum.

The key to diagnosing cough variant asthma is to demonstrate variable airflow obstruction, which may be related to episodes of coughing. Spirometry and reversibility testing or serial peak expiratory flow (PEF) monitoring may reveal characteristic patterns although they are often unhelpful. Demonstration of airway hyperresponsiveness by challenge testing is a more sensitive index of variable airflow obstruction and is often the only abnormal test in patients with cough variant asthma. Management of cough variant asthma should closely follow national and international guidelines for management of asthma.

Recently a group of patients with a cough and evidence on microscopic examination of the sputum of an eosinophilic bronchitis but no objective evidence of variable airflow obstruction have been described. How commonly eosinophilic bronchitis causes chronic cough is unclear but preliminary studies suggest that it may be responsible for up to 15% of cases. It is an important condition to recognise since, as with cough variant asthma the cough responds well to corticosteroid therapy.

Gastro-oesophageal reflux

Upper airway symptoms such as cough and hoarseness are well recognised in patients with symptomatic gastro-oesophageal reflux. It has become clear that patients can experience similar symptoms with sub-clinical reflux and recent studies show that up to a third of patients with cough due to gastro-oesophageal reflux do not have oesophageal symptoms. The mechanism is likely to involve sensitisation or direct stimulation of pharyngeal, laryngeal and even tracheal cough receptors by aspirated gastric acid although an oesophageal-tracheobronchial reflex has been proposed on the basis of studies showing that cough can be triggered by perfusion of the distal oesophagus with acid.

Gastro-oesophageal reflux associated cough can be elegantly demonstrated by combined oesophageal pressure and pH monitoring. Typically monitoring shows characteristic changes in the oesophageal pressure due to cough shortly after episodes of gastro-oesophageal reflux (Figure 1). Standard anti-reflux advice, acid suppression and occasionally pro-kinetic agents are usually effective in the treatment of the cough.

Post viral cough

Community studies show that the cough associated with upper respiratory tract infection has resolved or improved by two weeks in 77% of patients. The rest develop a more prolonged cough and in a small minority this persists for months. In some patients with a persistent post-infective cough an alternative explanation for the cough can be found, but there is undoubtedly a group of patients where this is not the case and where a diagnosis of post-viral cough is made by default. The cough is often dry and it is associated with a heightened cough reflex. In most cases the cough spontaneously improves. Patients are often empirically treated with inhaled corticosteroids although there is no good evidence that these help.

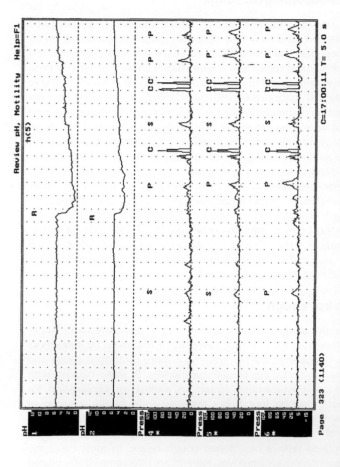

Figure 1. 24 hour oesophageal manometry and pH readings showing cough following episodes of gastrooesophageal reflux. Panel 1=Oesophageal pH 5 cm above lower oesophageal sphincter; panel 2=oesophageal pH 10 cm above lower oesophageal sphincter; panel 4,5 and 6=oesophageal pressure 15,10 and 5 cm above lower oesophageal sphincter (mmHg). C=cough; S=simultaneous wave; P=peristaltic wave; R=reflux

Angiotensin converting enzyme (ACE) inhibitor associated cough

Up to 10% of patients treated with ACE inhibitor develop a dry cough. The risk appears to be dose related and is shared equally by all drugs. Angiotensin receptor antagonists do not cause dry cough. The cough reflex is heightened in patients with ACE inhibitor associated cough and it returns to normal after the drug is stopped. Interestingly this is also the case in patients treated with ACE inhibitors who do not develop a cough. The cough and increased cough reflex are thought to be related to increased airway concentration of tussive mediators such as bradykinin and prostaglandins. Small clinical trials have shown that ACE inhibitor associated cough is inhibited by cyclo-oxygenase inhibitors, thromboxane receptor antagonists and by inhaled sodium cromoglycate although these drugs are not widely used in clinical practise. ACE inhibitor associated cough resolves quickly after withdrawal of the drug and this is nearly always the most appropriate management. Persistence of the cough might indicate asthma, the onset of which has been associated with ACE-inhibitor therapy.

An Approach to Diagnosis and Management of Chronic Cough

A detailed history and physical examination is of paramount importance with particular attention paid to the circumstances at the onset of the cough. All patients should have a detailed examination of their upper airway, chest X-ray, spirogram and if appropriate reversibility studies and a period of home PEF monitoring. Allergen skin prick testing can be useful in establishing risk and may provide information that may be useful in the future management of the patient. Further investigations can then be arranged on an individual patient basis and may be influenced by the patients age and co-morbid conditions. Our diagnostic algorithm is illustrated in Figure 2.

A detailed discussion of the diagnosis and treatment of individual causes of chronic persistent cough is outside the scope of this chapter but some guidance can be found in Table 2. The following general points on diagnosis and management are particularly important:

- the characteristics of the cough are of limited value in establishing the cause. A morning cough productive of sputum is typical of

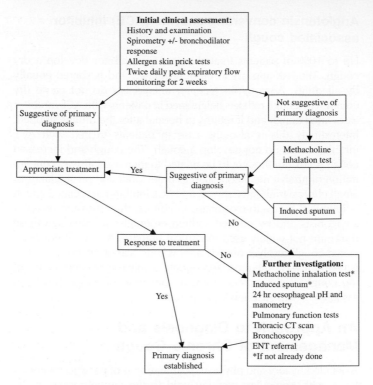

Figure 2. **Suggested diagnostic algorithm for patients with chronic persistent cough**

bronchitis and a cough productive of copious sputum suggests bronchiectasis although there is considerable overlap

- cough is due to multiple causes in up to a fifth of patients. The combination of asthma, rhinitis and/or gastro-oesophageal reflux is particularly common. Cough may only respond to treatment aimed at all causes

- although a trial of treatment is appropriate in some circumstances, in general objective confirmation of disease is preferable before starting treatment. This is particularly important in patients without suggestive symptoms. Pre-treatment investigations can provide a useful baseline against which the effects of specific treatment can be judged

- invasive and/or expensive investigations (ie bronchoscopy and high resolution CT scanning) have a low diagnostic yield and should be reserved for patients with suggestive symptoms, signs or chest X-ray findings, or in those with no objective evidence of the commoner causes of chronic cough

- treatment should be aimed at the cause of the cough. Non-specific anti-tussive agents have only a limited role although a small minority of patients with unexplained severe cough benefit from opiate cough supressants or nebulised lignocaine
- prolonged and aggressive treatment may be necessary before the cough improves
- treatment failure may be due to failure to control the correctly identified cause of the cough or to an incorrect diagnosis. Attempt to validate the effects of treatment before coming to the latter conclusion

Future Research

Although the anatomic diagnostic protocol results in identification of the cause and successful treatment of the majority of cases of chronic cough, important problems remain. Assessment of patients with chronic persistent cough is hampered by the absence of a reliable method for quantifying cough, which would allow verification of the diagnosis and validation the effects of treatment. Cough reflex sensitivity measured using capsaicin is usually abnormal in patients with chronic persistent cough and can be used to verify an abnormal cough response and to demonstrate improvement with treatment. Oesophageal manometry has promise as an objective means of quantifying cough (see Figure 1) although normal ranges have not been established and questions such as whether the presence of the pressure probe in the upper airway triggers cough have not been addressed.

Medical opinion box

History
Cough onset, duration, character. Associated symptoms, particularly upper airway symptoms, reflux, symptoms suggesting variable airflow obstruction. Atopic background, drug history.

Examination
Upper airway, signs of airflow obstruction.

Investigation
Spirogram, CXR, serial peak expiratory flow, full blood count and eosinophil differential.

Optional investigations
Methacholine airway responsiveness, sinus X-ray or preferably CT, allergen skin prick testing and sputum and nasal differential inflammatory cell counts helpful in most patients. Oesophageal manometry and pH monitoring, CT thorax and bronchoscopy in selected patients.

Treatment
Directed at cause or causes.

In an important minority of patients with chronic persistent cough (variously estimated at between 2 and 20%) no cause can be found. Studies suggest that such patients have subtle alterations in the airway neural sensory system and bronchoscopic evidence of chronic airway inflammation but these abnormalities have not been well defined nor is the specificity of the findings well established. There is a need for more detailed study of this group. Until more is known about the pathophysiology of idiopathic chronic persistent cough management is problematic. A better understanding of the physiology and pharmacological manipulation of the cough reflex might lead to more effective and selective anti-tussive agents for these patients and for the wider population with a distressing cough.

Further Reading

1. Irwin RS, Corrao WM, Pratter MR. Chronic persistent cough in the adult: the spectrum and frequency of causes and successful outcome of specific therapy. *Am Rev Respir Dis* 1981;**123**:413–417

2. Irwin RS, Curley FJ, French CL. Chronic cough. The spectrum and frequency of causes, key components of the diagnostic evaluation, and outcome of specific therapy. *Am Rev Respir Dis* 1990;**141**:640–647

3. Corrao WM, Braman SS, Irwin RS. Chronic cough as the sole presenting manifestation of bronchial asthma. *N Engl J Med* 1979;**300**:633–637

4. Irwin RS, Zawacki JK, Curley FJ, French CL, Hoffman PJ. Chronic cough as the sole presenting feature of gastroesophageal reflux. *Am Rev Respir Dis* 1989;**140**:1294–1300

5. Chung KF, Lalloo UG. Diagnosis and management of chronic persistent dry cough. *Postgrad Med J* 1996;**72**:594–598

6. Gibson PG, Dolovich J, Denburg J, Ramsdale EH, Hargreave FE. Chronic cough: eosinophilic bronchitis without asthma. *Lancet* 1989;**I**:1346–1348

7. O'Connor F, Thomas VE, Pride NB, Fuller RW. Capsaicin cough sensitivity decreases with successful treatment of chronic cough. *Am J Respir Crit Care Med* 1994;**150**:374–380

8. Boulet L-P, Milot J, Boutet M, St. Georges F, Laviolette M. Airway inflammation in non-asthmatic subjects with chronic cough. *Am J Respir Crit Care Med* 1994;**149**:482–489

25

Pulmonary Disease in Pregnancy

J Paul Dilworth

Normal pregnancies are characterised by a variety of changes in the lung and respiratory conditions frequently complicate pregnancy. This chapter describes the commonly encountered pulmonary problems associated with pregnancy.

The Lung in Normal Pregnancy

Anatomy during pregnancy

- elevation of the diaphragm by up to 4cms although its excursion is not impaired
- an increase in transverse and antero-posterior diameter occurs with a consequent increase in the subcostal angle and up to 7cms increase in chest circumference
- capillary enlargement throughout the respiratory tract with increased mucosal oedema and hyperaemia

Important endocrine changes

- increased progesterone leading to hyper-ventilation
- increased free cortisol; possibly disease modifying (eg; sarcoid)

Physiological abnormalities

- a 20% increase in oxygen consumption and 15% increase in maternal metabolic rate is compensated for by an increased tidal volume (VT = amount of air moved in one normal respiratory cycle) without an increase in respiratory rate

- hence minute volume (amount air moved/minute) increases by up to 40%

Pulmonary function

- TLC and VC normal as diaphragm excursion remains normal
- FRC and RV reduced by about 20% later in pregnancy
- pCO_2 reduced with a compensatory fall in bicarbonate and mild respiratory alkalosis
- pO_2 reduced in supine position only in third trimester (hence measure ABG sitting)

Symptoms

- dyspnoea is experienced by 60–70% during pregnancy especially in the second trimester probably secondary to progesterone induced hyperventilation and mechanical factors
- nasal congestion and sneezing are common due to hyperaemia and mucosal oedema

Radiation

Radiation doses resulting from most routine diagnostic procedures present no substantial risk of causing foetal death or malformation or impairment of mental development. It is judged that there is no contraindication to performing chest radiographs (mean dose to foetus <0.01mGy) if clinically indicated and **with patient consent**. A CT thorax (mean dose to foetus 0.06mGy) may also be performed if strongly indicated. 99mTc ventilation perfusion scans (usual mean dose to foetus 0.2mGy for perfusion scan and 0.3mGy for the ventilation scan) can be used but nuclear medicine departments will normally perform a half dose perfusion scan and proceed to a ventilation scan if abnormal. **Appropriate abdominal shielding should be utilised for all radiological procedures**.

Specific Respiratory Conditions in Pregnancy

Pulmonary embolism (PE)

Introduction

The incidence of pregnancy related PE is 0.3% (DVT 1.2%). It is the second most important cause of maternal death in the UK. The enlarged uterus and activation of clotting to prepare for placental separation are precipitating factors. Risk increases with age, parity, caesarian section and instrumentation.

Management

In suspected PE the benefits of chest radiography and ventilation-perfusion scanning outweigh the risk of radiation. The presence of normal arterial blood gases and a normal ventilation-perfusion scan virtually excludes PE. Where diagnostic doubt remains a leg ultrasound and echocardiogram may be helpful. Pulmonary angiography or spiral CT with appropriate abdominal shielding is possible.

Heparin does not cross the placenta and may be used to anticoagulate. Initial unfractionated heparin followed by once a day low molecular weight heparin is now the treatment of choice

Warfarin crosses the placenta and may cause foetal abnormalities and foetal haemorrhage. It should be avoided if possible but is used occasionally between the 12th and 38th week of gestation in especially difficult patients (eg; artificial heart valves). Generally alternatives are available.

There are few data on thrombolysis in pregnancy but it is probably contra-indicated. Inferior vena-caval filters are an alternative where the risks of anticoagulation are high (eg; labour and the immediate post-partum period.

Breast feeding

There is no contra-indication to heparin or warfarin. After a V/Q scan there should be no breast feeding for 24 hours.

Asthma

Introduction

Asthma is a significant complicating factor in 1% of all pregnancies.

Effect of pregnancy on asthma

This is unpredictable. Approximately one half are unchanged, one quarter improved and one quarter deteriorate. Previously mild asthmatics tend to improve and previously severe tend to worsen. A similar course is often found in each pregnancy. Exacerbations tend to occur between 24 and 36 weeks and symptoms tend to revert to normal within the first 3 months post-partum.

Effect of asthma on pregnancy

There is a risk of foetal growth retardation if severe chronic hypoxaemia is present and uncontrolled disease worsens maternal and foetal outcome. Well controlled asthma should not be associated with increased morbidity or mortality.

Management

Education about the benefits of good control and compliance with asthma treatment should be a part of early ante-natal care. The use of a home peak flow chart with a self-management plan is recommended.

There is no contra-indication to most first line treatments for asthma in pregnancy. Trigger factors including tobacco should be avoided. There is limited evidence on the use of long acting beta-2-agonists and newer inhaled corticosteroids in pregnancy. It seems sensible not to commence these agents during pregnancy but if they are required for good asthma control they should not be stopped. Prednisolone crosses the placenta poorly and is the steroid of choice but monitoring of maternal glucose should be undertaken. Monitoring of theophylline levels to avoid values in the toxic or high therapeutic range is appropriate.

Around the time of labour patients who have been on regular steroids may require hydrocortisone cover. Ergotamine and PGF2 may cause bronchoconstriction but the latter may be required for control of haemorrhage; the former is contra-indicated. Systemic beta agonists may inhibit labour. Adrenaline is correlated with congenital abnormalities and should be avoided.

Breast feeding

Generally no change in therapy is required and although it has been suggested that theophyllines may cause infantile irritability they are not contra-indicated. There is some evidence that breast feeding may reduce the risk of atopy.

Tuberculosis

Effect of tuberculosis on pregnancy

There is an increased complication rate in maternal tuberculosis. Standard treatment with an isoniazid (INH) and rifampicin based regimen is advised using quadruple therapy where appropriate.

Data on pyrazinamide are scanty but ethambutol appears free from problems and some physicians would substitute ethambutol for pyrazinamide as the third agent if treatment is required in the first trimester and triple therapy is adequate although if this is done therapy should continue for 9 months. There is some evidence that INH induced hepatitis is commoner in pregnancy and monitoring of liver function is sensible. The safety of rifampicin has previously been questioned but the risk of inadequately treated TB is greater.

Streptomycin is ototoxic with a 17% incidence of foetal eighth nerve palsy. It is contraindicated.

The tuberculin test (PPD) is not affected by pregnancy and has no adverse effects on outcome. In a mother who is found to be tuberculin test positive during pregnancy a respiratory history and chest X-ray should be performed. INH prophylaxis should be given but deferred until 3–6 months after delivery unless she is a recent converter, has been in close contact with smear positive TB, is in a high risk group or is immunocompromised.

Antituberculous treatment of infants born to mothers with TB or suspected TB during pregnancy should be considered in some situations. If the mother had already received treatment for over 3 months at delivery then the infant should have PPD testing followed by BCG if necessary but no therapy. If the mother had been treated for less than 3 months or is still culture positive at the time of delivery then the infant should have a chest radiograph and if clear receive INH prophylaxis.

There are little useful data on multi-drug resistance in pregnancy but the teratogenicity of many agents is unknown.

Rib fractures

Due to the altered alignment of the thoracic cavity the incidence of cough fractures is greater than normal and should enter the differential for chest pain.

Sarcoidosis

There is evidence that active sarcoidosis may regress during pregnancy perhaps due to increased free cortisol.

Pneumonia

Pneumonia is no commoner in pregnancy but is a serious complication requiring prompt treatment. Amoxicillin (due to increased renal clearance 500mg tds should be used), cephalosporins and erythromycin are safe. Quinolones, tetracyclines and trimethoprim are contra-indicated.

Cystic fibrosis

Counseling of prospective parents is essential as the chance of a child having CF will be between 1:20 and 1:44 if the father status is unknown. Maternal mortality is up to 12% and perinatal mortality up to 11%. The risk is related to the degree of maternal hypoxia and pulmonary hypertension.

Amniotic fluid embolism

Up to 10% of maternal deaths have been attributed to amniotic fluid embolism in some series. There is an 80% mortality; over half in the first few hours. Presentation is during labour with breathlessness, collapse, seizures or DIC. The differential includes aspiration (in which bronchospasm is commoner and the onset of DIC later), pulmonary embolism and haemorrhagic shock. Precipitating factors include a complicated labour, use of intrauterine stimulants, meconium stained amniotic fluid, higher maternal age, multiparity and intrauterine foetal death. The chest X-ray is usually abnormal (eg; pulmonary oedema, effusions cardiomegaly), ECG may indicate right heart strain pattern and ventilation-perfusion scans may show multiple defects. Treatment is immediate evacuation of the uterus and supportive care.

Acute respiratory failure

The commonest respiratory complication of labour is aspiration. Starving once labour is established and use of regular antacids may reduce the incidence. Other causes of breathlessness include PE, ARDS, amniotic fluid embolism, asthma, cardiogenic pulmonary oedema, pneumothorax, shock secondary to haemorrhage or infection and anaphylaxis

Further Reading

Miller JM (ed). Pulmonary diseases in pregnancy. *Clinical Obstetrics and Gynaecology* 1996;**39**(1):3–154

26

Perioperative Pulmonary Assessment and Treatment

J Paul Dilworth

Although chest infections are less common than wound and urinary tract infections postoperatively they have a much higher morbidity with increased length of hospital stay. The risk of postoperative pulmonary complications increases the closer to the thorax the site of surgery. Some degree of hypoxaemia and diminished lung volumes after upper abdominal or thoracic surgery is invariable. The mean fall in vital capacity after upper abdominal surgery is 55%, after major lower abdominal surgery 40% and after limb surgery only 0.5%. pO_2 falls by a mean of 25% after upper abdominal surgery.[1] Atelectasis occurs in 100% of patients after upper abdominal incision and chest infection occurs in up to 20%. Common postoperative pulmonary complications are listed in Table 1.

Table 1. Common post operative pulmonary complications

- Ventilatory failure
- Atelectasis
- Infection
- Pulmonary oedema
- ARDS
- Fluid overload/LVF
- Pulmonary embolism

Table 2.   Risk factors assessment and management for post-operative pulmonary complications

Thoracic/upper abdominal site
Smoked >20 pack years
Pre-existing lung disease   →   If any factors present
Current respiratory symptoms   consider spirometry with
Morbid obesity   reversibility and estimation
Anaesthetic >4 hrs duration   of oxygen saturation/ABG
Poor pre-operative performance status

↓   ↓   ↓

If any of the above clinical features or significant abnormality in spirometry or ABG

Very high risk if FEV_1 <800ml or hypercapnoea
Reconsider benefits of surgery
Consider postoperative ITU bed

IF RISK FACTORS PRESENT CONSIDER

Pre-op   Stop smoking
          Good nutrition
          Optimise lung function (eg; bronchodilators ± corticosteroids)
          Physiotherapy/Educate on deep breathing
          Review anaesthetic regimen
          Review surgical incision
          Document risk and plan

Post-op   Review analgesic and sedative regimen
          Physiotherapy/incentive spirometry
          Early mobilisation/nurse sitting
          Bronchodilators ± Corticosteroids
          Careful observation for signs of infection/atelectasis
          Oxygen
          Avoid aspiration

Preoperative evaluation

The aim of preoperative assessment is to identify those at risk of complications and those where the risk of surgery is greater than the potential benefits. Risk is dependent primarily on the **site of surgery** and the presence of **pre-existing respiratory disease** (Table 2). Those undergoing thoracic or upper abdominal surgery,

Table 3. Guidelines for pre-operative chest X-rays

- If risk factors for post-operative pulmonary complications
- If no available film for last 12 months and over age 65 years
- Recent immigrants
- High likelihood of requiring post-operative film
- Acute respiratory symptoms
- Malignant disease/possible metastases
- **If you order the film look at it!**

current or previous moderate or heavy **smokers** (>20 pack years over age 40 years) and those with known pre-existing lung disease (eg; asthma, COPD, neuromuscular disorders) are particularly at risk.[2] Severe **obesity** and **duration of anaesthetic** greater than 3.5 hours may also be risk factors.[3] It is unclear if age is an independent variable but many older patients will have ischaemic heart disease and other **co-morbidity** or lack motivation to undergo and recover from major surgery.

Patients risk can, therefore, be categorised initially by a simple smoking and respiratory history and physical examination. If any of the above factors are present then spirometry ± reversibility with estimation of oxygen saturation (arterial blood gases (ABG) if SaO_2 <93%) should be considered.[4] Greater than 90% of those developing complications will have had abnormal preoperative spirometry or blood gases. The presence of preoperative hypercapnoea or an FEV1 <0.8ml should precipitate re-evaluation of the benefits of surgery. The value of other lung function tests (eg; gas transfer) is less clear but may be helpful in those undergoing lung resection. Guidelines for pre-operative chest X-rays are given in Table 3.

Regimen advised in patients with risk factors

Cessation of smoking prior to operation may be of benefit by reducing mucous production. Good nutrition may improve postoperative respiratory muscle function. Patients lung function should be optimised for several days prior to surgery on occasion by early admission. In those with reversibility high dose inhaled or oral corticosteroids may be appropriate with high dose inhaled bronchodilators to assist in reversing airflow limitation and increasing mucociliary clearance.

The anaesthetic regimen should be tailored to reduce risk with the judicious use of regional anaesthesia. Postoperative analgesia should provide good pain relief without depression of ventilation or lung function and alternatives to opiate analgesics should be considered. A physiotherapist should advise pre-operatively and treatment continued after surgery. Although the most beneficial forms of physiotherapy intervention are unclear there is some evidence to support the use of incentive spirometry.[5] Early mobilisation should be strongly encouraged preceded by nursing in a sitting position. Bronchodilators by nebuliser or large volume spacer should be prescribed post-operatively in those with any degree of reversibility.

Careful postoperative observation with prompt antibiotics for lower respiratory tract infections may prevent life-threatening pneumonia. The oropharyngeal flora is altered postoperatively to include more gram negative bacteria and, therefore, the antibiotic chosen for post-operative lower respiratory tract infections should cover a different spectrum than for community acquired pneumonia (eg; co-amoxiclav or a second/third generation cephalosporin ± metronidazole).

Assessment for lung resection

Decisions about lung resection should be taken by a multidisciplinary team and with due consideration of co-morbidity. The following principles may be helpful. The above precautions for patients with risk factors described above are essential. In addition there is the a greater danger of ventilatory insufficiency. Lung function should be performed once it has been optimised pre-operatively. The proportion of lung to be removed should be calculated by segments.

ie; Pre-op FEV_1 × (no remaining segments/18)
= post-op FEV_1 after full recovery.

If the postoperative FEV1 will be below 0.8l then resection is relatively contraindicated. However, at the time of surgery on occasion it will be necessary to perform a larger procedure (eg; pneumonectomy) and conversely if the segments to be resected were playing no part in pre-operative ventilation then they should not be included in the calculations and a lung ventilation-perfusion scan may be helpful to assess this further.

Pulmonary embolism

The diagnosis and management of PE is described elsewhere but prophylaxis for pulmonary embolism should be considered when performing a pre-operative respiratory assessment and in a postoperative patient with fever, breathlessness, chest pain or unexplained radiographic change the possibility of pulmonary embolism should always be examined.

References

1. Hansen G, Drablos PA, Steinert R Pulmonary complications, ventilation and blood gases after upper abdominal surgery. *Acta Anaesth Scand* 1977;**21**:211–15

2. Dilworth JP, White RJ. Postoperative chest infection after upper abdominal surgery: an important problem for smokers. *Respiratory Med* 1992;**86**:205–210

3. Garibaldi R, Britt MR, Coleman ML, Reading JC, Pace NL. Risk factors for postoperative pneumonia. *Am J Med* 1980;**68**:219–23

4. Hayhurst MD. Preoperative pulmonary function testing. *Respiratory Med* 1993;**87**:161–63

5. Richardson J, Sabanathan S. Prevention of respiratory complications after abdominal surgery: a randomised clinical trial. *Br Med J* 1996;**312**:148–53

27

Physiotherapy

Tracey Hughes

Introduction

The objectives of this chapter are to provide a brief overview of physiotherapy practice in respiratory care and provide guidelines for medical staff in order to facilitate appropriate and speedy referral for treatment.

Guidelines can indicate whether physiotherapy intervention may or may not be appropriate, but they can never be absolute. For example, initially it may appear that physiotherapy is inappropriate for certain conditions but further examination of the problems may indicate that the application of physical intervention, such as pain relief, positioning, etc, can indirectly influence the outcome of treatment. Physiotherapy must therefore, be problem orientated. Application can be divided into four main sections.

Treatment

This includes treatment for acute and exacerbations of chronic problems.

Prophylaxis

Patients with chronic lung disease are taught to manage their own chest condition. This involves being able, independently and effectively, to clear excess secretions from their chest on a regular basis and to be in control of their breathing. Patients are also given advice on lifestyle and exercise.

Education, advice and monitoring are also important during periods of immobility such as with some neurological diseases, intubation, trauma/injury to the thorax, etc.

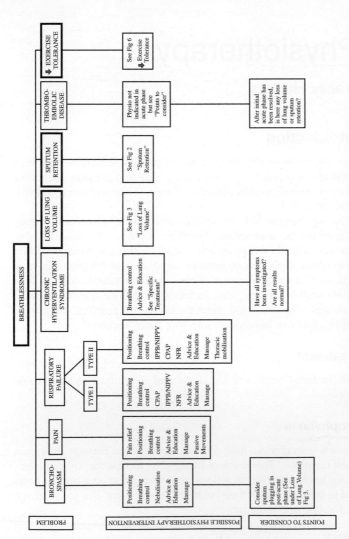

Figure 1.   Problem related indications for physiotherapy

Rehabilitation

The aim of rehabilitation is to restore maximum function of an individual within the limitations of their disease. It is integral to the care of the patient in a wide variety of problems for example, disordered breathing patterns such as demonstrated in Hyperventilation Syndrome and Vocal Cord Dysfunction, patients suffering with chronic obstructive or restrictive lung disease and also following an acute crisis e.g. pneumonia.

Other

This includes diagnostic testing i.e. induced sputum, assessment i.e. exercise tolerance testing, and the care of the terminally ill patient.

Most techniques are simple to perform but expertise is important in assessment and evaluation, enabling a correct diagnosis to be made and appropriate planning of treatment with an understanding of the physiological response to intervention.

Treatment Techniques

Positioning

Correct positioning is central to the performance of good chest physiotherapy because it can have dramatic effects on respiratory and cardiovascular function. The position may be dictated by the type of lung pathology, the extent to which a patient will tolerate some positions and whether or not the patient is intubated and receiving positive pressure ventilation. Examples where correct positioning is essential are given below.

- patients who have decreased functional residual capacity (FRC) e.g. post-operative patients or patients with neuromuscular disease will benefit from being positioned in an upright sitting position which will result in an increased lung volume and reduce the work of breathing
- patients with increased FRC, e.g. emphysema, will often instinctively assume a position which aids their breathing but others may need advice
- patients with severe hypoxaemia can be positioned to optimise ventilation/perfusion
- to aid removal of secretions (see Postural Drainage).

Breathing Exercises

Breathing exercises are used to control breathlessness at rest and during exertion and also to remove secretions.

Breathing control

This is relaxed, gentle tidal volume breathing which can be used to decrease anxiety associated with breathlessness or in conjunction with other physiotherapy techniques to allow for rests and restore equilibrium. It should always be used during exertion. Patients who are limited by breathlessness on exertion, can be taught to increase the tidal volume during exercise which has been shown to minimise desaturation. It is also helpful for these patients to develop a rhythmical breathing pattern e.g. when walking inspire for one step and exhale for two steps. Another example might be to exhale on effort and stretching e.g. reaching an object from a high shelf and then inhale on bringing the object down.

Patients with chronically hyperinflated chests may need to recruit accessory muscles of respiration to achieve adequate ventilation due to the diaphragm being shortened. This should not be discouraged. These patients must be shown positions to optimise their breathing which support and fixate the shoulder girdle to reduce the work of breathing (see Positioning).

Assuming the mechanics of breathing are not abnormal and the diaphragm is fully functional, the patient can be encouraged to breathe using the lower chest, with the upper chest and shoulders relaxed.

Deep breathing exercises

Deep breathing employs slow deep inspiration with thoracic expansion and passive expiration. The aim is to improve ventilation and to assist the removal of secretions when present. A maximum of five consecutive breaths is followed by relaxed breathing control.

Forced expiratory technique (FET)

Forced expiration with an open glottis, or huffing, can aid the clearance of secretions. When one or two huffs are followed by relaxed breathing, it is referred to as FET. Care must be taken not to induce coughing bouts and bronchospasm due to a prolonged expiratory manoeuvre.

Active cycle of breathing techniques (ACBT)

ACBT is a combination of deep breathing techniques, huffing and breathing control.[4]

Autogenic Drainage (AD)

This technique was first developed in Belgium for use in children with cystic fibrosis. AD requires concentration and commitment from the patient but for those who can master the art, it is an effective method of sputum clearance.

The treatment aims to generate high flow through the airways which helps to dislodge secretions but without causing airway collapse. In the first phase, 'the unstick phase', there is tidal breathing at low lung volume which aims to mobilise secretions in the small airways. In the second phase, 'the collect phase' the patient breathes at mid lung volumes to move secretions to large generation bronchi. In phase three 'evacuate phase' the patient is encouraged to breath at high lung volume to clear the secretions. It is important that cough is delayed until the patients can feel their secretions are loose enough to expectorate easily.

AD allows the patient independence with treatment but can be time consuming. It is indicated in patients with copious sputum.

Postural Drainage

Postural drainage promotes gravity-assisted drainage of secretions and is only effective when secretions are copious and thin enough to be affected by gravity. It employs specific body positions to drain different lobes and segments of the lung. It is often combined with other methods which promote sputum clearance including ACBT, autogenic drainage, manual techniques, PEP masks and flutter valves.

It is useful in the treatment of bronchiectasis and it is sometimes used in purulent chest infections including open lung abscesses and also in cases of acute aspiration.

Because postural drainage may increase the work of breathing and decrease function residual capacity, it may cause a temporary fall in oxygen saturation. Caution is, therefore, required in patients who have undergone surgery, have cardiovascular instability and also in pregnancy.

Manual Techniques

Manual techniques include percussion, vibration and shaking. The principle action is to loosen secretions and hence aid expectoration of sputum. They are commonly performed in conjunction with other physiotherapy techniques such as postural drainage and breathing exercises.

In percussion, rhythmic clapping with cupped hands is applied to the chest over the involved area of lung. The precise technique will depend on that which is found to be most effective and which the patient prefers. In vibration and shaking, there is intermittent chest wall compression which is either fine (vibration) or coarse (shaking).

These techniques are most useful in patients who need to clear large volumes of sputum but also in those who are too ill or weak to perform any independent chest clearance techniques. The techniques should be used with caution in cases of osteoporosis, rib fracture or thoracic pain, haemoptysis or lung cancer, pulmonary tuberculosis and patients with cardiovascular instability.

Positive Expiratory Pressure (PEP)

The PEP set consists of an anaesthetic type mask or mouthpiece and a one way valve to which a resistor is added. A manometer is included in the circuit and the patient is encouraged to expire actively to achieve a pressure of 10–15 cm of water. After 10–15 breaths, the patient should remove the mask and then after a short period of relaxed breathing, perform a forced expiration to clear secretions.

PEP mask treatment allows the expiratory time to be lengthened, delays airway closure, and aids movement of sputum proximally.[2]

The technique is indicated in patients with increased sputum production and retention and post operatively to prevent atelectasis. It should be used with caution in airways obstruction, facial injury or trauma and haemoptysis.

Flutter

The flutter is shaped like a tobacco pipe and has a stainless steel ball which sits inside a cone, inside the bowl of the pipe. On expiration, pressure is built up behind the ball which forces it up the side of the cone. As pressure falls, the ball drops back down into the cone and the cycle is repeated giving rise to the oscillatory

effect. It is hypothesised that the oscillating pressure waves generated by the pipe increase the diameter of the airways due to the
principles of pulmonary elastic resonance, and help prevent airway
collapse.

The number of oscillations, and therefore amount of positive
pressure produced on expiration can be altered by slightly changing
the inclination of the Flutter pipe. The amount of positive pressure
created is between 10–25cm H_2O and the resonance that is created
is felt as vibrations inside the chest. Therapeutic effect of the device
is considered optimal when the patient experiences the strongest
vibrations.

The Flutter is normally used in a sitting position but could also
be used in modified postural drainage positions, providing the
correct angle of tilt can be achieved.

The Flutter is indicated in patients producing copious sputum.
It should not be used in cases of pneumothorax or haemoptysis
and used with caution in patients with bronchospasm and severe
cardiovascular disease.

Humidification and Nebulisation

Humidification is indicated in patients where the normal mechanism provided by the upper airway has been bypassed or
compromised e.g. intubated patients or those with tracheostomies,
patients receiving FiO_2 greater than 0.35 or continuous positive
airways pressure. Ideally the humidifier should have a heating
element especially if there is a history of asthma. It is especially
important if the patient also has tenacious secretions. However,
thick secretions maybe a consequence of poor hydration in which
case oral or intravenous fluids are indicated.

Nebulisers delivering bronchodilators are most effective if the
particle size is between 2–5 µm. Ultrasonic nebulisers are more
efficient at delivering a densely saturated mist of the required
particle size and may be more effective but the patient must be
closely observed for signs of bronchospasm.

Non-invasive Ventilation

Intermittent positive pressure breathing (IPPB)

The Bird Mark 7 is the most commonly used machine and delivers
positive airway pressure up to 35 cm of water on inspiration and
allows passive expiration. It can be patient triggered or manually

controlled and driven by air or 35–40% oxygen. The principle effect is to improve tidal volume and decrease the work of breathing. The device can administer the pressure either by a face mask or mouth piece and must include a nebuliser to deliver saline or bronchodilators to counteract the drying effect of the high flow gas. For this reason, IPPB is only suitable for short-term use.

The device has a variety of settings which can be tailored to suit the individual patient. It is indicated in patients with poor tidal volume e.g. neuromuscular disease, patients with chronic respiratory disease who are fatigued and have retained secretions and those with chest wall deformity and acute chest infection.

Contra-indications and precautions are the same as for any IPPV device: undrained pneumothorax, large bullae, pulmonary carcinoma, facial injury, bronchopulmonary fistula, surgical emphysema and recent bronchial or oesophageal surgery.

Non-Invasive positive pressure ventilation (NIPPV)

Newer machines which are adapted for use with full face masks or more commonly nasal masks, can be used for longer periods of time than the IPPB devices. Research in the clinical setting has shown a more rapid reversal of type II respiratory failure using NIPPV than with conventional treatment.

For contra-indications, see IPPB.

Continuous positive airways pressure (CPAP)

CPAP causes an elevation in FRC, reduces the work of breathing and improves gas exchange.

It is indicated for use in patients with atelectasis or sputum retention. Contra-indications are as for IPPB but with the addition of severe heart failure. Hypercapnia may worsen.

Manual Hyperinflation (MHI)

In intubated patients, the practice of manually introducing a volume of air or air-oxygen mix into the lungs via a Waters bag can assist physiotherapy. The technique improves sputum clearance and has been shown to improve pulmonary compliance. Slow inspiration is thought to aid the inflation of alveoli, a short hold encourages recruitment of collateral channels of ventilation and quick release enhances the elastic recoil of the lungs to promote mobilisation of

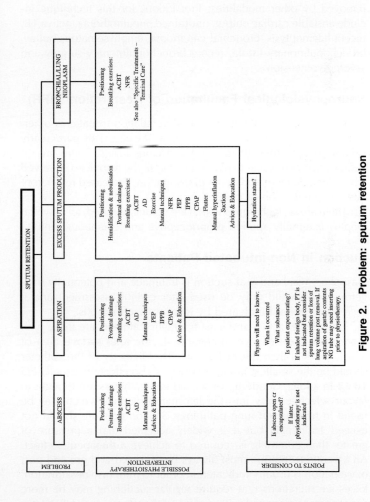

Figure 2. Problem: sputum retention

secretions into more proximal airways. Care must be taken not to induce baro or volutrauma.

The principle indications are atelectasis due to sputum plugging and decreased volume, and excess secretions which are not easily removed by other modalities. Precautions for this technique include unstable cardiac output, undrained pneumothorax, active TB, recent haemoptysis, bronchial carcinoma, emphysematous bullae, bronchopulmonary fistula, recent bronchopulmonary surgery and severe hypotension.

Neurophysiological Facilitation of Respiration (NFR)

These techniques facilitate increased ventilation in patients otherwise unable to co-operate with treatment. The effects are particularly striking in patients with reduced conscious levels. There are no definitive physiological explanations for all the responses observed which include increased depth of inspiration, decreased respiratory rate and stimulation of cough.[7]

There are six techniques which are commonly used, all of which employ externally applied proprioceptive and cutaneous stimuli.

Suction in Non-intubated Patients

Nasopharyngeal and oral suction is traumatic and potentially dangerous and should only be used after careful assessment and if secretions cannot be cleared by less invasive methods.

The most effective and least traumatic catheters are those with more than one side eye (preferably 4), the total surface area of which are less than the distal hole. The diameter of the catheter should be the smallest possible which is also effective, usually FG 10-12 in adults. Coudé tip or angled end catheters are thought to favour selective entry into the left main bronchus which may be useful in treating left lung pathology. Suction pressure should not exceed 160mmHg but it is widely accepted that a pressure of greater than 80mmHg is required to achieve a therapeutic effect. An asceptic technique must always be observed and pre and post oxygenation is usually indicated in order to minimise desaturation. Excessive secretions that require regular suctioning may be more appropriately managed with a mini-tracheostomy or intubation.

Contra-indications include tracheo-oesophageal fistula, recent pneumonectomy or oesophageal surgery, bronchial or high oesophageal tumour, severe bronchospasm or stridor. The technique should be used with some caution where there is nasal pathology, a history of recent pulmonary oedema or bleeding diathesis and recent head injury or brain surgery.

Passive Movements

Passive movements to the joints combined with muscle stretches ease the pain and stiffness of immobility. Gentle movement also encourages circulation and, in conjunction with regular position change, helps prevent bedsores.

Passive movements are indicated in patients who suffer mobility problems due to end-stage disease, neuro-muscular disease, chronic breathlessness or in unconscious or sedated patients. They should be used with caution in patients with friable skin, osteoporosis, musculoskeletal injuries and bony metastases.

Massage

Massage is useful to promote relaxation and decrease anxiety. The techniques are modified to accommodate the patient's disability and position. It is particularly useful in patient's with acute, controlled and chronic breathlessness, and in end stage respiratory disease.

Lymphoedema bandaging

Lymphoedema is both distressing and painful. Physiotherapy, although not a cure, can be useful in alleviating symptoms associated with the gross swelling. Treatment involves massage and the application of compression garments.

Thoracic Mobilization

The majority of patients with chronic airflow limitation present with varying degrees of immobility in the cervical and thoracic spine. This has been demonstrated even in young children and patients who are otherwise reasonably fit and active. Reduced range of movement in the spine leads to shortening of the ligaments, tendons, intercostal muscles and contraction of joint capsules etc. Any slight movement causes pain which further restricts mobility.

A variety of manual techniques can be applied to mobilise and manipulate joints of the cervical and thoracic spine through full passive and accessory ranges of movement. Research has demonstrated that lung function, thoracic spine mobility and rib movement will all improve even after one session but in order for this to be sustained, regular treatment is necessary.

The technique is contraindicated in patients with bony metastases, severe osteoporosis, rheumatoid and juvenile arthritis and prolapsed intervertebral disc.

Exercise

Exercise has many benefits including improved endurance, increased efficiency and strength of muscles, improved joint suppleness, increased respiratory rate, tidal volume and minute ventilation, as well as improved general fitness. It will also aid mobilisation of secretions in the chest. Physiotherapy treatment plans will incorporate an exercise regime which will be tailored to the individual patient. It is important to remember that in many cases the patients will be limited by their ventilatory rather than cardio-vascular capacity.

Exercise testing in the clinical setting

Exercise tolerance tests may be a more appropriate way of assessing the functional ability of a patient than lung function testing.

Two tests are commonly used.

The Shuttle Walking Test is an externally paced incremental test which correlates very well with maximum oxygen uptake.

The Six Minute Walking Distance (6MWD) permits rests when necessary providing the patient continues to perform maximally. At least three practice walks are required to ensure reproducibility.

The shuttle walking test is the preferred method in most research studies because it is less open to learning effects.

Pain Relief

Transcutaneous electrical nerve stimulation (TENS)

The TENS machine is a small portable device which uses 2–4 small electrodes which can be placed over the site of pain, over corresponding acupuncture points or over the relevant nerve trunk and dermatome. The analgesic effect is thought to be produced by saturating the pain-gate mechanism or possibly by releasing endorphins.[8]

The technique is particularly useful in rib fractures, post thoracotomy pain and other causes of chest wall pain. The machine should not be used on the thorax if the patient has a pace-maker and it should not be placed over the carotid sinus. It should be used with caution in patients with myocardial disease or pregnant women.

Entonox

Entonox is useful for post-operative pain, in palliative care and in chest trauma. It should not be used in cases of pneumothorax, lung abscess or large bullae and can cause nausea. Patients with type II respiratory failure may also be made worse by entonox even though it's duration of analgesic action is only 1–2 minutes.

Acupuncture/Shiatsu

This can be helpful in the management of pain but requires specialist training.

Specific Treatment and Rehabilitation

Chronic Hyperventilation Syndrome (CHVS)

Hyperventilation is a normal response to certain stimuli and is only a problem if it becomes habitual.

Patients with CHVS are not usually aware of the developing problem as symptoms can begin insidiously.

An altered breathing pattern can cause chronic hypocapnia to which the body adapts and finally accepts as normal, so that even a minute drop in $PaCO_2$ can cause the catastrophic symptoms experienced by some patients. These include headaches, visual impairment, G-I tract disturbances, chest pain, musculoskeletal problems, paraesthesia in upper limbs and face, rapid respiratory rate and associated bronchospasm, frequent sighing and gasping etc. A common comment is 'I can't get enough air into my chest'.

Patients are often frightened that their symptoms are indicative of a heart attack or cancer and the ensuing anxiety can compound the problems. They undergo numerous investigations, all of which are negative and often leads the patient and/or doctor to believe that their problems are psychological.

In addition to investigating the presenting signs and symptoms, all organic causes of disease that could result in hypocapnia must be ruled out eg, anaemia, pneumonia, depression, alcoholism. Once a diagnosis of CHVS has been established, referral should be made to a respiratory physiotherapist.

Physiotherapy assessment

This must include a detailed history which will often highlight a trigger point ie traumatic event or illness.

Frequency and severity of all signs and symptoms should be documented. A simple tool for this is the Nijmegen questionnaire[5] which has a tick box formula and if the scores exceed 23/64, a positive diagnosis of CHVS can be made.

Objective data is also important: $PaCO_2$, Sat O_2 (not usually a problem but perceived to be by the patient), respiratory rate and breathing pattern. The latter is not usually presented as an obvious panting or over-breathing but is more likely to be an abnormal pattern showing little or no diaphragmatic excursion but use of the upper chest and accessory muscles.

Treatment

This must begin with a simplified explanation of respiratory alkalosis leading to the symptoms that the patient is experiencing. Treatment is a gradual re-education of breathing pattern which can take up to a year to complete. Initially the patient is seen 2–3 times a week and additional practice of correct breathing control at home is essential until it becomes an automatic response.

The patient usually reports that breathing feels unnatural and uncomfortable at first but with perseverance can master the art.

Because CHVS is a vicious cycle, the patients are often deconditioned and unfit. Therefore, once a good breathing pattern has been established they are usually keen to commence an exercise training programme.

Vocal Cord Dysfunction (VCD)

Patients with VCD may be referred for physiotherapy either in conjunction with speech therapy for re-education of breathing pattern or because they demonstrate associated chronic hyperventilation syndrome (CHVS).

The connection between VCD and CHVS is not well documented but may be due to the fact that similar personalities are

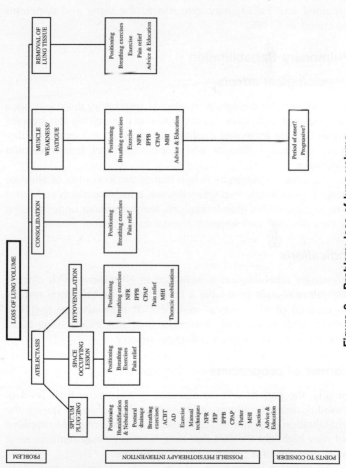

Figure 3. Problem: loss of lung volume

susceptible to both conditions i.e. those with depression, anxiety, psychological problems and perfectionists.

Secondly, it has been demonstrated that in people with VCD, a larger volume of air is expended during speech than is normal.[1] As this condition is likely to persist on a long-term basis, the sustained low $PaCO_2$ may give rise to the signs and symptoms described in CHVS.

Pulmonary Rehabilitation

Physiological effects

Rehabilitation for patients with chronic respiratory disease is not a new concept and there is much research extolling the benefits which include increased quality of life, improved exercise tolerance, decreased anxiety and depression and fewer hospital admissions.

The aims of Pulmonary Rehabilitation are to control or alleviate symptoms of chronic respiratory disease, educate patients and carers how to cope within their limitations, teach a greater understanding of their disease[6] and improve mental and physical fitness.

Indications

Pulmonary rehabilitation is indicated in all patients with chronic respiratory disease who have a limited exercise tolerance and are on optimal pharmaceutical treatment. It may also be useful in patients both before and after major lung surgery e.g. lung transplantation or lung volume reduction surgery.

Format of programme

Initially, the patient will be assessed to determine their level of disability, main problems, and goals to be achieved during the rehabilitation programme. Lung function is not expected to improve but may highlight the fact that lung function measurements are a poor indicator of a patient's physical ability.

An exercise programme which combines aerobic-endurance and strength resistance components is devised for each patient. Intensity can be calculated as a percentage of maximum exercise tolerance test performed, and work rate related to a perceived exertion score such as the Borg scale. A level walking programme

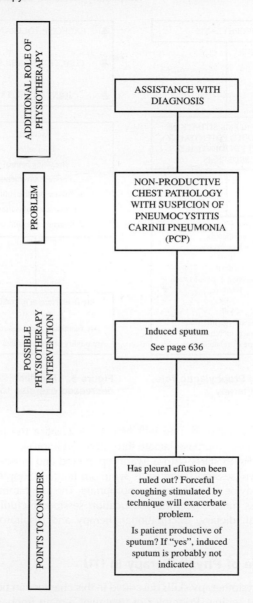

ASSISTANCE WITH
DIAGNOSIS

NON-PRODUCTIVE
CHEST PATHOLOGY
WITH SUSPICION OF
PNEUMOCYSTITIS
CARINII PNEUMONIA
(PCP)

Induced sputum
See page 636

Has pleural effusion been
ruled out? Forceful
coughing stimulated by
technique will exacerbate
problem.

Is patient productive of
sputum? If "yes", induced
sputum is probably not
indicated

ADDITIONAL ROLE OF
PHYSIOTHERAPY

PROBLEM

POSSIBLE
PHYSIOTHERAPY
INTERVENTION

POINTS TO CONSIDER

Figure 4. Assistance with diagnosis

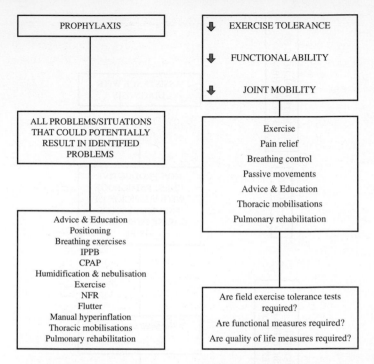

**Figure 5. Prophylactic role
of physiotherapy**

**Figure 6. Problem:
decreased exercise tolerance**

at sub-maximal work-rate will help to desensitise the patient to breathlessness, increase lactate threshold and improve endurance.

The session starts with a 'warm up' period and finishes with a 'cool down' session. Exercise is symptom limited. Supplementary oxygen may be administered if appropriate. The programme should encompass multi-disciplinary education sessions including pharmaceutical, dietary, occupational therapy and respiratory nurse input.

The Role of Physiotherapy in ITU

All the physiotherapy skills described in this chapter can be applied in the ITU setting. Principles of treatment remain unchanged but due to the severity of the condition and multiple problems, techniques need to be modified accordingly.

Terminal Care/End Stage Disease

The aims of treatment in the terminal care setting are to maintain patient dignity and comfort, ease the distress of breathlessness or excessive secretions and relieve or prevent pain. This will involve many physiotherapy techniques.

Sputum Induction for Diagnosis of Pneumocystis Carinii Pneumonia (PCP)

This may assist with diagnosis of PCP in the immuno-compromised host and is less invasive than broncho-alveolar lavage.

The technique may also be useful to detect eosinophils in sputum.

Technique

- The patient should, ideally, fast overnight to avoid food contamination of the specimen
- 30mls hypertonic saline (3%), to be nebulised via an ultrasonic nebuliser, needs to be prescribed
- the laboratory needs to be informed when to expect specimen as immediate investigation is necessary

The procedure MUST be performed in a well ventilated, single room as the nebulisation and coughing can cause spread of other infections.

The physiotherapist MUST take all necessary infection control precautions and follow strict protocol for induction of sputum – refer to local policy.

Side effects may include bronchospasm, breathlessness, oxygen desaturation and nausea. Bronchospasm may be decreased by delivering a nebulised bronchodilator prior to the procedure. Secretions obtained should be clear and non-purulent. The sample must be clearly labelled 'Biohazard' and sent to the laboratory immediately.

The absolute contra-indication is pleural effusion.

Conclusion

Physiotherapy is an integral part of the management of patients presenting with respiratory problems. In order for treatment to be optimised, referral needs to be appropriate and immediate. Over the past few decades Respiratory Physiotherapy has tried to dispel the traditional image of 'tip, tap and cough', and has developed into a highly specialised field which offers a wide range of modalities to both aid the recovery of patients with respiratory problems and prevent problems occurring in high risk patients.

The aim of physiotherapy is to rehabilitate the patient to the highest possible level of function within the limits of their disease or situation.

Physiotherapy intervention consists of a detailed assessment of the patient, analysis of the findings, short and long-term objective setting, plan of appropriate treatment, evaluation of intervention and ongoing assessment of the patient with modification of treatment if necessary.

It is essential that medical staff and physiotherapists communicate well and work together for the benefit of the patient.

Acknowledgements

I would like to thank the following people for their invaluable help in writing this chapter: Julia Bott, Julie Reeves, Alison Maddigan, Tim Harrison and Simon Range.

References

1. Sapienza CM, Stathopoulos T, Brown WS Jr. Speech breathing during reading in women with vocal nodules. *J of Voice* 1997; **11**(2):195–201

2. Falk M, Kelstrup M, Andersen JB et al. Improving the ketchup bottle method with positive expiratory pressure, PEP in cystic fibrosis. *Europ J of Respir Dis* 1984;**65**:423–432

3. Singh S, Morgan MDL, Scott S et al. The development of the Shuttle Walking Test of disability in patients with chronic airways obstruction. *Thorax* 1992;**47**:1019–1024

4. Webber BA, Pryor JA. The Active Cycle of Breathing Techniques. In: Webber BA, Pryor JA, eds. Physiotherapy for Respiratory and Cardiac Problems, pp 116–122. Churchill Livingstone 1993

5. Vansteenkiste J, Rochette F, Demedts M et al. Diagnostic tests of hyperventilation syndrome. *Eur Resp J* 1991;**4**:393–399

6. American Thoracic Society. Official Statement on Pulmonary Rehabilitation. *Am Rev Res Dis* 1981;**124**:663–66

7. Bethune DD. Neurophysiological facilitation of respiration. In: JA Pryor, ed. Respiratory Care, pp 121–45. Edinburgh: Churchill Livingstone 1991

8. Melzack R, Wall PD. Pain mechanisms: a new theory. *Science* 1965;**150**:971–978

28

Flying, Diving and Climbing

Kevin Peter McKinlay

Introduction

Patients with respiratory disorders may ask for advice on flying, diving or climbing in the following circumstances:

- to undertake commercial air travel for holiday or business
- to participate in sports diving or recreational climbing
- for occupational reasons, either to apply for or to continue employment in the aviation or professional diving fields

This chapter will deal with the physiological effects of both flying and diving as they relate to the commercial air traveller, the professional aviator, the sports diver and professional divers. Advice on climbing will also be covered. The decision as to whether an individual with respiratory disease is fit or otherwise to undertake such activities is based on a combination of factors:

- the correct diagnosis of the underlying problem
- an accurate clinical assessment of the condition and any co-morbidity
- an understanding of the activity the individual wishes to pursue, including the physiology and pathophysiology
- objective measurement of pulmonary function testing, chest radiology and arterial blood gas analysis as appropriate
- an accurate risk assessment based on points above

Commercial Air Travel

Flight in a commercial airliner imposes a number of stresses on an individual with respiratory disease:

- the aircraft cabin is pressurised to produce a cabin altitude between 5000 and 8000 feet whist the aircraft attains a cruising altitude between 30 000 and 40 000 feet. At a cabin altitude of 8000 feet the inspired oxygen concentration is 15%
- the cabin air is recirculated leading to a small rise in the partial pressure of inspired carbon dioxide. In addition, there is exposure to aero-allergens and inhalation of airborne pathogens. Dependent upon the duration of the flight there may be a total air exchange from outside which will lessen these exposures
- the cabin humidity is low leading to increased insensible fluid losses and a consequent risk of venous thrombo-embolism, especially when combined with long periods of immobility. This may compound underlying problems such as secondary polycythaemia or the increased thrombotic risk associated with bronchial carcinoma
- the ambient air pressure at altitude is reduced. Thus in accordance with Boyle's Law (pressure × volume = constant) any air within a non-communicating intra-thoracic cavity will expand in volume. At 8000 feet any air under such conditions will expand by a further 30% from its ground level volume. This heightens the risk of pneumothorax or pneumo-mediastinum in individuals with intra-thoracic trapped air, especially those with bullae, those who have undergone recent thoracic surgery and those with a recent history of pneumothorax. As a general rule, it is advisable that patients should not fly for a minimum of six weeks post thoracic surgery, including thoracoscopic procedures, and after a pneumothorax. Radiological assessment to identify bullae where suspected should be undertaken combined with body box measurements of static lung volumes. There are no strict rules on what level of residual volume can be regarded as hazardous and where there is bullous lung disease a clinical judgement needs to be made based on the PaO_2, degree of airflow obstruction, residual volume and the residual volume/total lung capacity ratio. Those with severe airflow obstruction ($FEV_1 < 50\%$ predicted) and an increased residual volume of >130% predicted are probably those most at risk.

Hypoxia and Fitness to Fly Testing

An individual with a normal PaO_2 at sea level of 12 kPa will, at a cabin altitude of 8000 ft, have a PaO_2 of 8 kPa. At this level the individual will function normally but there will be impairment in the ability to learn new tasks. Consequently, if the patient is hypoxic at sea level then this will worsen at altitude. Thus those respiratory patients with a lowered PaO_2 will need careful assessment before air travel. In general a $PaO_2 < 9.5$kPa or an inability to walk further than 50m on the flat would indicate the need for assessment. This is best done by the use of a fitness to fly test, also known as a High Altitude Simulation Test (HAST):

1. Measure arterial blood gases on room air
2. Administer 15%O_2 to the subject through a venturi mask for 30 minutes with monitoring of pulse oximetry
3. Recheck arterial blood gases at 30 minutes on 15%O_2

If the PaO_2 on $F_1O_2 = 0.15$ is less than 8kPa then supplemental oxygen will be required during flight.

Commercial airlines will provide supplemental oxygen during flight. It is necessary to order this at the time of booking and the decision to allow air travel in such circumstances lies with the airline's medical advisor. Some airlines charge for this service whilst others provide it free.

Professional Air Travel

You may be asked to advise individuals who wish to become civilian or military aircrew with a history of, or current, respiratory disease. Medical assessment of such individuals is usually made by either the Civil Aviation Authority or by the Defence Medical Services for military recruits. These organisations have strict rules and guidelines. It is of paramount importance when dealing with these individuals that the diagnosis is correct and that any medication justified. This becomes even more important if you see trained aircrew who may lose their careers if they develop chronic respiratory illness.

Military aircrew work within a hazardous environment. As one ascends to altitudes above 10000 ft, one encounters problems of hypoxia, reduced ambient pressure and reduced temperature compounded by the effects of positive acceleration (+Gz) forces. Respiratory physiology is stretched to the limit and any impairment may lead to significant problems. For example, an individual with a history of childhood or current asthma will not be allowed to undertake pilot training. A trained pilot who develops asthma may, under certain circumstances, be allowed to continue flying duties if asymptomatic and well controlled at step 2 of the BTS guidelines. Pilots who develop sarcoidosis are permanently disqualified, independent of the stage of respiratory disease, because of the perceived risk of cardiac involvement. A pilot who suffers a single spontaneous pneumothorax will need to undergo pleurectomy before resuming flying duties because of the increased risk of subsequent pneumothoraces in flight (up to a 30% increased risk of a second pneumothorax within 18 months). Candidates for military aircrew with a history of pneumothorax are expected to undergo open pleurectomy before taking up flying training. These examples highlight some of the management problems and the appropriate professional medical bodies should be advised in such circumstances.

Diving: Physiological Problems

The respiratory problems associated with diving relate to the adverse environment as water has a greater density than air and is virtually incompressible. The ambient pressure rises linearly with depth, at nearly 1 atmosphere for every 10 metres descent. Therefore at a depth of 10 metres the external ambient pressure is 2 atmospheres. Immersion in water causes a redistribution of circulating blood volume and there is an increase in circulating volume leading to a diuresis, which reduces the intrathoracic blood volume. When the individual gets out of the water he may become hypovolaemic due to the redistribution of blood volume. To descend to depth, a diver will breath-hold. Owing to the rise of pressure with depth, the intra-thoracic gas volume is reduced (Boyle's Law). When the diver ascends again, the gas will re-expand to its original volume. If the diver is using an air source at depth, he may increase the volume of intrathoracic gas to such an extent that, when he resurfaces, this volume may expand sufficiently to cause rupture (barotrauma) unless this air is vented. The bursting pressure of the lung is 75mmHg (1 metre sea water). Intrapulmonary rupture leads to either mediastinal emphysema or a pneumothorax. This increases the risk of air entering the circulation leading to air embolism. Other physiological problems associated with both sports and professional diving include nitrogen narcosis, decompression sickness and oxygen toxicity. Other problems facing professional divers relate to the greater depth encountered and preventing damage from exposure to very low temperatures.

Sport Diving

You may be asked to advise on fitness for diving, usually SCUBA (Self Contained Underwater Breathing Apparatus). Individuals wishing to undertake scuba diving have to undergo an assessment by a doctor recognised by the British diving authorities. The equipment worn by scuba divers has a demand regulator and provides about one hour of gas. Problems relate to the increased ambient pressure as detailed above. Patients with airflow obstruction are at increased risk of pulmonary barotrauma and in general patients with asthma are advised not to dive. Similarly those with bullous lung disease, a history of pneumothorax or recent thoracic surgery should not dive. Diving should be avoided in the twenty four hours before flying owing to an increased risk of decompression sickness.

Professional Divers

Professional divers work in hazardous environments in a physically demanding role. In the UK they undergo mandatory annual medical examinations by recognised doctors. Most chronic respiratory conditions are disqualifying. As with professional aircrew advice should be sought from the recognised authorities.

Climbing

Patients who wish to undertake recreational climbing face similar problems with altitude as discussed above. Climbing requires a high degree of physical fitness. Patients with respiratory disease are likely to encounter problems related to the lower ambient oxygen concentration experienced at altitude. At 2000m the pO_2 for a healthy individual will fall to 7.3kPa. Those with impaired oxygenation will experience problems at lower altitudes. The main risk is from acute mountain sickness with the individual experiencing headache and vomiting. This may lead to high altitude pulmonary oedema or high altitude cerebral oedema. Other risks include acute myocardial infarction, pulmonary venous thrombo-embolism and retinal haemorrhage. Those considered at risk include patients with diseases limiting ventilation (kyphoscoliosis, alveolar hypoventilation), pulmonary fibrosis, heart failure and anaemia. Thus assessment of cardio-respiratory fitness is essential in these patients with lung function tests, chest radiography, electrocardiography and an exercise test.

Further Reading

Ernsting J, Nicholson AN, Rainford DJ (eds). Aviation Medicine, 3rd edition. Butterworth Heinemann 1999

Weatherall DJ, Ledingham JGG, Warrell DA. Oxford Textbook of Medicine, 3rd edition. Aerospace Medicine Section 8.5.5(e), p 1193–1204

Diving Medicine, Section 8.5.5(f), p 1204–1210

Diseases of high terrestrial altitudes, 8.5.5 (d), p 1185–1193

Denison DM. Respiratory Problems in Adverse Environments. In: Brewis RAL, Corrin B, Geddes DM, Gibson GJ (eds). Respiratory Medicine, 2nd edition. WB Saunders Co Ltd 1995

29

Palliative Care

Andrew Wilcock

It is the right of every patient to receive palliative care: It is the responsibility of every doctor to provide it. A medical review based on open sensitive communication with all concerned will help to identify the physical and also the psychological, social or spiritual needs of the patient and their carers. This will allow support to be offered by the appropriate member(s) of the multidisciplinary team. Achieving the best possible quality of life in the circumstances is the focus of this holistic approach.

Introduction and definitions

Palliative care is the oldest form of health care. Despite recent advances, for the majority of patients with cancer and other chronic life-threatening diseases treatment is palliative rather than curative. All health care professionals have a responsiblitiy to provide good palliative care for their patients (whatever their diagnosis) by applying the palliative care approach (Box 1).

- **to successfully support a patient and their carers from the time of diagnosis through to death and in their bereavement can be a most rewarding professional and personal experience.**

Specialist Palliative Care Services (Box 2) act as a resource in order to help you to achieve this or to take a greater role in the care of the patient when distressing symptoms and other complex needs

Box 1

The *palliative care approach* is based upon palliative care principles:

- the focus is on quality of life which includes good symptom control
- there is a whole-person approach (i.e. the physical, psychological, social and spiritual needs)
- the care encompasses both the patient and those who matter to them
- there is respect for patients' autonomy and choice
- the emphasis is on open and sensitive communication between patients, informal carers and professional colleagues.

Box 2

Specialist Palliative Care is the active total care of patients with progressive, advanced disease and limited prognosis and their families by a multiprofessional team (e.g. doctor, nurse, social worker, chaplain, physiotherapist, occupational therapist, pharmacist etc.) who have undergone recognised specialist palliative care training. It is provided directly in a variety of settings — inpatient, outpatient, day care or home care and indirectly by the giving of advice (e.g. by hospital and community Macmillan nurses/support teams)

are not readily being relieved/met or when such difficulties are anticipated. The full range of specialist services are usually only available to patients with cancer but check this with your local service.

Palliative care is not synonymous with terminal care. This relates to the care of the patient during their last few days or weeks of life when it is clear that they have entered a phase of progressive decline.

The importance of a whole-person approach is illustrated by the mix of physical and emotional symptoms reported by patients with lung cancer at presentation (Box 3).

> ### Box 3. Common symptoms in patients with lung cancer at presentation
>
> - tiredness
> - lack of energy
> - shortness of breath
> - cough
> - worrying
> - lack of appetite
> - difficulty sleeping
> - anxious feelings
> - chest pain

Open and sensitive communication together with effective team working are the main components of the whole-person approach:

- **professionals generally underestimate what a patient already knows**
- **find out what the patient knows and what they want to know — most will want further information and the opportunity to ask questions**
- **continually check that the information is being given in a way that is understood**
- **use open questions to enable the patient to lead the conversation**
- **try to elicit the patients feelings and concerns**
- **never lie to a patient. Tell the truth gently. e.g. not "things are getting worse" but "things don't seem to be so good this week"**
- **be confident in using silence, in exploring and allowing the expression of emotions and to say "I don't know"**
- **document important information shared with the patient or carers in the patients notes and inform other relevant professionals within the hospital and community**
- **remember you cannot be all things to every patient. Recognise the contribution that other members of the multiprofessional team can make and involve them as appropriate in the care of the patient**
- **acknowledge that caring for patients can have an emotional cost for health care professionals. Using a team approach helps support the patient and the professional.**

Psychological support

The aim is to help the patient (and carers) to adjust to the situation in the best way possible for them. This often involves coming to terms with a series of losses which is associated with emotional responses such as:

- **shock**
- **numbness**
- **denial**
- **anger**
- **anxiety**
- **guilt**
- **grief**
- **resignation or acceptance**

Good communication skills will help the patient and carers to identify and vent their feelings. This may open the way for other important issues to be discussed with professionals, partners or family. Help them to identify areas of support and useful coping strategies. Be on the look out for marked anxiety or depression that may need specific treatment.

Spiritual needs are human needs and common to us all. A religious belief is one way of helping to address such needs. Whilst the provision of spiritual care is often seen as the responsibility of the clergy, all professionals (being human!) can help with spiritual issues which commonly revolve around relationships (the need to love and be loved/cared for) and the meaning and purpose of life.

Symptom control

- **the essential first step in symptom control is to identify the cause. The most effective palliation is usually obtained by directly treating or modifying the effects of the underlying disease process.** (Box 4)

When this is no longer possible or becomes inappropriate other methods can be tried although evidence supporting their use can be limited. This chapter deals primarily with these other methods of symptom control in patients with cancer although some approaches are applicable to patients with other chronic lung diseases (e.g. the relief of terminal breathlessness).

Box 4.   General strategy for symptom control

It is useful to consider the following questions:

- what is the cause of the symptom?
  Whilst this is often the cancer do not automatically assume this. The history, clinical examination together with appropriate investigations may identify non-cancer related cause(s) for which treatment should be given or existing therapies maximised. Seek the advice of colleagues if there is any doubt as to the best current treatment

- can the cancer be modified?
  This may include radiotherapy (including brachytherapy), chemotherapy, hormone therapy, immunotherapy, surgery, cryotherapy or LASER therapy. Obtain advice from your local oncology team

- can the effects the cancer produces be modified?
  This includes for example the use of corticosteroids, drainage of pleural/pericardial effusions or ascities and the insertion of endobronchial or superior vena cava stents

- have I explained the situation to the patient?
  Explanation of the cause of the symptom, its meaning and what can be done about it in terms the patient understands is an important part of symptom control. The fear of the known is usually less than the fear of the unknown. Encourage questions

Breathlessness (dyspnoea)

- **'an unpleasant or uncomfortable awareness of breathing or need to breathe.' The overall experience includes the perception of difficult breathing and the physical, emotional and behavioural response to it.**

In disease, breathlessness on exercise may be a result of disturbance in the circulatory system or the respiratory system; this may be insufficient ventilatory capacity or increased ventilatory drive on exertion or both. For the patient it is the sensation of breathlessness (and/or fatigue) which ultimately limits their ability to exercise.

Breathlessness appears related to the degree of reflex stimulation of brainstem structures concerned with the automatic control of breathing. Higher centres that impinge upon the brainstem centre appear important possibly explaining why the threshold and tolerance to breathlessness appears to vary between individuals; why exercise tolerance is reduced by low mood or anxiety and increased by encouragement; and how breathlessness can occur in several psychiatric disorders in patients who are otherwise healthy.

• **it is vital to appreciate that in addition to the physical consequences, breathlessness can impact upon the patients psychological, social and spiritual well-being which in turn may modify their perception and response to breathlessness**

Chronic breathlessness is common in patients with respiratory disease. In the UK an estimated 750 000 patients with COPD are breathless when walking on the flat and breathlessness is likely to have been present in the 25 000 patients who die from COPD each year in England and Wales.

Breathlessness occurs in 70% of patients with cancer in the last six weeks of life. It is more likely in patients with primary or secondary lung cancer, pleural disease and pre-existing cardiopulmonary disease although in some patients generalised muscle weakness resulting from cancer cachexia may be the only apparent factor.

The prevalence and severity of breathlessness increases as death approaches with 25% describing their breathlessness as 'severe' or 'horrible' in the last week of life. Breathlessness is an independent predictor of survival second only to performance status.

Aetiology

The commoner causes of breathlessness in patients with cancer are listed in Table 1.

Management

Consider the general strategy for symptom control (Box 4). Breathlessness is difficult to treat and so it is vital to identify any of causes that may be partially or fully reversible. For example, a study of patients with lung cancer attending a chest clinic found that half had airflow obstruction which was associated with more severe breathlessness. Of these, only 14% were taking bronchodilator therapy. A trial of bronchodilator therapy improved breathlessness in 60% of the previously untreated patients.

Table 1. Causes of breathlessness in patients with cancer

Cancer related

 primary and secondary lung cancer causing:
  airway obstruction (+/– collapse), mass effect, lung infiltration,
  tumour emboli, lymphangitis carcinomatosis
 generalised weakness
  loss of 'fitness', respiratory muscle weakness
 pleural effusion
 superior vena cava obstruction
 pericardial effusion
 phrenic nerve palsy
 splinting of the diaphragm
  ascites, hepatomegaly
 chest wall infiltration
 chest wall pain
 anaemia
  of chronic disease, due to marrow infiltration

Treatment related

 cancer treatments
 surgery
  lobectomy, pneumonectomy
 radiotherapy (usually with higher doses)
  pneumonitis leading to fibrosis
 chemotherapy
  e.g. methotrexate — pneumonitis; cyclophosphamide — fibrosis
 non-cancer treatments
 drugs precipitating fluid retention or bronchospasm

Other causes

 psychological factors
  e.g. anxiety, fear, anger, frustration, isolation, depression
 infection
  bacterial, viral, fungal
 chronic respiratory disease
  e.g. COPD, asthma
 chronic cardiac disease
  e.g. ischaemic heart disease, congestive cardiac failure
 pulmonary oedema
 pneumothorax
 pulmonary embolism
 cardiac arrhythmia

A full assessment of the breathless patient involves the consideration of the following:

- **exploration of the patients and carers understanding about breathlessness and the emotions it produces**

It is a common belief that the heart or lungs are being further damaged by becoming breathless and many fear that they might die suddenly during an episode of breathlessness. Activities are subsequently curtailed or avoided and many become socially isolated. It is important to stress that becoming breathless in itself is not dangerous and to encourage patients to remain as active as possible. Patients with lung cancer describe emotions such as anger, helplessness, depression, loss of strength, agitation, anxiety, fear of suffocating and nervousness during episodes of breathlessness. In patients with COPD and cancer, increasingly severe breathlessness is accompanied by higher levels of anxiety and depression; addressing this may lead to an improvement in breathlessness.

- **identify symptoms suggestive of hyperventilation** (Box 5)

Box 5.   Symptoms suggestive of hyperventilation

- poor relationship of breathlessness to exertion
- presence of episodic breathlessness
- breathlessness at rest
- rapid fluctuations in breathlessness within minutes
- fear of sudden death during an attack
- breathlessness varying with social situations

Hyperventilation is a common accompaniment in patients with breathlessness 'disproportionate' to the severity of their pulmonary disease. Explanation of the cause of the symptoms is the most effective treatment and allows the introduction of breathing control/relaxation exercises that aim to give the patient a greater understanding and feeling of control over their breathing. Underlying anxiety or depression requiring specific treatment should be excluded.

- **consider the practical implications of being breathlessness for the patient**

The impact of breathlessness on the patient can be observed by asking the patient to carry out a set task. This may reveal hyperventilation which can be highlighted to the patient. Alternatively, beneficial coping strategies that the patient uses can be reinforced. It also provides a baseline against which to monitor progress. The home situation, the use of practical aids, the presence of carers (family, friends or professional) and other sources of support should be identified.

Treatment strategy

It is useful to consider the treatment of breathlessness in three clinical settings that relate to the prognosis of the patient:

* breathlessness on exertion (months to years). This is a normal 'physiological' experience. It becomes pathological when it limits a patient's activities, their degree of independence or is associated with disabling anxiety
* breathlessness at rest (weeks to months)
* terminal breathlessness (last days of life). Distressing breathlessness in the last days of life can almost always be relieved.
  The approach can be divided into:
* non-pharmacological and
* pharmacological (the use of drugs to specifically reduce the sensation of breathlessness)

Both approaches are important but the relative value of their contribution varies according to the patients prognosis e.g. non-pharmacological methods are more useful than pharmacological ones in patients breathless on exertion; the converse is true for patients in the terminal phase (Figure 1).

Non-pharmacological approaches

The non-pharmacological approach requires the input of the whole multidisciplinary team in what is the palliative care equivalent of pulmonary rehabilitation. The approach includes exploring the patient's experience and understanding of their breathlessness in the context of their disease and prognosis; maximising their function; maximising their feeling of control over their breathlessness and addressing any feelings of personal or social isolation (Table 2).

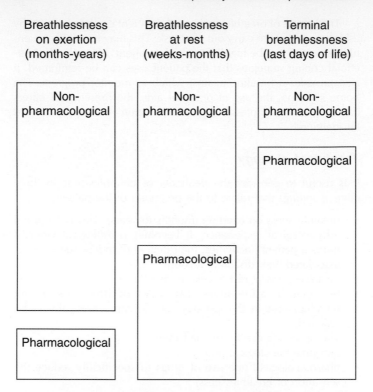

| Breathlessness on exertion (months-years) | Breathlessness at rest (weeks-months) | Terminal breathlessness (last days of life) |

Figure 1. The relative contributions of pharmacological and non-pharmacological approaches for the management of breathlessness in patients with cancer according to the severity of the breathlessness and the patient's prognosis. N.B. episodes of hyperventilation (panic attacks) are most appropriately managed by a predominantly non-pharmacological approach.

Pharmacological approaches

Opioids, oxygen, benzodiazepines and phenothiazines have been recommended for the relief of breathlessness in patients with cancer.

Opioids

Opioids act centrally to diminish ventilatory drive stimulated by hypercapnia, hypoxia and exercise. Depression of ventilation

Table 2. Non-pharmacological management of breathlessness

Exploring the perception of the patient and carers

exploration of anxieties — e.g. fear of sudden death when breathless
explanation of symptoms and meaning
informing patient and carers that breathlessness in itself is not dangerous
what is/is not likely to happen — "you won't choke or suffocate to death"
help to come to terms with deteriorating condition
    help to cope with and adjust to 'losses' (of role, abilities etc)

Maximizing functional ability

encourage exertion to breathlessness
    increase tolerance to breathlessness
    maintain fitness
exercise advice
    assessment by physiotherapist
aids for daily living
    home assessment by occupational therapist
social sevice input / benefits advice
    social worker assessment

Maximizing the feeling of control over breathlessness

breathing control advice
relaxation techniques
plan of action for acute episodes
    simple written instructions — step by step plan
    increase confidence in coping with acute episodes
use of fan
use of complementary therapies
    beneficial for some patients

Reduce feelings of personal and social isolation

meet others in similar situation
attendance at a day centre
respite admissions
self help groups (e.g. British Lung Foundation — 'Breathe Easy')

occurs in a dose dependent manner largely by a reduction in tidal volume with a more variable reduction in respiratory rate making it a less reliable index of respiratory depression.

In patients with COPD:

- various opioids have been examined in different schedules and have been found to be effective and well tolerated, effective but poorly tolerated or ineffective and poorly tolerated
- the bulk of the evidence does not support a beneficial effect of nebulized opioids
- overall, they are not seen as a routine therapy in this group of patients.

In patients with cancer:

- opioids are recommended for the relief of breathlessness in patients with cancer and are widely used even though the small number of studies carried out in patients with cancer have given conflicting results
- opioids may help some (but not all) patients breathless on exertion. Side effects may be troublesome
- opioids appear to reduce breathlessness at rest. The duration of relief of breathlessness may be shorter than that for pain
- despite numerous anecdotal and uncontrolled reports of the effectiveness of nebulized opioids the only randomized double-blind placebo controlled trial did not support the use of nebulized morphine (5–50mg). The results also suggested that nebulized morphine was having a central rather than a local effect upon the lung that had been postulated. If this is the case then the nebulized route is an inefficient way of delivering morphine systemically
- much is unknown about the use of opioids for breathlessness and further research is required.

Use of morphine in the clinical setting

- for opioid naive patients use small doses initially (e.g. 2.5mg oral morphine q4–6h) and titrate the dose according to response and side effects
- for patients already receiving opioids, observe whether the patient gains benefit from an additional dose. If so increase the regular opioid as one would for pain in steps of 30–50%. If no improvement is obtained or side effects occur then reduce the dose

- in the authors experience a continuous subcutaneous infusion of opioid can be tolerated better and be more effective for some patients — possibly by avoiding the peaks (with side effects) and troughs (with loss of effect) of oral medication.

Oxygen

There is great variation between individuals in the response to oxygen which can not be predicted by the level of oxygen saturation at rest or the degree of desaturation on exercise. Due to the emotive aspects of oxygen therapy an improvement is sometimes considered a placebo effect although a flow of cooling air against the face or through the nose can reduce breathlessness by stimulating facial and nasal receptors of the trigeminal nerve.

In patients with COPD:

- supplemental oxygen has been shown to improve exercise tolerance and prolong life in patients with COPD who are severely hypoxic ($PaO_2 < 9$ kPa)
- the role of oxygen in less hypoxic patients has been more difficult to determine
  In patients with cancer:

- severely hypoxic patients (oxygen saturation <90%) benefit from oxygen compared to air
- in less hypoxic patients both oxygen (4 l/min) and air reduce breathlessness
- overall oxygen is probably under used in Palliative Care Units in the UK due to the reliance on opioids and other therapies, the desire to avoid the 'medicalization of death' and the practical difficulties of relying on cylinders (few if any hospices will have piped oxygen).

The use of oxygen in the clinical setting

- an electric fan to deliver a cool breeze on the face may be useful
- oxygen therapy should be available to severely hypoxic patients
- in those less hypoxic a trial of oxygen therapy can be given via nasal cannulae for an agreed period of time. If on review the patient has persisted in using the oxygen and has found it useful it can be continued. If the patient has any doubts to its efficacy then it should be discontinued

- oxygen can be delivered at home via cylinders or an oxygen concentrator. These are more convenient but can be limited by their maximal flow rate (4 l/min). If necessary tubing from two machines can be joined by a T-piece to deliver higher flow rates
- helium (80%) — oxygen (20%) mixtures are less dense and viscous than room air which helps to reduce the respiratory work required to overcome upper airway obstruction. It should be seen as a temporary measure whilst definitive therapy is being arranged.

Benzodiazepines, phenothiazines and other anxiolytics

The use of benzodiazepines in patients with pulmonary disease has required caution following reports of ventilatory depression although this has not been a universal finding.

In patients with COPD:

- benzodiazepines reduce breathlessnes by relieving coexistent anxiety; patients without psychiatric morbidity do not benefit

In patients with cancer:

- anecdotal benefit from benzodiazepines is reported but there have been no studies. In view of the findings in patients with COPD they should not routinely be prescribed as a treatment for breathlessness in patients without coexistent anxiety
- chlorpromazine is used by some for the relief of terminal breathlessness in patients with cancer
- buspirone is an anxiolytic acting predominantly via serotonin receptors (5-HT$_{1A}$) which is free of sedative or respiratory depressant effects and as effective as diazepam in the relief of anxiety. In some but not all patients with COPD buspirone improved anxiety levels, along with breathlessness and exercise tolerance. It may be a useful alternative to diazepam when sedation is troublesome or concern exists about the risk of ventilatory depression.

Use of anxiolytics in the clinical setting

- oral benzodiazepine of choice is diazepam initially 2–5mg t.i.d., reducing within several days (as levels of active metabolites rise) to a maintenance dose of 2–5mg at night

- sublingual lorazepam (0.5–2mg) with a rapid onset of action is often suggested for the management of an episode of acute breathlessness. Note however its long halflife (10–20 hours)
- parenteral benzodiazepine of choice is midazolam initially 10–30mg per 24 h by subcutaneous infusion. If the patient is agitated or confused midazolam should be combined with haloperidol or methotrimeprazine (levomepromazine).

Terminal breathlessness

Patients often fear suffocating to death and it is important that we are positive to the patient, their family and to colleagues about our ability to relieve terminal breathlessness:

- **no** patient should die with distressing breathlessness
- failure to control is a failure to utilise drug therapy **correctly**
- combination of an opioid with a sedative anxiolytic such as midazolam is effective (Box 6).

Box 6. Drugs used in the treatment of terminal breathlessness

Drug	Starting dose	Upper dose range	Route
diamorphine	10mg/24 hours (opioid naive)	Titrate according to symptoms	SC infusion
midazolam	10–30mg/ 24 hours	200–260mg/ 24 hours	SC infusion
chlorpromazine	12.5mg IV q4h 25mg PR b-t.i.d.	300–900mg/ 24 hours	IV rectal
methotrimeprazine (levomepromazine)	25–50mg/ 24 hours	200–300mg/ 24 hours	SC infusion

IV = intravenous, SC = subcutaneous, q4h = four hourly, b.i.d. = twelve hourly, t.i.d. = eight hourly

---

Usually, due to distress, inability to sleep and exhaustion patients (and their carers) accept that treatment to make them more comfortable may make them more drowsy. Sedation is not the primary aim of therapy (unless there is overwhelming distress) and some patients often become 'brighter' with improvement in their symptoms. However, as increasing drowsiness is usually a feature of their deteriorating condition it is important to explain clearly to the relatives the aims of treatment and the gravity of the situation. The evidence for such an approach is largely anecdotal although a continuous infusion of intravenous morphine in patients with cancer was found to relieve terminal breathlessness in the majority of patients.

Stridor

Upper airway compression should be considered when the patient complains of increasing breathlessness accompianied by a harsh inspiratory wheeze. Corticosteroids are usually given whilst urgently arranging definitive therapy e.g. radiotherapy, tracheobronchial stents. Helium and oxygen mixtures may help. Acute stridor occuring as a terminal event should be treated as for massive haemoptysis.

Death rattle

About 40% of dying patients develop noisy retained secretions (due to salivary, bronchial or refluxing gastric secretions). Usually, the patient is unconscious and the most important part of the management is to reassure those in attendence (relatives, friends and other

---

Box 7. Antimuscarinic drugs given subcutaneously for the relief of 'death rattle'.

Drug	Dose		Notes
	Stat	CSCI/24 hours	
hyoscine hydrobromide	0.4–0.6mg	1.2–2.4mg	sedative, occasionally triggers aggitation
hyoscine butylbromide	20mg	20–60mg	non-sedative
glycopyrollate	0.2–0.4mg	0.6mg	non-sedative

CSCI — continuous subcutaneous infusion

patients) that the patient is not distressed by the secretions. Even with a structured approach including changes in position, antimuscarinic drugs (Box 7) and suction the noise may only be relieved in 60% of patients. If a patient is conscious and distressed by retained secretions a combination of an opioid (to suppress an ineffective cough (if present)) and a sedative (e.g. midazolam) may be required.

Cough

Cough is a physiological reflex that clears the central airways of foreign material and secretions. It becomes pathological when excessive, ineffective or persistent when it disrupts sleep, rest, eating or social functioning. It may lead to muscular strain and discomfort, rib or vertebral fracture, syncope, headache or retinal haemorrhage. Cough occurs in 80% of patients with lung cancer.

Aetiology

The commonest cause of acute cough is respiratory tract infection. For causes of chronic cough in patients with cancer see Table 3.

Management

It is useful to divide cough into 'wet' or 'dry'. A wet cough serves a purpose and expectoration should be encouraged. Conversely, a dry cough serves no purpose and should be suppressed. A wet cough distressing a dying patient too weak to expectorate should also be suppressed (Figure 2).

Treatment of a wet cough

Avoid cough suppressants if possible:

- encourage the expectoration of mucus with the use of: physiotherapy, steam inhalations, nebulized normal saline (2.5ml, prior to physiotherapy or on demand)
- evidence does not support the routine use of expectorants (to increase the volume of secretions e.g. ipecacuanha) or mucolytics (to reduce the viscosity of secretions e.g. carbocisteine)
- selected patients may benefit from mucolytics and a therapeutic trial could be considered (e.g. carbocisteine 750mg t.i.d.) if all other approaches have failed.

Table 3. Causes of cough in patients with cancer

Cancer related

Primary or secondary cancer causing:
airway
infiltration
compression
distortion
obstruction, leading to collapse +/− infection
pulmonary infiltration
pleural infiltration
pericardial infiltration
tracheo-oesophageal fistula
mucus retention
ineffective cough due to:
generalised weakness
vocal cord palsy
pain on coughing

Treatment related

cancer treatments
pulmonary infiltration /fibrosis related to:
chemotherapy e.g. methotrexate, cyclophosphamide,
radiotherapy
non-cancer treatments
e.g. ACE inhibitors — increase cough reflex
beta-blockers — induce bronchoconstriction

Other causes

infection
'smoker's cough'
COPD
asthma
post-infection increased cough reflex
lung abscess
bronchiectasis
post nasal drip syndrome
due to: sinusitis, rhinitis
gastro-oesophageal reflux
pulmonary oedema
pulmonary infarction
recurrent aspiration

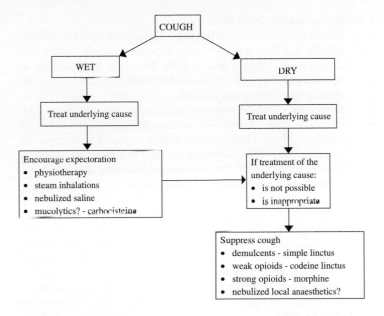

Figure 2. The treatment of cough

Treatment of a dry cough

- demulcents (first line)
  Contain soothing substances such as syrup or glycerol. The high sugar content stimulates the production of saliva and soothes the oropharynx. The associated swallowing may interfere with the cough reflex. The effect is short-lived and there is no evidence that compound preparations offer any advantage over simple linctus BP (5ml t-q.i.d.).
- weak opioids (second line)
  Opioids suppress the cough reflex centre in the brainstem. Codeine and dextromethorphan are common ingredients in compound cough preparations. Their effective dose is greater than the dose typically recommended by manufacturers of compound preparations. The benefit of compound preparations thus may reside mainly in the sugar content. The use of codeine linctus 5–10ml (15–30mg t-q.i.d.) is therefore recommended. If ineffective use a strong opioid. If a patient is already receiving a strong opioid it is nonsense to prescribe codeine as well.

- strong opioids (third line)

  Morphine solution can be used instead of codeine linctus, initially 2.5–5mg q.d.s. — q4h, or when codeine linctus fails to relieve, 5–10mg q.d.s. — q4h. The dose is titrated up as necessary or until unacceptable adverse effects occur. For patients already receiving strong opioids, if an 'as needed' dose relieves the cough, continue to use in this way or increase the regular morphine dose. If there is no benefit from a p.r.n. dose of morphine, there is little point in further regular dose increments. Some patients with cough but no pain benefit from a bedtime dose of morphine to prevent cough disturbing sleep

- nebulized local anaesthetics (fourth line)

  Nebulized local anaesthetics inhibit afferent nerve endings that trigger cough. They should only be considered when other avenues have failed; suggested doses are 2% lignocaine (5ml) or 0.25% bupivacaine (5ml) every 6 to 8 hours. Their use may be limited by their unpleasant taste, oropharyngeal numbness, risk of bronchoconstriction and their short 10–30 minute duration of action (although there are reports of single applications of nebulized lignocaine 400mg relieving cough for periods of one to eight weeks).

Cancer Pain

Pain is what the patient says hurts. Always believe the patient, remembering that patients in chronic severe pain often behave differently (i.e. may appear withdrawn and depressed) than those with acute pain. Cancer pain can be controlled in the majority of patients by:

- careful assessment of the cause (e.g. the cancer, its treatment, a concurrent disorder or debility) from the history, examination and appropriate investigations
- applying the general strategy (Box 4). For example, radiotherapy is the treatment of choice for painful bone metastases
- appreciating how psychosocial and spiritual concerns may influence pain
- use of appropriate pharmacological, non-pharmacological and other approaches tailored to the individual (Box 8)
- regular supervision
- seeking the advice of a specialist palliative care team, available in most hospitals headed by Macmillan nurses or consultants in palliative medicine (Box 9).

Box 8. Other methods of managing pain in patients with cancer

Pharmacological
  Analgesics
    non-opioids
    opioids
  Adjuvant analgesics
    corticosteroids
    antidepressants
    anticonvulsants
    muscle relaxants

Non-pharmacological
  Physical
    heat, TENS
  Psychological
    relaxation
    cognitive-behavioural therapy

Interuption of pain pathways
  Local nerve blocks
  Spinal analgesia

Modification of life style
  Mobility aids
  Additional physical help
  Immobilization

Pharmacological approaches

WHO guidelines

• by the mouth — the preferred route
• by the clock — treat chronic pain with regular analgesia
• by the ladder (Figure 3) — for mild to moderate pain start at step one and quickly (within 24–48 hours) move up a step if the pain is unrelieved. For severe pain go straight to step 3.

Use of morphine in clinical practice

The prescription of morphine always raises issues for the patient and family and time is required to listen, clarify, explain and reassure them about these.

Box 9.   When to involve specialist palliative care services

Refer for advice on the management of pain if:

- you are in anyway unclear or uncertain of what you are doing
- pain persists despite following the WHO analgesic guidelines (i.e. pain appears morphine poorly responsive — neuropathic pain, incident pain etc)
- you are considering the use of an alternative strong opioid to morphine
- you are considering the use of adjuvant analgesics
- the patient (or family) has psychological, social or spiritual issues that are adversely impacting upon the pain. An holistic approach that considers all such factors that contribute to the 'total pain experience' for the patient is vital.

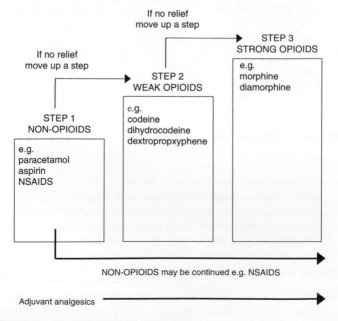

Figure 3.   The WHO analgesic ladder

Starting dose

- usually 10mg immediate release morphine (e.g. morphine solution (oramorph) or tablets (sevredol)) every four hours. In the elderly or those with renal impairment 2.5–5mg every 6–8 hours may suffice.

Dose increase

- titrate the dose (by 30–50%) against the pain every 24 hours (or 3–4 days in the elderly or those with renal impairment). In outpatients give the patient clearly written instructions on when and how to increase their dose of morphine or ask them to visit their GP to help them with this. Ideally update the GP by telephone beforehand and/or provide the patient with a handwritten note to take to the GP.

Breakthrough dose

- always instruct the patient what to do for breakthrough pain
- dose is usually equivalent to the to the 4 hourly dose of morphine
- if needing 2 or more breakthrough doses regularly increase dose of regular opioid.

Incident pain — patient is pain free at rest but experiences pain on movement.

- usually due to destruction of weight bearing bone +/– involvement of nerve tissue
- consider impending fracture of bone (long bone or vertebra) and treat appropriately
- consider spinal cord, cauda equina or nerve root impingement and treat appropriately
- increasing regular opioid to an effective dose often leads to unacceptable side effects (e.g. drowsiness)
- give breakthrough dose of morphine 30 minutes prior to movement or nitrous oxide.

Management of the adverse effects of morphine

- nausea +/– vomiting. Over 50% of patients require an antiemetic for the first 3–4 days (e.g. haloperidol 1.5–3mg nocte). If persistent, gastric stasis may be a factor requiring the prescription of a prokinetic (e.g. metoclopramide 10mg q.i.d.)

- constipation. Always prescribe a laxative. A combination of a softener and a stimulant is usually required (e.g. co-danthramer)
- drowsiness. Warn patient. Usually subsides over a few days
- psychological dependence. The patients (and professionals) fear of addiction is unfounded and should not limit the use of strong opioids for cancer pain. Caution in this respect should be reserved for patients with a present or past history of substance abuse; even then strong opioids should be used when there is a clinical need
- physical dependence can occur but does not prevent a reduction in the dose of a strong opioid if the patient's pain ameliorates, e.g. as a result of radiotherapy or a nerve block
- other side effects. e.g. delirium, hallucinations, myoclonus, pruritus. Reduce dose of morphine. Consider using an alternative strong opioid.

By applying the WHO ladder you should be able to relieve cancer pain quite easily in the majority of your patients. If the pain is not improving with increasing doses of morphine it may be that you need to reassess the cause of the pain, that you are dealing with an opioid poorly responsive pain (e.g. neuropathic pain) or you are underestimating the emotional aspects of the patients pain experience.

Adjuvant analgesics

Adjuvant or secondary analgesics are drugs that are not marketed primarily as analgesics but which can contribute to the relief of pain (Box 10). They are used when pain is poorly responsive to opioid analgesics (e.g. neuropathic pain, muscle spasm).

Haemoptysis

Usually only small amounts of blood are expectorated but rarely large bleeds occur sometimes with little or no warning. Death is by asphyxiation due to airway obstruction or by exanguination. In bronchogenic carcinoma approximately one third of patients experience haemoptysis with a mortality rate of 3%. Massive fatal haemoptysis is most likely to be due to squamous cell tumours (83%) that are located centrally or causing cavitation (48%).

In metastatic lung disease haemoptysis is usually due to endobronchial disease most commonly from cancer of the breast, colon,

Box 10. Examples of adjuvant (secondary) analgesics

Class of drug	Example	Possible analgesic benefits in
corticosteroids	dexamethasone	neuropathic pain, bone pain, painful hepatomegally
antidepressants	amitriptyline	neuropathic pain
anticonvulsants	gabapentin	neuropathic pain
cardiac antiarrhythmics	mexilitine	neuropathic pain
muscle relaxants:		
antimuscarinics (smooth muscle)	hyoscine butylbromide	intestinal colic
benzodiazepines (skeletal muscle)	diazepam	muscle spasm

kidney, and melanoma. Oesophageal carcinoma may extend directly into the tracheobronchial tree to cause massive haemoptysis.

In haematological malignancy pulmonary haemorrhage with or without haemoptysis is strongly associated with fungal infection. Other risk factors in this group of patients are thrombocytopenia and diffuse alveolar damage associated with certain chemotherapy agents, radiotherapy, bacterial or viral infection.

Aetiology

Some of the commoner causes of haemoptysis are listed in Table 4.

Management of haemoptysis

Apply the general principles in Box 4. Investigations appropriate to the clinical condition of the patient depend upon the causes being considered and the severity of the haemoptysis.

Submassive haemoptysis

- radiotherapy is the treatment of choice leading to prolonged relief in 85% of patients. The dose given is often palliative

Table 4. Common causes of heamoptysis and massive haemoptysis (*)

Cancer related

primary lung cancer (squamous cell*)
secondary lung cancer
bronchial carcinoid

Treatment related

aspirin/NSAID
anticoagulation
thrombocytopenia

Other

- infection
  viral, bacterial, fungal, parasitic infection
  lung abscess*
  tuberculosis*
  aspergilloma*

- pulmonary
  COPD
  pulmonary embolism
  bronchopleural fistula
  bronchiectasis*
  cystic fibrosis*

- cardiovascular
  pulmonary hypertension
  mitral stenosis
  tricuspid endocarditis

- haematological
  coagulopathy
  platelet dysfunction
  thrombocytopenia
  disseminated intravascular coagulation

- systemic disease
  Goodpastures syndrome
  systemic lupus erythematosus
  vasculitis
  sarcoid

allowing the treatment to be repeated if the symptom recurs
- when further external beam irradiation is not possible alternative options (depending on local access to specialist services) include brachytherapy, cryotherapy and laser therapy. Central airway tumours causing obstruction in addition to haemoptysis are most suited to these approaches
- it may help to discontinue drugs with antiplatelet effects (e.g. aspirin, NSAIDS). If this is not possible the NSAID could be substituted for paracetamol or by a non-acetylated salicylate NSAID (e.g. Diflunisal) which does not interfere with platelet function
- tranexamic acid (1–1.5g b–q.i.d.) is an antifibrinolytic agent which inhibits the activation of plasminogen to plasmin. Ethamsylate (500mg q.i.d.) is a haemostatic agent that inhibits the synthesis of prostaglandins that cause platelet disaggregation, vasodilatation and increased capillary permeability. Both appear effective in reducing blood loss in a number of conditions. Although sometimes given to reduce haemoptysis this role has not been formally evaluated.

Massive haemoptysis — appropriate to resuscitate patient

See Respiratory Emergencies chapter.

Massive haemoptysis — resuscitation inappropriate

This is a rare but frightening experience for both the patient, family and professionals in attendance. Try to stay calm. Resuscitation is not usually appropriate in a patient with advanced disease who has received previous anticancer treatment and has a poor performance status.

- stay with the patient and use blankets or towels to catch the blood
- lay the patient in a lateral position tumour side down if the site is known
- in the meantime someone else should be obtaining diamorphine (at least 10mg) along with a sedative such as midazolam 10mg if available. Give the medication intravenously or by deep intramuscular injection whichever is quickest
- death often occurs rapidly before any medication can be given

- if such an event is predicted have a syringe containing these drugs available for immediate use
- maintain sedation by repeating the combination of drugs as required or by continuous infusion (preferably i.v.).

Further Reading

Ahmedzai S. Palliation of respiratory symptoms. In: Doyle D, Hanks GWC, MacDonald N eds. Oxford textbook of palliative medicine, pp 583–616. Oxford: Oxford Medical Publications 1998

Ahmedzai S and Davis C. Nebulized drugs in palliative care. *Thorax* 1997;**52** (suppl 2):s75–s77

Faull C, Carter Y, Woof R. Handbook of palliative care. Oxford: Blackwell Science 1998

Twycross RG. Pain relief in advanced cancer. Edinburgh: Churchill Livingstone 1994

Twycross R. Introducing palliative care. Oxford: Radcliffe Medical Press 1999

Twycross R. Symptom management in advanced cancer. Oxford: Radcliffe Medical Press 1997

Twycross R, Wilcock A, Thorp S. Palliative care formulary. Oxford: Radcliffe Medical Press 1998

World Health Organization. Cancer pain relief. Geneva: WHO 1986

30

Teaching, Learning and Assessing

Venetia M France

Although the term students is used throughout this text the following principles can be applied to teaching in any situation from medical undergraduates to consultants and other health professionals.

Teaching is satisfying when done well. Time needs to be found; time to plan each individual session and time to review, when changes can be considered with the session fresh in mind.

Students need to acquire knowledge, skills and attitudes. Realistic situations — around the bedside or with families — provide the best practise for acquiring professional attitudes. Rapid feedback is integral to the development of appropriate attitudes, knowledge and skills.

Different people learn in different ways. Most of us (about 65%) learn better from visual rather than auditory or mathematical cues. Learning strategies may be categorised as deep, surface or strategic or a mixture. Some students search for meaning and structure their tasks (characteristic of deep learning). Others learn by rote without developing an organisational or conceptual structure for tasks. Still others aim simply to obtain high grades by managing their time and effort and predicting examination questions. Passing examinations is essential but may not be the only condition for effective practice. Teaching and assessment styles influence student learning strategies.

The Job of the Teacher

Setting goals

The first activity may be to make a chart relating your goals to those of the overall curriculum. This allows gaps to be seen and makes your rationale clear. Your task will be to set a goal for each session and to work out a series of steps to get there.

Setting objectives

It is particularly useful to write a set of objectives, perhaps three to six for each teaching session and for students directed self-learning between sessions. Objectives should be testable and show students what they need to know. Well-written objectives cannot be misinterpreted. They may be performance objectives, like demonstrating to a tutor, SHO or examiner a defined level of ability in a technical skill. Or they may be learning objectives e.g. list three reasons for using X instead of Y to treat Z. Higher-level objectives can be used to test a students underlying knowledge and their understanding of how knowledge should be applied in a particular context. For example "make a differential diagnosis for patient A whose case notes are supplied". Such objectives can be assessed using Modified Essay Questions (MEQ) where information is given in stages.

Setting up student learning groups

Much learning occurs outside teaching sessions. Your guidance is helpful in establishing self-help groups of four to six students who meet regularly to report to each other on ward work, prepare case presentations and, evaluate each others performance against objectives you provide. Groups flourish when given a sense of independence and achievement. If you call on individual students as experts in their topic, they will respond, motivating and helping others.

Structuring sessions to enhance learning

This is your main task. The structure must be built to achieve the session goal and objectives. At the end, students must be clear that they have learnt the relevant matter and acquired the skills set by the objectives. The more students participate, the more they will learn. After the session set questions for homework and test next time.

At the bedside

Patients and simulated patients provide the best opportunities for learning in context. Problems may arise if students feel anxious, under pressure to perform in front of an audience. Letting students take responsibility, making tasks very clear, breaking tasks into manageable sections, and keeping group size small all helps. If teachers encourage, commend success and refrain from criticism in the presence of the patient and staff, students will learn well. A supportive atmosphere dispels fear and allows students to concentrate on their activities. Feedback should be given individually *en route* to the seminar room where general points can be made and the more formal teaching take place.

In lectures

Active learning works well in lectures of 200 as well as in smaller groups. Based on a concentration span of 20–30 minutes, aim to break up a lecture, seminar or group session into two or three sections, letting pairs of students problem-solve between each section whilst you walk around. Groups might be analysing cases, slides of data or pathology, doing blood gas calculations, critically reviewing proposed procedures or peer assessing with marking schemes. Your role is to set the context and draw conclusions from students' results, using these to extend and consolidate the topic before setting a new task. Any questions come best from the groups rather than individuals in a large class.

Asking students questions checks learning, but in large classes rhetorical questions or questions to which students write down an answer are easiest to handle. For questions to groups of 15 or more, one strategy is to ask everyone to write an answer and then discuss ideas with a neighbour. Then call on one pair, or put up alternatives on the overhead. Ask for a show of hands, noting the results, before discussing each possibility in turn without necessarily giving the answer. Students check for understanding and problems can be discussed with their neighbours before you summarise.

If you intend to show slides or a video clip, focus attention by giving students two to three questions to consider before the show. Afterwards they discuss their responses in pairs then you summarise.

Table 1.   Learning is often better when

- the student knows what to learn and why s/he needs to learn it
  Provide a list of your goals and objectives for the session

- student learning is active/participatory

- the student knows what s/he has learned
  Incorporate frequent, short, informal assessments into sessions

- students practice the application of their learning
  Short sections of theory with immediate application in small groups of 2–4 in the lecture theatre, and peer feedback; skills are practised with observation

- errors are diagnosed rapidly. Correction offered quickly by peers or tutor

- the pace is suited to the individual
  Working in pairs at their own pace helps slower students to catch up

Points to consider when planning teaching are in Table 1.

Assessment

Assessment should be used to clarify goals and objectives of the course. Assessment can be:

- *formative* — giving rapid feedback to learners and teachers
- *summative* — determining progression to the next stage

Using formative assessment frequently is helpful. Peer marking, by redistributing work with a clear, detailed marking scheme, is an excellent way of embedding assessment criteria. If students see the marking criteria, they understand what you want them to learn.

Feedback is an effective tool for student and staff development. For example it is helpful to ask the presenter what they did well, invite positive comments from observers and then ask if the presenter would change anything next time and decide on action points for the future.

Table 2 gives ideas of ways to provide variety in assessment tasks and Table 3 gives a summary of assessment guidelines.

Table 2.   Assessment tools

The ideas below are mainly for formative assessment. They are easy and allow teachers to match learning or performance objectives to assessment.

Mastery learning
Set a standard (eg; 80%). Every member of the class must reach this standard before the class proceeds. Students in small groups will tutor each other in order that the whole group can proceed. This is well suited to computer-based testing or 'spot' slides. Provide alternate forms of the tests to enable students to be assessed on the same material at the second or third attempt.

Contracts
Students write themselves contracts for the week, specify what they will achieve (eg; 'I contract to read A and B and see six patients with X and Y ...') and how they will demonstrate that they have fulfilled their contract. In groups/pairs students look at each other's contracts. At the end of the week the same groups assess each other.

Spot tests
Give students unexpected tests; use the results for feedback to show students what they have learnt and what they have not. Get the students to mark each other's work using an answer sheet.

Staff marking exercises
Ask all your colleagues to mark the same piece of student work. Discuss your views and comments. Try to arrive at a set of criteria which explain how you have marked the work. Write them out so that the students can see what they are supposed to be aiming for. This exercise can be important on team taught courses.

Student marking exercises
As above, but the students mark the piece of work and try to arrive at shared criteria. Ask the students to set themselves directions; "next time I do a piece of work like this I am going to try to ..."

Doing it better
Take an anonymised laboratory report or patient case notes. Ask students to draw up a list of do's and dont's.

Quiz
Divide students into two to three teams to devise questions. Teams each nominate a judge. Judges vet the questions, chair the quiz, judge whether questions have been answered and keep the score.

Table 3. Assessment quidelines

- use assessment to direct students' attention to what matters
- use a variety of assessment methods
- encourage deep learning and understanding by your assessments
- tell students the criteria you are using for the assessment
- marking is subjective and unreliable
- give feedback promptly; make it positive
- encourage students to assess themselves formally and informally

Summary

1. STRUCTURE ALL SESSIONS FOR ACTIVE LEARNING. This includes lectures, seminars and bedside sessions on skills, knowledge and attitudes.

2. SET A GOAL AND OBJECTIVES for every teaching session.

3. REVIEW your teaching session and note things to change next time.

4. USE FEEDBACK to help students understand what they need to improve and how to go about it. Get their feedback on your teaching.

5. USE FREQUENT FORMATIVE ASSESSMENTS AND PEER MARKING to show students what you want them to learn.

6. DISCUSS TEACHING WITH COLLEAGUES. Make sure your contributions fit into the whole.

Reference

Gibbs G, Habeshaw T. 253 ideas for your teaching. Bristol, UK: Technical and Educational Services Ltd 1988

31

Preparation for Research

David A Lomas and Michael Plotnick

So you are almost there. You have learnt about the role of HRCT in the diagnosis of interstitial lung disease and even the veil of mystery that pervades pulmonary vasculitis is beginning to lift. Why bother reading this chapter? Why even think about research? It takes about five years after becoming a consultant to assimilate to knowledge required to see you through thirty years of clinical practice. There will be the odd rarity that will be worthy of a trawl through the journals but, on the whole, little will change in thirty years. A change of nomenclature perhaps, a new method of imaging, but a similar clinical outcome. How will you find the intellectual fulfilment that is the pre-requisite to job satisfaction? Private practice, the paperwork and bureaucracy of medical politics or endless rounds of golf? The glaringly obvious answer to the question is research. You don't have to sit on the sidelines watching others but can bring about major changes in your own working practices and influence the direction of your chosen profession.

Like all clinical training, a period of time in research needs to be carefully planned and there is a well recognised path to gain research experience that will hold you in good stead for the future.

When to do Research?

There is no right or wrong time to spend a period of time in research. Some students in Cambridge undertake a PhD as part of their undergraduate training. UK graduates might prefer to do research before entering the specialist registrar (SpR) grade, after two to three years of SpR clinical work or after obtaining a CCST. As you will need to identify a supervisor, plan carefully and apply for funds, it is this that is likely to dictate the timing of your entry into research. If you start too early you may have to break a winning run of results to complete clinical training, too late and there may be no buffer of SpR work to catch you if the funding does not materialise. It is important to start thinking about research projects as soon as you are appointed to an SpR scheme. Make an appointment with the University representative to discuss options both within your rotation and elsewhere in the UK.

In the USA, combined MD, PhD programmes provide the opportunity to begin training as a physician and scientist concurrently. Such combined degree programmes typically are completed after seven years, instead of the four years required to complete a standard medical school curriculum. Since funding is often available to combined degree candidates, the costs incurred can be significantly less than those from a four-year MD programme. Medical school applicants who are interested in pursuing a career as a physician-scientist are advised to consider undertaking a combined degree programme. A second opportunity for extensive research training is often available as part of subspecialty fellowship training in respiratory medicine. In fact, most of the top fellowship programmes require two years of full-time research training in addition to the clinical years.

Where to do Research?

There are many groups in the USA and UK carrying out excellent research in respiratory medicine. Many of these will be headed by respiratory physicians, but others are basic science units working on other subjects that can be related to respiratory disease. In some cases in the USA, the respiratory fellowship programme requires (or strongly urges) that you work under the supervision of a respiratory division member. Otherwise, you should be adventurous. There are great advantages of being a lone physician in a basic science group or in being one of the few who undertake formal training in epidemiological studies.

The most satisfying research experiences will involve an area in which you are interested, and undertaken in a cutting edge laboratory. Therefore, choose carefully, consult the journals and look for groups who publish in high impact journals and who are funded by nationally competitive grants. In the UK, these groups are being continually assessed and ranked as part of peer review and University research assessment exercises. If they have nationally awarded funds they must have competed well in the national and international arena and hence you will have a better chance of obtaining funding to work with them for a PhD or MD Avoid short-term pharmaceutical studies unless it is a clear means to an end. For example it may be worth undertaking such studies to fund you to work in a lab, as a spring-board to a new post or to undertake a taught MSc course.

MD or PhD or MD, PhD?

In the UK and USA there are some differences in the terminology. In the UK, a PhD results from a supervised structured project and requires payment of University fees. An MD is theoretically a thesis carried out without supervision by a medically qualified graduate. It is submitted to your *alma mater* and, as such, there is often a registration fee but no recurring charge. Unless you are outstanding or have a well-defined project in an area on which you are an authority, it is probably best not to embark on an MD without supervision. An MD can be undertaken whilst pursuing other clinical duties but this is often stressful and removes the enjoyment of research which, for many people, is time away from the daily grind to think about new projects and broaden their horizons. In the long term, registrars who wish to pursue a career in academic medicine are probably best advised to undertake a PhD as this is often considered to represent more rigorous scientific training. Moreover funding bodies often ask that a candidate registers for a PhD as a condition of awarding a three year training fellowship.

In the USA an MD (or DO) is the degree awarded following completion of the curriculum of an accredited medical school (osteopath school) and does not require research experience or a thesis. An MD or DO is required to practice medicine in the USA A PhD is awarded for the successful completion of a graduate programme and the writing of a doctoral thesis. As in the UK, PhD graduates are considered to have undertaken the most rigorous scientific training programmes. The combined MD, PhD degree requires completion of both medical and PhD programmes. The admissions process for combined degree programmes is usually more competitive than for standard medical school. It should be mentioned, however, that while there are financial benefits to a combined degree, with respect to medical school costs, it is unclear whether obtaining a PhD significantly increases the likelihood of success in an academic medical career. Currently, it appears that both MDs and MD, PhDs interested in pursuing a physician-scientist position will have to survive at least four years as a research fellow (post-doctoral fellow) following completion of clinical training.

Funding?

This is a thorny issue. In the UK the Medical Research Council (MRC), Wellcome Trust, Action Research and the cancer charities all offer competitive training fellowships to work in units where it is anticipated you will be well trained and will work on a relevant project. There are advantages to work in MRC, Imperial Cancer Research Fund (ICRF) or Cancer Research Council (CRC) basic science, clinical science or epidemiology units if you can tie in your project with their broad skills. Don't be too dogmatic about what you want to do, take advice from your proposed supervisor and ask him or her to help you write the project. No matter how well-read you are, you require someone at the cutting edge to write a coherent project that will stand up well to peer review and scrutiny by an interview panel. Virtually all training fellows are interviewed for funding and it will be an advantage, but not a prerequisite, if you have a BSc degree, honours, prizes or publications. Many SpRs underrate their chances of gaining a fellowship and do not apply. If an application for three year funding is unsuccessful, start-up funding can sometimes be obtained for one year from Health Authorities. This will provide work experience and a springboard for national applications. Remember if you do obtain funding for research it will be at a salary that is significantly higher than the other non-clinical PhD students or post-doctoral fellows who will often teach you techniques or give you advice on the project. This is a sensitive issue which needs to be handled with tact and humility.

Generally, research fellowships in the USA are funded for the first two years as part of fellowship training and are sponsored by the National Institutes of Health (NIH). Funds are typically awarded to the academic institution as training grants. Such NIH sponsored research fellowships contain a payback clause, i.e. for each year of NIH sponsorship you must commit to a year of academic medicine or you must pay back the cost of the grant. Since many respiratory training programmes only commit to supporting research fellows for two years, it is usually your responsibility to obtain funding for further training. Fortunately, there are multiple sources available from the NIH, private organisations, and pharmaceutical companies that provide grants for an additional two to five years of research training. Your mentor should help you decide when and where grant proposals should be submitted.

Some respiratory fellowships in the USA now provide an opportunity to obtain formal training in statistics/epidemiology. If you are interested in pursuing a career in clinical research, it would be advisable to look for such training programmes when applying for respiratory fellowships.

To go Abroad?

If the PhD or MD goes well it would be worth applying for fellowships to go abroad and work in key units in other parts of the world. Some departments run exchange fellowships in the USA or Commonwealth countries. Training for a career as a physician-scientist should be flexible and exciting and you are only constrained by your ambition.

Other Options

If you truly have no ambition to do research and know that you will not regret the lost opportunities you may consider taking a year out to pursue other interests. Again we suggest that you be ambitious in whichever project you wish to pursue. This is a chance to broaden your horizons; an MSc in medieval architecture, an MBA, medical officer at the Antarctic survey or writing novels are all possibilities. Whatever you decide, you must plan early and liaise closely with the programme manager to plan your exit from, and re-entry into, clinical medicine.

In summary this is an exciting time of your life. Your decisions will have an impact on your own future, your personal development and also on the future of respiratory medicine. Research is fun but a little time spent in planning in the early stages will make a huge difference to the end when you want to apply for project and programme grants, senior fellowships and even research professorships. Go on, look beyond the next clinical post, take the plunge into a new future!

Index

^{67}Ga scanning 33–34
^{99m}Tc-pentetic acid (DTPA)
  scanning 34

acid-base balance 1
acid-maltase deficiency 160
actinomycosis 295
activated partial thromboplastin
  time (APTT) 231
acute allergic alveolitis 483
acute extrinsic allergic alveolitis
  445
acute interstitial pneumonia (AIP)
  444
acute respiratory distress syndrome
    (ARDS) 527–543
  arterial blood gas analysis
    532–533
  broncho-alveolar lavage 534
  chest X-ray 532
  CT 534
  diagnosis 531–534
  exudative phase 529–530
  fibrotic phase 530
  haemodynamic monitoring
    533
  haemodynamic support
    537–538
  infection control 538–539
  lung injury assessment
    534–535
  management 535–541
  nutritional support 538

pathogenesis 530–531
pathology 528–530
pathophysiology 531
pharmacological therapies
  539–540
proliferative phase 520
pulmonary function recovery
  541–542
ventilation 535–537
acute severe asthma, 104–106
adenocarcinoma 235, 236
  growth rate 237
adenosquamous carcinoma 236
adult respiratory distress syndrome
  (ARDS) 446, 509
AIDS 296–297, 311, 318, 383–406
  anti-retroviral drugs 387–388
  background 383–384
  bacterial pneumonia 390–391
  bronchoscopy 402
  CDC classification 384
  clinical features 384–386
  CT 402
  failure to improve on therapy
    401–402
  fungal pneumonias 399–401
  Kaposi's sarcoma 403–404
  lymphocytic   interstitial
    pneumonitis (LIP) 405–406
  lymphoma 404–405
  monitoring 386–387
  mycobacterial infection 396–
    401

mycobacterium avium
complex 398–399
non-infective respiratory
manifestations 403–406
non-specific interstitial
pneumonitis (NSIP)
405–406, 443, 444
open lung biopsy 403
pleural effusion 296–298
pneumothorax 296
pulmonary complications
388–396
testing 386, 387
treatment options 403
tuberculosis 396–398
viral pneumonia 401
air conditioner lung disease 486
air-space consolidation 43–45
airway
function 4–7
mechanics 19
patency tests 5
stenting 258, 260
trauma 575–577
allergen immunotherapy 92
allergic bronchopulmonary
aspergillosis 86–87, 445
allergic rhinitis 116–117
allergy 107–129
aluminium exposure 490
alveolar cell carcinoma 445
alveolar disease (air-space
consolidation) 43–45
alveolytis 49
ammonia exposure 492
amoebiasis 296
amyloidosis 285
anaphylaxis and anaphylactoid
reactions 121–125
differential diagnosis 123
incidence 121–122
management 124–125
mechanisms 122–123
angiography 34

angiotensin-converting enzyme
(ACE) 594, 599
inhibitors 503
anthrax 353, 489–493
anti-cholinergics 144–145
anticoagulant treatment 211, 230
antihistamines 117–118
antimony pneumoconiosis 473
anti-smoking strategies 141–143
aortic aneurism 41
aortic tears 578
Apert's syndrome 196
apical-lordotic projection 30
arterial blood gases 2, 207
arterial hypoxaemia 207
asbestos related diseases 443,
472–482
asbestosis 477–478
benign plural disease 481–482
and compensation 482
lung cancer 481
mesothelioma 478–481
ascending contrast venography 225
ascitic effusion 286
Aspergillus spp 273, 295
Aspergillus fumigatus 295
aspiration 30, 574
aspirin sensitivity 127–128
management 128
Association of Respiratory
Technicians and Physiologists
(ARTP) 2
asthma 11, 81–106, 311, 595,
596–597
acute severe 104–106
assessment 104
discharge 106
treatment 104–105
allergen avoidance 114–116
chronic stable 94–98
clinical features 83–91
examination 83
history 83
investigations 83–86

clinical management 109–113
    examination 110
    history 109–110
    investigations 110–113
corticosteroid resistant 101
deaths 82
inhaler devices 93–94
management 91–106
    drug treatment 93–94
    non-drug treatment 91–93
new treatments 98
occupational 88–91
    aetiology 88–89
    diagnosis 90
    management 90–91
osteoporosis linked 99, 100
pregnancy and 103, 607–608
self management 93
severe 98–101
steroid sparing agents 99–101,
    102
syndromes 86–88
atelectasis 274, 574

bacterial pneumonia 390–391
Bagassosis 485
baritosis 473
BCG vaccination 365
bee and wasp venom allergy
    125–126
bellows spirometer (Vitallograph) 5
Berylliosis 488
beta agonists 144
bilateral lung transplantation (BLT)
    548, 549–550
Bird fanciers lung 485
Blastomycosis dermatitides 295
blood gas analysis 12–14
blunt cardiac trauma 577
bone marrow transplantation
    (BMT) 351–352
bony injuries to the chest 570–571
botulism 12
brain stem cerebrovascular events
    160

breathlessness 649–661
aetiology 651
anxiolytics 658–659
death rattle 660–661
exertional 14
management 650–653
non-pharmacological
    approaches 653–654, 655
opioids 654–657
oxygen 657–658
pharmacological approaches
    654
physiotherapy for 618
stridor 660
terminal 659–660
British Thoracic Society (BTS) 2
bronchial biopsies 67–72
bronchial challenge testing 18–19
bronchial gland carcinoma 236
bronchial infections 331–333
    bronchitis 331–333
bronchial obstruction 311
bronchiectasis 159–160, 414–421
    antimicrobial chemotherapy
        419–420
    causes 416
    clinical features 414–415
    CT scanning 414, 415
    cystic fibrosis 416–417
    investigations 415–416, 418
    management 417–421
    medical treatment 417
    mucus clearance 419
    physiotherapy 419
    supportive treatment 420–421
    surgical treatment 421
    therapy 420
bronchiolitis 448–449
bronchiolitis obliterans organizing
    pneumonitis (BOOP) 45, 445,
    448
bronchitis 11, 331–333, 595
bronchodilators 143–144
bronchogenic carcinoma,
    radiological staging 54–57

bronchopleural fistula 318–319
bronchoscopy 65–73, 281, 402
    complications 72–73
    fibreoptic 66–67
        sampling techniques 67
    pathological appearances 67
    rigid 65–66
        sampling techniques
            68–71
bronchostenosis 41
brucellosis pneumonia 353, 489
Burkholderia cepacia 412–413
Byssinosis 488

cadmium exposure 490
carbon monoxide 9
carcinoid tumour 236, 256–257
cardiac failure 11
cardiac trauma
    blunt 577
    penetrating 577–578
cardiorespiratory failure indicators
            164–165
    management 165–166
cardiovascular system monitoring
            511
catamenial pneumothorax 318
CFA 11, 438–440
challenge testing 3
chemical pleurodesis 324–325, 326
chemotherapy 254, 302
chest radiography 29–31, 35–52,
            204–207, 270–272, 281
    acute cardiogenic pulmonary
        oedema 47
    aspiration 30, 574
    cryptogenic fibrosing
        alveolitis, see DPLD
    evaluation checklist 35
    hyperlucent lungs 49–52
    left upper lobe collapse 42
    left upper lobe pneumonia 39
    normal anatomy 36, 37
    pneumothorax 51–52
    pulmonary emphysema 50

right lower lobe pneumonia 39
right middle lobe collapse 44
right middle lobe pneumonia
            39
chest trauma 567–581
    airway 575–577
    assessment 568–569
    bony injuries 570–571
    cardiac injury 580
    deformity 580
    haemothorax 272, 305–306,
            572–573
    herniation 580
    obstructive defects 580
    pain 580
    parenchymal damage 580
    penetrating injuries 570
    pleura 571–572
    pulmonary function 580
    soft tissue injury 569
    thoracotomy 569
chest tube drainage 302–304
chest ultrasound 31
chest wall disease 158, 160
chest wall function 2, 11–12
chlamydia 489
chlorine exposure 492
chromium exposure 490
chronic allergic alveolitis
            483–484
chronic fibrosing alveolitis (CFA)
            444
chronic obstructive pulmonary
        disease (COPD) 131–154,
            213, 214, 239, 311, 317,
            466–467
    aetiology 132
    and air travel 150
    assisted ventilation 152–153
    case study 26–27
    clinical features 134–138
    definition 131
    drug therapy 143–147
    ECG and echocardiography
            140–141

epidemiology 131–132
exacerbation management
    136, 150–153
haematology 141
hypercapnic exacerbations
    161–163
investigations 138–141
management 141–150, 159
NIPPV therapy 168
oxygen 148–149
pathology 132–133
pathophysiology 133–134,
    156–157
psychological health 150
pulmonary rehabilitation 148
pulse oximetry 140
radiology 138–139
reversibility testing 139–140
spirometry 138
sputum culture 141
surgery 149–150
symptoms 134–136
vaccination 147
ventilatory failure 158–159
chronic stable asthma 94–98
Churg-Strauss syndrome 87–88,
    113, 447
chylothorax 272, 273, 306–310
aetiology 307–308
causes, 307
clinical presentation 308
investigations 308
management 308
non-traumatic 309
surgical 309
traumatic 309
circulatory collapse 218–219
cirrhosis 274
cobalt exposure 490
Coccidiodes immitus 295
coccidioidomycosis 353
collagen vascular diseases
    282–283
rheumatoid arthritis 282–283
systemic lupus erythematosus
    283

community acquired pneumonia
    (CAP) 333–343
aetiology 334
antibiotic therapy 340–342
clinical features 334–335
complications 342–343
general investigations 335–337
management 338–340
microbiological investigations
    337–338
complementary medicine, and
    asthma 92–93
computed tomography (CT) 31–32,
    53, 208, 226, 243–244, 272,
    402
congenital absence of respiratory
    drive 196–197
constrictive obliterative
    bronchiolitis (OB) 448
continuous hyperfractionated
    accelerated radiotherapy
    (CHART) 252
continuous mechanical ventilation
    506
continuous positive airway
    pressure (CPAP) 506
copper exposure 490
cor pulmonale 137, 213–214
causes 214
management 213
corticosteroids 147
cough 591–603
ACE 594, 599
aetiology 593–599, 661
anatomy and physiology
    592–593
asthma 595, 596–597
chronic bronchitis 595
diagnosis and management
    599–601, 661–664
eosinophilic bronchitis 594
future research 601–602
gastro-oesophageal reflux 594,
    597, 598
post viral 595, 597
rhinitis 593–596

Coxiella burnetii 295
Coxiella burnetti pneumonia, see
    Q fever
CREST syndrome 454
Creuzon's syndrome 196
Cryptococcus neoformans 295,
    297
cryptogenic bilateral fibrosing
    pleuritis 286
cryptogenic fibrosing alveolitis
    (CFA), see DPLD
    case study 25–26
cryptogenic organising pneumonia
    (COP), see BOOP
Cushing's syndrome 241
cystic fibrosis 311, 407–421
    adult symptoms 407
    airway therapy 410
    bronchiectasis 416–417
    cepacia syndrome 413
    childhood symptoms, 407
    clinical features 409
    diagnostic tests 408
    management 410–414
    monitoring 409–410
    pathophysiology 408
    sputum cultures 410
    transmembrane conductance
        regulator (CFTR) 407
    treatment 411–412
    viral infections 414

daytime somnolence 174, 191,
    192–194
decongestants 118
desquamative interstitial
    pneumonia (DIP) 444
diaphragm assessment 12
diaphragm rupture 578–579
diffuse alveolar haemorrhage (DAH)
    446
diffuse parenchymal lung disease
    (DPLD), 48, 423–455
    aetiology 428–429
    bronchoalveolar lavage (BAL)
        435

classification 424–426
CT 433
diagnostic problems 442–451
disease behaviour 424, 427
finger clubbing 427
history 426–427
inspiratory crackles 429
mid-inspiratory squawk 429
patient liaison 441–442
physical examination 427–426
severity 426–427
staging 427
therapeutic problems 451–455
treatment 437–440
diphtheria 353
diseases of the chest wall 214
diuretics 210
Doppler ultrasound 225–226
double-lung transplantation (DLT)
    548, 549–550
Down's syndrome 196
Dressler's syndrome 284
drowning 584–590
drug-induced respiratory disease
    (DRD) 499–504
    amiodarone 501–502
    angiotensin-converting
        enzyme (ACE) inhibitors
        503
    bronchospasm 503
    chemotherapy agents 501
    interstitial lung disease 500–502
Duchenne muscular dystrophy 167
dyspnoea 219

ECG 140
echocardiography 140–141, 208,
    227
Ehlers-Danlos 311
electrocardiogram (ECG) 207
emboli 574–575
emphysema 11, 49–51, 166–167,
    557–559
    case history 22–23
    -like changes (ELCs) 311
    subcutaneous 319

empyema 272, 273, 286, 290–292
  intercostal tube drainage
    290–291
  needle thoracentesis 290
  surgical drainage 291–292
  tuberculous 295
  unresolving 292
encephalitis 160
endobronchial obstruction 41
endobronchial therapy 73, 74,
    257–262
  airway stenting 258, 260
  radiotherapy 258, 260–262
  tumour debulking 258–260
end-stage lung disease 443
cosinophilic bronchitis 594
eosinophilic lung disease 45
eosinophilic pneumonia 445
Epworth sleepiness scale 175
European Respiratory Society (ERS)
    3
exercise testing 2, 3, 14–17
expiatory function test 5
extrinsic allergic alveolitis (EAA)
    483–487, see also DPLD
  investigations 484
  management 484
exudates 276–278

familial mediterrean fever 285
Farmers lung 485
fibreoptic bronchoscopy 242–243
fibrosing alveolitis 311, 443–444
fibrosis 47, 495–497
fibrothorax 158
Flenley diagram 13
flow-volume loop 5, 6, 8
follicular bronchiolitis 448
food allergy 126–127
forced expiratory volume in one
    second (FEV$_1$) 5
forced vital capacity (FVC) 5
functional residual capacity (FRC)
    7
fungal infections 295–296
fungal pneumonias 399–401

gas exchange 2, 9–10
gastro-oesophageal reflux 594, 597,
    598
glomerulonephritis 274
Gnathostomiasis 296
graft versus host disease (GVHT)
    351
granulocyte colony-stimulating
    factor (GCSF) 255
Guillain-Barre 12, 160

haemodynamic monitoring and
    support 511–512
Haemophilus influenzae 296,
    390, 419
haemoptysis 239–240, 241,
    581–582, 668–672
  aetiology 670
  management 649, 669–672
haemorrhage 45
haemothorax 272, 305–306,
    572–573
  non-traumatic 306
  traumatic 305–306
heart-lung transplantation (HLT)
    166–167, 212, 353, 421,
    547–549
heparin 230–231
hepatotoxicity management 368,
    369
high resolution CT (HRCT) 32
histiocytosis X 311
Histoplasma capsulatum 295, 297
Histoplasma capsulatum
    pneumonia 353
HIV 383–406
  anti-retroviral drugs 387–388
  background 383–384
  bacterial pneumonia 390–391
  bronchoscopy 402
  CDC classification 384
  clinical features 384–386
  CT 402
  failure to improve on therapy
    401–402
  fungal pneumonias 399–401

Kaposi's sarcoma 403–404
lymphocytic interstitial
  pneumonitis (LIP) 405–406
lymphoma 404–405
monitoring 386–387
mycobacterial infection
  396–401
mycobacterium avium
  complex 398–399
non-infective respiratory
  manifestations 403–406
non-specific interstitial
  pneumonitis (NSIP)
  405–406, 443, 444
open lung biopsy 403
pulmonary complications
  388–396
testing 386, 387
treatment options 403
tuberculosis 396–398
viral pneumonias 401
hospital acquired pneumonia
  (HAP) 343–347
aetiology 344
antibiotic therapy 347
clinical features 344–346
general investigations 346
management 347
microbiological investigations
  346–347
HRCT, 57–58
lymphagiomyomatosis 60
pulmonary fibrosis 59
pulmonary sarcoidosis 59
subacute extrinsic allergic
  alveolitis 60
Humidifier fever 488
Hunter's syndrome 196
Hurler's syndrome 196
hydatid 296
hydrogen sulphide exposure 492
hypercalcaemia 241
hypercapnia 160
hypersomnia 192–194
  idiopathic 194

post-traumatic 194
recurrent 194
hypoalbuminaemia 274
hypothyroidism 274
hypoventilation 9

iatrogenic trauma 579
idiopathic pulmonary fibrosis, see
  DPLD
imaging techniques, for thoracic
  disease 21, 29–34
immunocompromised associated
  pneumonia (IAP) 347–351
clinical features 348–350
general investigations 350
management 351
microbiological investigations
  350–351
infection control 3
inhaled agents 584, 586–589
inotropic support 514–516
intensive care 505–526
haemodynamic monitoring
  and support 511–512
inotropic support 514–516
mechanical ventilatory
  support 505–510
nutritional support 519–522
pneumonia 526
pulmonary artery flotation
  catheters 512–513
renal support 516–519
sepsis 522–525
shock 513–514
intercostal chest drain 314–316,
  320–323
intermittent positive pressure
  ventilation (IPPV) 152, 506
interstitial lung disease 46–48,
  500–502
interventional chest radiology
  58–62
intrathoracic lesion localisation
  35–38
ipatropium bromide 118

Kaposi's sarcoma 403–404
Kaposi's sarcoma associated virus
  (KSHV) lymphoma 297
kidney transplantation 352
Klebsiella spp 390
Kleine-Levin syndrome 194
Klippel-Feil syndrome 158

Langerhans cell histiocytosis 455
large cell undifferentiated
      carcinoma 236
    growth rate 237
laryngeal sleep apnoea 195
lateral decubitous projection 30
lateral projection 30
Legionella pneumonia 296, 333
leukotriene receptor antagonists
  (LTRAs) 118–119
liver transplantation 352–353
lobectomy 564
long term oxygen therapy (LTOT)
  166
lung, response to injury 574–575
lung cancer 235–267, 481
    brain metastases 256
    chemotherapy 254
    classification 235–238
    clinical features 238–240
      airway obstruction
        238–239
      haemoptysis 239–240
      paraneoplastic syndromes
        239
    CT scanning 243–244
    diagnosis 240–248
    early detection 263–264
    endobronchial therapy 257–262
    extra-thoracic disease 239
    fibreoptic bronchoscopy
      242–243
    fine needle aspiration 243
    laboratory investigations
      241–242
    local disease 239
    mediastinoscopy 244

pleural effusions 244–245
quality of life 262–263
radionuclide bone scanning
  244
radiotherapy 252–253
smokers 238
solitary pulmonary nodule
  245–247
sputum cytology 242
staging 248–251
standards of care 264–265
surgery 247–251
TNM definitions 249
lung cysts 311
lung function assessment 2, 4, 207
  interpretation 10–11
  oxygen prescription 18
  reference values 2
  surgery 17–18
  travel 18
lung infections 331–354
lung reduction surgery 166–167,
  557–559
lung transplantation 212, 421,
      454–455, 545–565
  assessment 552–553
  bilateral (BLT) 548, 549–550
  complications 555–556
  contra-indications 545–547
  donor selection 551–552
  double- (DLT) 548, 549–550
  future developments 557
  heart- (HLT) 166–167, 212,
      353, 421, 547–549
  indications 545–547, 548
  lobar 550–551
  long-term care 556–557
  management 554
  matching criteria 551–552
  preparation 553–554
  single- (SLT) 548, 550
  survival 556
lung trauma 574–579
  aspiration 574
  atelectasis 574

diaphragm rupture 578–579
emboli 574–575
iatrogenic 579
management 575
oedema 574
oesophageal 579
pulmonary contusion 573
pulmonary lacerations 573
thoracic duct 579
lung volume 2, 7–9
lung volume loss, physiotherapy
    for 631
lupus pleuritis 272
lymphadenopathy 41, 357, 361
lymphangioleiomyamatosis 311,
    455
lymphocytic interstitial
    pneumonitis (LIP) 405–406
lymphoma 49, 297, 404–405
lymphoproliferative disease 445

magnetic resonance imaging (MRI)
    32–33, 227–229
malignant pleural effusions
    298–305
chemotherapy 302
chest tube drainage 302–304
clinical features 299
observation 302
pleural fluid 300–301
pleurectomy 304
pleuro-peritoneal shunt
    304–305
radiology 299–300
radiotherapy 302
thoracentesis 302
thoracoscopy with talc
    poudrage 304
treatment 301–302
Malt workers lung 486
manganese exposure 490
Maple bark strippers disease 486
Marfan's syndromes 311
MDR-TB 370–371, 378

mechanical ventilatory support
    505–510
features 507–510
principles 505–507
weaning from 510
mediastinal tumour 41
mediastinoscopy 244
melioidosis 353
mercury exposure 491
mesothelioma 273, 478–481
Metal fume fever 488
methicillin resistant
    Staphylococcus aureus
    (MRSA) 522
microscopic polyangitis 447
mid expiatory flow rate (MMEF) 6
MIGET 20
Mill fever 488
mitral stenosis 446
Moraxella catarrhalis 390, 419
motor neurone disease 160, 167
mouth intermittent positive
    pressure ventilation (MIPPV)
    167–168
MRI 244
MRI image, left Pancoast tumour 55
muscular dystrophy 11
Mushroom workers lung 485
myaesthenia gravis 11, 161
mycobacterial infection 396–401
mycobacterium avium complex
    398–399
Mycoplasma spp 295
Mycoplasma pneumoniae 296,
    333
myxoedema 285

narcolepsy 192–193
nasal continuous positive airway
    pressure (nCPAP) 182–186
nasal surgery 187
nebulisers 145–146
nemaline myopathy 160
neuromuscular disease 158

nickel exposure 491
NIPPV 162–163
    in restrictive disease 163–164
nitrogen oxides exposure 492
Nocardia spp 390
Nocardia asteroides 296
Nocardiosis 295
nocturnal hypoxaemia 207
nocturnal laryngeal spasm 195–196
nocturnal oxygen saturation
    monitoring 207
non-allergic rhinitis with
    eosinophilia syndrome
    (NARES) 113
non-Hodgkin's lymphoma (NHL)
    297
non-invasive positive pressure
    ventilation (NIPPV) 152,
    168–170
non-invasive ventilation (NIV) 506
non-specific interstitial
    pneumonitis (NSIP) 405–406,
    443, 444
nutritional support 519–522

obesity 11
oblique projection 30
obliterative bronchiolitis 555–556
obstruction of extrathoracic
    airways 214
obstructive sleep apnoea 174–197
    cardiovascular consequences
        189–190
    central supine variant 195
    clinical assessment 174–180
    congenital absence of
        ventilatory drive 196–197
    consequences of 188–190
    daytime ventilatory failure
        189
    definition 174
    driving regulations 188–189
    haemodynamic effects 189
    management 180–186

    mandibular advancement
        device 182
    nasal continuous positive
        airway pressure (nCPAP)
        182–186
    out-patient assessment 190–192
    paediatric aspects 196–197
    pathophysiology 173
    physical examination 176–177
    prevalence 171–172
    respiratory pump inefficiency
        197
    sleep deprivation 188
    sleep study 177–180
    surgical treatment 187–188
    symptoms 176
    thyroid function test 180
    ventilatory drive instability
        197
occupational asthma 459–465
    aetiology 460
    clinical features 461–462
    compensation 465
    definition 459–460
    diagnosis 462
    diagnosis 464
    exposure 462
    history 462
    hyper-reactivity 463
    immunology 464
    management 464–465
    peak flow recordings 462–463
    predisposing factors 460–461
    prevalence, 460
    prognosis 465
    specific challenge 463
occupational lung disease 457–493
    anthrax 489–493
    asbestos 472–482
    brucellosis 489
    chlamydia 489
    COPD 466–467
    histoplasmosis 493
    Legionnaires disease 487

occupational alveolitides
483–487
particle inhalation 457–459
pneumoconiosis 467–472
Q fever 489
reactive airways dysfunction
syndrome (RADS) 466
TB 489
oedema 574
oesophageal trauma 272, 579
Ondine's curse 1196
open lung biopsy 209–210, 403
open pleural biopsy 281
organic dust toxic syndrome 487
OSA 207
oxygen therapy 210

palliative care
breathlessness 649–661
cough 661–664
definitions 645–647
haemoptysis 668–672
pain relief 664–668
psychological support 648
symptom control 648–649
paragonamiasis 296, 353
parapneumonic effusions 286–289
bacteriology 287–288
clinical features 288
complicated 289
imaging 288
management 288
uncomplicated 289
parasitic infections 296
particle inhalation 457–459
Pasteurella multocida pneumonia
353
peak expiratory flow (PEF) 6
peak expiratory flow rate (PEFR) 5
peak inspiratory flow (PIF) 6
penetrating cardiac trauma 577–578
penetrating chest injuries 570
percutaneous fine needle
aspiration 243
percutaneous transthoracic needle
biopsy 58–62

pericarditis 274
period movement of the legs (PMLS)
193
peritoneal dialysis 272
PET scanning 246
phosgene exposure 492
photodynamic therapy (PDT)
258–259
physiotherapy 617–638
active cycle of breathing
techniques (ACBT) 621
acupuncture 629
autogenic drainage (AD) 621
breathing exercises 620–621
chronic hyperventilation
syndrome (CHVS) 629–630
continuous positive airways
pressure (CPAP) 624
entonox 629
exercise 628
flutter 622–623
forced expiratory technique
(FET) 620
humidification and
nebulisation 623
intermittent positive pressure
breathing (IPPB) 623–624
ITU 636
lymphoedema bandaging 627
manual hyperinflation (MHI)
624–626
massage 627
neurophysiological facilitation
of respiration (NFR) 626
non-invasive positive pressure
ventilation (NIPPV) 624
non-invasive ventilation
623–624
pain relief 628–629
passive movements 627
positioning 619
positive expiratory pressure
(PEP) 622
postural drainage 621
pulmonary rehabilitation
632–636

sputum induction 636–637
suction 626–627
terminal care 636
thoracic mobilization 627–628
transcutaneous electrical
    nerve stimulation (TENS)
    628–629
vocal cord dysfunction (VCD)
    630–632
Pierre Robin syndrome 196
plague pneumonia 353
plasma D-dimer 227
pleural aspiration 319
pleural biopsy 319–320
pleural drainage 62
pleural effusion 244–245, 269–310
    chest X-ray 270–272
    CT 272
    diagnostic approach 273–282
    exudates 276–278
    imaging 270–272
    malignant 298–305
        chemotherapy 302
        chest tube drainage
            302–304
        clinical features 299
        observation 302
        pleural fluid 300–301
        pleurectomy 304
        pleuro-peritoneal shunt
            304–305
        radiology 299–300
        radiotherapy 302
        thoracentesis 302
        thoracoscopy with talc
            poudrage 304
        treatment 301–302
    patient observation 282
    signs 269–270
    subdiaphragmatic causes 284
    symptoms 269
    transudates 274–276
    ultrasound 271–272
    undiagnosed 280–282
eural fluid 272, 273
    al fluid diagnositic tests

278–280
    amylase 279
    glucose 278–279
    lactate dehydrogenase 278
    nucleated cells 279–280
    pH 279
    protein 278
pleural needle biopsy 281
pleural techniques 319–325
pleural trauma 571–572
pleural tumours, primary 305
pleurectomy 304
pleuro-peritoneal shunt 304–305
plombage 158
pneumoconiosis 49, 311, 467–472
    clinical features 468
    CT 469
    history 468
    lung function testing 469
    management 469
    pathogenesis 467–468
    pathology 469
    X-ray 468–469
Pneumocystis carinii 295, 296
Pneumocystis carinii pneumonia
    (PCP) 296, 311, 389, 391–396,
    446, 636–637
pneumonectomy 561–564
pneumonia 39, 40, 45, 333–353,
    526
    community acquired 333–343
pneumonitis 495–497
pneumothorax 51–52, 158,
    310–319
    flying 318
    management 328–329
    primary spontaneous (PSP)
        311–317
poliomyelitis 11
polymyositis 160, 161
post viral cough 595, 597
postero-anterior (PA) projection
    29
postoperative pulmonary
    complications 611–615
Prader-Willi syndrome 196

pregnancy 605–610
  acute respiratory failure 610
  amniotic fluid embolism 610
  anatomy 605
  asthma 103, 607–608
  cystic fibrosis 610
  endocrinology 605
  physiology 605–606
  pneumonia 609–610
  pulmonary embolism 233–234,
    606–607
  pulmonary function 605–610
  radiation 606
  rib fractures 609
  sarcoidosis 609
  tuberculosis 608–609
primary pulmonary hypertension
  aetiology 201–202
  clinical features 202–204
  epidemiology 201
  investigation 204–210
    arterial blood gases 207
    blood tests 204
    chest X-ray 204–207
    CT scan 208
    echocardiography 208
    electrocardiogram 207
    lung function tests 207
    nocturnal hypoxaemia
      207
    open lung biopsy
      209–210
    right heart catheterization
      208–209
    ventilation 208
  management 210–212
    anticoagulation 211
    diuretics 210
    lung transplantation 212
    oxygen therapy 210
    prostacyclin 211
    vasodilators 210–211
  pathology 202
primary spontaneous pneumothorax
  (PSP) 311–317
  aspiration 314

clinical presentation 312
imaging 312–313
intercostal tube drainage
  314–316
management 313–314
observation 314
recurrence 313
video assisted thoracoscopy
  (VAT) 316–317
prophylactic cranial irradiation (PCI)
  256
Prospective Investigation of
  Pulmonary Embolism
  Diagnosis (PIOPED) 220, 222
prostacyclin 211
pseudoalveolar disease 45
pseudochylothorax 310
Pseudomonas spp 390
Pseudomonas aeruginosa, 410,
  411–412
psittacosis 334
pulmonary alveolar proteinosis 45
pulmonary and chest wall
  compliance 19–20
pulmonary angiography 226–227
pulmonary artery flotation
  catheters 512–513
pulmonary capillary wedge
  pressure (PCWP) 512
pulmonary collapse 38–43
  causes 41
pulmonary contusion 573
pulmonary embolectomy 232–233
pulmonary embolism (PE) 214–234,
  282, 283–284
  angiography 226–227
  anticoagulation 230–232
  ascending contrast
    venography 225
  clinical features 217–218
  clinical likelihood 220
  clinical presentation 218–220
  CT scanning 226
  diagnosis 52–54, 217–230
  Doppler ultrasound 225–226
  echocardiography 227

lower limb vein assessment 224–226
magnetic resonance imaging 227–229
plasma D-dimer 227
predisposing factors 215–217
pregnancy 233–234
thrombolysis 231, 232
treatment 230–234
V/Q lung scan 220–224, 229–230
pulmonary fibrosis 59, 214
pulmonary function tests 1–27
pulmonary haemorrhage 219
pulmonary hypertension 137, 199–214
classification 200–201
primary 201–212
aetiology 201–202
clinical features 202–204
epidemiology 201
investigation 204–210
management 210–212
pathology 202
secondary 212–214
causes 212
cor pulmonale 213–214
pulmonary lacerations 573
pulmonary neurofibromatosis 311
pulmonary nodules 48–49
pulmonary oedema 45
pulmonary sarcoidosis 59, 451–454
pulmonary vasculitis 199–234, 446–447
pulse oximetry 140

Q fever 333, 489
quality of life 262–263

radiation pneumonitis 45
radio-allergo sorbent testing (RAST) 112–113
radiology 138–139
radionuclide bone scanning 244
radiotherapy 252–253, 302, 495–497

reactive airway dysfunction syndrome (RADS) 88, 466
regional lung function 20
renal failure 516–519
research 679–683
residual volume (RV) 7
respiratory disorders
and climbing 643–644
and commercial air travel 640
and fitness to fly testing 641
and professional air travel 641–642
and professional divers 643
and sport diving 643
respiratory drive 20
respiratory emergencies 581–590
drowning 584–590
haemoptysis 581–582
inhaled agents 584, 586–589
tension pneumothorax 582–583
upper airway obstruction 583–584
respiratory failure of central origin 214
restrictive defect 5
rheumatoid arthritis 282–283
rheumatoid nodules 49
rheumatoid pleurisy 272, 273
rhinitis 593–596
allergen avoidance 114–116
clinical management 109–113
examination 110
history 109–110
investigations 110–113
definition 109
immunotherapy 119–120
pathophysiology 108
pharmacotherapy 116–119
surgery 120–121
Rhodococcus equi 390
right bundle branch block (RBBB) 207
right heart catheterization 208–209
rolling seal spirometer 5

sarcoidosis 11, 49, 274, 285, 311, 364, 445,
scleroderma 59
scoliosis 11, 12, 158
scrufuloderma 357, 362
secondary pulmonary hypertension, causes 212
secondary pulmonary hypertension, cor pulmonale 213–214
secondary spontaneous pneumothorax 317–319
segmental resection 564
selenium exposure 491
sepsis 522–525
    definition 522–525
septicaemia, clinical features 524
septicaemia, complications 525
severe asthma 98
shuttle walk test (SWT) 15
siderosis 473
silicosis 469–471
simple coal workers pneumoconiosis (SCWP) 471–472
single breath nitrogen test 21
single-lung transplantation (SLT) 548, 550
six minute walk (SMWT) 15
skin prick testing 110–113
sleep apnoea syndrome 171–198
slow or relaxed vital capacity (SVC) 5
small cell carcinoma 236, 241, 248
    chemotherapy and radiotherapy 254–256
    growth rate 237
snoring 176, 191, 194–195
sodium cromoglycate 117
soft tissue injury to the chest 569
spirometry 5, 6, 138
spontaneous pneumothorax, secondary 317–319
sputum cytology 242
sputum induction 3

sputum retention, physiotherapy for 625
squamous cell carcinoma 235, 236, 240, 241
    growth rate 237
stannosis 473
staphylococcal pneumonia 311
Staphylococcus aureus 390, 412
Stenotrophomonas maltophilia 413–414
Streptococcus pneumoniae 296, 390
subcutaneous emphysema 319
Suberosis 486
sulphur dioxide exposure 492
superior sulcus (Pancoast) tumour 55
systemic inflammatory response syndrome (SIRS) 523
systemic lupus erythematosus 283

Takayasu's arteritis 447
TB meningitis 358, 362
teaching 673–678
tension pneumothorax 582–583
theophyllines 146–147
thoacroscopy, rigid 75
thoracentesis 302
thoracic duct trauma 579
thoracic idiopathic scoliosis 157, 158
thoracic imaging 29–63
thoracoplasty 12, 158
thoracoscopy 73–78, 281, 559–560
    complications 78
    procedure 73–75
    talc poudrage 304
    techniques 75–77
thrombolysis 231, 232
thyroidectomy 24
tidal volume (TV) 5
titanosis/titanocosis 473, 491
TLCO 3
total lung capacity (TLC) 7
total parenteral nutrition 519
Toxoplasma gondii 297

tracheal tumours 238
tracheostomy 187
transbronchial lung biopsies 72
transudates 274–276
tuberculosis 282, 355–382,
        396–398, 445, 489
    BCG vaccination 365
    chemoprophylaxis 378–381
    clinical features 356–357
    contact tracing 363, 366
    diabetes 374
    differential diagnosis 363
    drug dosages 372
    drug interactions 376
    drug reactions 375
    drug resistance 375–378
    HIV 368–370, 374
    infection control 367–368
    investigations 259–367
    liver function, 368, 374
    management 367
    non-respiratory 357–358,
            361–363
        abdominal 357
        bone/joint 357, 361
        central nervous system
            358, 362
        gastrointestinal 361–362
        genitourinary 358, 362
        lymphadenopathy 357,
            361
        miliary 358, 363
        pericardial 362
        skin 357, 362
    notification 367
    pregnancy 374
    pretreatment precautions 367
    referral 381
    renal disease 374
    respiratory 359–360
    testing 360, 365
    treatment regimens 371–373
tuberculous empyema 295
tuberculous pleural effusions
        293–295
    aspiration 294

    clinical features 293
    HIV 295
    investigations 293–294
    pleural biopsy 294
    radiology 293
    skin tests 293
    treatment 294–295
tuberculous pleurisy 272
tularaemic pneumonia 353

ultrasound 271–272
unusual interstitial pneumonia (UIP)
    444
upper airway obstruction 583–584
    case study 23–25
uraemia 285
urinothorax 272, 273, 274, 285
uvulopalatopharyngoplasty (UPPP)
    187–188

V/Q lung scan, 220–224, 229–230,
    281
vanadium exposure 491
vasculitis 446–447
vasodilators 210–211
ventilation 208
ventilation-perfusion radionuclide
    lung imaging 33
ventilatory insufficiency 155–170
video assisted thoracoscopy (VAT)
    316–317
viral pneumonias 401
vital capacity (VC) 5

warfarin 231–232
wasp and bee venom allergy
    125–126
    desensitization 126
    therapy 126
Wegener's granulomatosis 49, 445,
    447

yellow nail syndrome 285

zinc (chloride) exposure 491